Farm animal behaviour and welfare

Erratum

the following errors appeared in the last printing

page 163,	para3 line 8	for Gonyar, read Gonyou
page 260,	para2, line 16	for 7%, read 0.7%
page 371,	para3, line 3,	for egg population, read egg production
page 376,	para 2, last line:	for p.310, read p.309
page 378,	Fig.39.4	in the figure please delete 9m x 8m (should read "Divided sections to take 200 birds")
page 414,		for McGlore, read McGlone

The following references were omitted

Banks, E.M. (1982). Behavioural research to answer questions about animal welfare. *J. Anim. Sci.,* **54,** 434-46.

van Logestijn, J.G., Romme, A.M.T.C. and Eikelenboom, G. (1982). Losses caused by transport of slaughter pigs in the Netherlands. In *Transport of Animals Intended for Breeding, Production and Slaughter*, ed. R. Moss, *Curr. Top. vet. Med. Anim, Sci.,* **81,** 105-112.

Stott, G.H. (1981). What is animal stress and how is it measured? *J. Anim. Sci.,* **52,** 519-57.

Farm animal behaviour and welfare

Third edition

A.F. Fraser
Memorial University of Newfoundland, Canada

D.M. Broom
Colleen Macleod Professor of Animal Welfare,
University of Cambridge, UK

CABI *Publishing*

CABI *Publishing* **is a division of CAB** *International*

CABI Publishing
CAB International
Wallingford
Oxon OX10 8DE
UK

Tel: +44 (0)1491 832111
Fax: +44 (0)1491 833508
Email: cabi@cabi.org
Web site: http://www.cabi.org

CABI Publishing
10 E 40th Street
Suite 3203
New York, NY 10016
USA

Tel: +1 212 481 7018
Fax: +1 212 686 7993
Email: cabi-nao@cabi.org

A catalogue record for this book is available from the British Library, London, UK.

ISBN 0 85199 160 2

First Edition 1974
Second Edition 1980
This edition first published by Baillière Tindall 1990
Reprinted with corrections by CAB *International* 1997 (twice), 1998, 2001

Printed and bound in the UK by Bookcraft, Midsomer Norton, Avon.

Contents

Preface

Every farmer, every veterinary surgeon and indeed all those who have an interest in livestock production need to know about farm animal behaviour in order that they can carry out their jobs properly. All of these people and all consumers of farm animal products have to consider their moral stance in relation to farm animal welfare and require precise information about that welfare in order to do this. This book is a comprehensive guide to the behaviour of farm animals which provides practical information for those involved with farming and veterinary work. It also reviews the scientific information which is available concerning the assessment of animal welfare, and the evaluation of the effects on animals of different management methods and housing conditions. Such assessment necessarily involves measurement of physiology, disease state and production as well as behaviour.

Farm animals are very good subjects for behaviour studies so many important advances in our understanding of fundamental aspects of animal behaviour have come from farm animal behaviour studies. Concepts concerning social structure, behaviour development, parent–offspring relationships, sexual behaviour, and the role of behaviour in coping with adversity have depended greatly on evidence obtained from farm animal studies. If evolutionary questions are being asked the changes in the species during domestication must be taken into account, but farm animals have the same range of behaviour as wild animals. It is easy to obtain data about behaviour from farm animals; they are available in large numbers and are often genetically very similar to one another. Our understanding of farm animal behaviour and welfare, however, is much enhanced by ideas based on studies of the behaviour of wild animals, laboratory animals and man. This fact will be apparent to readers as this book refers to examples of important work on a variety of species where such information is necessary for adequate appreciation of the mechanisms underlying farm animal behaviour.

The number of research studies in progress now on the behaviour of farm animals is at least five times larger than the number which were underway when the first edition of *Farm Animal Behaviour* was published and such work is helping farming and veterinary practice in many ways. Precise scientific studies on animal welfare are now sufficient to form an important part of the evidence upon which laws can be based. In these circumstances, those who are learning about, keeping up to date with, or legislating upon livestock farming, veterinary medicine or applied biology need a source of information about the current state of our knowledge of farm animal behaviour and welfare. This text provides that information in a way which is easy for the beginner to understand but which includes discussion of complex topics and reference to the literature relevant to that area.

Hence, as well as being useful to farmers, agricultural advisors and veterinary surgeons, it is suited to a comprehensive university or college course on behaviour science applied to farm animals.

This book includes much new material which is not in the second edition of *Farm Animal Behaviour*. The first two sections are entirely new and deal with fundamental aspects of behaviour. They include a substantial chapter on describing and measuring behaviour. The next three sections concern the organisation of behaviour in the individual farm animal and the social, reproductive, developmental and parental behaviour of farm animals. The final section of twelve chapters on farm animal welfare is new and represents the most extensive review of this subject published to date. This section includes practical information on the humane control of livestock and on welfare and behaviour in relation to disease as well as details of the scientific assessment of animal welfare and comparisons of the welfare of cattle, pigs and poultry in different systems. The book is illustrated with many photographs and includes a comprehensive reference list and a glossary.

A.F. Fraser   MRCVS, MVSc, FIBiol
Professor of Surgery (Veterinary),
Memorial University of Newfoundland,
Canada

D.M. Broom   MA, PhD, FIBiol
Colleen Macleod Professor of Animal Welfare,
Department of Clinical Veterinary Medicine,
University of Cambridge,
U.K.

Acknowledgements

The many authors whose work forms the basis for this book are mentioned in the reference list but we should like to thank especially the following colleagues who have given encouragement to one or both of the authors: J.L. Albright, G.W. Arnold, A. Brownlee, I. Ekesbo, M.W. Fox, D. Fraser, H. Hastie, K. Johnson, A. Littlejohn, F. Loew, R. Stricklin, P.R. Wiepkema and D.G.M. Wood-Gush. We pay tribute especially to the late Ron Kilgour who was a pioneer and made important contributions to various aspects of farm animal ethology and to the late Alex Stolba for his work on pig behaviour and welfare.

We thank the following for providing illustrative material for use in the book or for advice or help concerning such material: A.M. Aitchison, B.A. Baldwin, D. Bieger, M. Bieger, C. George, T. Grandin, B. Payton, H.H. Sambraus, E. Shillito-Walser, T. Tennessen and C. Thorne. Efficient and considerable secretarial support was given to the authors by Mrs D. Dooley and Mrs E. Kirby and we thank them for their tolerance.

1 Introduction

The farming of animals has played an important part in the development of human civilisation. Food, clothing and transport are obtained by man from a wide variety of species (Broom, 1986a; Messent and Broom, 1986). In addition to being such a resource, farmed animals have long been treated as companions and viewed with affection by those whose job it was to care for them. The species which were domesticated had to be suitable for providing meat, milk, eggs, wool etc. but they also had to have certain behavioural characteristics in order that domestication was possible. The potential for showing reduced anti-predator responses to man, low aggression to man and effective reproduction in captivity were essential if the animals were to be farmed. Given this potential in their animals, the early domesticators and all those involved with animal husbandry ever since have had to be able to assess and interpret animal behaviour. Good stockmanship has always involved knowing how to respond to the behaviour of animals when handling them or identifying their problems.

By the start of the twentieth century, farm animal use had increased with the expansion of human needs. Animals began to be kept in concentrated populations and, before 1970, intensive animal husbandry had arrived in the form of close confinement for cattle, pigs and poultry under new husbandry systems. The innovations in management are principally characterised by larger livestock numbers kept together in markedly reduced space. Such conditions have effects on disease transmission and they require considerable physiological and behavioural adaptation. It has been assumed that the animals could adapt to the environmental restrictions but both adaptation and failure to adjust have come to be recognisable in the behaviour of animals. Substantial new knowledge of the behaviour of livestock under intensive husbandry systems is therefore needed to assess these systems of management. This knowledge can then be applied in the agriculture industry in order to improve production and welfare. Many of the current animal husbandry problems are not soluble by investigating nutrition, body physiology, or disease control but require investigations of the behaviour of the animals before progress can be made towards a solution.

The term ethology is often used for the observation and detailed description of behaviour with the objective of finding out how biological mechanisms function. The scientific study of animal behaviour has proceeded very rapidly during the last thirty years. There have been substantial recent advances in the precision of behaviour description and the understanding of the behaviour organisation in relation to physiological and evolutionary processes. Modern techniques in ethology and in experimental psychology mean that we now have a much more extensive knowledge of sensory analysis, motor control, hormonal effects, motivation, body maintenance behaviour in good and difficult conditions, reproductive behaviour and social structure. This knowledge and these techniques can be and are being applied to farm animals; a knowledge of animal behaviour is therefore essential for all those who have a part to play in livestock farming.

Behaviour and animal production

A major theme of this book is that farm animal behaviour research is relevant and necessary for animal production enterprises to be carried out effectively and economically. The stockman, the farm manager, the animal transporter, and the designer of animal accommodation and equipment have to be aware of well established facts and recent research on the ethology of farm animals.

An appreciation of how to handle animals necessitates knowledge of behaviour which in the past has been gradually acquired through personal experience. Some of this information can be taught and all of it is learned more easily if general principles of animal behaviour are known. Practical experience is still very important, however. Feeding behaviour is an example of an important topic for those who have to manage animals. The control of feeding, food selection at pasture or when composite feeds are offered, and learning about food and behaviour in competitive feeding situations are all relevant to intakes and food conversion efficiency.

Reproductive behaviour is of great importance to those managing a stock unit. Behaviour assessment is the major method of oestrus detection in dairy cows and pigs. Work on mating preferences and factors affecting libido are of critical importance in the management of sheep, goats, beef cattle and horses where a high proportion of successful matings is desired. Each animal whose offspring production fails, or is delayed, costs the farmer money. The frequency

with which maternal behaviour fails in sheep or other animals and problems with the survival of young piglets, lambs or calves can all be reduced by a knowledge of behaviour and consequential modifications of stockmanship.

Wherever animals have to be grouped or decisions have to be taken about the housing and density of animals, information about social behaviour is important. Farm animal management which leads to fighting, injury or extreme fear can result in reproductive failure, poor food conversion, reduced carcass value or increased mortality. Such losses can be substantially reduced if the long-standing knowledge of the good stockman and the results of research on social behaviour are utilised to improve animal management.

These very wide-ranging applications of behaviour study to farm animal production, together with the relevance of behaviour work to understanding animal welfare, emphasise the importance of including a lecture series and practical experience in courses on animal science, animal production and applied biology.

Behaviour and veterinary medicine

The practising veterinary surgeon uses knowledge of behaviour frequently but much of this knowledge is acquired after formal training is completed. Situations in which such expertise is important include: handling animals, using behaviour as a sign in diagnosis, advising on animal husbandry methods, dealing with behaviour problems and assessing welfare. Behaviour is also important as a part of the general biology of the animal so it is relevant when considering, for example, feeding responses to adverse temperature conditions, or disease transmission.

The importance to a veterinary surgeon intending to handle an animal, of recognising the signals which indicate that the animal is about to attack or will kick if handled, are obvious. It is also very beneficial to veterinary treatment if handling procedures can be modified according to observed behaviour in such a way that the animal is not adversely affected by the handling itself. Studies of behaviour are also especially relevant where it is necessary to move animals from place to place along races, up ramps, into vehicles or into strange rooms.

The working veterinarian is regularly presented with clinical cases having histories which are symptomatically behaviour-based. In fact, it is common for animal illness to be first manifested behaviourally, such as in loss of appetite, altered activity or diminished body care. Clinical veterinary work has a very real and special relationship with pathognomonic behaviour in animals. Those who practise professionally the art and science of clinical veterinary medicine and surgery acquire competence at the interfaces between illnesses and their behavioural signs through years of training, experience and witness.

Behavioural signs of impairment and histories of behavioural symptoms give invaluable help to the veterinary clinician in the initiation of a clinical appraisal of the animal's condition. With such orientation, further points are sought out for special investigation and detailed examination. On systematic examination, the behavioural feature of a veterinary problem often becomes seen as a screen over a generalised and mixed array of physical signs of illness. As substantive correlates of the behavioural manifestation are found in physiological and pathological factors, the behavioural picture fades into the background of the clinical problem. Treatment and restorative action then become focused physically on lesions and infections. The behavioural problem thus becomes resolved by a transformation through veterinary medical concepts into an identifiable clinical condition which can then be given appropriate case management and therapy.

When the internal milieu of the animal has become abnormal, the bodily feedbacks to the central nervous system are also abnormal and in consequence the homoeostatic integrity of the animal is impaired, with dynamic irregularities becoming evident. The veterinarian considers these for purposes of diagnosis and prognosis. Sometimes the animal's irregular behaviour does not translate into a physical condition as, for example, when physico-pathological correlates of the condition do not exist or are not identifiable. Varieties of hypopraxia (abnormally diminished activity) are good examples of this type of condition. Just as in man, some disorders are distinguishable only by their effects on behaviour whilst others are manifested in a variety of ways.

A necessary prerequisite to the recognition of abnormal behaviour, whether as a sign of pathogen presence or as an indicator of poor welfare which is not due to a pathogen, is a knowledge of normal behaviour. The concept of what is normal behaviour for a species can be taught to a limited extent, but requires practical experience in order that it can be formulated effectively.

If a horse is seen to be pacing in its stable and kicking at its belly, this is identifiable as a sign of colic, but someone with no experience of horse behaviour would not recognise it as such. More subtle signs such as the partially hunched posture adopted by a sheep with abdominal pain require clear observation of both the normal and affected animals (see Chapter 31).

The relevance of expertise in behaviour to animal husbandry and to the assessment of animal welfare are discussed in other sections in this chapter. Both are areas where the veterinary surgeon is expected to be able to give advice. Behaviour problems which affect the practicalities of managing animals are also frequently presented to the veterinary surgeon for solution. One area of general behavioural knowledge which helps in the explanation of such problems in both farm and companion animals, concerns the ways in which early experience affects behaviour development. Another area is learning. The veterinary surgeon should be able to advise on how to avoid behaviour problems and what training or other procedures to utilise in order to deal with them. The preparation which is required in order that every veterinary student has an adequate knowledge of the fundamental principles and veterinary applications of animal behaviour is a course of lectures in the subject and reference to specific techniques and literature at various points in the clinical part of the course.

Animal welfare: assessment and moral judgement

Animals have to contend with a complex environment and they have a variety of methods of attempting to cope with it. That environment includes physical conditions, social influences and any predators, parasites or pathogens which may attack the individual. The coping methods include physiological changes in the brain, adrenals and immune system and, linked to some of these, behavioural changes. Some factors which affect an animal may result in it having great difficulty in coping. It may fail to cope in that its fitness is reduced and either it dies, or it fails to grow or its ability to reproduce is reduced in some direct way. The welfare of an animal is its state as regards its attempts to cope with its environment (Broom, 1986c). Hence welfare is a characteristic of the individual animal which varies on a continuum from poor to good. The attempts to cope and the results of failure to cope can be measured. Hence welfare can be assessed in a precise scientific way using a variety of indicators.

The assessment of welfare can be carried out in an objective way which is quite independent of any moral considerations. Mortality rate, reproductive success, extent of adrenal activity, amount of abnormal behaviour, severity of injury, degree of immunosuppression, or level of disease incidence can all be measured. Our knowledge of each of these welfare indicators has improved rapidly in recent years as people with backgrounds in zoology, physiology, psychology, animal production and veterinary medicine have investigated the effects of difficult conditions on animals. Much remains to be learned but we are already in a position to apply recently gained knowledge to comparative studies on farm animals of different systems of management, designs of housing, methods of handling or transportation, and procedures in operations or in slaughter. In addition to measurements of poor welfare, it is possible to investigate the preferences of animals and the value which they place on various resources or other aspects of their environment. Such studies and a wide range of work on the basic biology of animals give information about the biological needs of animals. If these are not met there will often be indicators of poor welfare which can be measured, but in some circumstances we have not yet got the expertise to evaluate adverse psychological effects on animals.

When scientific evaluation of welfare has been carried out, there remains the moral question of how poor welfare should be before it is regarded as unacceptable. This is an issue where the farmer, the veterinary surgeon, the welfare research worker, or the member of the general public are equally entitled to have an opinion. One person might say that a certain degree of poor welfare in an individual farm animal is acceptable, given the human requirements involved, whilst another person might consider that degree of poor welfare to be unacceptable. Moral positions in such matters have changed as people have come to know more about the complexity of animal organisation, the sophistication of animal behaviour and the degree of similarity between farm animal species and man. Both recent research and media coverage of such research, have contributed to this change of attitude. The feeling that man has a moral obligation to ensure that the welfare of animals which are kept on farms is never very poor has become widespread. The idea that, when decisions are taken about methods in animal husbandry, animals should be considered as individuals and their responses to their environment should be evaluated and understood, is now held by many in the agriculture industry and the veterinary profession. This is an important part of the subject of veterinary ethics (Tannenbaum, 1989).

Questions about behaviour

There are two kinds of questions which can be asked when trying to understand a particular kind of behaviour. The first of these is "How does it work?" The answers to this question refer to the mechanisms underlying the behaviour which cause it to occur at the time of observation and with the form which is seen. What changes are occurring within the body of that animal which result in the movements which are shown? Some of these changes are physiological processes which we know quite a lot about, such as those involved in sensory reception, impulse conduction along nerves, or muscle contraction. Changes within the brain involving emotional variables, learning, decision making and control of actions have been extensively investigated, but we still have much to discover about them.

The second kind of question about behaviour is: "Why does it happen?". The answers to this question refer to the way in which this behaviour has arisen in the species under observation. In order to try to appreciate how the pattern and use of a behaviour have evolved it is necessary to consider what the selective advantage of the behaviour is. Put another way, in what way will the effects of a gene which affects behaviour promote the spread of that gene in the population? In practice, "why?" questions and "how?" questions are linked because questions about evolution depend upon a knowledge of the mechanism underlying a behaviour and questions about causation are often helped by an understanding of the evolutionary origins of the system. For both kinds of questions we need to consider behaviour in relation to the general biology of the animal.

Behaviour, like physiology and anatomy, is part of the general functioning of an animal. The various aspects of life can be classified into *functional systems* which include behaviour as a component (Broom, 1981, p. 4). These are: obtaining oxygen, osmoregulation, temperature regulation, cleaning the body surface, feeding, avoiding chemical hazards, avoiding physical hazards, predator avoidance, and reproduction. Behaviour often serves more than one function, for example exploration and establishing social relationships may be relevant to almost all of them so they become secondary objectives in themselves. The role of behaviour in each of these functional systems is discussed in detail in this book but the key to understanding the behaviour of an animal is an appreciation of how resources are apportioned and decisions taken about which activity to show and when. The study area which deals with decisions about the timing and nature of changes in behaviour is that of motivation. This important subject is essential to an understanding of all aspects of behaviour and also to questions about animal welfare. Many welfare problems result from frustration or environmental unpredictability and a knowledge of motivational state is needed in order that these can be recognised.

When trying to answer questions about how behaviour works, investigatory methods are used in which the experience of an animal is controlled and its effects are assessed. Some such studies are carried out during the development of the individual. Learning occurs when some experience modifies later behaviour. Learning has an effect on all aspects of life so some reference must be made to it in discussions of every aspect of behaviour. All systems develop in animals as a consequence of interactions between the genetic information in the animal and influences from the environment of that genotype. Since all behaviour depends on the genetic information in an animal and environmental factors will always affect the expression of genes, it is not useful to try to distinguish between instinctive or innate behaviour and that which is environmentally determined. The interesting questions concern how differences in genotype and in the environment result in differences in behaviour. Behaviour genetics and the processes which occur during behaviour development are both exciting topics which will be discussed in this book.

This book includes answers to the various

questions posed above but it does so with especial reference to the requirements of those who need to know about the management, housing, veterinary treatment and general biology of farm animals. Chapter 2 is about the techniques which can be used to obtain information about behaviour. Behaviour recording methodology has become much more sophisticated in recent years. Chapters 3 to 7 deal with fundamental processes in behaviour and relevant information about brain function, hormones and pheromones. The examples given in these chapters are of work which best illustrates the point which is being made, so they often refer to animals other than farm animals. Chapters 8 to 14 deal with the control of behaviour in individual animals and refer to eight of the functional systems listed above. There follow seven chapters on social and reproductive behaviour (Chapters 15 to 21) and six describing behaviour development and maternal behaviour (Chapters 22 to 27). The final section of the book is principally concerned with welfare. It commences with Chapters 28 and 29 on welfare concepts and measurement. These are followed by Chapters 30 to 36 on animal handling, welfare in relation to disease and abnormal behaviour, including reference to management methods. Finally Chapters 37 to 39 cover the welfare of cattle, pigs and poultry with sections explaining the problems and comparing different systems for management, housing and transport.

2 Describing, recording and measuring behaviour

This short chapter is not intended to be a comprehensive account of the subject. There is a useful book which concerns farm animals in particular (Jensen *et al.*, 1986) and a good book which refers to all animals (Martin and Bateson, 1986); the reader is referred to these for more detailed information.

Levels of description of behaviour

The words which are used to describe behaviour are a consequence of how people think about what they see or hear. Those words in their turn, however, may change the way of thinking of the person who uses them or the person who hears or reads them. This occurs especially when the word used to describe the behaviour implies something about the emotional state or intentions of the animal whose behaviour is described. Hence it is important to be accurate and cautious when describing. As an example of the problem, suppose that a hen is seen to move rapidly, flapping her wings, over a distance of three metres starting on the edge of one group of birds and finishing next to a wall where a single bird standing there moves away. An observer might describe this sequence of behaviour by saying that the hen is frightened or is angry, or is aggressive. In fact none of these descriptions is justified by the observation and none informs others about what has been observed. In order to communicate effectively with the listener or reader when describing behaviour, it is best to state what is seen in the manner of the descriptive sentence above.

Objective description of behaviour can be at various levels of detail. When considering the hen mentioned already, her behaviour could be described in terms of:

1. the contraction of each muscle;
2. the movement of each group of muscles;
3. the movement of one part of the body relative to another, e.g. the wing is flapped, or the legs are moved with a running gait;
4. the movement of the animal, or part of it, in relation to the environment, e.g. moving from point A to point B 3 m away or touching the wall;
5. an effect on the physical environment, e.g. flattening straw by stepping on it, or knocking over a food container, or pecking a key;
6. an effect on another individual, e.g. causing another bird to move, or eliciting a submissive posture, or a courtship display.

The decision as to whether to describe the structure of the behaviour, go into much detail or little detail, or describe the consequence of the behaviour, depends upon the aims of the observation.

In selecting measures for a particular study it is useful to know the array of behaviours which the animal is capable of showing. A largely complete description of such an array is called an *ethogram* and papers have been published which present an ethogram for a species. These papers are necessarily based on an extensive study of that species and they can be very useful if the behaviour description is precise enough. It is still necessary, however, for the observer to spend some time becoming familiar with the behavioural repertoire of the animal. It is likely that any detailed behavioural study will add to our knowledge of the repertoire and organisation of that animal's behaviour so no ethogram is ever complete. The actual selection of measures should take account of whether or not the measures are independent of one another, for example one activity may be necessarily preceded by another or may prevent the occurrence of another.

When considering the level of detail of description it becomes apparent that some behaviours like sleep are continuous, others like walking are a series of repeated movement sequences and others like displays or grooming are made up of sets of recognisable units. Rowell (1961) distinguished between *acts*, such as a finch bill-wiping "bending forward, wiping the bill on the perch and resuming an upright posture", or a step during walking, and *bouts* such as a sequence of walking with a gap before the next sequence. The question of how to decide, for activities such as walking, preening, eating or displaying, when a bout ends is discussed by Slater (1975), Machlis (1977) and Broom (1981, p. 59.) When acts can be grouped together into longer units, because they are frequently combined in a particular way, this probably reflects some neural control circuit and it is convenient to use a word for that unit. Many of our measures of behaviour are of this kind. The units might be movements in: prey-catching, other food acquisition, grooming,

courtship display, mating or parental behaviour and they are often referred to as *action patterns*. As discussed by Broom (1981, pp. 62–75) the term fixed action pattern has been used in the past, but careful studies show that the action pattern is not fixed in detail of sequence or in a genetic sense so the term is inappropriate. Barlow's (1977) term "modal action pattern" is more accurate but such a statistical descriptive word seems unnecessary so action pattern by itself is sufficient.

More prolonged sequences of individual behaviour by farm animals which require description on occasion are stereotypies and rhythms. The subject of stereotyped behaviour is extensively reviewed in Chapter 32. A *rhythm* is a series of events repeated in time at intervals whose distribution is approximately regular and the more precise term *periodicity* means a series of events separated by equal periods in a time series (Broom, 1980). Rhythmic activities include heart-beating, breathing, walking, flying, chewing, being active rather than resting, diurnal activity, oestrous behaviour and breeding. Some methods of detecting and analysing activity rhythms are reviewed by Broom (1979). Investigations of sequences of behaviour show that rhythms can be important variables affecting behaviour so they must be taken into account in certain sorts of behaviour investigation. For example, young domestic chicks showed periodicities in walking behaviour and heart rate with wavelengths of 24 h, 20–30 mins, 13–15 s and 1–2 s (Forrester, 1979; Broom, 1980).

Behaviour measures during veterinary examination

Behaviour is used during clinical appraisal and is generally qualitative, in that the presence or absence of a certain kind of behaviour is noted, rather than quantitative. The examination of the animal is more reliable if some previous information about that individual is available and if the reactions as well as the posture of animals or groups of animals can be assessed. The animal's attitude, disposition and temperament should be assessed before any handling is performed. Its alertness and apparent awareness of its general environment should be noted. In particular, the subject's appreciation of visual, auditory and positional stimuli must be determined. Eye movement, involving the lids and orbit, is an important feature. A high degree of exposure and mobility of the orbit suggests anxiety while a very fixed orbital position may indicate some distress.

Appraisal of the animal's willingness to move and the nature of its gait are important considerations. Evaluation must also be made of various reflex responses, both general, such as the response to sound, or specific, such as the response to a local stimulus, e.g. pressure on a given site on the body. Reflex responses to localised pain such as skin-pricking or pinching may also be noted if circumstances indicate a need to determine nerve function. Within a long examination period, acts of normal behaviour should become noticeable. These might include behavioural items of self-maintenance such as feeding (or response to an offering of food) and body care. The significance of acts of body care in a long behavioural examination is considerable since this behaviour often ceases as a first sign of sickness.

Common actions, or their absence, should be noted. For example, self-grooming and stretching commonly occur after rising in healthy stock but several factors, including illness in general, can inhibit grooming and stretching reflexes. In cattle, tonguing of the nostrils may be inhibited during illness. It has also been suggested that the eructation reflex in ruminants becomes inhibited in many illnesses and, as a consequence of this, distension of the rumen develops and leads to the condition of bloat which is seen associated with various illnesses in ruminants. Recognition of these minor reflexes in the normal behaviour of cattle is an indication of sound health and, consequently, their absence suggests that health is impaired.

In a study of posture, as an aid to behavioural appraisal, it must be remembered that many postural abnormalities are not shown unless the animal is at rest in its usual environment. For this reason, patient and quiet observation of the animal may be necessary before abnormalities of posture can be detected and appreciated.

Behavioural examinations are best performed in a quiet space or enclosure with limited light where distractions will be minimal. Tranquilisation should be avoided; parts of the examination which may tend to excite the animal should be postponed until the end. At the conclusion of the examination it may be apparent that further specialised clinical tests and specific medical examinations are required. In the course of convalescence, the behaviours of self-maintenance return to the animal's behavioural repertoire. An extended period of behavioural examination of the animal in its bedded premises is usually necessary for convalescence to be appraised by the behavioural method.

Behaviour signs of pathological state are reviewed in Chapter 31. In general the use of behaviour in clinical examinations has not utilised modern techniques of behaviour assessment. It is possible that, as we learn more about the relationship between health and behaviour, clinical appraisal will start to incorporate more sophisticated behavioural tests and aids such as the video-recorder which can tell the clinician about the behaviour of the animal when it is not being examined.

Design of experiments and observation procedures

Before commencing a behaviour study it is important to consider whether the design of the procedures to be used is adequate to allow reliable conclusions to be drawn from the results of the work. The first precaution concerns the effects of the presence of the observer on the behaviour of the animals. As mentioned above, an animal which is being examined may behave in a different way in the presence and absence of an observer. Small animals like chickens, unless handled frequently and gently from an early age, treat man as a dangerous predator. Hence their behaviour can be affected very substantially by the proximity of a person watching them. Larger farm animals are also affected by human presence so it is advisable, when watching any of these animals, to either observe from a hide or to carry out checks to ascertain how much behaviour is changed by the observer.

Behaviour observation can be accurately replicable if the definitions of measures and precision of recording are clear enough. It is desirable, if more than one observer is involved, however, for studies of inter-observer reliability to be carried out. The possibility of bias, deliberate or unintentional, should also be considered when designing observation procedures. If two treatments are being compared, wherever possible the observer should be "blind" in the sense that the treatment category to which each animal belongs is not known at the time of observation.

Wherever experiments are carried out one or more control situations should also be studied. For example, in a study of the effect of a hormone treatment on behaviour, a control group whose conditions are exactly the same as the experimental group but with an inert substance given to the animal in the same way as the hormone, should be used. Studies of behaviour often require replication since unknown variables can sometimes lead to spurious results. An illustration of such necessity is in the study of orders of movement of a group of animals from one place to another. The order of animals on one occasion, or in one situation, will be affected by chance and may be substantially changed by local conditions so orders should be recorded on several occasions and in several different situations before any conclusion about social relationships can be reached. Whenever sets of observations are replicated, the experimenter must be aware of any possible effects of learning on the results. No animal which has been exposed to experimental conditions can be assumed to be unaffected by them so its behaviour may be different during any repetition of these

conditions. In some studies these very changes are under investigation or, as in the case of regular movement orders, the situation is a very frequent one in the animals' lives so behaviour is not likely to change rapidly because of previous experience of that situation. In other studies, however, an unusual stimulus is presented to the animal and a subsequent response to the same stimulus may be either much less, due to habituation, or much greater, due to sensitisation.

Marking animals

A final, practical point about setting up experimental studies concerns the marking of animals. Much more information can be obtained from studies of behaviour where the identity of individuals is known. The idea that animals behave in a "species typical" way has been shown to be a gross over-simplification by observations of individuals. There is often considerable variation amongst individuals in how they respond to a particular situation and how they attempt to cope with difficult conditions. If the animals are in groups then some form of marking is needed. Animals such as dairy cows are often marked with a collar, an ear tag or a freeze brand. They might also be marked using methods which cause a certain amount of suffering, like an ear notch, or a great deal of suffering, like a hot-iron brand. Sometimes animals are sufficiently variable without additional marking. Friesian or Holstein cows, for example, can often be distinguished individually by coat pattern when there are not too many animals in the group. Horses are commonly described according to an internationally agreed procedure (Federation Equestre Internationale, 1981) and some of these markings are sufficient to allow recognition during behaviour observation.

Whenever animals are marked, care must be taken to discover whether the mark itself affects the outcome of the study. In a study by Burley *et al.* (1982) with zebra finches it was found that coloured plastic leg bands (or rings), put on to allow individual recognition, altered the attractiveness of the birds to the opposite sex. A red leg band made a male more attractive to females whilst a black leg band made a female more attractive to males. Birds wearing green or blue bands were avoided by members of the opposite sex. Other effects of marks on animals include the possibilities that the marking method or the mark may be painful, that the social status of the animal may be changed, or that the vulnerability of the animal to predators may be affected. In order to be aware of the possible effects of marks on the study which is being carried out, it is advisable to check such effects separately. If marks are used, either all of the animals should be marked or none of the animals should be marked.

The nature of the mark used will depend on the requirements of the observer. Animals which are watched only at feeding time may be identifiable from a small ear tag, but those ranging over a large area need a large mark on the sides and back. Where video-recording is used, a larger and clearer mark is needed than when direct observation only is carried out.

In some studies, a mark which persists throughout the life of the animal is needed. This can be a tattoo for pigs or horses; an ear tag for pigs, sheep, goats, buffalo or cattle; a freeze brand for cattle, buffalo or horses; or a leg ring or wing tag for poultry. Another identifier which can be used is a very small transponder which is small enough, (10 mm × 3 mm) to be implanted beneath the skin and which can be recognised later using the correct identifying equipment. This transponder is useful only when the animal is being handled or is close to the identifying equipment. However, this equipment can be located in the animal accommodation and can operate gates, for example at the entrances to an electronic sow feeder, a boar pen, or a farrowing area (R. Buré, personal communication).

Temporary marking of animals can be carried out using leg rings or feather dyes for poultry and hair dyes, paint, collars, or coat-clipping for mammals. Paints and dyes are available commercially as many farmers need to mark animals. Some dyes or paints last for only a short time because the mark itself fades quickly or because the animals rub or lick it off themselves or one another. The life of the mark in the experimental situation should be checked before the investigation proper is initiated. It is possible to use numbers or letters as marks on farm animals but it is easy to confuse some of these if they might become indistinct. Letters are better than numbers as there are more of them, even after confusingly similar letters have been excluded. An example of heifers marked in this way is shown in Fig. 2.1. If wear or other effects might reduce clarity it is better to use combinations of simple marks. Figure 2.2 shows an example of marks on poultry which are distinguishable even if feathers are ruffled or some loss of mark occurs. The presence or absence of each of these marks in four positions gives 15 possible combinations excluding complete absence of marks. Spots or bars can also be used on pigs or other mammals. Collars are suitable for cattle, buffalo, goats and some sheep, but there is a risk that they will come off so a permanent mark is necessary too.

Sampling and measuring

Several decisions have to be taken when

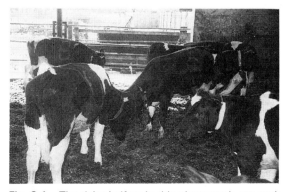

Fig. 2.1 The dairy heifers in this photograph are each marked with a letter to facilitate individual recognition in a study of social interactions (photograph by D.M. Broom).

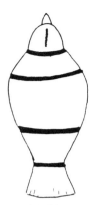

Fig. 2.2   One example of how poultry may be marked with spray colour. By painting lines across the backs of the birds, one or more of the four positions may be used, giving a large number of possible combinations. The symbols are easily recognised, even when the plumage is ruffled (after Jensen *et al.*, 1986).

behaviour is to be measured and these are inter-related in that they are limited by the capabilities of the observer and greater detail in one aspect means potentially less detail in another aspect. The first decision concerns which animals to observe. If much detail from direct observation is required then it will be possible to observe only one animal at a time. This may be an individual in its own pen or it may be a focal animal which can move around within a group. With appropriate sampling methods, data on several or many animals at once can be collected by scanning them but information about each individual is lost by sampling.

The information about one kind of behaviour which can be obtained from observation and recording is:

1. the presence or absence of the particular activity;
2. the frequency of occurrence of each activity during the observation period;
3. the duration of each bout of each activity;
4. the intensity of the activity at each occurrence;
5. the latency of occurrence of the activity after some stimulus or previous action;

6. the timing and nature of subsequent activities;
7. the timing and nature of behaviour changes in relation to physiological changes.

For further discussion of how to devise appropriate measures of each of these see Chapter 3 of Martin and Bateson (1986).

Continuous recording of behaviour can be difficult if many measures are used and recording aids (next section) are often needed, but it offers opportunities for all the different methods of analysis. Sampling behaviour makes possible the collection of data on more than one individual and it allows an estimate of the duration of activities in situations where continuous recording is not possible. There are three sorts of sampling which can be used, two sorts of time sampling and behaviour sampling (Fig. 2.3).

Behaviour sampling or "conspicuous behaviour recording" involves continuous observation of animals but recording of certain kinds of behaviour only. For example, a group of cows may be watched and all occasions where one animal mounts another recorded in detail. Behaviour sampling may also occur automatically in that a single action, such as pecking a key by a chicken, may be automatically recorded but all other actions are ignored. This method is particularly useful for rare behaviour patterns which might otherwise be missed.

Point sampling which is also known by the name "instantaneous sampling" or by the less clear name "interval recording", involves observing animals at regular, predetermined points in time and recording whether or not each of a range of behaviours is being shown at that instant. As shown in Fig. 2.3, a useful estimate of duration of the more common activities is obtained if the observation period lasts long enough and if the interval between the samples is not too long. Rare activities might be missed altogether, however. It is essential that the observer does make an instantaneous observation in order that an accurate estimate of duration is obtained. This is a problem of the

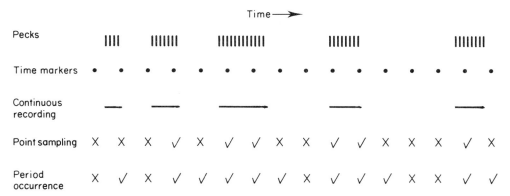

Fig. 2.3 Comparison of behaviour recording methods. A series of pecks by a chick are shown as if produced by an event-recorder moving at a constant speed. If Continuous Recording were used, lines like those shown, or precise times of stopping and starting each bout of pecking, would be produced. Point Sampling and Period Occurrence would produce Yes or No answers at each time mark as shown.

method in that observers tend to try to include activities which do not actually occur at the moment of sampling. A further problem is that some activities take some time to recognise. For example when a cow is ruminating it takes a few seconds to be sure of this since the characteristic jaw movement takes time to identify and the animal might be swallowing just at the moment of sampling. The major advantage of this method is that it can be used when many individuals are scanned so one person can collect much information.

Period occurrence recording, (Broom, 1968b, 1969a) often rather confusingly called "one-zero sampling" (Altmann, 1974) is another form of time sampling in which the events which have occurred during a predetermined time period are recorded at the end of the period. Several animals can be observed simultaneously because the data do not have to be recorded continuously. As is apparent from Fig. 2.3, this method has the advantage that even rare events are not missed, but its important disadvantage is that the figure obtained is not a true representation of the actual duration of each behaviour. If the period between samples is short in relation to the activity bout length, however, then the figures obtained are quite good estimates of activity duration. Period occurrence recording is much easier than continuous recording. Now that recording aids such as computers are available, continuous recording or time sampling are generally preferable to period occurrence recording but there are some circumstances where period occurrence is the only possible recording method or where the scores provided are more useful than measures of frequency or duration (Martin and Bateson, 1986, p. 62).

When social behaviour is described it is often desirable to produce data on general activity and on specific kinds of interactions. In these circumstances more than one method of behaviour measurement can be used simultaneously. In a herd of cows, general activity can be recorded by point sampling whilst rare events such as fights or mutual grooming can be recorded by behaviour sampling. The data from such behaviour sampling is produced as a list of initiators and targets of attacks, or winners and losers of fights, or groomers and groomed, or pairs of individuals associating. These data are best studied further by putting them in a matrix with each animal in the group represented along each margin. Further analysis of such matrices and analysis of sequences of behaviour are discussed further in Jensen *et al.* (1986, pp. 49 and 59) and in Martin and Bateson (1986, pp. 109 and 63).

Table 2.1
Summary of statistical tests which are useful in behaviour studies. Tests are non-parametric if not marked or are parametric if marked with an asterisk

Question 1	Does the sample come from a specified population? (Tests of goodness of fit for single samples) *Chi square test* for one sample (nominal data) *Binomial test* (nominal data) *Kolmogorov–Smirnov* one sample test
Question 2	Is there a significant difference between the scores of two unrelated samples; for example, between the scores of two different groups of subjects? (Tests of difference between two unmatched samples.) *Chi square test* for two independent samples (nominal data) *Fisher* exact probability test (nominal data) *Mann-Whitney U test* *Student's t test* for unmatched samples ("*t* test")*
Question 3	Is there a significant difference between the scores of two related samples; for example, between the scores of the same subjects under two different conditions, or between siblings? (Tests of difference between two matched samples.) *Wilcoxon* matched-pairs signed ranks test *Student's t test* for matched samples ("matched-pairs *t* test")*
Question 4	Are there significant differences between the scores of several unrelated samples? (Tests of difference between *k* unmatched samples.) *Chi square test* for *k* independent samples (nominal data) *Kruskall–Wallis* one-way analysis of variance *Analysis of variance**
Question 5	Are there significant differences between the scores of several related samples; for example, between the scores of the same subjects measured under several different conditions? (Tests of difference between *k* matched samples.) *Friedman* two-way analysis of variance *Repeated measures analysis of variance**

Table 2.1 *Cont'd*

Question 6	Are two sets of scores associated? (Measures of correlation between two samples.) *Spearman* rank correlation coefficient *Kendall* rank correlation coefficient *Pearson* product–moment correlation coefficient ("correlation")*
Question 7	Are several sets of scores associated; for example, are the scores of one group of subjects consistent when measured several times, or is there an overall association between several different measures for the same set of subjects? (Test of concordance between *k* rankings of the same subjects.) *Kendall coefficient of concordance*

An important final stage of measuring behaviour is the statistical analysis of data. A survey of common statistical tests, modified after Martin and Bateson (1986) is summarised in Table 2.1

Recording aids

Behaviour recording is often difficult because events occur too quickly to write down both the nature of the event and the time at which it occurs. When making a written record of behaviour, much time is saved by using a single symbol abbreviation of the title of a measure. If a sampling procedure is used then a recording sheet can be prepared with spaces for writing symbols or ticks at the predetermined time intervals. For continuous recording the simplest method is to use a stopwatch on a board with squared paper on which a line across the page represents time, for example one minute or 30 s. The hand is moved across the page and symbols are written at a place on the line which represents a certain time. The duration of each activity can then be measured as the total distance on all the lines on the page where that activity was recorded. The next step from this is to use a moving paper event-recorder which is combined with a keyboard on which each key represents a different event. A further step is for the key-board to be connected to a computer with a real time clock so that the nature of the events and the time can be recorded. Such computer-linked recording systems are the best for many pur-poses but recording on squared paper or on a moving paper event-recorder are still useful because the data are visible. Hence in the early part of a study it may be best to use such methods before deciding on all the information which will be recorded using a computer system.

Where behaviour changes are very rapid, tape-recording and video-recording are of particular value. The study of bird song and many other detailed sequences of behaviour has been facilitated by the possibility that behaviour could be recorded and then slowed down. The data can also be played back repeatedly. A representation of a sound sequence can be produced using a sonograph. Video-recording also has the advantage that animals can be watched by a camera, rather than a person, so observer disturbance can be minimised. Time-lapse cine film or video-recording provides an opportunity for animals to be studied over a long period without the necessity for an observer to be present. For some sorts of behaviour recording, automatic systems which monitor switch closure or output from various forms of sensors can be used. Further detail about record-ing aids is provided by Jensen *et al.* (1986, p. 20) and Martin and Bateson (1986, p. 76).

Field studies

Studies of animals in a natural or semi-natural environment provide valuable information about their range of behaviour and how they allocate resources, but there is a considerable likelihood that behaviour will be altered by the presence of an observer. Hence if wild, feral or free-ranging animals are to be watched then aids to distant observation are needed. Binocu-lars, telescopes, telephoto lenses and parabolic reflectors for microphones may be required. Close observation requires the use of a hide

unless the animals are fully habituated to human presence. Experiments can be very valuable in field situations; for example animals can be pre-sented with food items, sounds, or odoriferous marks.

Test situations

Very many behavioural tests are possible and much of the experimental psychological litera-ture can provide ideas for farm animal behav-iour work. One kind of test which has provided information about the biological needs of ani-mals is the preference test. Any investigation of animals in a varied environment offers the opportunity to find out what animals choose to do but specific choice tests are also possible. Different foods, flooring, housing design, com-panions, temperatures, light levels, or air flow conditions can be presented. Preference tests may be simultaneous or successive. Simulta-neous testing situations need to be designed care-fully for they may be confusing to the animal. A choice may be the consequence of initial orienta-tion or an animal may appear to be liking one alternative when it is really withdrawing from the other alternative or the observer. Successive presentations of different stimuli may give con-fusing results because the animal is rapidly becoming less responsive to all stimuli. The order of presentation needs to be varied in a sys-tematic way. All preference tests require careful thought and good controls but they can provide very valuable information (Chapter 29).

Another procedure which is useful in behavioural research is to deprive the animal of some resource or ability in a controlled way and then to monitor behaviour when the deprivation period ends. Such studies often mimic depriva-tion which is normal on some farms. The effects of deprivation of, for example, particular foods, social contact, or space to flap wings for a long period or a short period can be assessed by recording immediate and long-term changes in behaviour. Deprivation is often used as a prelude to studies of learning. Farm animals perform very well in learning tasks provided that they are given adequate cues and the responses required are appropriate.

Other test situations (Fraser, 1978c) include exposure to a novel environment and tests associated with reproduction. If an animal is moved to a new pen it shows exploratory behaviour and may also be disturbed by the conditions so that responses associated with adrenal activity are shown. As a consequence the monitoring of behaviour in a novel test pen or arena, sometimes mis-named an "open field", is used as a measure of the effects of previous experience and of individual differences. Mating behaviour can be tested by presenting an individual with a potential partner or a model and parental behaviour can be tested by exposing the animal to young animals, sounds or models. The results of such experimental studies are mentioned frequently throughout this book.

3 Experience, learning and behaviour development

Experience

During development, the expression of genes and the synthetic processes which lead to the growth of cells and organs into a particular form are dependent upon environmental factors. In adulthood, many genes are still active and a wide range of bodily processes are modified by input from the rest of the body and the world outside the body. Behaviour is controlled by the nervous system and effected by muscles, bones, etc. within the body. The environment affects the development and continuing functioning of these. One consequence of this is, as mentioned in Chapter 1, that no behaviour is independent of the genetic information in the animal and no behaviour is independent of all environmental factors. Another consequence is that every interaction between an individual and its environment has a potential for modifying that individual.

An effect of the environment on behaviour may be mediated via sense organs or via other cells in the body. A change in environmental oxygen concentration might result in a change in behaviour without a sense organ being involved, for example. There is no fundamental reason for distinguishing between such an environmental effect and one which reaches the brain as a perceived stimulus. The animal might discover that if it goes to a certain place a wide variety of consequences, sensory or otherwise, due to lack of oxygen follow. If it goes to a second place a dangerous predator might be detected. Each of these could be considered to be part of the experience of the animal. People often imply, however, that some sensory perception has occurred when they say that something is experienced. An experience is thought of as a mental construct which results from some event in the environment, not just of the body but of the brain. Some experiences are a consequence of changes in hormone levels or of other aspects of the physical and chemical environment of the brain. Many other experiences are a result of sensory input. The input to the brain, however mediated, will usually result from some change outside the body. However it will sometimes result from physiological changes which are a consequence of previous changes outside the body or from changes which are entirely internal. An imaginary event might lead to adrenal activity which will itself result in a bodily change being experienced. *An experience is a change in the brain which results from information acquired from outside the brain.* Some experiences are very brief indeed whilst others are very long-lasting. Existing information in the brain affects whether or not they are long-lasting.

Learning

When learning occurs, an experience of some kind has led to a change in behaviour. This change must itself be a result of a process within the brain so a definition is as follows. *Learning is a change in the brain, which results in behaviour being modified for longer than a few seconds, as a consequence of information from outside the brain.* The reference to "a few seconds" excludes simple responses. The experience and the consequence might range from the effects of oxygen concentration on enzyme action during the development of a motor control mechanism to the effects of scarcely perceptible signs on the behaviour of an individual in a complex society. This wide range of learning means that it is involved in almost all aspects of behaviour. Learning experiments are important for people with a wide range of objectives in their research and no-one studying behaviour can ignore the effects of learning. It is important to realise that, as Hinde (1973) put it, "learning is not episodic but is occurring continuously, though not necessarily affecting behaviour immediately". Having said this, however, it is apparent that many events in the environment of an animal do not lead to any change in future behaviour. Some events are not detected by the animal, some do not reach decision-making centres as a consequence of sensory filtering mechanisms, but some are real *cues* in that the animal can detect them. A question of fundamental importance is how animals learn to ignore irrelevant cues (Mackintosh, 1973). Such learning occurs partly because animals have a predisposition to respond to certain cues, associating them with particular actions (Lorenz, 1965), and partly because responsiveness changes with the repetition of cues.

Predispositions to learn

The fact that, out of an array of detectable cues, animals are much more likely to learn to associate some of them than others with an action or another cue has been discussed at length by Bolles (1975). He points out that for rats, learning to respond to aversive stimuli, such as an electric shock, with an avoidance reaction is more likely to occur and is much faster than learning to respond to a signal indicating imminent food arrival by pressing a lever. This is explicable because rats which modify their behaviour quickly when a cue indicating danger is recognised will produce more offspring than rats which are less good at doing so. Hence genes which promote such an ability have spread in the rat population. In contrast, learning new activities to obtain food is rarer and it may be better if it is slow because of the necessity of avoiding novel objects which might be poisonous or otherwise hazardous. A similar kind of conclusion can be drawn from work of Shettleworth (1972, 1973) which shows that some sorts of responses are very difficult to associate with food whilst others are associated easily. Food was presented to hamsters on a series of occasions when they were carrying out some activity. The hamsters learned readily to associate some activities with food but did not learn as readily with other activities. Pressing a bar in the cage, rearing on their hind legs in the centre of the cage, scrabbling or digging were all increased in frequency if food was presented at the instant that they occurred. Washing their faces, scratching themselves with the hind leg, or scent-marking on the cage were not increased in frequency by food presentation. The activities which the hamsters did learn to associate with food were more like those involved in food finding and acquisition so it would seem that the possibility that the arrival of food might be contingent on such an activity was more credible to the hamster than that it should be contingent upon some body cleaning or social activity.

The examples given above are of learning to associate a cue with an action. Similar examples of predispositions to learn could also be given for other learning situations, for example habituation to cues which might be associated with a dangerous predator is less likely than habituation to minor disturbances or social signals of minor importance (see next section).

Predispositions to learn develop as a consequence of genetic and environmental factors, just like other behaviour controlling systems. Animals which had more effective predispositions would have produced more offspring so genes which promoted effective learning about predators would have spread in the population. In any individual, however, genetic and environmental factors will have interacted in developing its set of predispositions both in the general sense and in relation to particular actions. An act in the hamster's repertoire of behaviour, for example, might be incorporated in a grooming sequence and hence become difficult to associate with food, or in a digging sequence and be easy to associate with food.

Habituation and sensitisation

If a flock of sheep is moved from a quiet field to one near a road, they will show an escape response on the first occasion that they see or hear a motor vehicle pass along the road. Subsequent vehicles elicit less and less response until each member of the flock ceases to show any behavioural response; it habituates. *Habituation is the waning of a response, which could still be shown, to a repeated stimulus*. The repetition might be very frequent or as infrequent as once per day but habituation would still occur. The likelihood of habituation and its rate would depend upon the nature of the stimulus, its rate, its regularity and the state of the animal. A stimulus like the sound of a falling pine cone might elicit a startle response initially from a sheep but habituation would occur rapidly if pine cones fell every minute and less rapidly if they fell irregularly at a rate of five per day. The sheep would not be likely to habituate to the sight of a hunting wolf, however. Indeed the reverse might occur in that it would become sensitised. *Sensitisation is the increasing of a response to a repeated stimulus*. The wolf might elicit a greater response the second time it is seen than the first, or a sound like a cracking stick

could elicit little response the first time but more and more response when it recurred. In each of these examples the repetition might mean greater danger than a single stimulus so sensitisation is advantageous. Habituation is an even more important process for it saves energy which would be wasted on repeated response to a trivial stimulus and it may also prevent the animal from being detected by a predator during a response to a trivial event. As mentioned earlier in this chapter, habituation is an important means of ensuring that animals do not respond to too many of the events which occur in their environment.

Habituation could occur as a consequence of receptor fatigue or adaptation of a neuron in the brain pathway and it may be that such simple habituation does occur. It seems likely, however, that much habituation is just as complex as the various forms of associative learning because it is so specific. Sokolov (1960) describes the habituation of the startle response in dogs to a tone but the reappearance of the full response when these habituated dogs are presented with a tone which differs only slightly in frequency. Sokolov also demonstrated very specific habituation of the physiological startle response of dogs to the duration of a sound. Broom (1968a) carried out a similar experiment in which the behavioural response of young domestic chicks, to a light repeatedly switched on for 10 s and off for 20 s, habituated. When the light was switched on for only 5 s, so that it went off early, the chicks responded and when it was left on for 15 s they responded at 10 s when it should have gone off. Such studies demonstrate that the animal must be establishing a model of the environmental change in its brain and comparing each input with that model. This is much more elaborate a form of learning than mere neuronal adaptation.

Important practical aspects of habituation concern the waning of the responses of farm animals to handling procedures and housing conditions. If much handling is likely to be needed during an animal's lifetime, as it is for milking cows, breeding stock or show animals, then careful habituation of animals to handling procedures is necessary. Any new procedure or item of equipment may need further training. The sudden introduction of a different kind of vehicle for distributing food may result in escape responses but preliminary exposure and slow approach will allow rapid habituation. Similarly, a different item of clothing like a suit or white coat may elicit a response in an animal which has habituated to a person in an overall. This last point is especially important for animals taken to shows or markets, as is the necessity for animals to be exposed gradually to situations where there are many people and other novel stimuli.

Experimental learning studies

A high proportion of what is written about learning refers exclusively to learning tests in laboratory situations and this often misleads the reader into thinking that learning is scarcely relevant to real life. Nothing could be further from the truth as learning is involved in all of the functional systems. It is discussed, as it must be, in every chapter of this book. The animal which is efficient in its ability to learn about its physical environment, individuals of its own species, sources of danger and resources of various kinds, will survive and reproduce. Poor ability to learn such things means reduced fitness.

Experimental studies are of value for it is difficult to carry out controlled studies in the field. Experimental results are vulnerable to errors of interpretation, however, because in some studies animals fail to learn because they are frightened by the experimental situation, or because either the stimulus presented or the action required of them is inappropriate. A sheep will not work in a learning test if what it views as a dangerous predator is present or if its long-term companions are absent. Neither will it work readily for food which it does not want to eat or if it is required to perform an action like putting its foot on a lever. Examples of experimental situations which have been used for farm animals are classical conditioning, in which an animal learns to show an existing response to a new stimulus, operant conditioning in which the animal learns to perform an "operant" response in order to obtain a reward or avoid an aversive experience, and maze learning in which the animal learns to take a particular path in order to obtain a reward. These terms are consistent descriptions of procedures but it is likely that the changes which occur in the brain during learning are similar in different situations. In each situation, an environmental change which acts as a *positive reinforcer* or reward, increasing the likelihood of a response, or as a *negative reinforcer*, decreasing response likelihood is involved. Positive reinforcers include various correctors of homeostatic imbalance (see Chapter 4) such as food, water, temperature change, etc., and opportunities for social behaviour, sexual behaviour, or exploration. Negative reinforcers are painful events, frightening stimuli or extensions of homeostatic imbalance.

The best known consequence of *classical conditioning* on farms is milk let-down by dairy cows in response to the typical sounds of a milking parlour. Milk let-down is initiated by oxytocin release following stimulation of the teat by a calf attempting to suckle. Cows with calves soon start to release oxytocin when other stimuli from the calf are detected and cows milked using a milking machine may respond to other cues in the same way. There is variation amongst breeds of cattle with respect to how readily such conditioning can occur, and old breeds such as the Salers in France are much less ready to let down milk to stimuli other than real calves than are Friesians or Holsteins. Pavlov's original studies of classical conditioning involved dogs which show the unconditioned response of salivation to the unconditioned stimulus of detecting food. They started to salivate to the sound of a bell if the bell had been paired with food presentation on a number of occasions. The bell is referred to as a conditioned stimulus and the salivation as a conditioned response. Using these terms, milk let-down becomes a conditioned response to the

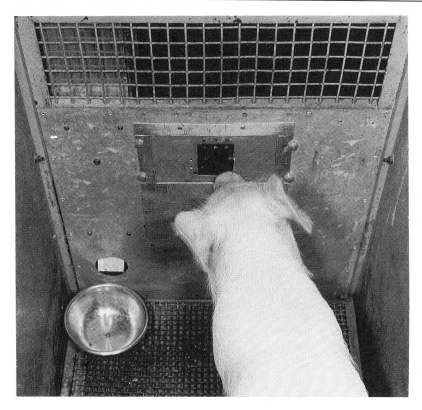

Fig. 3.1 This pig is about to push the black panel and thus operate a switch. Pigs learned to press for food, for a period of heat, or to switch lights on or off (from Baldwin, 1979, with the authors' permission).

conditioned stimulus of clanking noises etc. in the milk parlour. Farmers need to be aware of the fact that milk let-down in a parlour is a conditioned response and that such learning depends upon adequate training. If disturbing stimuli are present in the milking parlour the young animal may not learn and the older animal which is conditioned may be inhibited from showing the response. As Kilgour (1987) points out, any veterinary work which involves discomfort for the cow should not be carried out in the milking parlour but in a separate facility.

Another form of associative learning is *operant conditioning*. Sheep and pigs, studied by Baldwin (1972, 1979), learned to operate a switch for food, light or heat (Fig. 3.1). A sheep was able to switch on a heater over its pen by putting its nose in a slot and breaking a beam monitored by a photocell; it learned that when the ambient temperature was low it could warm itself by the operant behaviour of putting its nose in the slot. Sheep did not do this when they had a full fleece but only when they had been shorn. Very many studies of this kind have been carried out by experimental psychologists using rats pressing a lever, for a reinforcer such as food, in a "Skinner box" in which the lever pressing and food delivery are automatically monitored. Some experimentation has involved studying the effects of different schedules of reinforcement. If food is delivered every fifth time that the lever is pressed this is referred to as a fixed ratio of reinforcement (FR5). Animals still learn when the ratio is very high and this is not surprising because in wild conditions they might often need to carry out a food searching behaviour many times in order to obtain a food item. A consequence of this for farm animals is that they might repeat a movement which has resulted in reinforcement many times. A dog was trained to bark 33 times for small food rewards (Salzinger and Waller, 1962) and this explains why dogs which are occasionally fed scraps when their owners are eating and which sometimes bark in this situation, may associate barking with feeding and bark even more. The operant response of barking is effectively reinforced on a large, rather variable ratio of responses to rewards, but the dog still learns the association.

A quite different schedule of reinforcement is that where the reward follows the operant behaviour but only after a fixed interval. In a laboratory experiment the animal still has to press a lever in order to obtain food but lever-pressing has no effect except after the predetermined interval. If the interval is long enough, animals usually learn not to press the lever except when the time of reinforcement is close. The existence of quite accurate internal clocks is apparent from such studies, as it is from observation of animals on the farm. Cows use the operant response of bellowing when it is time for the farmer to collect them for milking and sows using an electronic sow feeder enter the feeder more often at the time that the daily feed cycle is about to begin.

Learning ability of farm animals

A form of associative learning in which several successive responses are associated with a reinforcer is involved in learning how to get from one place to another. Farm animals readily learn their way around the area available to them on farms so it is to be expected that they can learn to run mazes. Studies by Pollard *et al.* (1971) compared the performance of several species in a variable (Hebb–Williams) maze which involved a set of six different simple detours to reach an objective by walking. A score of 100% could be obtained if the animal solved the problem in the first four of eight runs given daily and slower learning resulted in a lower score. Kilgour (1987) repeated these trials using various farm animals, dogs, cats and man. The learning scores were 99 for children, 90–93 for dogs, cows, goats and pigs, 85 for sheep, 81 for cats and rats, 61–66 for hens and pigeons and 48–53 for mice and guinea pigs. Using a score based upon numbers of errors, sheep were as good as cows and dogs but pigs were less good. Some results in such experiments might be affected by variation in motivational state, especially being frightened, but it is clear that the farm animals performed very well. Comparative studies of apparent learning ability using many tasks, like those reviewed by Houpt and Wolski (1982, p. 227), are so dependent upon the motivational state that it is difficult to draw realistic conclusions. A wide range of other studies, however, show that farm animal species can learn simple and complex tasks with great rapidity. The maximum possible performance in any one of a wide range of learning situations is probably the best indicator of learning ability. Using such a criterion, cattle, sheep, goats and pigs learn at least as well as dogs. Horses may be slightly less good at learning but there are surprisingly few well-controlled studies on them. Domestic fowl perform somewhat less well but all of these species are very competent at various tasks. Measurements of brain size, or brain size in relation to body size, offer little additional information. For mammals, the degree of folding of the cerebral cortex may be related to intellectual ability. The ungulates such as sheep, cattle, goats, pigs and horses have more folding than most mammals, with only the primates and whales clearly showing more folding.

Observations of learning in the real world which farm animals encounter offers the most impressive evidence of their ability. Grazing animals are often thought to lead an uncomplicated life but recent research shows that this is certainly not so. As explained in Chapter 9, sheep and cattle are very selective about what they eat and they have to learn about all the different plants which they encounter. They also have to learn to identify patches of good grazing and to return to them after intervals so that they obtain adequate quantities of a good mix of plant material without wasting energy going to places which have not regrown after the last grazing. These animals live in groups with an elaborate social structure and they have to learn a lot about other individuals. The most complex tasks in the lives of animals are those associated with establishing and maintaining social relationships. Hence flock- and herd-living farm animals have to have a considerable intellect for this purpose alone. Farmers are accustomed to rapid learning by farm animals to the extent that they may not appreciate that much is being demanded of the animals. A simple form of con-ditioning with a negative reinforcer is learning to avoid an electric fence. Some individuals explore the fence and learn to avoid it after receiving a shock. Some learn, by watching others, that the fence has some unpleasant characteristics. A few discover that whilst a moist nose applied to the fence results in a substantial shock, a touch with a better insulated area has less effect, so they monitor the fence at intervals to check that it is still activated. The provision of food in troughs whose lids have to be lifted requires quite sophisticated operant conditioning, as does the use of Callan–Broadbent doors (Fig. 3.2, 3.3). One of these doors (or gates) opens only when the cow wearing the correct transponder comes close to it. Hence a cow which is newly equipped with such a transponder and then faced with a row of doors, has to learn that food is available to it when it pushes down with its head on one of the doors in this row. This very complex task is learned very quickly by most cows with little

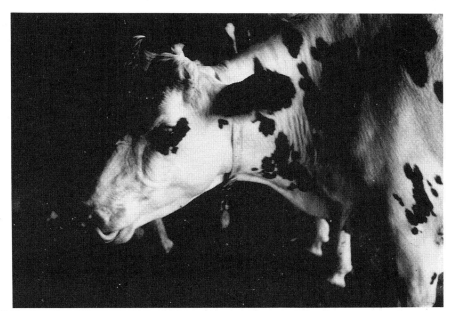

Fig. 3.2 Holstein cow with transponder which could be used for opening a Callan–Broadbent gate or for entry to a feeding stall. The transponder is recognised individually and an appropriate electrical response initiated (from colour slide by D.M. Broom).

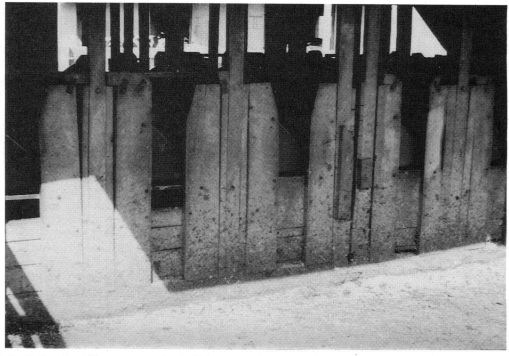

Fig. 3.3 Callan–Broadbent gates, each of which can be opened by an individual cow's transponder (from colour slide by D.M. Broom).

training. Another complex automatic feeder whose operation is readily learned is the electronic feeding stall for cattle or sows which again depends upon the wearing of a transponder but in which the operation is more complex. Problems associated with training animals to use these stalls are more to do with social contact with other cows or sows near the feeder than with the operation of the system. Not only do the animals learn to operate these feeders, but they learn how to beat the system and obtain extra food by chasing other animals out, or coming back in through the exit gate, or banging the food dispenser so that it delivers a few extra pellets of food. Many examples of the learning ability of farm animals are described in other chapters of this book.

Behaviour development

There are two kinds of problem for the young developing animal. The immediate problem is how to survive during the first period of life when it is very vulnerable to predation, to physical conditions and to the risk of not obtaining adequate nutrients. This is often a quite different problem from that of the adult because the young animal is smaller, less able to defend itself than are adults, subject to attack by predators which might not attack its parents and often requires different physical conditions and diet from adults. The other problem for the developing animal is how to change in such a way that it becomes an effective adult. There is often an assumption that most behaviour during development is directed towards the adult objectives but the very high incidence of early mortality in most species means that there is a high selection pressure promoting efficient survival mechanisms at this time.

Development of domestic chick behaviour

What does a young domestic chick have to do in order to survive, grow and eventually become a successful adult? In the early stages especially, it is not possible to understand how behaviour

changes without knowing about the development of body anatomy and the biochemistry and physiology of the brain. Developmental changes in behaviour start before hatching but increase dramatically in number and complexity after hatching. A summary of pre-hatching and early post-hatching changes is shown in Fig. 3.4. Some behavioural contact with the mother occurs before hatching by the chick calling and reacting to parental calls. Just before hatching the embryo chicks commence making clicking noises. Vince (1964, 1966, 1973) has demonstrated that the chicks in a clutch of eggs are

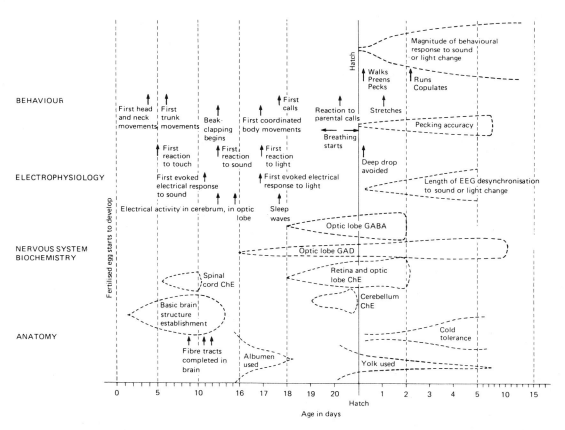

Fig. 3.4 Some changes in the domestic chick's anatomy, physiology and behaviour during development from fertilisation. Abbreviations in diagram: GABA, γ amino-butyric acid (a neurotransmitter); ChE, cholinesterase and GAD, glutamic acid decarboxylase (enzymes which break down neurotransmitters); EEG, electro-encephalogram (from Broom, 1981).

communicating with one another by this means. The clicks have the effect of accelerating hatching by some chicks and hence synchronising the hatching of the eggs in a clutch. A chick which hatches early or late is more vulnerable to predation so synchronisation is advantageous to all.

After hatching the young chick needs to recognise the mother, keep the mother close or follow her, make the mother do things which benefit the chick, recognise anything dangerous and respond in a way which minimises the danger. Within a short time after hatching the chick needs to develop an ability to look after itself. It must learn about feeding, body temperature regulation and many other aspects of life. The motor and sensory ability of the chick is quite good at hatching but both improve during the first few days of life (Kruijt, 1964). Pecking is an important way of investigating the environment and it improves in accuracy during the first week after hatching (Padilla, 1935). Dark-rearing only slightly impairs this improvement (Cruze, 1935) and corrections for distorted vision are possible (Rossi, 1968). The chick prefers to peck at objects which are small, shiny (Baeumer, 1955), three-dimensional (Fantz, 1957) and of certain colours (Hess, 1956; Kear, 1964, 1966). These preferences are modified by experience during the first few days of life (Dawkins, 1968). The chick has the sensory ability to see and hear the mother in the few hours after hatching. Newly hatched chicks, ducklings and goslings approach objects which are larger than themselves and which move at approximately walking speed (Lorenz, 1935; Fabricius, 1951; Hinde *et al.*, 1956). These do not have to be the mother and it is particular visual or auditory patterns which are attractive. A flashing light or a rotating disc could also be maximally effective visual stimuli in attracting chicks (James, 1959; Smith, 1962). In normal circumstances, the object which the chick sees with these characteristics is the mother. The chick rapidly learns her precise characteristics and is subsequently more likely to follow something with these characteristics (see Bateson, 1966, for a review of such studies). This period

of rapid learning is associated with particular structural and biochemical changes in the chick's brain (Horn, 1985). At the same time as learning about its mother, the chick is learning the characteristics of other aspects of its environment and starting to avoid the unfamiliar (Bateson, 1964). The chick must form a neural model of this familiar world in order that discrepancies can be recognised and avoided in case they are dangerous (Broom, 1969b). The manipulation of maternal behaviour by the chick is important for early survival. A cold chick calls loudly and thus encourages the mother to come and brood it. Chicks make twitter calls which encourage the mother to stay with them and they are able to copy her pecking movements. Hence they can learn from her as well as deriving protection from her.

Development in each functional system

The chick whose development is described above is very different from a sparrow or rabbit in its stage of development when it emerges into the complex and dangerous outside world. Animals which are well developed when they are born or when they hatch are precocial whereas those which are helpless are altricial (Fig. 3.5). There is a continuum between the two extremes, man being more altricial than precocial, but all of the major farm animal species are at the precocial end.

After birth or hatching the development of sensory systems is affected by experience. For example, animals reared in darkness have fewer cells and fewer synapses between neurons in the visual pathway. Studies of the functioning of the visual system show that various sophisticated analysers do not develop if the eyes are alternately covered or if the environment is limited to vertical stripes during early rearing (Blakemore and Cooper, 1970; Hirsch and Spinelli, 1970; Blakemore and van Sluyters, 1974). Such developmental changes will affect all aspects of behaviour, as will the development of ability to make certain movements. Altricial mammals do

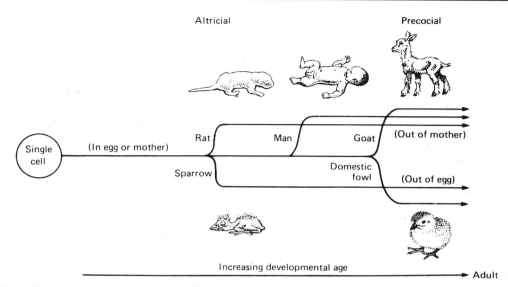

Fig. 3.5 Diagram of development from fertilised egg to adult showing that altricial animals emerge into the outside world at an earlier stage of development than do precocial animals. The origins of arrows show the point of hatching or birth (modified after Broom, 1981).

not avoid a cliff in the early stages of life but when perceptual and motor abilities are sufficiently developed they do avoid it. Young domestic chicks, on the other hand, avoid cliffs as early as 3 h after hatching. Their depth perception and awareness of danger are adequately developed by that age (Tallarico, 1961). The development of predator avoidance may be very unspecific initially, for example there is an increase with age in avoidance by young domestic chicks of anything which is unfamiliar (Broom, 1969a). Such general effects become more specific as the complexity of experience increases. Studies with rhesus monkeys, chimpanzees and domestic chicks showed that responses to relatively harmless novel stimuli were less if the animals had been reared in more complex early environments than if they had been kept in more barren environments (Harlow and Zimmermann, 1959; Menzel *et al.*, 1963; Broom, 1969b). The recognition of specific predators also depends upon experience. Lorenz (1939) and Goethe (1940) had reported that young precocial birds showed a flight response

to hawks or falcons but not to flying geese. Experiments by Schleidt (1961) showed that this difference could have been due to habituation to geese but not to hawks. Models of hawks and geese can be distinguished by ducklings and both elicit responses (Mueller and Parker, 1980), but extreme escape is more likely to be shown if other birds have been observed to show it. If an actual predator attack occurs, surviving individuals usually improve their ability to deal with such an attack as a result of this experience. This is apparent when deer are chased by wolves or larks are chased by falcons. The more experienced individuals have learned tricks which help them to escape.

Behavioural efficiency in other functional systems also develops with age and experience. Grazing time increases during the first four months in calves as rumen function develops (Chambers, 1959; Hutchison *et al.*, 1962). Young animals are, however, less efficient as grazers than are older animals. Preliminary evidence for this came from Hodgson and Wilkinson's (1969) observation that 12-month-old calves graze for 1 h per day more than heifers and 1.6 h per day more than 3½-year-old cows. This could be because calves are more selective or because of mouth size, but work on sheep suggests that it is largely because of their lower grazing efficiency. Arnold and Maller (1977) and Arnold and Dudzinski (1978) found that sheep reared with no grazing experience for three years grazed much less efficiently than experienced sheep (Fig. 3.6).

Communication and courtship behaviour are sometimes not very variable within a species but detailed studies show how much the final form depends upon experience during development. Although most bird calls develop normally when birds are reared in isolation (Marler and Hamilton, 1966) they depend upon the ability of birds to listen to themselves, for early deafened birds are abnormal (Nottebohm, 1967). Songs of birds like chaffinches (*Fringilla coelebs*) and white-crowned sparrows (*Zonotrichia leucophrys*) vary according to the sounds of singing birds heard during the juvenile period (Thorpe, 1958; Marler and Tamura, 1964) and the songs

of territorial rivals heard during adulthood (Jenkins, 1978; Baptista and Petrinovich, 1986). Developmental studies of sexual behaviour in the jungle fowl, the wild ancestor of the domestic fowl, show that movements involved in courtship and mating appear in the behavioural repertoire at an early age but become organised into sequences and used at appropriate times as the bird gets older and more experienced (Kruijt, 1964). Jungle fowl, guinea-pigs, rats, cats and rhesus monkeys reared with insufficient contact with social companions show abnormal courtship and mating behaviour. Incorrect orientation or atypical movements and sequences result in partly or wholly ineffectual mating.

Mate selection is substantially affected by early experience. The discriminations between potential mates are very subtle and many animals devote much energy to behaviour which maximises the chances of obtaining a high quality mate so that offspring are likely to be successful. Many studies of waterfowl have shown that birds reared by foster parents often directed courtship to that species when they became adult. For example, Schutz (1965) found that male mallard ducks, the most common domestic duck species, reared by their parents for 21 days but by another species from 21–49 days or later, showed most sexual behaviour when adult towards the other species. Studies of zebra finches (*Poephila castanotis*), exposed to their own and another finch species by Immelmann (1972, 1977) and ten Cate (1984), showed that the later mating preferences of males depend upon the species which is active as a parent during the rearing period, the species of the other young reared with them, the species with which they interact after fledging, their age at each of these contacts and the duration of the contacts. Cockerels, turkeys and doves reared alone by hand will court and attempt to mate with a human hand but prolonged contact with females of their own species usually reverses this (Schein, 1963; Schleidt, 1970; Klinghammer, 1967). Within a species, work on quail has demonstrated that the sexual partners chosen are those which are similar to but not identical

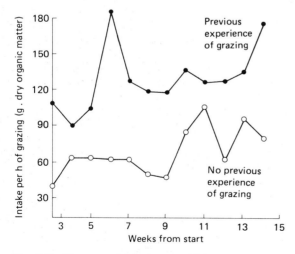

Fig. 3.6 Three-year-old sheep which have had no experience of grazing (open circles) are less efficient grazers than are sheep which have grazed (filled circles). Their performance improves after 10 weeks' practice (after Arnold and Dudzinski, 1978).

with the birds which were present during the first 35 days of rearing (Bateson, 1978). The age at which the characteristics of parents and siblings are learned varies from species to species, but it is clear that mates are selected which are familiar in their characteristics but discrepant to some degree from the parents and siblings (Bateson, 1980).

Much social behaviour, as mentioned already, is complex and difficult to learn, so it is not surprising that its development is slow, prolonged and greatly affected by experience. Isolation-rearing does not prevent the development of the motor patterns involved in fighting, threatening or caring for mate and offspring. It does alter the production of social signals and the timing of all behaviour during social interactions so that isolation-reared animals are socially incompetent. Mason (1960) and Harlow (1969) working with rhesus monkeys found that their social behaviour after six months of social isolation was drastically altered and they tended to avoid other members of their species when exposed to them. Monkeys, rodents and cattle did badly in social competition after isolation rearing (Mason, 1961; Rosen and Hart, 1963; Donaldson *et al.*, 1966; Broom and Leaver, 1978). The failure of isolation-reared monkeys to "acquire effective elementary communicative skills which serve to coordinate and control the form and direction of social interactions" is reported by Mason (1961). Broom (1981, p. 257, 1982)

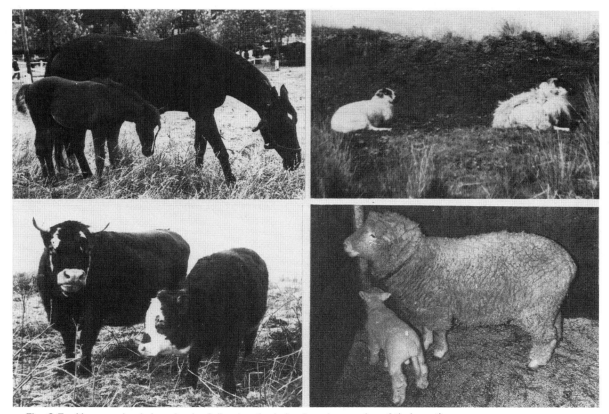

Fig. 3.7 Young animals learning by following the behavioural examples of their mothers.

describes how heifers which had been kept in individual pens over the eight months from birth to turnout to pasture in spring were quite inadequate in their social responses. In encounters with heifers experienced in social encounters they did not return the gaze, kept their ears back much more when approached, failed to retaliate if attacked and lost most competitive encounters. As a consequence they got less food in competitive feeding situations. These social inadequacies persisted for at least a year.

Social encounters during development help individuals to improve their performance in such encounters, but they also make other advantages possible. Farm animals, like monkeys and other social animals, learn from one another, especially from their mothers (Fig. 3.7). Some of the improvement in ability to forage effectively and manage other resources must come from observing efficient individuals and doing what they do. Predator avoidance improves with age and some of this is a consequence of being with and copying experienced individuals. Farmers know that once an animal in a group learns to open a gate, or manipulate a piece of equipment so as to get more food, or intimidate a stockman, that others in the group are likely to learn to do it too. We have much to learn about the role of social factors in the development of behaviour but it is important that we do know more about this. It will help to understand existing farm situations and to facilitate the use of new automatic systems on farms where the animal is required to control its own environmental conditions, food supply, milking or access to mates or parturition accommodation.

4 Motivation

When a pig awakens after lying asleep in the corner of a field or yard, what determines which movements it will then make and which functional system will be served by its behaviour? If a young domestic chick is observed and its behaviour categorised as shown in Fig. 4.1, what determines the nature and timing of each transition from one behaviour to another? These are questions about the motivation of the animal. *Motivation is the process within the brain controlling which behaviours and physiological changes occur and when.* An understanding of motivation is fundamental to all studies of behaviour and is especially relevant to most of the practical questions which farmers and veterinary surgeons ask about farm animal behaviour such as feeding, reproduction and handling. An appreciation of the subtleties of motivational systems is also necessary in order that behaviour can be used as an indicator of animal welfare.

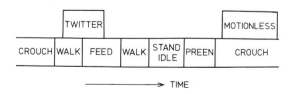

Fig. 4.1 Sequence of behaviour shown by young domestic chick.

Causal factors

The pig or the chick might initiate an activity which is likely to result in obtaining food, such as standing and walking to a place where food could be present or starting to peck at the ground in a particular place. A number of factors could affect whether or not these behaviours are shown. There might be *sensory input to the brain about the body's environment*, e.g when a food odour is detected or a possible food item is seen. There will be *internal input from* body monitors, such as those affected by gut distension or blood nutrient levels, which provide information about general or specific body deficiencies. There could be *internal input from oscillators* within the body which produce an output after a particular time and can indicate normal feeding time or interval since the last feed. Each of these factors has some direct relevance to the feeding functional system but the likelihood of food-searching will also be affected by inputs to the brain about other aspects of the animal's life. Possibilities include: *input about a skin irritation* which results in scratching and rubbing rather than food-searching; *input about the presence of a potential mate, rival or predator* which again leads to some other activity being given priority over food-searching; or various aspects of *hormonal state* which change the likelihood of occurrence of the various behaviours.

All of these factors mentioned above will be altered, in their effect on the probability of a particular behaviour being initiated, by the *previous experience* of that animal. Many kinds of previous experience might make a pig less likely to start food-searching behaviour. (1) An odour of food might be detected by the pig which has been experienced on numerous previous occasions and has never been followed by food being made available to the pig, perhaps because it is caused by farm staff eating their lunch. (2) The gut may be empty but experience shows that the gut has to be empty for several hours before food is forthcoming. (3) An oscillator could indicate feeding time but recent experience might be that a more dominant pig is always at the feeder at this time. The odour of a potential mate could be detected and the hormone level could be high on frequent occasions when a barrier to that mate is known to be present, but (4) if these factors are combined with the sound of two particular people talking, it could mean that it is worth delaying food-searching as serving could be imminent.

Each input to the brain must be interpreted in relation to previous experience. Some inputs will never reach the decision-making centre in the brain because the interpretation results in their relevance being assessed as zero. It seems likely that most inputs will reach the centre after modification. The actual inputs to the decision-making centre, which are interpretations of a wide variety of external changes and internal states of the body, are called *causal factors*. At any moment there will be very many different causal factors and the levels of these will determine what the individual actually does. Some causal factor levels will change very rapidly because they are altered by rapidly changing environmental events. Others, such as those which depend upon the levels of certain steroid hormones in the blood, change slowly.

All changes in behaviour are a manifestation of the animal's response to changes in causal factors. The experimental investigation of the relationships between causal factors and behaviour may involve either attempting to find out all the effects on behaviour of a single causal factor, or assessing the effects of variation in a wide range of causal factors on a single behaviour (Hinde, 1970). A difficulty of research in this area is that causal factors cannot be measured directly and some are very hard to estimate at all. Many valuable studies have been carried out, however, in which one activity or one experimental manipulator of causal factors has been studied in detail, for example, drinking or effects of water deprivation. In order to understand motivation in real life, however, work investigating situations where more than one experimentally modifiable set of causal factors is acting needs to be considered. This approach was pioneered by McFarland (1965, 1971) who worked initially on feeding and drinking in doves.

Motivational state

If a pig is deprived of water, after some time there will be input to the brain from (1) monitors of body fluids, (2) sensory receptors indicating a dry mouth, and probably from (3) oscillators which would normally prompt drinking and (4) other brain centres indicating that the animal is aware of the fact that drinking has not been possible for some time. The change in the state of the animal with respect to this group of causal factors is shown in Fig. 4.2. As the levels of these causal factors rise there will also be increases in the likelihood of drinking if the opportunity arises and the extent of activities which should result in water acquisition. If the pig were deprived of food as well, then its state with respect to another group of causal factors could be described and combined in a plot with the plot for water deprivation. In Fig. 4.3 a pig whose state has reached B is more likely to eat and to work in some way to get food than one whose state is at O, while an animal whose state is at A is more likely to drink than one whose state is at O. Plotting the state of the animal in this two-dimensional space allows interactions between the two sets of causal factors to become clear.

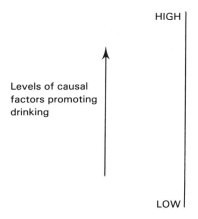

HIGH

Levels of causal factors promoting drinking

- e.g. many hours with no water

- e.g. few hours with no water, salty food eaten
- e.g. few hours with no water, hot sunny conditions

- e.g. few hours with no water, shade conditions

- e.g. animal which has just drunk

LOW

Fig. 4.2 Levels of causal factors which promote a particular action vary over a range and the state of the animal can be described in terms of these.

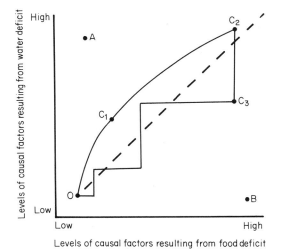

Levels of causal factors resulting from food deficit

Fig. 4.3 Motivational state of animals A, B and C in two-dimensional causal factor space. Animal A is most likely to drink whereas animal B is most likely to eat. The changes in state of animal C are explained in the text.

When a pig is deprived of water its state moves up towards A on the state space plot but it also moves to the right because pigs given no water cannot eat as much. The change in state of the animal as a consequence of water deprivation is shown as a trajectory from O to C_1. If this animal was then deprived of food as well as water, its state would move sharply to the right and up further to C_2.

The behaviour of an animal which is given the opportunity to either eat or drink will depend upon its state as represented in Fig. 4.3. A pig whose state is at C_2 is a little higher on the water deficit side so it might drink. This would bring its state down across the boundary line to C_3 at which time it might switch to eating, thus lowering the causal factors resulting from food deprivation. An example of a possible course of the animal back to O is shown. The actual paths chosen by animals whose state was manipulated in this way are described and the nature of the decision making mechanism explored in papers by Sibly (1975), McFarland and Sibly (1975) and Sibly and McCleery (1976). The position of the boundary line for switching from feeding to drinking could be altered by making the animal search harder for the food or use more energy to get the water (Larkin and McFarland, 1978).

In the state space plot shown, only two sets of causal factors are considered. In reality, the likelihood that the animal would eat or drink at any moment would be affected by many other causal factors as well. Each of these could be plotted in the same way so the motivational state of the animal is its position in a multidimensional causal factor space. Each of these causal factor levels might interact with others in the same way that those relating to food and water deficit interact. A simpler definition, however, is that *the motivational state of an animal is a combination of the levels of all causal factors*.

Motivation concepts

Early attempts to explain how it came about that animals showed a behaviour when they did referred to "instincts" which were thought of as some inherited property of an animal which made it act in an automatic way in certain circumstances. The term implied development without environmental influence, an idea now discredited, and detailed studies of behaviour showed that animals, especially vertebrates, are far from being automata, so the term is no longer used. It was replaced by the term "drive", which was thought by some people as a component of a homeostatic control system and by others as the agent causing a particular behaviour to occur. The idea of a thirst drive which caused drinking and an esploration drive which caused exploration was criticised by Hinde (1959, 1970), who said that "drive concepts can be useful if defined independently of the variations in behaviour which they are supposed to explain". Hinde follows Miller (1959) in suggesting that it could be useful to think of "thirst" as an intervening variable between effects on animals (independent variables) such as water deprivation and amount of dry food eaten, and behavioural responses (dependent variables) such as amount of water drunk and rate of pressing a bar for a water reward. Figure 4.4. shows relationships of "thirst" to six variables. When these relationships were measured, both bar pressing rate and amount of bitter quinine required to stop drinking had a linear relationship to the level of a dependent variable supposedly manipulating thirst, but the amount of water drunk had quite a different relationship. Hinde concludes that the single intervening variable idea is simplistic but Houston and McFarland (1976) point out that

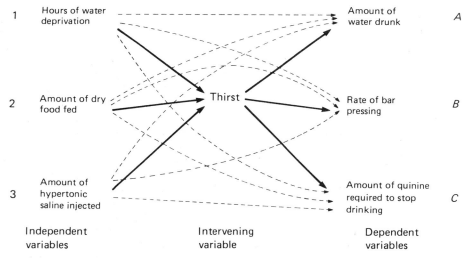

Fig. 4.4   The relationship among each of three independent and three dependent variables (see text) can be simplified if an intervening variable is considered. This diagram refers to experiments on the maintenance of water balance in a rat (from Broom, 1981, modified after Miller, 1959).

the scale of measurement has a big effect on such results. Toates (1986, pp. 33 and 161) emphasises the complexity of motivational systems which is demonstrated by such experiments but affirms that it is helpful to think of motivation as involving incentive objects or goals.

Another view of motivation which requires comment is that Lorenz (1966) who thought of motivation as an accumulation of action-specific energy which is released when the action occurs. However, energy is clearly an inappropriate term for the accumulated potential to perform an action and although the potential to carry out some actions may accumulate this does not happen for other actions. Hence the concept might be useful in certain situations but it is not a general model. Similarly, ideas about general arousal or activation (Duffy, 1962; Berlyne, 1967) are clearly important, for animals sometimes increase their responsiveness to a whole range of inputs, but they do not explain a high proportion of changes in behaviour. Levels of arousal, referring to a defined range of effects, are best thought of as causal factors which are combined with others in decision making.

Observations of the behaviour of rats learning operant responses in "Skinner Boxes" in which, for example, the animal presses a lever for a food reward, led to ideas of motivation as merely the link between a stimulus and a response. Many people assumed that behaviour could be explained as being the largely automatic response to a series of stimuli from the environment. Toates (1987) explains that the stimulus–response model is inadequate in important respects. "Contemporary theory sees the animal as being (a) intrinsically active rather than passive, even in the absence of impinging stimuli (b) goal-seeking, or, in other words, purposive, (c) flexible, (d) able to learn cognitions and (e) exploratory". The examples of motivational state already discussed make it clear that animals are very far from being automata and that they have complex concepts about their environment. An appreciation of an object or an event which is not directly detectable or is not actually occurring at the time is a *cognitive*

representation. A dog which searches for a thrown stick after it has lost sight or smell of it must have some representation of stick in its brain whilst it is looking. A cow whose calf has been removed has cognition of that calf during the period when she is showing distress and perhaps thereafter. Any animal which is working towards a goal is utilising cognitive processes in its behaviour control. An example of purposive behaviour which requires cognition is the burying, by a rat, of an object which delivers electric shocks (Pinel and Wilkie, 1983). Various behaviours have been recorded which have the effect of covering the aversive object with bedding so that the rat does not receive electric shocks from it. Many examples of cognition in farm animals will be apparent throughout this book.

Two other terms which have been used when referring to motivation are "conflict" and "displacement activity". The idea of motivational conflict arose when people were trying to explain situations where an animal was thought to have two important drives, each of which would make it carry out a different behaviour. Although the term conflict appeared to be necessary when it was thought that one drive operated at a time, it is of much less value in modern thinking. Where there are very many different causal factors, in a sense there is conflict all of the time for several different causal factors will always be competing for the animal's time and energy. The situation where two activities are both very likely because of the levels of the causal factors which promote them is of great interest, but it is different only in degree from all other motivational states.

When ethologists observed animals in situations where two actions were likely they sometimes saw that a third action was performed. For example, van Iersel and Bol (1958) observed a tern (*Sterna*) landing near its nest after being alarmed and preening before reaching the nest. The observers considered that incubation and anti-predator behaviour were the most likely activities so preening seemed to be inappropriate. As the preening behaviour was unexpected and it was difficult to see what its function was, the authors followed Tinbergen (1940) and others in calling it a displacement activity. The observation by van Iersel and Bol that terns with wet feathers were more likely to preen, however, suggests that plumage maintenance might be of more importance than they expected, even in the situation described. Animals do carry out actions during behaviour sequences which appear irrelevant to a human observer but there seems to be little value in ascribing the name "displacement activity" to such an action. Work investigating such activities, however, has been important in helping our understanding of behaviour sequences and their control.

Monitoring motivation

Although causal factor levels cannot be measured directly, some estimate of the likely levels of certain causal factors can be made by direct physiological measurement. Blood sugar and hormones can be assayed, for example. Most estimates of motivational state, however, come from behaviour observation, especially where the change in state is rapid. Brain recording and brain chemistry assessment can also be used. Both sorts of measurement can be misleading because, firstly, many activities and brain states are common to a wide variety of motivational states, and secondly, many causal factor levels may be high without there being any evidence of this from current activity. Additional information about motivational state can be obtained from experiments in which behaviour is interrupted, stimuli are presented and brain activity is artificially modified (Broom, 1981, p. 90; Colgan 1989, Chapter 2).

There is a large literature on a wide variety of animals in which sequences of activities are studied whilst various attempts are made to manipulate motivational state. It is clear from such work that changes from one behaviour to another may depend much more on some causal factors than on others. Sometimes a particular causal factor has much urgency, for example when a predator is suddenly detected, so the fact that this input overrides any others in determining behaviour is not surprising because of the survival advantage. Experimental studies have shown that activities such as feeding and courtship sometimes seem to have a higher priority than other activities such as grooming or nest repair. Hence it seems that the input to the decision-making centre must include a weighting which evaluates the importance and urgency of that input. These importance or urgency ratings might therefore be regarded as causal factors for they will certainly change according to the conditions of the individual's life. Grooming could be very important if it is the eyes which require grooming and the situation is dangerous.

A useful tool in investigating motivation is the experiment in which an animal has been trained to carry out an operant response and the amount of work which it will do can be related to particular positive or negative reinforcers (Chapter 3). Using such experiments, an animal can be asked about its own criteria of what is important at that time. Animals will work for food, water and comfortable physical conditions. They will also work for access to social companions, for opportunities to manipulate bedding material and for certain kinds of novel stimulation. Experiments of this kind are mentioned in various chapters of this book. In some situations it is clear that positive reinforcers can be behaviours as well as objects or physical changes. For example, de Wilt (1985) described how young calves try hard to suck at teats as well as to obtain milk. He and Waterhouse (1979) showed that artificial teats are sucked by young calves, even after milk has been drunk to satiation. The sucking behaviour itself is a reinforcer. Herrnstein (1977) suggests that stalking and capturing prey is a reinforcer for a predator which is additional to the reinforcers which result from the ingestion of the prey. Comparisons of various reinforcers are made by Hogan and Roper (1978). These ideas about what constitutes a reinforcer are important for our general understanding of farm animal behaviour and, since absence of important positive reinforcers can cause difficulties for an animal, for appreciation of welfare.

Motivational control systems

Body state is maintained within a tolerable range of temperature, osmotic state, nutrient level, etc. by a set of *homeostatic* control systems. The concept of the tolerable range as that within which the animal seeks to maintain itself is fundamental in biology. It implies that there are upper and lower set points beyond which remedial action is taken. Some of the regulatory actions are physiological, such as sweating or changing blood vessel dilation, but many are behavioural. Some of the variations in state can easily be described in terms of body physics and chemistry, as in temperature or blood sodium level. Others, which might be just as important to the animal, are not easy to describe in that way, for example level of total sensory input or degree of reassurance from parental contact by a young animal.

One sort of control mechanism works by *negative feedback* (Fig. 4.5). As displacement from an initial state within the tolerable range occurs, this change is monitored and, as soon as a set point is reached, some corrective action is

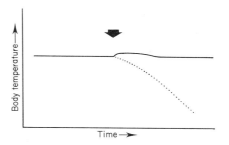

Fig. 4.6 In feedforward control a change in state is predicted and corrective action taken *before* it can occur so that the state changes little from its former condition. In the example shown a drop in body temperature is predicted and behavioural or physiological action (marked by arrow) is taken. The dotted line shows how the state would change if no correction occurred.

taken. Another form of control which is similar but needs no sensory feedback is that where a body variable such as blood glucose is automatically prevented from passing a certain level by a mechanism such as storage. The major alternative to negative feedback is *feedforward control* (Fig. 4.6), in which a displacement from the tolerable range is predicted and a correction is made *before* the state changes. As a consequence of many detailed studies of body biochemistry and physiology, the importance of negative feedback control has been apparent for some time. A decline or an increase in causal factors can often result in a sufficient change in motivational state for a corrective behaviour or physiological response to be made. Research on animal behaviour is providing more and more evidence of feedforward control in operation. Animals use a variety of cues and previous experience to predict that the state will depart from the tolerable range and they act in a way which prevents this from happening. When feedforward control is very efficient an observer may be unaware that any change in state would have occurred because the action compensates for it exactly.

The realisation that animals do a lot of predicting of likely changes in body temperature, body nutrient levels or social actions has

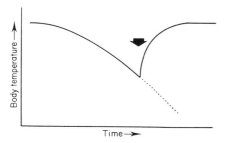

Fig. 4.5 In negative feedback control a correction is made after the state of the animal has changed which restores the state to the former condition. In the example shown here a drop in body temperature is detected and corrective behavioural or physiological action (marked by arrow) is taken. The dotted line shows how the state would change if no correction occurred.

resulted in our view of animals changing to one of cognitive beings aware of the complexities of their environment. Animals are information processing systems which utilise information about how their environment is in relation to how it should be. The idea that animals have a "should-be value" or *Sollwert* for each important aspect of their environment and that they compare this with an "actual value" or *Istwert* has been presented by Wiepkema (1985, 1987). The *Sollwert* is the animal's neural construct of the tolerable range. Related to this is the animal's expectation of what input it will receive when it performs a certain action. It is essential for simple movement control for animals to have a model of the expected input following actions with which they can compare actual input (Broom, 1981, p. 75). With more complex actions too the animal is continually predicting changes in input and comparing actual and expected input. Many responses to perceived environmental changes are not just related to that change but also involve predictions about what will happen next. Studies of animals in learning situations show that they not only associate successive events, but also assess the probability that events will occur (Dickinson, 1985). Rats running in a maze show clearly their expectation of a food reward at the end if that reward is not present or inadequate. Pigs fed at a particular time of day change their behaviour in the hour before feeding and cattle show reponses if their feed gate does not work. Previous unpleasant experiences also result in expectation so that a cow which has experienced unpleasant veterinary treatment in a crush may be unwilling to enter it later (Broom, 1987a) and a sheep which has been roughly or painfully treated at the end of a race will be difficult to drive into and along that race on subsequent occasions (Rushen, 1986).

If animals live in a world which they organise so that many of the events in it are predictable and the state of the animal is closely regulated, then it is logical to ask whether unpredictability is especially aversive to those animals. Work by Overmier *et al.* (1980) has shown that rats and dogs show a clear preference for prediction and control over unpredictability and lack of control. Predictable shocks cause fewer ulcers in rats than unpredictable shocks (Weiss, 1971; Gliner, 1972), and unpredictability in feeding after previous regular feeding leads to increases in adrenal cortex activity (Levine *et al.*, 1972). If aversive events are predictable, animals can prepare for them behaviourally or by activating the analgesic brain opiate system (Fanselow, 1979). They can also prepare for events which are not aversive and inability to prepare makes body regulation more difficult. The problems associated with unpredictability are discussed further by Broom (1985) and Toates (1987). The general conclusions are that, whilst certain events are aversive whatever the degree of predictability and the absence of a predicted painful event is a relief, unpredictability of a wide range of events is hard for animals to cope with and can lead to adverse effects.

One kind of situation where there is no match between expected and actual input leads to frustration. If the levels of most of the causal factors which promote a behaviour are high enough for the occurrence of the behaviour to be very likely, but because of the absence of a key stimulus or the presence of some physical or social barrier the behaviour cannot occur, the animal is said to be *frustrated* (Broom, 1985). For example, Duncan and Wood-Gush (1971, 1972) thwarted hens about to feed by covering their food dish with a transparent perspex cover. They showed stereotyped pacing and increased aggression. Feeding is often frustrated by the presence of stronger rivals in group-housing situations. Some frustration must be of trivial importance in the life of the animal but frustration can be so frequent and involve so fundamental an activity that the fitness of the animal is impaired.

5 Evolution and optimality

The mechanisms which control behaviour have evolved by natural selection like any other characteristic of living organisms. This fact is sometimes overlooked by those studying farm animals, but a realisation of it helps to explain some of the present attributes of these animals. Farm animals still have systems for defence against predation, for example, and these have important effects on a wide range of their activities. Domestication has changed the animals but it has changed a relatively small proportion of their behaviour. Evolution has continued during domestication; new environments and active selection by man have been important factors. Even so, although many evolutionary adaptations of the animals have occurred during the period of human management, most have not occurred because of human selection during breeding. Man has looked for certain characteristics but very many other characteristics have changed during the generations and some of these are not beneficial to man.

The way in which behaviour control mechanisms must have evolved will be emphasised in many of the chapters in this book, but it is useful to refer first to some general principles concerning the evolution of behaviour. This subject area has received a great deal of attention in the ethological literature in recent years and has changed ideas about social behaviour, the organisation of feeding, and all other functional systems. The major writings which have stimulated this explosion of research activity have been those of W.D. Hamilton (1963, 1964a, b) and E.O. Wilson (1975).

Variation, heritability and selection

There is much variation in behaviour amongst the individuals of a species and some of this variation is a consequence of genetic differences. Much of the research which has investigated the genetic aspects of behaviour has been carried out on fruit flies, other insects, fish or birds. Variation amongst species of ducks in the displays which they perform during courtship were described by Lorenz (1941) and used to classify the duck species. McKinney (1978) described how certain displays of ducks, such as the "head-up tail-up", are common to several closely related species but absent from others. It is likely that the mechanism for showing the behaviour has been inherited from a common ancestor. An example of a study of variation and heritability of behaviour within a species is that of Scott and Fuller (1965) on the behaviour of two breeds of dogs. Attempts to restrain Cocker Spaniel puppies result in little struggling but similar attempts to restrain Basenji puppies led to much struggling, avoidance and vocalisation. When Scott and Fuller crossed the two breeds, the F_1 hybrids behaved like the Basenji parent and back-crosses indicated that a single dominant gene influences this behaviour in Basenjis. Other behavioural characteristics are clearly affected by more than one gene. Behavioural differences amongst breeds are also well known in farm animals, for example Le Neindre (1989) showed various consistent differences in behaviour between Salers and Friesian cattle. These differences are important when recommendations about management procedures are being made, as the best method for one breed may not be suitable for another.

Natural selection acts on animals so as to increase the proportion of some genes in the population at the expense of others. If a gene's action is such that an animal shows a particular kind of display during courtship and this display is more effective at attracting a mate and hence producing offspring than that shown if a different gene is present, then the bearers of the first gene will be more common in the next generation. There are many examples of genetic variations in behaviour which are less successful than the norm; one such example comes from the work of Bentley and Hoy (1972), who studied the songs of male crickets *Teleogryllus*. These songs are produced by scraping one wing over another and are a consequence of nerve impulse output from central ganglia. If there is a genetic difference which is such that the song has too many or too few pulses in it, females are much less likely to approach the singing male. Hybrids between two cricket species were produced. The males were intermediate between the parents in normal output and song characteristics and less attractive to females of the parent species.

In all aspects of life, some characteristics will result in more offspring being produced than others. Genetic variation can lead to more or less efficient food-finding, predator avoidance, poison avoidance, etc. and those genes which, on average, result in better survival and offspring production will become more common in succeeding generations. A gene will survive and spread if its effects promote that spreading and survival. Sometimes behaviour can affect the survival of other, related

individuals and it is the overall spread of the gene, in whatever individual, which is important. This point, first made clearly by Hamilton (1964a, b) and followed up by Wilson (1975), Maynard Smith (1978, 1982) and Dawkins (1976, 1982, 1986), has explained how natural selection has led to many aspects of social and other behaviour. A behaviour which promotes the survival of a close relative, including brothers, nieces, etc. as well as offspring, can be selected for in that genes which promote it can spread in the population. Since it is easier to consider individuals bearing genes than the genes themselves, Hamilton (1964a) introduced the term "inclusive fitness" to refer to gene frequency in terms of the effects of that gene on individuals. The idea has been discussed in more detail by Grafen (1982, 1984). Some genes affect the survival of the bearer only, so individual fitness refers to the number of offspring of that individual which themselves survive to breed. Other genes affect relatives, so the inclusive fitness must take account of this. Close relatives, such as offspring and siblings whose coefficient of relatedness is 0.5, must count for more than distant relatives, such as cousins, for which the coefficient is 0.125, in this calculation. However as Grafen points out, when considering the effects of a particular gene which results in helping relatives, only those individuals who are actually helped should be included in the calculation of inclusive fitness. In practice the number of offspring which survive to adulthood is generally the best estimate of inclusive fitness.

A final important point concerning the action of natural selection in relation to behaviour, or any other characteristic, is that all evolutionary changes can be explained in terms of gene survival. The idea that a characteristic might be present in an individual solely for "the good of the species" is now shown to be incorrect. The problems of how social behaviour might have evolved are explicable using Hamilton's ideas and group selection ideas are unnecessary.

Ideas about optimality and efficiency

The consequences of natural selection have been a gradual removal of inefficient methods for achieving objectives in life. As a consequence of arguments about the changes which have occurred during evolution, MacArthur and Pianka (1966) proposed that animals are likely to have mechanisms for "the optimal allocation of time and energy expenditures". The "currency" which they proposed in order to assess what was optimal was energy, e.g. for feeding behaviour this would be the energy obtained from food or utilised during attempts to obtain food. Later studies have made it clear that energy measurements are relevant in certain circumstances but not in others. Energetically efficient food acquisition would be of no use if the individual concerned was then much more likely to be eaten by a predator or much less likely to ever obtain a mate. Where optimal refers to the whole life of an animal it should be measured in terms of the fitness of the animal, and for behaviours which affect relatives, in inclusive fitness. For behaviours such as foraging for food, energetic efficiency is of particular interest provided that it is remembered that being able to achieve a good energy balance is only one of the things that an animal has to do. The energetic approach will be discussed in Chapter 9 but it is useful to consider the evolution of motivation in order to appreciate what behaviour might be optimal at some particular time.

As emphasised in Chapter 4, at all times individual animals have to decide to which functional system they will allocate time and energy. For example once they have decided that they must try to obtain water, they also have to decide how to do it, so this is a second level of decision taking. The initiation of behaviour which serves a new function will also involve the termination of a previous behaviour, even if this is only resting. A cow which has given birth to a calf has to decide when to stop tending the calf, by licking it and staying near it, and go off to find a patch of pasture and graze. Genes which

increased the chances that a cow would leave her calf too early, before adequate licking and a meal of colostrum, or too late, so that the cow lost weight and could not lactate adequately, would be less likely to survive in the population than those which facilitated an accurate assessment of biological priorities. Another kind of decision is that for an animal which must choose whether to forage for food in a risky place where there is much food or a much less risky place where there is less food. For an animal which behaves in a rational way the decision should depend upon the actual risk involved and the advantages of obtaining more food as regards consequences for individual survival and production. Again, a gene which promotes good decision making in this situation should survive better in the population than one which leads to poor decisions, and thus motivational systems evolve. As a consequence of evolution acting on motivational mechanisms, animals should make rational decisions and sequences of decisions about which behaviour to show (Sibly and McFarland, 1976; McCleery, 1978; Broom, 1981, p. 78). Where we are able to assess all the relevant factors effectively it is clear that animals do behave in a rational way. There will, of course, be much individual variation in decision making and every individual will depend upon its own experience in the development of its motivational systems.

The evolution of social behaviour

If the distribution of a population of a farm animal species which is free to move about is studied, the individuals are almost always seen to be clumped rather than spaced out. One individual remains with another because it chooses to be near it and not just because of the place where it is. Once associated they show sophisticated interactions and establish a complex social structure (Chapters 15–17). These farm animals, like many others, show social behaviour, but how might this have evolved in the species? There are disadvantages associated with being close to others with the same requirements for there might be competition for food, resting places, or a mate and predators might be attracted by an aggregation of animals. Presumably any advantages outweigh these disadvantages or social behaviour would not have evolved in so many species. The arguments summarised here are discussed in detail by Broom (1981, p. 176).

Individuals might benefit from being in a group in that their local environment is modified by the others of their own species. Small grazing animals such as rabbits and prairie dogs have difficulty feeding in long grass but can graze readily in areas kept short by others. Termites, ants and bees can collectively change their physical environment substantially by building nests and social animals of any species can huddle together to reduce heat loss.

Food finding can be facilitated by watching others and this may be very important to individuals, especially when food is scarce. A hungry individual bird in a roost or mammal in a resting place may be able to find food by following others more knowledgeable than itself at a time when an isolated individual might find little or no food. Feeding methods can be learned by watching others so young birds derive advantage from flocking with others who know more about how to feed efficiently and older animals may benefit from others if new foods become available. Once found, food may be acquired more readily if others are present. Packs of wolves can catch prey which single animals could not catch and pelicans synchronising scoops into the water for fish catch more than single pelicans. Groups of animals are less likely to return to a depleted food source. Favre (1975) found that sheep in alpine pastures did not return too early to areas which they had grazed and this was probably facilitated by the presence of experienced ewes who controlled flock movements. Groups of animals may also be able to defend a food source.

Predator attack is a major selective factor in the evolution of behaviour. Individuals can reduce the risk to themselves simply by insuring that another individual is between themselves and any predator. Animals can hide within a group when no predator is present and can move into the centre when danger threatens. Colonially nesting birds do better if they position their nest in the central part of a colony. Living in a group also allows the possibility of responding to alarm signals given by others. For some species, collaboration in defence is possible.

Reproduction may be facilitated by group-living. Mates are much more readily found in a group but this must be balanced against the necessity to compete for them. For females, males can be more readily tested if they are forced to compete with others before they will be accepted. In some species which live in groups there is collaboration in rearing young, the most extreme examples coming from the social insects.

The relative importance to group-living of the various advantages and disadvantages will vary from species to species. The first step in the origins of social behaviour might have been either aggregation in localities where food was abundant or shelter was good, or parents and offspring failing to separate. The possible sequences of events are illustrated in Fig. 5.1. If aggregation was at a food source, individuals might subsequently stay together in order to reduce predation or to find food more effectively. Individual offspring benefit in various ways by staying longer with the parents and in some species the parents might tolerate this if the presence of the older offspring increases the survival chances of the next set of offspring. The possibility that altruism might be shown to relatives other than offspring or parents is explicable following Hamilton's (1964a) and Dawkins' (1978) arguments that selection acts on the replicators and a gene which promotes a kin-helping action could survive if enough kin bearing the same gene are helped. Altruism can also be directed at individuals which are not relatives. If this is done it must be reciprocal in order that genes promoting it will survive. There are many examples of reciprocal altruism in human society and some in other species. Packer

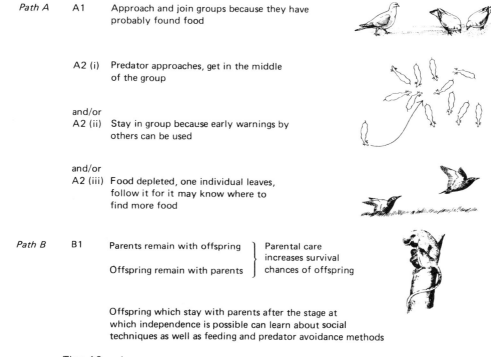

Path A   A1   Approach and join groups because they have probably found food

A2 (i)   Predator approaches, get in the middle of the group

and/or
A2 (ii)   Stay in group because early warnings by others can be used

and/or
A2 (iii)   Food depleted, one individual leaves, follow it for it may know where to find more food

Path B   B1   Parents remain with offspring   ⎫ Parental care increases survival chances of offspring

Offspring remain with parents   ⎭

Offspring which stay with parents after the stage at which independence is possible can learn about social techniques as well as feeding and predator avoidance methods

Then A2 as above

? B2 Animal stays in group because close relatives survive better if it stays

Fig. 5.1   Possible origins of social behaviour and steps in its evolution. (From Broom, 1981.)

(1977) reported that two sub-dominant baboons took it in turn to engage the dominant male in fighting or chasing whilst the other mated with females. There are also many examples of allo-grooming, first by animal A on animal B and then the reverse, amongst primates and ungulates, for example the work of Benham (1984) on cattle and of Hart and Hart (1989) on impala.

6 Neuroethology

In order to concentrate on the functions of behaviour it was necessary for early ethologists to consider the brain, as the controlling mechanism, to be in the nature of a "black box". As a result of this approach the external features of behaviour organisation could be freely studied in detail and models relating to these could be created and modified. Such an approach revealed in much detail the natures of many general behavioural phenomena and many specific behavioural characteristics of species, sexes, ages and types. In the course of this, ethology became a well-established scientific discipline and subsequently a highly applied discipline. The view of brain mechanisms as being those of a "black box" was evidently profitable and justified in ethology during its formative years at a time when neurobiology was largely concerned with excitable tissues. For many questions now, however, it is necessary to consider behaviour and brain processes together. Dramatic advances in neurobiology have occurred so the links with behaviour are becoming easier and easier to forge.

As a result of correlation of behaviour with neural events, the field of comparative neurobiology opened up and its relevance to ethology became increasingly acknowledged. This has involved a change of emphasis in matters of interest for people in both disciplines. The neurobiologist was quick to recognise the value in studying the neural substrate of many finite features of behaviour, such as perception and items of locomotion, and in due course acknowledged that neuroethology was the study of the overall neural control of behaviour.

The chemistry of transmission in the mammalian central nervous system has been studied to great effect in the last two decades with discoveries of biogenic amines and an increasing list of neuropeptides. The array of transmitter substances within the nervous system greatly improves our comprehension of brain metabolism and sheds light on the chemical basis of behaviour. At the present time, approximately 30 neuropeptides with a transmitter function have been identified and many others are active in the nervous system. Although neurophysiology may have far to go, it has already harvested such a quantity of valuable information that it is now in a position to support other disciplines such as ethology. To some extent neurobiology was the lateral expansion of neurophysiology in which its workers took the findings of neuron function into the mixed circumstances of animal life. Many new observations were made and many old ones were evaluated, resulting in an impressive body of information regarding newly discovered catecholamines and the role of amino acids as transmitters in the central nervous system. Transmitter substances have been found with characteristic patterns of distribution in the brain. Such substances include noradrenaline (= norepinephrine), dopamine, serotonin (= 5 hydroxy tryptamine) and acetycholine. The role of the biogenic amines in behaviour begins to clarify the way in which sundry items of behaviour are in fact not a miscellany, but a family of activities. Families of many forms of behaviour find common kinship in neurochemistry.

Neuroethology is now launched as a concept with the publication of several texts, entitled *Neuroethology*, by Ewert (1980), by Guthrie (1980) and by Camhi (1984). To some extent the text on *Comparative Neurobiology*, by Mill (1982) is in the same category. As a massive support for such relevant literature is *Motivation* by Satinoff and Teitelbaum (1983) and *Principles of Neural Science* by Kandel and Schwartz (1981). It is clear that neuroethology has a strong literary base although it is a young discipline. The precise area to which current neuroethology is devoted is that which is concerned with the physiological processes involved in the release and control of behaviour. Neuroethology deals with neuron function, stimulation, neural network chemistry, neural circuits, sensory discrimination, motivation, learning, the inheritance of neural traits, release and control of action patterns and processes.

Sufficient progress has been made in some of these areas to allow neurophysiological knowledge to mesh with behaviour. Studies on the neural determinants of sleep and trophism rationalise the bulk of behavioural observations on these features. Studies of the neural control of ingestion, aggression and courtship also rationalise the behaviour studies which have gone into these areas. Neuroethological studies reveal a complex interplay between sensory information and the action of localised groups of cells and their broadcast fibres in the central nervous system. The integrity of action is assured in many circumstances by neurosecretory and endocrine cells and by the secretions of aminergic tracts. Such revelations improve comprehension and establish behavioural knowledge on a satisfactory foundation. Furthermore, in the course of explaining the basis of behaviour which is normal, neuroethology begins to reveal the probable basis of behaviour which is aberrant. Aberrances increasingly perplex applied ethologists but their comprehension is vital to the credibility of the applied ethologist who must now seek this comprehension in neuroethology.

For the ethologist the challenge has been great. Whereas the neurobiologist moved step-by-step with the developments in neuron physiology, the ethologist must suddenly challenge behavioural theory with the body of information concerning structure and function of the nervous system. This situation requires the ethologist to set aside cherished models of behavioural organisation in order to pursue the knowledge which now exists regarding the ways in which behaviour is actually organised. It may mean tearing down some ethological prefabrications and starting to build, in their place, enduring structures based on neurophysiology. The specific sequences of activities which compose pieces of behaviour are determined by the way in which central neurons interact. Their interactions, in turn, are prescribed by laws of layout and chemical specificity. Searching out these laws and applying them to behaviour is the general methodology of neuroethology.

Neural structure

Neuroethology has been concerned principally with invertebrates but we shall consider attempts to study the behaviour of vertebrates in which complex brain structures have evolved. These are animals whose central nervous system consists of the following principal items:

(a) a spinal cord and brainstem;
(b) a highly organised cerebellum connected with the spinal cord;
(c) basal ganglia and their links with the brainstem;
(d) a diencephalon linked to the pituitary and other endocrine glands via the autonomic system;

(e) a limbic system connecting and interacting with several brain structures such as hypothalamus, hippocampus, amygdala, mammillary bodies, thalamus and cortex; and

(f) a thalamo-cortical system mediating both specific and nonspecific sensory influences.

Neurons which conduct information towards the central nervous system are classically called sensory or afferent neurons; those which conduct information out from the central nervous system are called motor or efferent neurons; while those which are contained completely within the central nervous system and whose function it is to distribute and integrate information within the latter are termed interneurons or internuncial neurons. Implicit in this definition of interneurons is that they both receive information from, and transmit it to, other neurons.

The nervous system's essential function of electrical communication depends on signalling properties of neurons through their long processes. These signalling properties express primary attributes of protoplasm, namely, irritability and conductivity. Patterns of electrical messages are conducted from sensory organs, acting as receivers, to recipient aggregations and associations of neurons. Mediated via chemical transmitter substances, these evoke additional electrical patterns which mobilise the organism and establish conscious experience. Such is the electrical principle of behaviour.

The cellular basis of neuroethology

Of basic importance in neuroethology is the fact that there are two main classes of neurons. In the first class are cells with apparently invariant morphology. These are the large, principal neurons of the brain whose long axons constitute the main nerve-fibre tracts. They have been called macroneurons. The second class consists of highly variable interneurons. They are present in all parts of the nervous system, but are particularly prominent in areas of the brain, such as the cerebral cortex, that are known to be involved in modifiable behaviour. Cells of this type have been called microneurons. These two classes of neurons differ not only in their morphology but also in their ontogeny. As a rule, the macroneurons are formed first in each part of the brain, and the microneurons are formed later. This generalisation applies to all parts of the nervous system of vertebrates.

The fact that these two classes of neurons arise at different times in development is evidence of a fundamental difference between them. The large neurons originate and complete their development at a time when the embryo is still protected from the variability of the extra-uterine environment. Macroneuronal development and differentiation therefore appear to be largely controlled by intrinsic ontogenetic mechanisms. In contrast, the microneurons mainly originate and undergo their differentiation postnatally, when the animal is exposed to massive environmental influences. The small, variable interneuron cells are apprently responsive to environmental influences and are thus responsible for the plastic or modifiable aspects of mature behaviour. Such exogenous influences must still operate, however, within the constraints imposed by intrinsic ontogenetic mechanisms, i.e. by the inheritance.

Developing neurons pass through a series of stages of differentiation involving the outgrowth of various cellular processes comprising the axons and dendrites. In the case of the large macroneurons the axons grow along well-circumscribed routes or trajectories which eventually constitute the nerve-fibre tracts that are among the most invariant features of neuroanatomy. Neuron processes terminate at characteristic positions in the nervous system and in many instances appear to make synaptic connections with selected cells. Neuronal circuits develop in this way by the formation of selective connections between different groups of neurons, or between neurons and sensory receptors or muscle fibres.

The axonal process must make appropriate connections once it reaches its predetermined target region, as a rule, where the axon terminal undergoes extensive branching. Most of these branches will eventually disappear, leaving behind those which were able to establish permanent connections. This suggests that the axonal process makes tentative contact within its target area, maintaining only those branches and terminals which turn out to be functionally suitable and tenable. By this theory of tenability, tentative neuronal connections could be confirmed by the quality of activity generated in the developing nerve circuits. This could allow external factors dependent upon the animal's interactions with its environment to be involved in the selection of those neuronal interconnections which best serve the functional requirements of the nervous system. This would be a means of using information from the external environment to optimise the organism's ability to function within that environment. This validation of tentative connections would have to occur at the appropriate stage of development so it must be governed by an appropriate, presumably genetically controlled, timetable. Selection of the appropriate connections from among the excess that had been created embryologically would have to be delayed until the animal's first exposure to the external environment. One would, therefore, expect environmental factors to have their effect on the developing nervous system during some postnatal "critical period". Herein lies the neuroethological basis of "imprinting" (see Horn, 1985).

The dendritic processes must also develop and establish contact with the proper axonal terminals to complete the developing neuronal interconnections. Differentiation of dendritic processes also follows precise timetables. However, in the sequence in which dendrites mature in the different regions of the brain, the differentiation of dendrites of large macroneurons occurs before that of smaller microneurons. Furthermore, there is a tendency for nerve cells in the motor fields of the nervous system to develop their dendrites before those of cells located in sensory fields. Significantly an operant capability is established before a sensory one. Prior to establishing connections, dendritic processes undergo extensive branching and many of these branches disappear before the animal reaches adulthood. In such instances, sensory stimulation apparently plays a role in determining the final destiny of the dendritic processes.

Neuronal variability

The most prominent neurons of the brain are the principal large neurons with long axons linking the various parts of the nervous system which evidently are laid down by developmental programmes operating under genetic control. These programmes ensure the development of an invariant neural framework which is a prerequisite for orderly nervous functioning and species-specific behaviour.

Such an invariant structure, capable of a degree of modification and variation as a result of learning, is able to use information from the environment to determine behaviour in the interests of survival. This involves interpretation and transformation of sensory information as it is presented to the central nervous system by its numerous converging input pathways and as it is executed by the pathways directing efferent outflow. The necessary flexibility in such information-processing ability of the nervous system is evidently provided by the variable connectivity of the countless short-axon interneurons found throughout the brain, particularly where complex information processing occurs. The branching of their axons and dendrites and their distribution show that these microneurons serve as the variable components of the nervous system.

These variable components of the nervous system exert their influence by modifying— either facilitating or inhibiting—the pattern of activity generated by neurons comprising the invariant framework of the nervous system. The small, short axon microneurons seem ideally suited for introducing local changes in the activity patterns generated by larger macroneurons, and they might be thought of as local circuit neurons.

Neurophysiological studies show that sensory stimulation plays an active role in the final differentiation of the neurons and is necessary for the normal development of neuronal organisation. Although the information necessary for tracts to connect with the appropriate part of the brain is supplied by intrinsic developmental programmes rather than by the animal's experience, such experience, or exposure history, during early postnatal development exerts a powerful influence on neuronal capability in the cortex. These effects are long-lasting since they persist after years of overlying experience. Environmental conditions introduce variability into the developing nervous system and establish another rule of neuroethology.

The chemical basis of transmission in neuroethology

Neurons are distinguished from other cells by their molecular properties. Their characteristic properties are responsible for their signalling activities. Such activities include:

(a) responding to specific chemical transmitter substances by altering membrane permeability to common ions (Na^+, Cl^-, K^+, Ca^{2+});
(b) conducting electrical impulses; and
(c) communicating with other, postsynaptic cells by the process of synaptic transmission.

Basic to each of these three physiological functions are the neuron's specific responsiveness to certain substances resulting from various intrinsic membrane proteins called receptors. Membranes of different neurons contain different receptors and this creates neuronal diversity.

The release of transmitter substances from presynaptic axon terminals is another physiological function that is composed of many biochemical processes some of which are characteristic of specific neuron cells, whereas others relate to pathways of numerous cells. Chemical transmission can be divided into four steps:

(1) synthesis of transmitter substance;
(2) storage and release of the transmitter;
(3) interaction of the transmitter with a receptor in the postsynaptic membrane; and
(4) removal of the transmitter from the synaptic cleft.

Even though synaptic transmission occurs at nerve terminals, it is important to realize that other parts of a neuron contribute significantly to the process. The terminal is dependent upon the cell body for the macromolecular components needed for transmission. These components are rapidly exported after being synthesised in the cell body and move along axons to nerve terminals by either fast or slow axonal transportation. Transmitters are substances that are released synaptically by neurons and affect other neurons or effector organs in a specific manner. Several substances clearly function as transmitters, but there are many other chemical substances with similar functions. The four types of transmitter substances are as follows:

1. Acetylcholine
2. Biogenic amines, including:
   dopamine
   norepinephrine (= noradrenaline)
   serotonin (= 5 hydroxy tryptamine)
   histamine.
3. Amino acids:
   γ-aminobutyric acid (GABA)
   glycine
   glutamate
4. Neuropeptides.

Each transmitter has the following four essential characteristics:

(a) It is synthesized in the neuron.
(b) It is presented in the presynaptic terminal

and is released in order to exert its action on the receptive neuron or effector organ.

(c) It mimics exactly the biological action of the endogenous transmitter when applied exogenously (as in a drug).

(d) It has a specific mechanism for removing it from the synaptic cleft, its site of action.

Nerve cells have been characterised according to their transmitter biochemistry and the important generalisation has emerged that a mature neuron makes use of the same transmitter substance at all of its synapses. The majority of neurons use only one transmitter substance and this is neuronal specificity. A specific set of biosynthetic enzymes in a neuron is the determinant of transmitter specificity. An enzymatic step exists in all transmitter pathways where the overall synthesis of the transmitter is regulated. This enzyme step is characteristic of the neuron and therefore endows it with the property of being cholinergic, norepinephrinergic (noradrenergic), dopaminergic, serotonergic, etc.

Acetylcholine

Acetylcholine (ACh) is the transmitter used by the motor neurons of the spinal cord and operates therefore at all nerve–skeletal muscle junctions in vertebrates. ACh is diffusely localised throughout the brain, but is highly concentrated in neurons of the basal ganglia. It is important in the autonomic nervous system, being the transmitter for the parasympathetic neurons.

Amine transmitters

Dopamine and noradrenaline (norepinephrine) are two important transmitter substances which are synthesised in common pathways. In the central nervous system, noradrenaline-containing nerve cell bodies are prominent in the locus coeruleus, a nucleus of the brain stem concerned with arousal. These neurons project diffusely throughout the cortex, cerebellum and spinal cord. In the peripheral nervous system noradrenaline is the transmitter in the postganglionic neurons and is thus the transmitter for the sympathetic nervous system.

Dopamine-containing cells are located in three regions: the substantia nigra, where the cells project to the striatum; the midbrain, where they project to the limbic cortex; and the hypothalamus, where they project to the pituitary stalk.

Serotonergic cell bodies are found in the midline of the brain stem. These cells (like the noradrenaline cells of the locus coeruleus) send fibres throughout the brain and spinal cord. Histamine is concentrated in the hypothalamus. Noradrenaline and dopamine are catecholamines and serotonin is an indoleamine. Catecholamines, indoleamines and histamine are all referred to as "biogenic amines" and have much effect on behaviour (Mason, 1984).

Amino acid transmitters

Acetylcholine and the biogenic amines are substances that are not intermediates in general biochemical pathways; their production occurs only in certain neurons only. In contrast, a group of amino acids released as neurotransmitters are universal cellular constituents. Glycine and glutamate are two of the 20 common amino acids that are incorporated into the proteins of all cells; glutamate and γ-aminobutyric acid (GABA) also serve as substrates of intermediary metabolism. Glutamate is a transmitter in the cerebellum and the spinal cord. Glycine is an inhibitory transmitter in spinal cord interneurons. GABA is present in neurons in the basal ganglia which project to the substantia nigra; cells of the cerebellum are GABA-minergic, as are certain inhibitory interneurons in the spinal cord. Transmitter glutamate is kept separate from metabolic glutamate by compartmentalisation of the amino acid transmitters. With ACh and the biogenic amines it has been demonstrated that the transmitter substances are packaged in specific membranous vesicles. Similar vesicles are present in neurons that use the amino acid transmitters. The biogenic amines move into aminergic vesicles because of a "chemiosmotic" mechanism. Apparently vesicles constitute the transmitter compartment.

Neuroactive peptides

More than 25 short peptides have been found to be localised in neurons and to be pharmacologically very active, causing inhibition, excitation, or both. Some of these peptides were previously identified as hormones with known targets outside the brain—for example, angiotensin—or as products of neurosecretion—for example, oxytocin, vasopressin, somatostatin, luteinising hormone (LH) and thyrotropin-releasing hormone (TRH). In addition to being hormones in some tissues these peptides may act as neurotransmitters in other tissues. These neuroactive peptides are localised in regions of the brain thought to be involved in the perception of pain, pleasure and emotion. Two classes of peptides possess opiate-like actions—the endorphins and the enkephalins. These opioid peptides are involved in a variety of functions including the modulation of pain.

Three pharmacologically active endorphins exist, namely α, β, γ. All of these, and the enkephalins, are derived from a large peptide with 91 amino acids pro-opiomelanocortin. The most active is β-endorphin, which is synthesised in the hypothalamus, as well as in the pituitary. The enkephalins are two pentapeptides, namely metenkephalin and leuenkephalin. The enkephalins are synthesised in cell body ribosomes and transported within secretory vesicles to nerve terminals. Enkephalin molecules are produced during this transportation. Unlike β-endorphin, the enkephalins are widely distributed in the brain. The distribution matches that of the opiate receptors.

Substance P is a peptide concentrated in certain neurons of the dorsal root ganglia, basal ganglia, hypothalamus and cerebral cortex. It has been proposed as the transmitter for sensory fibres involved in mediating pain. Substance P is a transmitter involved in the modulation of motor movement.

Transportation of transmitters may be fast or slow. The outstanding slow transmitters are the catecholamines, noradrenaline and dopamine. Acetylcholine is the well-known fast chemical messenger.

Hormone-dependent neural function and behaviour

With the recognition that there is chemical specificity among neurons, it is clear that there must exist neuronal circuits which can produce behavioural potential but which may not be in regular use if the appropriate chemical message is not provided. The principal chemical messengers are neuropeptides and hormones.

Following the discovery of chemospecific neuron tracts in the central nervous system, their special importance as conduction routes must be recognised, together with the special neurochemical factors which must be involved. These special intraneuronal messengers employ chemospecific pathways in the transneuronal transport of behaviour potential throughout the nervous system. It would appear that neuropeptides act on nervous tissue by energising the production of neuronal output in these neuronal systems which are programmed to function in the presence of the given chemistry.

It becomes necessary to recognise that, in the ethograms of animals, two main categories of behaviour production take place. One of these is the phasic production of continuing "maintenance" behaviour. This vegetative-expressive behaviour represents the bulk of the behaviour of animals and is the behaviour concerned with such activities as ingestion, locomotion, certain physiological needs such as resting, body care, thermoregulation and some social activities. In addition, occasional forms of behaviour can be recognised. These are the behavioural processes which are needed for dealing with occasional, specific and often critical circumstances. These instances include such things as the new role of the maternal animal, the new role of an animal post-puberty, the new role of animals following the start of the breeding season, etc. Since many "new role" circumstances operate through the production of hormones it can be seen that, in all probability, the purpose of such hormones is to activate neuronal systems which are not involved in routine maintenance behaviour. These new roles, or any emergency roles of behaviour, must nevertheless be established in the neuromechanism of the individual animal, to be called upon only when circumstances require their activation. In some circumstances their activation may never be necessary in the entire life of the animal.

It may be necessary to reflect on the subdivision of behaviour into that which is produced in the normally extant chemistry of the body and other behaviour which are is produced in the presence of short-lived chemical agents in the form of hormones. It will be obvious that the neuronal circuits will be laid down in embryonic stages of development. It will also be obvious that because of this the circuits will be present and the same in individuals of both sexes. For this reason the sex hormones will only activate those neuronal circuits appropriate to their chemistry. This implies that neuronal circuits for the alternate sexual behaviour exist but are not normally called into play in the lifetime of the animal. When abnormal circumstances occur, e.g. the presence of a gonadal tumour, the alternate neuronal system of sexual behaviour may then be motivated. This will result in the manifestations of behaviour patterns of the opposite sex. In the case of female animals the behaviour will be "virilistic". In the case of male animals the behaviour will be "feministic". It will be obvious that virilistic behaviour as shown by female animals in the presence of androgens are produced under clinical circumstances.

The neuronal circuit for sexual behaviour of the alternate gender evidently does not lose potential merely because it is never called into play during the lifetime of the animal. The explanation of this is that the lifetime of the neuron equals the lifetime of the individual animal.

Nervous organisation

The nervous system's main parts are the central nervous system and the peripheral nerves. The central system has its own major divisions, namely, the brain and spinal cord. The cerebrum, cerebellum and brain stem are, of course, the main parts of the brain. In addition there are special parts such as the cerebral cortex, the basal ganglia, the reticular formation and a range of regions, such as the hypothalamus. Specialised nuclei, such as the locus coeruleus, are also recognised in abundance. One notable system which is a collection of specialised brain parts is the limbic system.

Nuclei are collections of allied nerve cells, or neurons, usually concerned with finite aspects of neural business. Usually, nuclei have incoming and outgoing tracts or pathways made up of filamentous extension, or arborisation, of the nerve cell body. The filaments convey electrical charges and pass their electrical signals across terminations of output filaments, or axons, at their synaptic junctions with the input filaments, or dendrites. The chemistry at synaptic junctions dictates transmission as a result of nerve cell secretion. Neurosecretion and transmission are necessary for the physiological communication of sensory information.

In spite of the diversity of regions and centres in the brain, the variety of tracts in the spinal cord and the array of peripheral nerves, the nervous system functions as a whole and all parts are connected to all other parts through neuron linkage. It is estimated that no more than seven nerve cells are required to link any one part with any other (Hockman and Bieger, 1976). The brain stem is an important bottleneck in the processing and integration of behaviour. Its notable structure is the reticular formation.

Reticular formation and connections

The reticular formation's functions include the production of general arousal in the central nervous system. The reticular formation embodies a mechanism by which states throughout the central nervous system are regulated. Some of these regulations are diurnal. For example, one state is sleep, another is wakefulness. Between these two are many degrees of alertness and inattentiveness. All are expressions of some pattern of activity in the reticular formation.

The reticular formation is a place of convergence for information of widespread origin. This is the role of the reticular formation in ascending systems and also in a context of descent. Neurons in the rhombencephalic reticular formation can respond to inputs from secondary sensory cell groups in the spinal cord. They may also respond to a message from the cerebellum, or from the neocortex. A large number of heterogeneous inputs converge on the reticular formation which must integrate this variety of neural afflux, ascending and descending in the brain, and then dispatch impulses over reticulospinal fibres that terminate on immediate neurons or on motor neurons directly.

Cerebral cortex

The cerebral cortex, although acting as a unit, has certain localised regions where sensory impulses are received and subjected to redirection. These specialised areas of the cortex are primary sites for sensory reception, the nervous activity subsequently spreading over a greater area. The cortex has a multitude of cells and neural paths, each one communicating with many others. This extremely complex relay system permits tremendous variability in the way that nerve impulses may be channeled.

The cerebral cortex possesses four main sensory areas into which projectory fibres discharge. These are:

1. the somaesthetic or body sense area;
2. the visual area;
3. the auditory area; and
4. the olfactory area.

All of these are important in the reception and interpretation of nerve signals, and are fundamental in determining behaviour.

Somaesthetic area

This area is sited in the parietal lobe of the cortex and receives nerve impulses from many parts of the body including its surface.

Visual area

Nerve fibres are collected from the retina of the eye into the optic nerves and are distributed, within the cortex, to the extensive visual area at the occipital part of the cerebrum. Recognition of patterns and releasers takes place in the visual area (Diamond, 1982).

Auditory area

This is located in the temporal lobe of the cerebral cortex. The area receives nerve impulses concerned with auditory sensations from the thalamus. The fibres of the hearing nerve end in the pons, from which region other fibres pass to the thalamus and then to the cortex.

Olfactory area

The sensory area dealing with smell plays a much more important role in breeding behaviour than has generally been recognised. An olfactory region is located in the hippocampus which receives projection fibres from the centre in the olfactory bulb. This centre deals with olfactory reflexes. The fibres of the olfactory system originate with nerve cells located in the mucous membrane of the nasal passages and terminate within the olfactory bulbs.

It seems that areas of the cortex are designed to correlate dynamically with receptive areas on the body's surface. The neural importance of the superficial area and central nervous areas changes according to the major activities of an animal; for example, it seems that the appropriate area of the cortex is more receptive to stimulation from the genitalia during breeding times than at other times.

The limbic system

The limbic system is a determinant and integrator of strategic and tactical functions (Isaacson, 1982). Physiological evidence points to the involvement of the limbic system in displays of emotional behaviour. The limbic system is conceptually seen as the central representative of the autonomic system, and to consist functionally of an interconnected group of brain structures within the cerebral borders (limbus: a border); it includes portions of the frontal lobe cortex, temporal lobe, thalamus and hypothalamus, together with certain midbrain parts which act as functional generators. Linking neuron pathways connect all these brain regions in segmental integration. The component parts of the limbic system, therefore, have many connections with each other and with other parts of the central nervous system. Information from the different afferent and efferent routes influences the limbic system and its peripheral arm, the autonomic system (Figs. 6.1 and 6.2).

Activity of the limbic system can result in a wide variety of autonomic responses and of body movements which comprise purposeful behaviour. In the hypothalamus—the main output stage of the limbic system—a rage response can also be caused by destruction of certain parts. Experimental stimulation of certain other hypothalamic areas elicits behaviour in animals which seems to have a strong

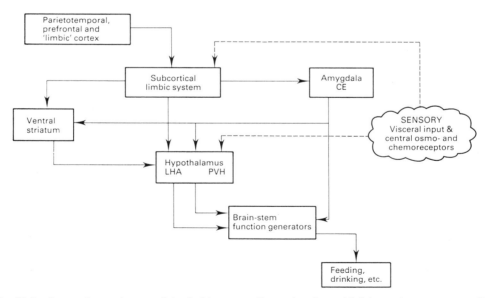

Fig. 6.1 Major descending pathways of the limbic system illustrating the multiplicity and convergence of inputs to function generators. Note: arrows symbolise main throughput pathways. All structures are connected reciprocally by parallel, horizontal and ascending connections, most of which are omitted for clarity. (Figure courtesy of D. Bieger.)

"emotional" component. For example, the medial hypothalamus exerts inhibition on the circuits producing fight-or-flight behaviour. Upon receipt of appropriate environmental stimuli, the temporal lobe inhibits the medial hypothalamus, allowing activity in the integrated limbic system to increase, with resulting emotional behaviour. The structures involved in the control of emotional behaviour are therefore predominantly located throughout the limbic system, and the main controlling centres for consummatory, or drive, behaviour are located there, and within the hypothalamus in particular. Much consummatory behaviour, of course, relates to maintenance, the ongoing operation of which relates to behavioural homeostasis. Limbic matters therefore clearly relate to homeostasis which is the essential business of self-maintenance. Much of the behaviour of domesticated animals is concerned with self-maintenance. Various parts of the forebrain convey neural activities to the hypothalamus through the limbic system, either directly or after interruptions, so that by one route or another it is in receipt of impulses from optic, olfactory, acoustic, tactile and internal sources. The limbic system apparently contains neural centres such as the amygdala which control aggressive behaviour in its various forms (Adamec, 1978).

Portions of the neocortex may speed up the processing of information, at least of some types of information. Experimental stimulation of the temporal neocortex in animals can alter the activity from uninterested to attentive. By implication, this temporal neocortex can be thought of as regulating the excitability and the processing time of the primary sensory systems. Neocortex information, such as memory, is very diffusely stored; memories may not even be localised uniquely in the neocortex (Nicholls, 1976). The frontal cortical areas may play a role in coordinating the signals from the limbic system that are to be integrated with the activities of the "cognitive brain", that is, the majority of the neocortical surface (Lindsley, 1972).

A puzzling feature of brain organisation relates to the ways in which interactions may occur between the limbic system and motor systems, since the anatomical relationships between the limbic system and the basal ganglia are sparse. Recently, however, work on the projections from limbic system to the nucleus accumbens and the ventral tegmental area has made the limbic basal ganglia association clearer. The association is functional and the nucleus accumbens can be thought of as a limbic striatum.

The limbic system, or the paleomammalian brain, represents a device for providing the animals with better means of coping with the environment. Parts of the limbic system are concerned with primal activities related to food and sex; others are related to emotions and feelings; and still others combine messages from the external world. One way to conceptualise the limbic system may be to see it as a regulator of survival business. On the basis of behavioural analysis, this regulation seems to be inhibitory in nature. Stimulation of the limbic system often produces a suppression of ongoing behaviours, and lesions of other disruptions made within often seem to "release" various activities. Each limbic system structure may be sensitive to its own effects on the whole system's manifestation. Each of the limbic system structures is highly specialised, and is tuned to specific changes of the internal or external environment. The hypothesis is that however specialised the structures of the limbic system may be, their end product is the regulation of basic, even primitive, activities (Heimer, 1978).

The limbic system, acting through suppressive mechanisms, tends to allow new directions in behaviour to occur. The circumstances under which the hippocampus acts to regulate the activities of other brain regions seem to be conditions of uncertainty. Life becomes uncertain when old patterns of responding fail to produce the anticipated rewards, when old habits fail to pay off. This suppression prevents the animal from continuing in its old ways of responding and from over-reacting in general. An animal with damage to the amygdala, on the other hand, reveals quite a different sort of behavioural syndrome. It is slow to initiate new responses and seems characterised by a reduction in reactive quality.

The view has been taken by some that a concept of limbic permeability requires to be seen as the basis of differences in animal "disposition". This permeability relates to the phenomenon of "kindling" in which a repeated stimulation leads to a build-up in neuroenergy or neurophysiological output in general. The limbic system, more than any other brain part, gives the animal's own characteristic output of emotionally-tuned behaviour (Stark-Adamec, 1983).

Basal ganglia

Three large subcortical nuclear groups—(1) the caudate nucleus, (2) the putamen, and (3) the pallidum—are collectively called the basal ganglia. Together they account for 5% of the brain mass. The basal ganglia and several associated subthalamic and midbrain structures are referred to as the extra-pyramidal system. These nuclei participate in the control of movements together with the cerebellum, the corticospinal system and other descending motor systems. Although part of the motor system, the basal ganglia do not project directly to the spinal cord.

The basal ganglia play an important role in the initiation and control of movement (Evarts, 1973). Many neurons of the basal ganglia change their activity during movement of a specific body part. These neurons are typically clustered close together, forming a somatotopic representation of the body. Neurons whose activity relates to movements of the forelimbs are found ventral to those whose activity relates to hindleg movements. Characteristically the changes in activity of these neurons takes place before the movement of the body, indicating that they play a role in the initiation of movement. Disorder of the basal ganglia can be characterised by abnormal movements including oscillatory

movements of a body part, chorea (twitching movements of the limbs and facial muscles) and abnormal patterns of action. The presumptive basis of some pathological motor patterns is the dopaminergic projection from the substantia nigra to basal ganglia such as the pallidum. Dopamine constitutes about one-half of the catecholamine in the brain and 80% of it is localised in the basal ganglia.

Hypothalamus

It is at the level of the hypothalamus that patterns of nervous activities become integrated and regulated so as to establish the adaptive reactions of the animal. Even behaviour which is largely dependent upon experience and learning in the animal is seldom, if ever, completely free of control by the primitive mechanisms established in the hypothalamus and in the subcortex generally. The neural links involving the subcortex, and the links between the hypothalamus and the surrounding brain in particular, remain the principal integrators of most behavioural processes.

The working units of the hypothalamus are neurons which are grouped into "nuclei" These nuclei operate together in a fashion resembling a computer. The information from various levels of the brain is received and processed by these nuclei before signals are subsequently reissued to more specialised parts of the body, which are geared to function under the control of the hypothalamus (Fig. 6.3). Much of the influence of hypothalamic activity is directed at the production of hormones in the subjacent pituitary gland. The pituitary is the principal endocrine gland in the body and its hormonal production is all-important in the maintenance of the bulk of the body's activities, including behaviour. Even the central hypothalamus is responsive to some of the endocrine activity for which it is initially responsible. Quite recently it has become clear that there is probably a considerable amount of hormonal control over the hypothalamus. The receipt of afferent stimulation gives the hypothalamus the role of maintaining and regulating the activity of the pituitary gland since it is clear that the hypothalamus is characterised by its glandular appendage—the pituitary. It is also, of course, continuous in the forward direction with the septum, a structure that is part of the limbic system.

Accordingly, most or all of the activities of the hypothalamus should be capable of modification by manipulations of the limbic system. The limbic system makes possible the suppression of the traditional ways of responding in order to allow behavioural modifications based on information from the internal environment as directed by the neocortical tissue. Both the limbic system and the neocortex become elaborated in mammals and usually work in concert.

Autonomic system

In the autonomic circuitry, fibres passing without interruption from the hypothalamus to the autonomic motor neurons of the spinal cord's grey matter constitute a small minority of the outgoing hypothalamic fibres. The hypothalamus appears in large measure to project no further than the midbrain, where neurons of the reticular formation take over. The pathways descending to autonomic motor neurons are interrupted at numerous levels. At each interruption further instructions enter the descending lines. The convergence of information on motor neurons is as characteristic of the autonomic nervous system as it is of the somatic nervous system. The major influence exerted on the hypothalamus from the cerebral hemisphere derives from the hippocampus and the amygdala, two principal components of the limbic system. Other limbic components include the fornix at the free edge of the cerebral mantle. Some fibres leaving the hippocampus extend into the hypothalamus directly while others establish their synapses in the septum, from which fibres are extended again to the hypothalamus. The hippocampus is a destination for sequential projections that span the neocortical sheet.

It is increasingly recognised that the autonomic system acts as a behavioural integrator: its full role is in modulating the intensities of behavioural responses in general, and in particular the emotional component of behaviour. The autonomic system, known from the first century A. D. as the nervous system of sympathetic feeling, is now known to affect and mould all states, reactions and behaviour. It integrates glandular function and somatic behaviour. Since it is a moulder of reaction, it plays a part in determining the nature of behaviour and of emotive states associated with behaviour. Through this system, conditioned reactions determine the nature of future responsiveness, for autonomic conditioning may last for years and require little reinforcement. Any reinforcement to this system is powerful and may even occur in anticipation of a set of circumstances without them necessarily occurring.

The autonomic conditioned reactions are in many cases triggered by telereceptors and even in anticipation of what may occur. The reactions are very fast and precede somatic components of defence, alerting, fight-or-flight. Autonomic innervation improves the acuity of olfaction, taste and possible hearing. The same is true of touch and proprioception. In animal life, the autonomic system is involved in agonistic reactions, self-determinations, survival efforts, comfort seeking and preparation for future circumstances. All this supports an ancient and modern view that the autonomic system carries the social senses and responses essential to society. Certainly, it is the system by which modulations are dictated to behaviour, so that the subject meets the requirements of the environment and its society (Brooks, 1981).

Cord

Functionally, the spinal cord and brain are extensions of each other. Specific tracts coursing through the cord to and from the brain exemplify this scheme. The role of the spinal cord is sometimes autonomous, as in certain reflex mechanisms. Simple reflexes such as limb withdrawal in response to a local stimulus have cord organisation. The scratch reflex is the outstanding example of coordinated cord reflex action. Spinal reflexes are quite numerous; although their role is major in birds they have much less influence on mammalian behaviour.

Two types of arrangements serve reflex spinal activity. A sensory neuron entering the dorsal root can give rise to branches running up and down beyond this level of entry into the cord. Some of the branches run to synapse with motor neurons in the ventral column, but these direct synapses are restricted to the same level of the cord at which the sensory nerves enter. In some other situations a dorsal root ganglion neuron branches to run both rostrally and caudally synapsing with a second nerve cell (not to be confused with the second order sensory neuron). The second nerve cell distributes to segments above and below, synapsing with motor neurons at many spinal segmental levels.

Various degrees of cord involvement are manifest by the rising complexity of behaviour patterns from the lower to the higher vertebrates (Macphail, 1982). Fish behaviour owes more to spinal cord control than does mammal behaviour. In birds, eliminative acts are generally spinally controlled and are not embodied in multi-purpose eliminative behaviour patterns. However birds do defaecate more in certain kinds of frightening situations. The idea that bird behaviour is more rigid than that of mammals is correct for a limited number of situations but birds are very adaptable in other situations and their learning ability can be very impressive. Brain organisation is different but parallels with mammalian brain centres are generally found when they are sought.

Each spinal segment has something in the order of 0.3 million neuronal cell bodies in the grey matter of the cord, approximately 10 000 sensory fibres entering by the dorsal roots and half this number of motor fibres leaving by the ventral roots. This also means that the interneurons comprise approximately 84% of the total population. The possibilities for multisynaptic pathways are tremendous due to the interneurons. Such flexibility of responses is advantageous to adaptation in the face of environmental variability. Low reflex spinal arcs are by no means eliminated or replaced but, in domesticated mammals for example, they are modified and controlled by superior reflex arcs involving the cerebrum. For example, a high order of control of defecation is seen in the eliminative behaviour of pigs and horses in which patterns of defecating behaviour are often elaborate and specialised. At the same time, such patterns are not always operant. For example, if the horse is being worked, the demands of this work engage the cerebrum sufficiently to return the control of defecation to the appropriate spinal centres. This example again demonstrates that lower levels of CNS control are never eliminated or replaced by higher ones. They are only made subordinate in the hierarchical order as it has evolved. Complicated yet coordinated motor behaviour such as occurs in the scratch reflex can be seen in terms of these cord mechanisms and reflex pathways. The whole nervous system can enter into innumerable varieties of coordination giving behaviour its continuum which is directed at homeostasis.

Circuits of homeostasis

The circuitry which is the basal organisation of homeostatic behaviour is mapped out in Figures 6.1, 6.2 and 6.3. These show the complex, but programmed, neural circuits which are basic to maintain activities and the establishment of drive states (Bieger, personal communication). Several direct inputs into the function generators of the brain stem can be identified (Fig. 6.1). This figure indicates the circuitry to the function generators of the brain stem which control such homeostatic activities as feeding and drinking. In this organisation one particular

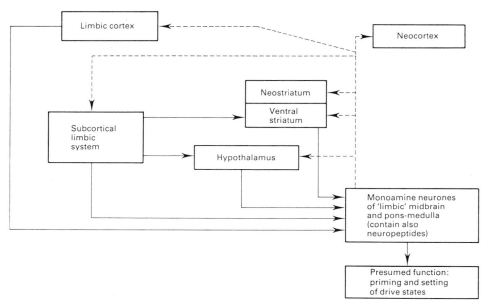

Fig. 6.2   Monoamine neurons as an integral part of the ascending connections of the limbic system. (Figure courtesy of D. Bieger.)

input arises from the central nucleus of the amygdala which gives a direct input into the function generators. This arrangement is evident in the case of oral activities and swallowing. The circuitry exists as a descending projection from other brain regions existing as a direct link of cascades. These cascades do not go to one point only, e.g. the lowest point, but go also to successive, serially connected points which are connected again to the lowest point.

The main inputs into the amygdala can be tracked back as its main afferents. The immediate input comes from the rest of the amygdala which of course is a part of the subcortical limbic system (the limbic system having cortical and subcortical components). The subcortical structures of the limbic system have circuitry in the form of descending connections leading to the hypothalamus, and thence to the brain stem. Although these components are reciprocally connected they are presented in Fig. 6.2 as a flow chart of hypothalamic links with brain stem (and its function generators). It is known that there are at least two direct links which are important

in the control of ingestive behaviour. It would be an over-simplification to recognise the hypothalamus as the control station for such behaviour, but there is no doubt that this region is more than a bottleneck for fibre systems that pass through; it contains neurons in their own proper constellations. These are sites of integration. As a result the hypothalamic area receives input, not only from various sources of the limbic region, notably the subcortical limbic region, but also from the ventral striatum. The ventral striatum, however, receives—like the amygdala—input from the subcortical limbic system (this arrangement sets it apart from the rest of the basic ganglia).

Figure 6.3 shows a more detailed flow chart indicating the specific connections of the limbic system controlling maintenance behaviour. This figure also shows the complexity of feedback connections between the cortical level and the hypothalamus. Obviously there is some general integration based on the reception of visceral inputs and hormonal–humoral signals. The hypothalamus has the means to deal with such

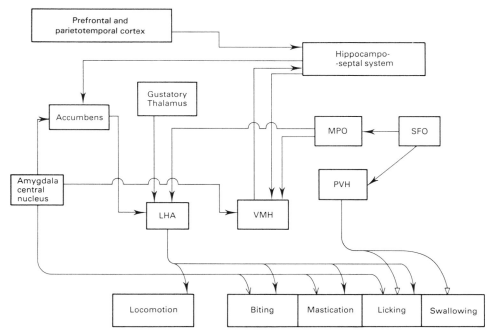

Fig. 6.3 Main output connections of limbic system controlling maintenance behaviour. VMH, ventromedial hypothalamus; LHA, lateral hypothalamic area; MPO, medical preoptic area; SFO, subfornical organ; PVH, paraventricular nucleus of hypothalamus. (Figure courtesy of D. Bieger.)

inputs and signals but the latter also reach the subcortical system rather directly.

The overall, suprahypothalamic level of processing provides a global organisation which activates the function generators of the brain stem. By this, there is activation of the complex sequences relating to each piece of maintenance behaviour. For example, grazing involves exploration, locomotion, oral action and monitoring the environment in addition to ingestive activities such as prehension. The circuits are concerned in this integration in a function that has been referred to as ''motivational time sharing''. This refers to the setting of priorities in which these various behavioural processes are enacted.

Neuroethological organisation

Progress in the acquisition of knowledge and

understanding about brain organisation and behaviour in animals is substantial. Despite the recent advances that have been made, however, the brain–behaviour frontier awaits countless discoveries.

The goal of neuroethology is to understand the nature, mechanisms and role of the parts, regions and finite aspects of the nervous system in the integration and regulation of behaviour, particularly in animals. This is an ambition unlikely to be quickly or easily attained except through cumulative contributions and achievements by which some progress has been made within recent years. In the past two decades there has been world-wide growth in the number of workers from varied disciplines who have focused their attentions and interest on phenomena and problems related to the central nervous system and the behaviour of the utilised animals. Many scientists have found common interests and mutual cooperation in newly formed national, and international societies amalgamated under the multi-discipline of applied ethology.

It has been said that the roles of the nervous system in health and disease, and particularly the understanding of its mechanisms for facilitating plasticity and adaptation to the environment of the organism it subserves, together with psychological functions of perception, learning, memory, thinking, problem solving and performance in the higher organisms, are so important that every logically conceivable scientific approach should be utilised to solve this problem. It should not be merely a matter of simple versus complex organisms, but rather what contribution both can make to overall problems. Anomalous behaviour in farm animals is a growing problem calling for modern understanding. Neuroethology can be a fresh approach to the problem. Some of the chemistry of neuroethology is given below for those in applied ethology who wish to look at this prospect.

Aminergic neurotransmitters in behavioural illnesses

Synaptic neurotransmitters must be either inactivated or removed from the synaptic cleft for the process of neurotransmission to continue. The major part of the amino neurotransmitter is removed by active, energy-dependent re-uptake and storage by the presynaptic neuron. In some forms of depression, turnover of noradrenaline (norepinephrine) in brain tissue is diminished.

Noradrenaline inhibits the release of corticotrophin releasing factor (CRF) from the hypothalamus. Diminished functional central noradrenaline activity might, therefore, increase CRF release, which results in increased ACTH release, which in turn results in increased release of glucocorticoids such as corticosterone or cortisol into the vascular system. It has been found that some depressed cases have a relatively continuous release of large amounts of cortisol. This finding is increasingly confirmed in animals such as pigs with depressed behaviour.

The amine hypothesis of affective behavioural disorders has suggested that a deficiency of central amines, especially noradrenaline or serotonin, is associated with depressive symptomatology, whereas an excess of catecholamine, particularly noradrenaline, is associated with stereotypies and mania. There is diminished central noradrenaline turnover in depressive states, and depressive symptoms appear to be well correlated with diminished noradrenaline metabolism. Dopamine-receptor-blocking agents, such as the neuroleptic drugs, are effective in the treatment of manias and manic symptoms can be temporarily ameliorated by the use of physostigmine, which raises the level of acetylcholine within the central nervous system.

Critical balances among neurotransmitter systems exist within the brain. Such critical balances can be destroyed in some circumstances of chronic environmental stress. Agitation and stereotyped behavioural disorders may result from dopamine predominance. Perhaps this can take place as a result of deficiencies in cholinergic function or perhaps it can occur as a result of actual dopamine excess. Current data suggest that, although diminished noradrenaline may be associated with depressive symptomatology, other abnormalities associated with relative predominance of dopamine systems may be associated with manic, stereotyped characteristics in behaviour (Fraser, 1985). Neurophysiological studies show that there is increased dopamine turnover in the frontal cortex of the limbic system as a common first response to stressors. As a result, dopamine over-synthesis has become an established neurochemical indicator of stress. Hyperdopaminergic behaviours can therefore also serve as markers of stress. Not only do they serve as markers of husbandry stress, but they are indicators of behavioural illnesses. In them, there now exist new groups of illness, behaviourally manifest, which call for recognition, differential diagnosis and rational management.

7 Hormones and pheromones

The nervous system and the endocrine system are clearly adapted for different roles, but contact between them is essential in their full function since they are interdependent. The two systems cooperate with each other through the processes of neural secretion and through the priming effects of hormones on the brain. Hormone secretion is subject to the influence of many forms of stimulation. Endocrinologists now recognise an elaborate system of interactions between the animal's own activity, the external stimuli which it receives and its internal physiological state. Any of these three factors—behaviour, environment and internal state—can alter so as to cause a change in others. This elaborate apparatus clearly creates a potentially complex situation of chemical dependence.

Neuropeptides, hormones and pheromones, which convey information to other individuals by olfactory means, are active in the business of chemical communication. Such communication advises and instructs the organism's parts on the physiological status and requirements of the whole. An outline of the system of chemical messengers is therefore essential to an appreciation of behavioural scenery in general.

The physiology of hormones

The generation of cyclic AMP (adenosine monophosphate) is the common biochemical action of most hormones. In spite of this common denominator, different target organ cells vary in their abilities to be activated by different hormones. This is a result of qualitative differences in membrane receptor sites in different tissues. Consideration of hormone physiology can be based on the roles and effects of the endocrine system by hormone production sites.

Hypothalamus

The role of the hypothalamus in endocrine affairs is considerable (Mess *et al.*, 1970). It is responsible for controlling the secretions of both anterior and posterior pituitary lobes. In addition, the production of releasing and inhibiting factors, the operation of feedback mechanisms and the control of rhythmic phenomena and sexual behaviour are major endocrine roles of the hypothalamus (McCann, 1970).

Endocrine stimulation through the output of releasing factors under hypothalamic control is notable (Blackwell and Guillemin, 1973). Such control of pituitary secretion has some effect on eventual behaviour. As an example, the gonadotrophin releasing hormone acts on the anterior pituitary gland causing it to produce and release dual hormones: the luteinising hormone (LH) and the follicle stimulating hormone (FSH) (Flerko, 1970). The gonado-trophins on their pituitary release operate cyclic ovarian activity and related behaviour (King and Miller, 1980).

One hypothalamic–hypophysiotropic hor-mone requires special appreciation, namely the corticotrophin releasing hormone (CRH). As a result of the action of this hormone, ACTH (adrenocorticotrophic hormone) is put into the circulation from the anterior pituitary. Signifi-cantly increased ACTH secretion is involved in glycogenolysis and some stresses have been shown to deplete the glycogen content of the median eminence and the anterior pituitary. This, in turn, leads to the output of adrenal cor-tisol (Motta *et al.*, 1970) (see Fig. 7.1).

Anterior pituitary

Thyroid stimulating hormone (TSH) is pro-duced by the anterior pituitary which is anatomi-cally equivalent to the adenohypophysis. This hormone initiates thyroxine output, which determines metabolic rates, energy provision and thermal homeostasis. It is also concerned with reproductive behaviour in general since many reproductive acts require suddenly increased energy output (Li, 1972).

The adrenocorticotrophic hormone, or ACTH, works in controlling other endocrine glands. This hormone, often termed corticotro-phin, causes the adrenal cortex to enlarge and produce a variety of glucocorticoids, character-ised by cortisol. The increased blood levels of cortisol under stress is the result of increased ACTH activity. Sometimes circadian rhythms of cortisol output in farm animals can be dis-arranged, or dissociated, as a result of irregular-ities in ACTH output resulting from major husbandry disturbances. ACTH is sometimes termed the adaptive hormone to unusual cir-cumstances since it is notably secreted during adaptation, or attempted adaptation (Williams, 1974).

The output of gonadotrophic hormones from the anterior pituitary is of fundamental importance in reproductive behaviour (Beach, 1970). The two gonadotrophins luteinising hormone (LH) and follicle stimulating hormone (FSH) are produced in concert with one another in both sexes. In the female the levels vary while the production of gonadotrophins in the male appears to be level and continuous. In both sexes the follicle stimulating hormone supports the production of the gametes—spermatozoa and ova. Again in both sexes luteinising hormone promotes activity of gonadal cells—the inter-stitial testicular cells in the testis and the ovary; that is, LH can stimulate steroidogenesis in both ovary and testis. High levels of either androgens or oestrogens can inhibit the secretion of both FSH and LH by a feedback effect through the hypothalamus.

Prolactin is a further hormone concerned with the reproductive function which is produced by the anterior pituitary (Pasteels, 1970). It is considered to be the hormone which evokes the maternal drive. However, maternal behaviour does not entirely depend on prolactin, some maternal behaviour being governed by the ratio

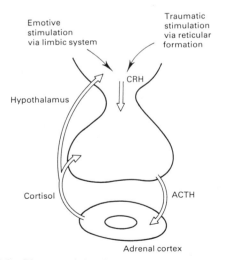

Fig. 7.1 Diagram of the closely connected relationship between the hypothalamus, the pituitary (hypophysis) and the adrenal cortex showing routes of outgoing stimu-lation and the feedback arrangements.

of progesterone to oestrogen typically occurring in the post-partum period. Prolactin also promotes grooming behaviour.

Posterior pituitary

The posterior pituitary which corresponds anatomically to the neurohypophysis, issues the hormones oxytocin and vasopressin. In terms of reproductive behaviour oxytocin is more commonly known as "the let-down hormone"—the hormone which encourages the free out-flow of milk at suckling and also plays a predominant part in labour. It is produced promptly in response to appropriate signals of stimulatory behaviour by the nursing animal. This usually occurs as local physical stimulation of the mammary region by the nursling.

Vasopressin is associated with ACTH and its output and therefore participates in stress responses. Vasopressin, as a neuropeptide, is now known to function as a neurotransmitter. Certain hypothalamic cells rely on vasopressin to signal to other brain cells and clearly this neurohormone has a role in the initiation of some behavioural activities. Vasopressin output aids memory and improves attention and learning. Training episodes which evidently involve increased blood pressure, through vasopressin output, increase the animal's acquisition of improved performance. Vasopressin, among its various roles, may serve to signal that the survival of the animal is challenged (Brownstein *et al.*, 1980). Conversely, its absence may indicate that the animal is currently safe.

Pineal gland

The pineal is a small singular rounded gland of solid consistency located within the brain, in midline at a point above the thalamus. In mammals the pineal gland is influenced by the stimulus of environmental lighting via the visual system. The only nerve supply to this gland is by sympathetic fibres. Stimulation of the pineal results in the release of noradrenaline (= norepinephrine) which has the ability to increase the amount of cyclic AMP, which in turn is involved with pineal metabolism (Wurtman, 1970). Hydroxyindole-*O*-methyl transferase (HIOMT) which is found in the pineal body, exerts enzymatic action from which melatonin is produced. Melatonin is evidently secreted from the pineal gland into the general circulation so that the pineal is a true neuroendocrine gland (Fraschini and Martini, 1970). Melatonin output is influenced by the photoperiod and is basic to the operation of numerous cyclic and seasonal phenomena in animals. Much remains to be learned about the role of melatonin in diurnal and seasonal cyclic behaviour.

Thyroid gland

Many active functions acquire the function of the thyroid gland and its secretion of thyroxine. The thyroid hormone influences energetic behaviour by affecting the metabolic pool of nitrogen and available energy. Thyroxine influences the activity of the gonads in synergism with the gonadotrophins and influences the maintenance of lactation. As proof of this, aberrations of the oestrous cycle have appeared in both hypothyroid and hyperthyroid animals in many spices. These effects may appear as lengthening, irregularity or complete disappearance of the cycles. In cattle thyroidectomy has caused heifers to show an absence of the usual signs of oestrous, a condition of "silent" oestrus occurring in these animals. Reversal of these results follows replacement therapy.

The testis

Testosterone is produced by the Leydig interstitial cells of the adult animal under the influence of LH from the anterior pituitary. Testosterone is responsible for typical male behaviour but the testosterone blood level only partially determines the level of male sex drive or libido. Male sex drive is not fully displayed in the absence of testosterone. Excessive output of testosterone by the testes will affect the pituitary through a feedback mechanism in such a way that there will be a reduction in gonadotrophic output which, in turn, reduces the production of testosterone.

In those species where there is seasonal fluctuation in the expression of male sex drive, e.g. the horse and sheep, it has been found that there is a corresponding fluctuation in the production of testosterone. In most cases investigated a reduction or cessation of testosterone output is associated with a reduction in size of the interstitial testicular cells. Leydig cells apparently shrink annually in seasonal breeders. In the ram, with its seasonal variation in libido, it has been found difficult to identify Leydig cells histologically comparable to these that occur in the bull, which has an almost constant reproductive drive throughout the year.

The ovary

Both the interstitial cells and the follicles of the ovary produce hormones. As the follicles mature with the rapid pro-oestrus growth, their output of oestrogen, the female sex hormone, increases sharply. As the threshold level is attained it affects the animal's behavioural responses and the signs of oestrous typical for that species will occur. Apparently pre-ovulatory progesterone is needed to synergise with oestrogen to produce all the features of oestrus. Oestrous behaviour is maintained for a period, while the follicle is at the peak of its maturity on the ovary. With follicular arrest there is a short drop in oestrogen output. The resulting disappearance of oestrogen in the general circulation is responsible for the termination of oestrous behaviour. It is evident, therefore, that the female sex drive will only be manifest normally during the time when there is a ripe follicle on the ovary, a condition which is of short and only periodic occurrence. This

contrasts with the male sex drive which is maintained over a long period of time by the continued output of testosterone by permanent interstitial cells. Although the corpus luteum initiates the endocrine functions in pregnancy, hormonal production by cells in the placenta soon occurs so that the corpus luteum becomes dispensable as a temporary endocrine gland.

The placenta

During pregnancy the placenta synthesises the steroid hormones of progesterone and oestrogen (Boyd and Hamilton, 1970). Increasing amounts of progesterone and oestrogens are found in the placental tissue and in maternal blood and urine as gestation progresses.

It appears that the placenta also contains a very high concentration of β-endorphin. It is believed that uterine physiology during parturition evokes the release of β-endorphin from the placenta permitting its uptake by the maternal circulation, thereby inducing an opioid state to block some of the pain of parturition.

Adrenal gland

From an endocrine perspective, each adrenal gland consists of an outer portion, the cortex, and an inner portion, the medulla, with the entire gland enclosed in one tissue capsule (Mason, 1972).

Cortex

Various steroid compounds occur in the adrenal cortex including adrenal cortical hormones which have glycogenic activity (glucocorticoids) and male sex hormones (androgens). The most active glucocorticoid is cortisol in ungulates (e.g. cattle, sheep, pigs) and man, but in rodents and poultry corticosterone is the most active. Under the influence of cortisol or corticosterone the effects of various stressors are reduced. The hormones are able to activate carbohydrate metabolism so as to increase blood sugar for the needs of sudden energy demands.

Medulla

The adrenal medulla is sometimes likened to an oversized sympathetic ganglion which releases its active substance directly into the bloodstream in the way of an endocrine gland (Bloom and Fawcett, 1968). The hormonal output of the adrenal medulla is adrenaline (epinephrine) which is biologically similar to noradrenaline (norepinephrine).

The adrenal medulla (as a general reinforcer, or booster, of sympathetic activity) comes under the close control of the limbic system, and of the hypothalamus in particular. The effects on the body of adrenaline are complex and various. In principle this hormone prepares the animal for gross physical activity in situations of emergency. It is particularly responsible for temporary increase in blood pressure in response to stressful stimulation. Sudden increases in adrenaline output are associated with agonistic events in general and specific forms of it in particular such as male fighting and maternal protection. Adrenaline also provides the basis for alarm responses in general.

Other hormones

Many other hormones not mentioned above are produced in the body and there are some whose secretion is controlled, at least in part, by completely distinct mechanisms. These include aldosterone from the adrenal cortex, insulin and glucagon from the pancreas, parathyroid hormone, several kidney hormones and gastro-intestinal hormones. The direct behavioural significances of these miscellaneous hormones is not thought to be great and description of their mechanisms is omitted here in this general sketch of polypeptide organisations.

The physiology of pheromones

Many animals communicate by olfactory substances, frequently conveyed through their secretions. The basic arrangements for this mode of communication are: (i) a source of odour, such as a skin gland, (ii) a signal of odour —usually as a secretion containing complex molecules, (iii) the olfactory mucous membranes of the nasal cavity acting as a receptor; and (iv) the rhinencephalon, or old "nose-brain", operating as the executive organ. Further components are: (v) the stimulated centre in the olfactory part of the telencephalon; (vi) the olfactory sphere of consciousness located in the cerebral cortex; and eventually (vii) the form of behaviour reactively produced. A substance responsible for such a chain reaction is termed a pheromone. More definitively, a pheromone is a substance produced by one animal which conveys information to other individuals by olfactory means.

There is variation amongst species in the sources of pheromones. Some animals have scent glands within which the secretion of specific chemicals occurs. Often the secretions are held for some time so the final composition and odour of glandular products depends upon bacterial action. Many different substances will be present in the odoriferous product. Other sources of pheromones are body products such as urine, faeces and saliva. The effects of pheromones may be the rapid initiation of action, as in alarm pheromones, or the production of sustained behavioural responses.

The important effect of pheromones is the stimulation of olfactory centres in the brain so pheromone detection depends on macrosmatics, which is the possession of keenness of smell, to an extremely high degree. Most animals' olfactory centres are more differentiated than are those of man, who is microsmatic, and the olfactory portion of the telencephalon of cattle and sheep is about twenty times larger than in the human. A special organ apparently involved with pheromone reception, through its mucous membrane, is the vomero-nasal, or Jacobson's organ. This organ is an olfactory receiver in the form of a pair of blind-end tubes located within the nasal cavity and linked to the roof of the mouth. It is connected to the centres of olfaction in the brain with its own mechanism of conduction and its own reactive behaviour. It is instrumental in an olfactory reflex act which is known as flehmen. In flehmen the head is elevated and extended, the upper lip is curled up with the mouth slightly open and the nostrils constricted. The flehmen reaction (Fig. 7.2) indicates that the male is testing the urine of the female. The concentration of pheromones can reflect levels of sex hormones in the individual and in this case the male is monitoring the oestrous state of the female. Oestrus synchronisation in female mammals can result from common olfactory urine checking. Male urine can also provide olfactory information about hormone levels. Urine is used for territory

markers in some mammalian species, such as badgers, and some animals mix faeces, urine and scent gland products in acquiring a distinctive individual odour.

The two types of scent-producing glands are sebaceous glands, such as the ventral gland of the Mongolian gerbil which is used for territory ownership marking, and apocrine glands. The two types of glands are often mixed in glandular areas. The axillary glands in man produce pheromones whose release is facilitated by both the presence of axillary hair which provide a larger surface area and by the action of arm raising. Pigs, ruminants and horses possess specialised gland complexes located in the skin. The skin as the primary protector of the body surface is covered with glands serving temperature control, excretion, greasing and maintaining the pH in fending off microorganisms. This, in its totality, produces a specific body odour. In these animals the convoluted type of skin glands, with their apocrine excretions, produce a volatile substance which is moved to the skin's surface and mixed in a product which is particularly suited to contain, or bond, odoriferous substances. The occurrence and location of skin regions which produce odour relate to certain forms of behaviour (Vandenbergh, 1983).

Widely studied glands include those of many insects and mammals. The chin gland of rabbits is used to mark territory, to warn others and to mark young for recognition. Dogs and their relatives have anal glands and the secretion in the female fox contains twelve volatile components including trimethylamine and several fatty acids. The chemical inducing sexual behaviour in dogs is *para*-methyl hydroxy benzoate. Cats have glands on the side of the face and at the base of the tail. They use these to mark objects in their environment including their ''owners''. When cats rub their head and tail base against you they may well be merely establishing their ownership of you! Deer have elaborate glands, that of the musk deer containing as much as 120 g of sebum. The tarsal tuft on the leg of the black-tailed deer has specially adapted hairs which trap volatile substances from the tarsal

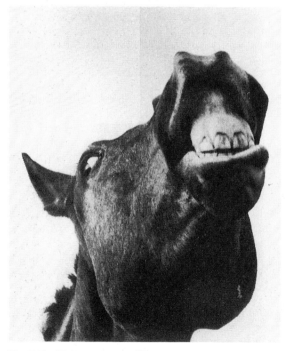

Fig. 7.2 Flehmen in a stallion.

gland and from urine which is deposited on the tuft (Müller-Schwarze, 1977). The odours from the tarsal gland in this species and from the metatarsal gland in the roe deer (Broom and Johnson, 1980) attract much attention from other members of the species and probably allow individual recognition.

Many wild ruminants are endowed with interdigital glands on all four feet, particularly below the dew claws. The skin around these interdigital glands is richly endowed with convoluted glands, which produce a mixed secretion of pheromones. It appears that an alarm pheromone is produced and stored there as a colloid. The domestic ruminants have remnants of analogous glands which may still function as sources of specific odours.

Saliva can be involved in chemical communication and behavioural evidence of this is notable in the pig in pre-mating and nursing situations and in social events in the horse. Experimentally, saliva has been found to play a part in organising the suckling behaviour of the rat and the aggressive behaviour of mice. Rat pups reportedly engage in long periods of licking and nuzzling the mother's oral region and this suggests that a chemical mechanism operates via saliva in regulating nursing interactions. Sows and their young piglets show essentially similar nosing of the maternal oral area. Young animals show a tendency to pursue olfactory examination of the mouths of associating adults and of their mothers' mouths particularly (Fig. 7.3).

Experimentally, juvenile gerbils were found

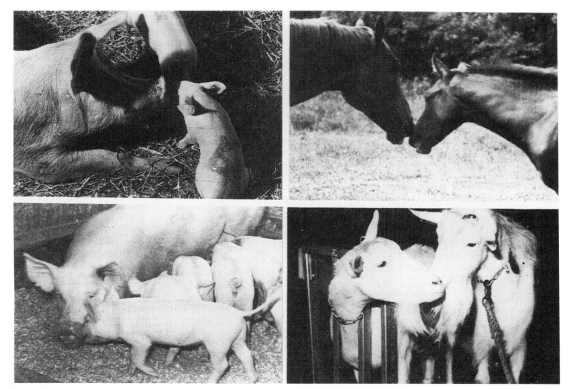

Fig. 7.3 Close nose-to-mouth contacts between young animals and adults and between sexes. This behaviour is strong circumstantial evidence of the role of salivary chemicals acting as pheromones in farm animals in the way that studies on experimental animals have shown.

to respond preferentially to females carrying their littermate's saliva rather than to those carrying non-littermate saliva. Adult male gerbils spend more time contacting the facial regions of recipients carrying saliva from an oestrous female. They exhibited no difference in their contact times with the ventral scent glands or anogenital regions. Social preferences were evident in the behaviour following salivary exposures. These findings suggest that saliva-related cues may act as chemosignals in all stages of social behaviour in gerbils (Block *et al.*, 1981). Such salivary factors probably function in other animals including farm livestock. Among farm animals many social interactions take the form of nose-to-mouth contacts in which it is likely that salivary cues of identity, and possible status, are communicated. This has been noted in the horse and sheep and it seems that salivary pheromones may affect social behaviour in animals to extents not appreciated before. Many so-called "naso–nasal" contacts are in fact found to be nose-to-mouth contacts when carefully studied.

The production and the effects of phero-mones have been noted in the pig (Signoret *et al.*, 1975). The boar produces a chemical substance called muskone which appears to have a releaser effect on sows during oestrus so that they show the rigid mating posture more readily after they have been exposed to the male pheromone. The boar's pheromone is apparently produced in the submaxillary salivary gland. There is copious production of saliva, in frothy form, during the natural pre-mating activities between boar and sow. During these activities nose-to-mouth con-tacts are clearly shown. Pheromone excretion in the boar also occurs via the prepuce. Proof of this has been shown in large-scale, experimen-tal studies in pig artificial insemination work. Small quantities of boar seminal fluid dropped onto the snout of a sow showing dubious or incomplete signs of oestrus causes the complete oestrous display to be reflexly shown in many instances, with resolution of the problem—one way or the other—concerning the oestrous state of the sow.

The phenomenon of sexual responsiveness, particularly in the female to male presence, has been termed bio-stimulation (Fraser, 1968). It would appear that much of the substrate of bio-stimulation is pheromonal communication (Lindsay, 1965). Much more study remains to be done on this to determine the details of the phenomenon. Evidence of bio-stimulation in all the farm animals has been accumulated in abun-dance and it clearly has a major effect on vital reproductive behaviour (Fletcher and Lindsay, 1971).

8 Reactivity to predators and social stimuli

As a very broad category of behaviour reactivity refers to the likelihood of showing some response to a wide variety of stimuli. Some of the most important stimuli which an individual encounters during its lifetime are those emanating from predators. Other sensory inputs come from conspecific animals or from other aspects of the animal's environment. Sensory input modifies existing motivational state and may or may not result in a motor output. The term output usually implies muscle action but it can also involve glandular action.

Motor output

Motor output is highly organised in the central nervous system using specialised neural pathways descending throughout the spinal cord and dominated by sets of neurons in the motor cortex and cerebellum. From the area of the sensorimotor cortex there is a descending partnership of pyramidal and extra-pyramidal neurons initiating motor activity. In regard to motor output in general, it ranges from reflex activity at the spinal cord level to a whole series of conative acts resulting from sensory information processed at the cortical level. Conation, or willpower, is involved in many environmental reactions such as choosing feed and shelter.

Much reactivity is influenced by the autonomic nervous system, conveniently considered as the peripheral arm of the limbic system.

The chief role of the autonomic nervous system is to maintain internal homeostasis, or physiological stability of the internal organs. As a rule the effects of sympathetic stimulation relate to active "fight-or-flight" states of the body and its organs. Parasympathetic stimulation generally induces relaxed vegetative activities and conditions. The effects of the two divisions typically tend to be opposite and the two subsystems are therefore antagonistic. The antagonism is due to the chemistry of the two divisions.

In the "fight-or-flight" state the physiological changes favour great muscular effort of either fighting or fleeing, depending on the resolved decision of the animal. These physiological changes, resulting from sympathetic stimulation, include: increased heart rate, increased blood pressure, expansion of the bronchial tubes and suppression of alimentary activity. All of these ensure good oxygenation of musculature. Parasympathetic stimulation produces the opposite effects of slower heart rate, lowered blood pressure, constriction of bronchi and increased activity of the gut.

Most sympathetic nerve endings release the neurotransmitter substance noradrenaline (norepinephrine) which is chemically very similar to adrenaline (epinephrine) produced by the medulla of the adrenal gland. The nerve fibres creating such chemistry are therefore termed adrenergic. After release of noradrenaline at the adrenergic nerve fibre termination it becomes altered to *O*-methyl transferase, an enzyme which the nerve ending can reabsorb.

Most parasympathetic nerve endings release acetylcholine at synapses and nerve endings so they are therefore termed cholinergic. After its synaptic release, acetylcholine may be inactivated by cholinesterase or may be reabsorbed by the nerve ending.

A gamut of physiological changes resembling the activation of the sympathetic nervous system's basic responses of fear or rage, fight or flight occur in association with reactivity to aversive stimulation and pain. These physiological changes include increases in heart rate, blood pressure, blood sugar and adrenaline secretion; reduction occurs in gastric motility and blood flow to the internal organs. In particular, the experience of pain includes some emotional components of fear, anxiety and unpleasantness. The complex nature of pain is due to the combination of a sensory experience plus a reaction to it. *Pain is defined as a sensation which is itself extremely aversive.* This definition excludes sensory inputs which are aversive by association, such as those which occur when a predator is detected. Pain is a form of suffering and so is an important cause of poor welfare in animals (see Chapter 29).

Anti-predator strategies

All wild animals are subject to attack by predators and parasites and the selection pressures promoting efficient means of countering these attacks are very great. Domestic animals still have these anti-predator and anti-parasite mechanisms so everyone involved with animals on farms needs to know about them. The principles of anti-predator behaviour summarised here

are discussed at greater length by Broom (1981, p. 157). Exploration is also important in anti-predator behaviour and is discussed in Chapter 12. The two basic types of defensive mechanisms are primary defence mechanisms, which operate regardless of whether or not there is a predator in the vicinity, and secondary defence mechanisms, which operate during an encounter with a predator (Edmunds, 1974).

Primary defence mechanisms include (Broom, 1981):

1. hiding in holes, e.g. rabbits resting in holes;
2. the use of crypsis, e.g. moths which are difficult to see on a tree trunk or mammalian prey species which minimise their body odours;
3. mimicry of inedible objects, e.g. caterpillars which look like bird droppings;
4. exhibition of a warning of danger to predators, e.g. skunk coloration;
5. mimicry of individuals in category (4), e.g. flies which look like bees;
6. timing activities so as to minimise the chance of detection by a predator, e.g. being active at night;
7. remaining in a situation where any predator attack is likely to be unsuccessful because of possibilities for secondary defence, e.g. rabbits feeding near their holes or small antelope grazing near thorn bushes;
8. maintaining vigilance so as to maximise the chance of detecting the advent of a predator, e.g. sheep spending time looking, sniffing and listening for predators.

Secondary defence mechanisms are used when a predator is detected, or when detection is supposed, or when an actual attack occurs. Types of active secondary defence include (Broom, 1981):

1. exaggerating primary defence, e.g. a camouflaged caterpillar remaining entirely motionless when a predator approaches;
2. withdrawal to a safe retreat, e.g. a rabbit running to its burrow or an armadillo curling up;

3. flight and evasion, e.g. a hare running and jinking when pursued by a dog;
4. use of a display which deters attack, e.g. moths moving wings to reveal large eye spots;
5. feigning death, e.g. American oppossums and many birds including chickens;
6. behaviour which deflects attack, e.g. some butterfly eye marks which deflect bird pecks away from body and broken wing displays by plovers which deflect predators away from the nest;
7. retaliation, e.g. biting, butting, or chemical secretions.

Varieties of reactive behaviour

All reactive behaviours are organised responses using neural circuits which range from simple spinal arcs, involving only two large neurons, to elaborate internuncial networks of many small neurons localised in higher brain centres. Among the various forms of behavioural reactions several major classes of reactivity can be recognised including: (1) reflex action, (2) vocal communication (3) responses to specific environmental (including seasonal) factors, (4) avoidance reactions, (5) reproductive reactions, and (6) agonistic reactions. Some reactions involve combinations of these categories (Table 8.1).

Table 8.1
Some classes of reactivity

Class	Examples
Reflexes	Moving when startled
Orientation	Turning towards or away from intruder
Vocalisation	Distress call (chick)
Displays	Threatening head lowering (bull)
Agonistic actions	Butting (ram)
Social, non-agonistic action	Mutual grooming (cow)
Defensive action	Retreat
Initiate maintenance behaviour	Feed at sunrise

Reflex behaviour

Many forms of reactive behaviour occur as simple reflexes, such as reflexes involving extension or withdrawal of a limb in response to various stimuli, locally applied. Limb reflexes have protective or postural functions. Reflex evacuation, involving sudden defaecation or urination, is common in cattle and sheep following the stimulus of invaded individual space.

Vocal communication

Those involved with farm animals sometimes fail to appreciate the complexity of vocal communication which they show. Particularly in circumstances of social reactivity, vocal sound is a major feature of communication. For example, vocal signals occur as exchanges between mother and neonate, between breeding male and female, and by socially bonded individuals when separated. As reactivity increases, vocalisation tends to increase in volume, quantity and complexity. Deep vocal sounds often accompany the threat displays of mature males. Many vocalisations are incorporated into responses concerned with alarm and threat.

Specific sounds relate to specific circumstances. Hunger generates much vocalisation, notably among young animals such as piglets and calves, but hunger in all age groups of farm animals causes hunger calls. Again, changes in phonation, from major to minor key, take place at oestrus in cattle. Stallions are actively vocal in the breeding season; rams are particularly guttural in autumn; bleating is almost continuous in female goats during oestrus. Innumerable examples of specific vocalisations occur in the usual circumstances of animal farming.

An animal's vocal and other reactions to its environment are often related to temperament. The subject's appreciation of sensations of vision, sound and position is qualitatively affected by its temperament and this is reflected in vocalisations. It has been suggested that the horse makes three basic sounds: a neigh, a grunt and a high-pitched crying noise. These sounds vary in their degree of intensity and duration and also show variations according to sex and age and the particular stimulus which elicits them. There are also specific sounds which are variations of the three basic ones. The neigh is the loudest phonation of the horse. It is often heard when a mare is separated from her foal or when a horse is curious about events outside its range of vision, or when it is seeking to communicate with other horses. Horses grunt, most commonly just prior to feeding. Grunts are emitted by stallions at the beginning of a sexual encounter and by mares when they have cause to worry about their foals. The squealing sound can vary in volume and is usually heard during aggressive encounters as a part of threat in fighting or in instances of aggressive sexual rejection. Additional forms of vocalisation include trumpeting in the male and the throaty gurgling of general satisfaction.

In the mating season, rams emit a hoarse "baaing" sound when approaching ewes. Vocalisation also plays an important part in the maintenance of communication between members of the flock. If a mother is separated from her young she will "baa" until they are brought together and the young do the same. When adult members of the flock become disengaged from the others, they become more animated in attempts to locate the main flock and increase vocalisation. Increased vocalisation has been shown generally to be accompanied by increased mobility. Other studies of vocalisations include: domestic fowl (Collias and Joos, 1953), ungulates in general (Kiley, 1972) and horse (Ödberg, 1974).

Environmental reactions

The animal's willingness to move to use its environment is an important aspect of reactivity. Seasonal and daily changes in reactivity are sometimes evident in major changes in behavioural routines. In the seasonally breeding animals, such as sheep, horses and goats, the introduction of reproductive activities affects other routine behaviours, modifying some of their priorities. Male animals, in their breeding season, show increased aggression. Seasonal changes occur in grazing behaviour. For example, sheep show progressively more active grazing throughout the day in winter, reaching the height of the diurnal activity prior to evening twilight. This grazing pattern does not contain the active phases of early morning grazing, characteristic of summer behaviour. Behavioural responses to weather occur but in many parts of the world they vary greatly according to the season.

Older animals under free-range conditions can transfer information about routes, good pasture areas and watering points to their progeny by example (Arnold, 1977). In this way, home-range areas can be established and perpetuated. Sheep in pastures of 100 ha may establish up to three separate home-range areas and subgroups of the whole flock work with minimal overlap in these regions. In smaller pastures, dairy bulls over four years of age under set-stocking conditions set up small territories which they defend. Sudden attacks of dairy bulls on their handlers might be caused by this territorial reactivity.

Avoidance and submissive reactivity

As the main instrument of their group negotiations, sheep, cattle and horses maintain visual contact with associates while pigs, which are more body-contact animals, use vision less but keep in auditory communication with conspecifics. If disturbed, sheep and horses first bunch and then run from the source of disturbance while pigs and cattle move in a looser group. To facilitate reactivity, sheep orient themselves to one another at a visual angle of approximately 100 to 120 degrees.

During the bunching of animal groups in natural or high-density situations, individuals may be forced to violate the individual spaces of others. Reactivity at such close quarters depends on the hierarchical positions of the animals. Hierarchical orders, when stable, require in each member: (a) a recognition of individual animals, (b) an initial encounter when the social position is first established, and (c) a durable memory that enables each animal to react to the other according to its established social status.

The most obvious avoidance reaction is flight, which may be socially controlled or uncontrolled. When herd flight is controlled, the animals flee in their normal travelling order (Sato, 1982) in which a high rank individual female is usually the leader. When panic occurs there is uncontrolled flight without commitment to any order. Schafer (1975) ascribes the promptness of flight in horses to their original habitat on the plains where it served as a vital survival tactic. In addition, it has been pointed out that, although horses can be frightened by sound, the visual impression is more important than the audible one. It is certainly common knowledge that suddenly visible stimuli are more likely to cause an alarm reaction in the horse than strange sounds.

Avoidance reactions of cattle in response to threatening approach can be passive or active. Avoidance of an exchange in the form of social submission has characteristic gestures and postures. These may vary from the most common one of slight head depression with deviation away from the stimulus, to the gross display of hypotonic submission in which the animal assumes recumbency and refuses to rise. This latter behaviour is a confusing condition in the presence of a concurrent illness contributing to recumbency. The characteristic feature of such submission in cattle is vigorous, low extension of the head and neck when aversive stimulation is given. The recognition of submissive reactions is essential in handling sick or "fallen" livestock of all species, to ensure that their condition is given appropriate consideration. The general inertia of submission is a common feature which is characterised by an abnormally low level of reactivity of such stimuli which usually cause some change of position or posture.

Social dominance, avoidance and submission may have effects which can be important in cases of high stocking densities (Squires and Daws, 1975). Inadequate space in indoor housing, lack of feeders or trough space can mean that dominant animals command resources at the expense of subordinate animals. When the latter practise extreme avoidance or submission they suffer in health and general production. Documented examples of this include the higher internal parasite load carried in subordinates and the higher death rate during droughts when limited food becomes commandeered by dominant stock. For optimum reactive functions there may be an upper limit to the number of group members. The conspecific numbers that can be recognised or remembered by one individual could be 50 to 70 in cattle and 20 to 30 in pigs.

Reproductive reactivity

Reactivity is often greater during reproductive periods. Threat displays are most frequently produced as reactions to man by animals in reproductive states. Such displays often represent a physiological state of fight-or-flight and are most readily shown by mature males. In this state a bull hunches his shoulders, flexes his neck and shows protrusion of the eyeballs and erection of hair along the dorsum. During the threat display the bull turns shoulder-on towards the threatened object. In the stallion the threat display involves rearing on the hind legs. The boar in a threat display turns his side towards the threatened object, holds his head down, erects hair on the back and emits barking sounds. Threat displays are occasionally shown by rams towards humans or other potential aggressors and in these circumstances the display usually involves vigorous stamping with a forefoot.

Oestrogen-primed females exhibit oestrous displays, often in reaction to male stimulation. Although these displays are state dependent, basically they are usually elicited as reactions which are stimulus dependent. Mature animals, such as bulls, boars and stallions, have a high level of aggressive reactivity in their behaviour.

This is often displayed as prompt reaction to violation of individual space. Evidently testosterone is a chemical primer for reactive behaviour relating to instances of territorial threat, when threat displays are aggressive reactivity. A notable form of reactive behaviour occurs between rams in autumn. At the onset of their breeding season, rams in their existing bachelor groups engage in running towards one another and butting. They crowd together and may buffet each other with their shoulders. In this pre-breeding behaviour they engage in close, concentric bunching and show intermittent running activities. When stationary they occasionally emit snorting sounds and paw the earth with their forefeet. The unsettled nature of ram groupings, with regard to their composition of the group, which occurs in autumn is a result of rams wandering from one location to another. Shepherds note that the morning is the time when rams are likely to stray from their own breeding territories (Wilson, 1929).

Agonistic reactivity

Aggressive behaviour is most seen when groups of pigs, cattle or horses are first formed. Production of milk and other physiological responses can be affected for several days while aggressive social interactions are taking place (Dietrich *et al.*, 1965). Although sheep seldom show fighting behaviour, rams compete at the start of each breeding season and sheep may show aggressive butting if intensive husbandry conditions increase competition over food or bedded areas. Butting in cattle and sheep, biting of the mane or withers in the horse, and rooting, pushing and biting in pigs are common forms of agonistic behaviour. Retaliation, avoidance, flight and submission are the dependent reactivities (Fig. 8.1).

Agonistic behaviour embodies many of the behavioural activities of fight-or-flight and those of aggressive and passive behaviour. Agonistic behaviour includes all forms of behaviour by an animal which is in conflict with another animal. Such activities are principally involved in self-determination in relation to social hierarchies and feature both acts of positive aggression and equivalent acts of avoidance or negative reaction (Dickson *et al.*, 1967). Aggressive acts are most evident when the aggression of the initiating animal is countered with equivalent aggression. This is common in exchanges between individuals closely matched in dominance status (Fig. 8.2).

When one bovine animal makes an intention approach towards another, a mild reactive threat by the latter may often be enough to discourage engagement in physical contact. If, however, the approached animal is slow to react it may be butted, often from the rear. The up-swinging motion of the butt may cause injury, particularly if the attacking animal has horns. In an active approach by one animal towards another, the initiator makes a deliberate threat to the one encountered. If the latter animal resents this approach, its resentment is indicated by the lowering of its head as in aggressive behaviour; the animal's forehead is directed to the ground with the neck flexed and arched. If the animal being threatened in its turn displays threatening behaviour, fighting ensues. In some cases the two opponents stand a few metres apart with their heads lowered, hind legs drawn forward, eyes on each other. The threat position of females is essentially similar to the fight-or-flight posture of males, though less pronounced. Threat is shown in cattle when an animal paws at the ground and rubs its head and neck on the loosened ground (Fig. 8.3).

The form of *fighting* varies from species to species. Horses are often unpredictable in the way in which they react aggressively. Their response to alarm or threat may be flight or attempted flight on the one hand, or attack on the other, depending largely on temperament. It is thought that aggressive acts in horses maintained in isolation may be the result of over-excitement. Horses attack using their teeth and hind feet. Equine combat behaviour and flight are well documented (Schafer, 1975). As foals mature, the fighting element in their behaviour

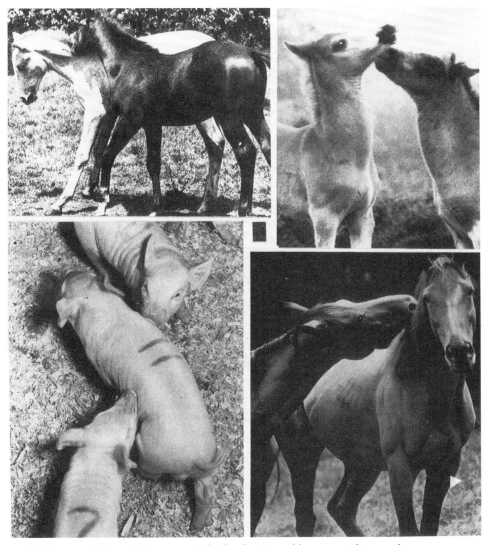

Fig. 8.1   Initiating agonistic acts in horses and pigs leading to positive or negative reactions.

emerges clearly and the speed of fighting reaction increases gradually. Sparring matches and real fights occur among young stallions. In sparring there is skirmishing in which they circle, sniff each other, and stamp with a forefoot. In the fight each tries to force his opponent to the ground. In reaction to this the defending animal uses neck movements to ward off the attack. Attempts are made to bite the opponent's muzzle, forelegs, neck, shoulder and ribs while whirling round, rearing and kneeling. Serious fights begin without skirmishing and start by

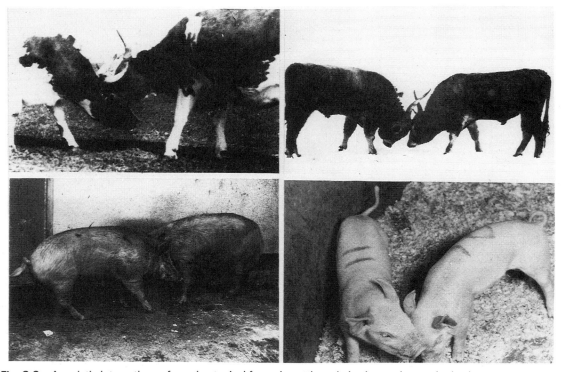

Fig. 8.2   Agonistic interactions of species-typical forms in cattle and pigs in evenly matched pairs.

attempting to bite, rear up and strike out with the forefeet. When an animal is losing a fight he takes flight, defending himself as he does so by kicking out with the hind feet. In stallion fights, loud bellowing vocalisations are made.

To minimise aggressive events, horses maintain large individual distances. Horses, like other livestock, react within set distances, such as the flight distance, the individual and "critical" distance. Each of these distances, then, is the point at which the given distance between the animal and the advancing subject has been so reduced that the approached animal must react. The individual distance is that at which some response to the advancing animal is made. In the case of the "critical distance" the animal will be more likely to attack than take flight. These distances vary according to the typical reactivity of the animal resulting from its

inherent temperament, its experience, domesticated training, competition, housing, feeding, and so on. Differences are recognised between horse breeds and types in regard to aggressiveness and speed of fight reaction. Horses of oriental blood, i.e. hot and "warm" blooded horses, such as Arabs and throughbreds, are more reactive than "cold" blooded horses, such as draught breeds. Mares with young foals are particularly reactive towards the approach of strange individuals.

Fighting between pigs is most severe among adults. Mixing adult pigs together, therefore, is an operation which must be carried out with care. If a strange sow is introduced to an established group of sows, the collective aggressive behaviour of the group directed at the stranger can be so severe that physical injuries may result in death. When two strange boars are first put

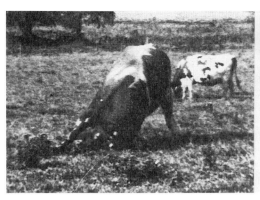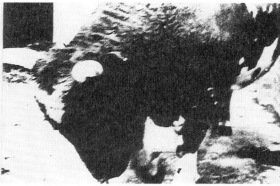

Fig. 8.3   The threat display of the bull involves (left) horning the ground and (right) pawing with the head lowered and directed obliquely at the stimulus.

together, they circle around and sniff each other and in some cases may paw the ground. Deep-throated barking grunts may be made and jaw-snapping engaged in as fighting starts. The opponents adopt a shoulder-to-shoulder position, applying side pressure against each other. Boars tend to use the side of the face permitting the upwardly-directed, lower tusks to be brought into use as weapons. Boars attack the sides of their opponents' bodies in this fashion. Fighting may continue for an hour before submission in one animal. The loser then disengages from the conflict and runs away squealing loudly. With the other's dominance thus established, the encounter ends.

When fighting begins in cattle the animals fight with their heads and horns. They try to butt each other's flanks. If one animal manoeuvres itself into a position where it can butt the flank of the other, the second animal turns round to defend itself and attempts a similar attack. Fighting sessions do not normally last longer than a few minutes, but in cases where the animals are equally matched the "clinch" move may be repeatedly employed. This is a move where the animal being attacked from the side turns itself parallel to the other and pushes its head and horns into the region of the other's lower flank. This often arrests fighting for several minutes before action is resumed. When one animal submits, it turns and runs from the other which may assert its dominance by chasing after it for a short distance. If neither animal submits, fighting may continue until both tire.

As a feature of social reactivity, *mock fighting* is seen as a variant of play (Reinhardt and Reinhardt, 1982). Mock fighting occurs in all the species of farm animals when they are grouped. As might be expected as a variety of play, mock fighting occurs more often in young animals than in adults. While some mock fighting may occur in adult female stock as cows, it is not recognised as normally occurring between older males.

The form of mock fighting is somewhat ritualised. The initial activity is one of solicitation. This usually takes the form of the approaching animal bounding towards the associate animal with jerky head movements. In cattle there is head lowering and tail raising. In horses and pigs there is biting of the neck of the associate. The following phase in mock fighting is usually in the form of a contest in which one animal pushes or applies weight to the other. During this it is common for the animals to circle. Such circling motions are a feature of mock fight behaviour in calves and piglets reacting to associates. Head butting also takes place. The termination of mock fights is usually without consequence and does not lead to a rout or chasing. Mock fighting is more often seen in male calves than in heifers. Young female animals are less inclined to respond to pushing contests initiated by males, particularly as the age of sexual maturity is reached when male mock fighting becomes common.

Apart from causing physical injury, fighting between cows can result in a reduction of milk yield since the inhibited subjects may not feed properly in a restricted area of grazing. It is advised practice to keep new cows in a field adjacent to the main herd at first, before introducing the animals in pairs to the other members, thus allowing all individuals to become familiar with each other. Limited fighting may occur as the new animals struggle for self-determination in the social hierarchy of the whole herd.

Defensive reactions to man by farm animals

Man was a dangerous predator to the ancestors of our farm animals and people are often treated as a source of potential danger by present-day farm animals. This fact is often ignored by those who work on farms but competent stockmen learn to recognise such responses and to treat the animals in a way which minimises their occurrence. If a person enters an animal house rapidly and noisily the animals may show a violent escape response. This can occur in a calf, pig or poultry house but the response of poultry can be the most damaging. A wave of escape behaviour, often called hysteria, can pass down the house and result in a pile-up of birds against the wall of cages or of the house. Many birds may die in this situation. If entering is preceded by a knock and unexpected movements and noises are avoided such problems can be minimised.

The qualities of a good stockman include the avoidance of causing panic, as described above, and an ability to act calmly and predictably when coming close to animals. Early studies on stockman behaviour and effects referred especially to dairy cows. Baryshnikov and Kokorina (1959) showed that milk let-down occurred faster if the cows saw the familiar milker and Seabrook (1977) showed that milk yield was higher if the cowman moved in a deliberate, calm way, talked quietly to the cows and followed a regular routine. Management efficiency and milk production have been improved by studies of defensive behaviour of cows to cowmen and to disturbing aspects of milking parlour design (Albright, 1979). Recent studies of stockmanship emphasise the advantages of the good stockman, both for animal welfare and for production efficiency (Metz, 1987; Seabrook, 1987).

9 Feeding

Feeding involves a complex series of decisions and depends upon an elaborate array of mental, motor and digestive abilities. Wild animals, or free-ranging farm animals, need to find the right sort of habitat and then to find concentrations, or patches, of food before they can start looking for particular food items. Finding the food source is also important for young animals which have to find their mother's teats or another food source which they have not seen before. The word *foraging* is used to refer to *the behaviour of animals when they are moving around in such a way that they are likely to encounter and acquire food for themselves or their offspring* (Broom, 1981, p. 124).

The initiation of feeding behaviour can be affected by diurnal rhythms and social factors but inputs from monitors of body state are of particular importance. Signals reported to be of importance in several species include visual input, input from taste receptors, input resulting from stomach contractions, insulin effects, plasma glucose detector input and fat store monitor inputs (Mogenson and Calaresu, 1978). Stimulation of the lateral hypothalamus can lead to eating by rats or cattle but the lateral hypothalamus is not essential for eating to occur. Glucose levels are clearly of little importance to feeding in ruminants (Baile and Forbes, 1974). Once food is found the rate of ingestion will limit intake. This will depend upon: (1) oral mechanics and other abilities of

the animal; (2) the physical and mechanical properties of the food; (3) the availability of water; (4) the nutrient qualities of the food; and (5) the effects of disturbances such as those due to danger of predation, attacks by insects, or competition from other members of the species. Both the efficiency of finding food and the various effects on the rate of ingestion will be modified according to the previous experience of the individual. The point at which ingestion of a meal ceases will depend on gut size and input to the brain from sensory receptors, such as those which signal that the gut is full. Booth (1978) has proposed that eating occurs when the flow of energy from absorption becomes too small and disappears again when absorptive flow becomes adequate. Such explanations, whether or not referring to satiety centres in the hypothalamus, cannot explain the many different situations in which feeding is initiated or terminated.

During the delay before the next meal, the food is processed. The rate of processing, which depends on gut cross-sectional area, enzyme activity in the gut and food quality, will often be a major factor limiting food intake. The next meal may be delayed more than the digestion time if there is input to the brain which indicates that the general metabolic state as indicated by, for example, the fat store level, is such that no further meal is needed. If extra food is needed due to metabolic needs, e.g. external temperature is low, then the onset of the next meal is accelerated. Another important factor which can affect the delay before the next meal is the quality of the ingested food. If this is insufficient then the animal may move to a better place before recommencing eating. The efficiency of digestion can be impaired by illness, parasites or by adverse conditions which lead to adrenal activity, as well as by the quality of food, so any of these factors can have an effect on intake.

Physiological facts alone do not explain all about feeding behaviour. Feeding behaviour is strongly influenced by reinforcement, both positive and negative, from food palatability and by the environmental and social associations of feeding. It is necessary then, for example, for the concepts of motivation and reinforcement to be incorporated into any comprehensive view of food intake control. One current scientific conclusion is that as the animal develops, drinking and feeding may occur as natural complements of each other, and they may occur frequently and in modest amounts, not because the animal is compelled to restore accumulated deficits, but because it anticipates the pleasures of ingestion and thereby avoids the deficits entirely (Epstein, 1983). Studies of various animals with food continuously available, including rats (Le Magnen, 1971) and cattle (Metz, 1975), show that meal size is more often correlated with the interval before the following meal than with the interval since the last meal. Hence the animals are not compensating for an accumulated deficit but are using a feedforward control system. They must have learned that food has a certain effect so they consume enough for a certain future period duration.

The remainder of this chapter will deal with grazing behaviour as an example of how feeding is organised, finding food, the ability to obtain food, meal size and food selection, the effects of disturbance on feeding, social facilitation, competition and feeding behaviour, and then some specific details about feeding in cattle, sheep, horses, pigs and poultry.

Grazing behaviour

From consideration of this range of factors it will be apparent already that feeding is complex behaviourally and physiologically. Any animal which wishes to feed must take a series of decisions about how to behave so as to find, ingest and digest food (Broom, 1981, p. 124). A grazing cow, for example, must first find a suitable patch of herbage on which to graze. In doing this it will need to remember where such a patch may be found and it will do best if it returns to a patch which has been allowed to regrow since it was last harvested. There is evidence from the work of Favre (1975), on sheep grazing on mountain pastures, that the flocks return to small areas of pasture at intervals which would allow effective regrowth. When a grazer is standing in utilisable pasture it does not eat all green material at random but must still take a series of decisions which will allow it to harvest the food effectively (Broom, 1981, p. 150). The grazer must assess the herbage and decide whether to lower the head and take a bite, how large a bite to take, at what rate to bite, whether to stop biting and chew or otherwise manipulate the grass in the mouth, whether to swing the head to one side, whether to take one or more steps forwards, and whether to raise the head and carry out some other behaviour. Then it must decide when to start grazing again.

Diurnal patterns of eating are characteristic of grazing behaviour in horses, cattle and sheep (Fig. 9.1). Distribution patterns of grazing periods are correlated with hours of darkness and light. The actual duration of active eating is influenced by food quality and availability. Grazing activity is largely confined to the daytime and the onset of active grazing is closely correlated with the time of sunrise. Most of the daylight hours are occupied with grazing periods. These periods usually add up to more than half of total daylight time, but some night grazing is also practised. The most active grazing season coincides with spring in most regions. The ratio of day to night grazing is affected by

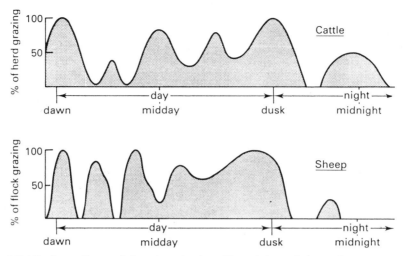

Fig. 9.1 Typical distribution patterns of diurnal grazing in cattle and sheep during spring, summer and autumn. The daily dips in activity are more noticeable in summer and disappear in winter.

very hot weather in summer when more night grazing occurs. Cold and wet spells of weather in winter can reduce grazing, but they do not have a very significant effect upon the ratio of day to night grazing. In winter, horses spend most of their time grazing while less time is spent grazing during very warm weather. Summer grazing behaviour in both cattle and horses is adversely affected by heat and fly attacks. Both of these circumstances demand a behavioural switch to body care activities which preclude grazing.

On arid ranges sheep and horses have been observed to travel long distances each day to water. It is likely that usable range is determined by the furthest distance from available water that livestock are able to travel on a daily basis. Grazing animals can ingest snow as an alternative to water if the latter is difficult to reach, or is frozen, in winter (Fig. 9.2). Range grazing animals, in the presence of snow, can afford to forage outside the usual watered territory. Cattle drink twice daily, on average, in warm weather, but once-daily drinking is more common in winter.

Grazing involves travel in addition to time. The nature of the grazing territory, and its quality, influence grazing travel. Horses may travel 3–10 km (2–6 miles) per day and spend about 2–3 h in grazing travel. Cattle move from 2–8 km (1–5 miles) daily in grazing travel distance and spend about 2 h in grazing travel time. Sheep on range travel about 6 km (4 miles) per day and spend 2 h on this travel. On good pasture land, sheep may only travel about 1 km per day. Range livestock also travel considerable distances regularly to salt lick locations which should, therefore, be strategically and adequately sited.

The grazing activities of milking cows are synchronised and arranged around the milking times. Very active grazing usually follows each milking session. Active grazing bouts are usually followed by rumination in sternal recumbency. Synchronised grazing occurs in response to environmental cues such as dawn, dusk and rain. It may also be a consequence of management methods and is influenced by social factors.

The investigation of grazing behaviour is greatly facilitated by the use of automatic recording methods. The rate at which grazers bite at the herbage and the duration of grazing

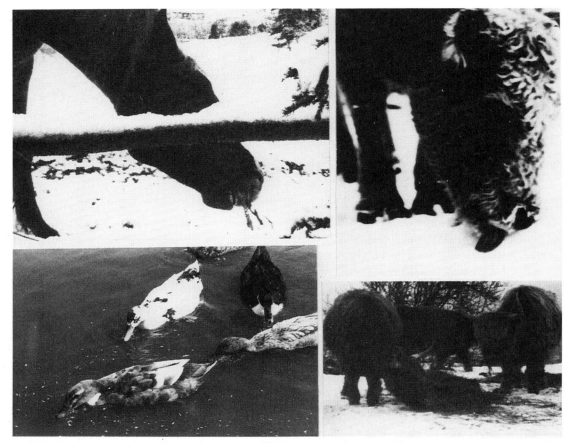

Fig. 9.2   Feeding adaptations. Top: eating stems and licking snow — horse and Hereford bull. Bottom: surface feeding of supplemental feed — ducks and Highland cattle.

and ruminating can be determined using a recorder like that developed by Penning. The stretching of an elastic tube placed around the jaw of the animal can be monitored and records like that in Fig. 9.3 produced. Biting, rumination and swallowing are distinguishable and can be recorded on a recorder carried by the animal or telemetrically (Penning *et al.*, 1984).

Finding food

Sheep, goats or cattle on sparse pasture often

have to use much energy searching for plant material which is worth harvesting. They may have to travel long distances and remember where suitable patches of pasture are to be found. Since less suitable plants may be more readily available, foraging in such conditions may involve selection and is considered under that heading. On some occasions, however, suitable food is present but at very low density. Sheep in Australia may have so little green material available that it is worthwhile for them to dig in the ground for the shoots and seeds of subterranean clover *Trifolium subterraneum*.

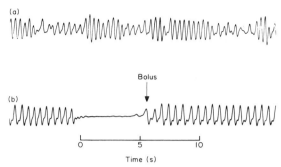

Fig. 9.3 Traces produced by the jaw movements of a sheep with a thin elastic tube, containing carbon fibre, around its jaws. The stretching or contracting of the tube changes electrical resistance and this is converted to up and down pen movements. Trace (a) shows jaw movements during grazing, which can be distinguished readily from (b), the characteristic trace during ruminating and swallowing (after Penning *et al.*, 1984).

Grazers may also turn to browsing on plants which are normally avoided.

When a calf is born and left with its mother it is important for its disease resistance that it obtains the colostrum, or first milk, from the mother. Dairy cows which have had several calves have large, pendulous udders and fat teats and this causes difficulty for the young calf when it makes searching movements which would result in teat finding if the teats were higher and smaller (Selman *et al.*, 1970; Edwards and Broom, 1979). In a study of 161 calvings, 80% of heifers' calves were successful in finding a teat and ingesting colostrum within 6 h but 50% of calves of cows three or more years old failed to find a teat in this time (Edwards, 1982). Hence it is important for cowmen to put the calves of older dairy cows on to a teat, preferably within 3 h of birth, as colostrum production and the ability of calves to absorb immunoglobulins from colostrum both decline rapidly after birth (Broom, 1983a).

There is seldom any teat-finding problem for calves of beef cows or for other farm animals. Lambs may, however, be deserted by their mothers and hence fail to obtain colostrum or milk. This problem is worse if twin lambs are born and is much greater in some breeds, such as Merinos, than in other breeds. Piglets are usually able to find the udder unless they are very weak at birth but there may not be enough functional teats if the litter is very large. Due to the very brief milk ejection period and the competition between piglets for teats, piglets which are weak at birth, overlain by the sow, or which become separated from the sow may fail to suckle. The problem of finding the food source may be even greater for young animals fed artificially. A young calf, lamb or kid will often not drink milk from a bucket unless actively trained to do so. Calves fed from artificial teats sometimes do not suck from these. In a study of dairy calves reared in groups from 24 h of age, an artificial teat was put in the mouth of each calf but some calves were not readily stimulated to go to the teat and drink. Such problems are discussed further in the section on social facilitation.

Ability to obtain food

It is easy for a chicken to obtain a food grain, once it has found it, but the harvesting of pasture plants is more difficult because of the structure of the plants. Vincent (1982, 1983) has shown that grass leaves cannot be broken by the propagation of a crack across the leaf, following local damage, but require a considerable amount of force as many fibres have to be broken. As a consequence of the relatively large amount of energy and time which is needed each time the grass, or other pasture plant, must be broken, short pasture is less worthwhile energetically to the grazer, than longer pasture. Even if the animal is offered cut fodder, larger particles may be more profitable energetically than smaller particles, of the same digestibility, for cattle prefer unchopped silage to chopped silage (Duckworth and Shirlaw, 1958). Presumably the larger amount of material per mouthful which can be obtained is the reason for this. The ease of harvesting food is clearly a factor which the ruminant takes into account when deciding how and what to eat.

The mechanical difficulties associated with breaking growing plant material, the movements involved in gathering the food and the manipulations necessary before swallowing, set limits on the rates at which animals can eat. Such rates are of importance where animals are required to eat quickly, for example a cow in a milking parlour. A cow requires 2–4 min to eat 1 kg of grain or manufactured concentrates. Hence high-producing cows which are fed most or all concentrates during the milking period may have difficulty in consuming their ration before they are required to leave.

The efficiency of feeding by animals is altered by experience. In studies of developing domestic chicks Cruze (1935) showed that accuracy of pecking at food grains improved as the chicks matured but the practice had a considerable effect on pecking accuracy (Fig. 9.4). The efficiency of grazing in young sheep also improves with experience. Arnold and Maller (1977) reared sheep without grazing experience for three years and then found that their intakes were considerably lower than those of experienced grazers on the same pastures (Fig. 3.6). Farm animals usually learn very fast when food is provided in a new place or when a new procedure for obtaining food is required of them. Modern methods for individual feeding are examples of such situations. There are systems where cows, calves or pigs wear a transponder around their necks which is recognised electronically and causes a door to open or food to be provided. The Callan–Broadbent gate system for dairy cows involves individual mangers being accessible through a movable, hinged gate which opens and allows the cow to lower its head into the manger only if the transponder on the cow's neck is recognised. Hence cows have to learn which gate is theirs and most do this very quickly. Systems where rations are provided on a daily basis at a single feeder when a cow, calf or pig approaches and its transponder is recognised, are also readily learned. Farm animals are also remarkably adept at learning how to gain food when the stockman does not intend that they should do so!

Meal size and food selection

Many studies of animal feeding show that animals can recognise the energetic value of foods and can take account of the energetic cost of obtaining food when organising their feeding behaviour. Animals so often select food of high energy value and utilise optimal foraging techniques, which are energetically efficient, that it is clear that they have an appetite for energy. This does not mean that energy intake is always paramount in determining how feeding will occur, however. Nutrient quality, other functional systems including water balance, predator avoidance and social factors also influence feeding.

The amount of food eaten over a period of several days by a full grown individual with free access to food, is generally just sufficient to maintain body weight. The energy value of the intake, which we would measure in joules, is that

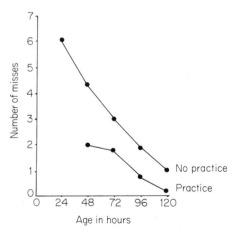

Fig. 9.4 The number of pecks which missed the grain declined with maturation of young chicks given no pecking practice, but at each age chicks given 12 h practice were more accurate (data from Cruze, 1935).

which keeps the body fat stores at a set point (Baile and Forbes, 1974, p. 264). If a pig, for example, is given food diluted with low energy material, it eats more so that the energy intake remains constant (Owen and Ridgman, 1967; Miller *et al.*, 1974). The energy intake is reduced, however, after a period of forced feeding when intakes are higher than normal. The establishment of the set point occurs during rearing so animals which are starved early in life may remain thin when adult, even if abundant food is present, and young animals which are overfed may become obese adults. One consequence of the operation of the system which controls intake is that changing nutritional demands, such as those due to pregnancy or lactation, can be allowed for if adequate food is available, as can extra energy requirements due to adverse climatic conditions. A period of deprivation may not be compensated for, however. When chickens are deprived of food for 24 or 48 h, for example, their rate of pecking is the same and their intake during the period soon after deprivation is the same (Wood-Gush, 1983). For a discussion of the control of feeding in relation to energetics (see Baile and Forbes, 1974).

Farm animals require a variety of nutrients and they can obtain different nutrients from different sorts of food. As mentioned above, there is much evidence of animals choosing food which gives the best net energy return and the energetic content of food usually corresponds well with the animal's requirements if food is available ad libitum. A constant question, relevant to ingestive behaviour, is whether homeostatic mechanisms exist to stimulate consumption of specific and essential nutrients, in proportion to their need by the body. The answer appears to be in two parts. Firstly, regulatory systems exist for water and sodium, creating thirst and salt appetites (Fitzsimmons, 1979). There is also evidence for a specific calcium appetite in birds. Secondly, nutritional deficiencies in general do not have specific homeostatic methods of self-correction. Centres mediating thirst are located in the hypothalamus (Anderson, 1971; Almli and Weiss, 1974). Pigs,

sheep and cattle which are made sodium deficient will consume appropriate amounts of solutions containing sodium ions (Denton, 1967; Lustgarten *et al.*, 1973) and can be trained to show an operant response for a sodium reward (Abraham *et al.*, 1973; Sly and Bell, 1979). An ability to recognise a body calcium deficit is present in domestic fowl, for calcium-deprived hens will choose a calcium-enriched diet even if that same diet without the calcium would be rejected as unpalatable (Hughes and Wood-Gush, 1971).

Salt deficiency results in freely available salt licks for animals being put to full use. They provide one way of supplying trace elements which might not be ingested, even if made equally freely available in another mixture. Sometimes a salt appetite in farm animals can be very acute and can lead groups into long searches for salt. In pigs, for example, voluntary salt ingestion can be excessive enough to create salt poisoning. Grazing animals with access to the seashore can be seen foraging on the shore below the high tide line, where they will frequently ingest seaweeds and will lick and chew other salted material.

There are no regulatory ingestive systems for specific deficiencies of minerals or essential organic substances but animals can learn that certain foods reduce illness. Garcia *et al.* (1967) found that thiamine-deficient rats learn to eat more of thiamine-rich foods. Animals can compensate for deficiencies and provide for special needs, e.g. during pregnancy, by trying a variety of foods not normally eaten and continuing to eat foods which have beneficial effects. The absence of most nutrients in the diet of farm animals is not recognised directly and the animals must use trial and error learning to attempt to compensate for dietary deficiencies. The consequence of this is that the food selected by farm animals may fulfil nutrient requirements but, especially when the food is manufactured, the wrong amounts of various nutrients may be taken. Tribe (1950) found that sheep offered linseed cake meal consumed twice as much protein as necessary but if the protein was in the form of fish meal they took less than the necessary amount. Growing pigs offered a protein-free or adequate protein diet by Devilat *et al.* (1970) ingested the amount of protein which resulted in a maximal weight gain, but pigs offered different protein-containing and non-protein diets by Robinson (1975) chose the non-protein diet. Similar results have been obtained during studies using other nutrients.

Mineral deficiencies can lead to "depraved appetites" in farm animals. Depraved appetite, or pica, is a notable feature of phosphorus deficiency in cattle. It involves the chewing of wood, bones, soil, etc. At first glance it would appear to be a homeostatic ingestive behaviour, but this is misleading. Even when given free access to bonemeal, deficient animals still do not change the pica to selective ingestion of the appropriate foodstuff. When phosphorus-deficient cattle can eat such bonemeal they seldom eat enough to correct completely a deficiency great enough to have caused the pica. Horses have been found incapable of correcting mineral deficiency when given free access to a digestible mixture rich in the necessary mineral.

In obtaining food, animals not only have to obtain sufficient energy and nutrients but they have to contend with the defences of the food animals and plants. Natural selection has acted on both plants and animals so as to minimise the chances that they will be eaten. Physical defences include weapons and mechanical defence. The weapons of a group of buffalo menaced by a lion are obvious but the thorns of an acacia or bramble and the irritant chemicals of a nettle or poison ivy are just as effective. Some animals have tough hides or bony plates to protect them and plants can also have tough outer layers. Grasses and other pasture plants have developed rows of parallel fibres within their tissue which makes the leaf and stem very difficult to break (Vincent, 1982). Plants often have chemical defences (Arnold and Hill, 1972; Harborne, 1982) and may change their growth form so as to make grazing on them more difficult (Broom and Arnold, 1986). Animals deal with poisons by recognising that a poison has been ingested and getting rid of it from the gut, developing enzyme detoxification mechanisms or by learning to avoid consuming an amount which poisons them (Freeland and Janzen, 1974). It is important to the majority of animal species to be able to deal with poisons. The desirable behavioural characteristics are: (1) consume only small quantities of new food; (2) have a good memory for different food characteristics; (3) be able to seek out special foods; (4) sample foods whilst eating staple foods; (5) prefer familiar foods; (6) prefer foods with small amounts of toxic compounds; (7) have a searching strategy which compromises between maximising variety and maximising intake.

Food preferences can also serve a useful function in that they allow animals to avoid foods with toxins in them. Foods may be avoided when first encountered because of their taste or other characteristics. It is also possible, however, that farm animals could learn that certain foods lead to later illness. Laboratory experiments on rats show that foods containing poisons which took up to 12 h to cause effects were subsequently avoided by rats (Garcia *et al.*, 1966; Rozin, 1968, 1976). Studies on cattle, sheep, goats and horses by Zahorik and Houpt (1981) demonstrated that novel food whose consumption was followed by sickness and discomfort within 15 min was avoided subsequently, but if the delay before the discomfort was 30 min the animals did not seem to associate that discomfort with the novel food and that food was not avoided subsequently. When animals are grazing they do very often show clear rejection of plants with toxins in them and in many cases this must be a consequence of learning from the effects, perhaps immediate, of eating the plants. Chemicals whose presence led to rejection include tannins, coumarins, isoflavones and alkaloids (Arnold and Dudzinski, 1978, p. 106). Grazers also avoid pasture contaminated by their own dung, a behaviour which reduces the likelihood of parasite or disease transmission. Since dung, especially slurry from cow sheds, is important as a fertiliser for pasture, this avoidance behaviour is important.

Cattle offered clean pasture or pastures treated seven weeks earlier with slurry preferred to eat the clean pasture (Broom *et al.*, 1975). If the only pasture available was slurry treated the cows ate only the tops of the grass. They stopped grazing and walked more often than on clean pasture and they were involved in more competitive encounters (Pain *et al.*, 1974; Pain and Broom, 1978).

Given the opportunity, all grazers are selective in their diet (Watkin and Clements, 1978), but this selection depends upon net energy return from each plant species as well as on any toxic substances which might be present. Preferences for particular plants over others occur both when food is plentiful and when herbage availability is low, for example in sheep grazing annual pastures in Western Australia (Broom and Arnold, 1986). The senses used in selection of plants from pasture are sight, touch on the lips, taste and smell (Arnold and Dudzinski, 1978, p. 102) but sight seems to be the least important sense, in this respect, for Merino sheep. Taste and smell are of great importance when housed animals are choosing amongst food items. Many diets include several different components and animals will take some of these preferentially and hence will not consume the supposedly balanced diet which is provided for them. Many experiments have been carried out on the preferences of farm animals for substances which can be added to manufactured foods. For example pigs show a clear preference for sweet substances (Kennedy and Baldwin, 1972) as do goats (Bell, 1959), but cattle reject 20% sucrose and sheep reject sucrose stronger than 5% (Goatcher and Church, 1970). For a review of such studies on various domestic animals, see Houpt and Wolski (1982, p. 263).

If young pigs obtain a flavour from their mother's milk they will accept food with that flavour more readily when they are older (Campbell, 1976). Similarly, Chinese farmers have found that piglets fed water hyacinth shortly before weaning will eat more of it later (Kilgour 1978). Early experience can have a considerable effect on food preferences. Arnold and

Maller (1977) found that sheep reared on rangeland areas of Australia had different preferences from those reared on sown pastures. Similar factors can result in animals refusing to accept foods which would be beneficial to them. Lynch (1980) found that up to 82% of cattle totally rejected food supplements. Arnold and Maller (1974) showed that the reluctance of sheep to eat grain early in life was reduced if they were fed it when they were lambs. Keogh and Lynch (1982) found that a similar improvement in adult grain consumption could be obtained if lambs observed their mothers eating grain, even if they themselves did not eat it.

The effects of disturbance

The times of starting and stopping feeding and the rate of feeding will depend principally on the feeding control system in ideal conditions, but feeding behaviour can be considerably affected by climatic conditions, predators, insects and competitors. The effects of competitors are considered in a later section. Animals may refrain from eating during the hottest part of the day because they must seek shade at this time (Bennett *et al.*, 1985; Johnson, 1987) or may cease eating during heavy rain or high wind because the normal feeding movements are difficult in these conditions. If an animal detects the presence of a predator it will stop feeding and all domestic animals maintain some vigilance for potential predators. A chicken or a sheep which spends much of its time looking out for possible predator attack may be unable to consume an adequate amount of food and may feed in a different way when it does feed. Man is often treated as a predator by farm animals and disturbance by people may have considerable effects on feeding. Animals may not feed normally when they have to come close to people to obtain food and precise records of normal feeding behaviour are often not obtained by experimenters for this reason.

Insect attack may have very large effects on feeding behaviour. Cattle attacked by warble flies *Hypoderma* and sheep attacked by the sheep-bot fly *Oestrus* may show panic reactions which certainly affect feeding behaviour (Edwards *et al.*, 1939). Biting flies may also have considerable effects on where and when animals feed as well as on the number of interruptions during feeding. The stable fly *Stomoxys calcitrans* and other flies which bite or cause annoyance to cattle can impair growth rates or milk production (Bruce and Decker, 1958; Cheng, 1958). This may be due to decreased intake or increased energy demands caused by fly attack. These flies and others such as the headfly *Hydrotaea irritans* which transmit disease, attack specific parts of the body of the animal (Hillerton *et al.*, 1983, 1984). Their attacks can be reduced considerably by the use of insecticidal ear tags (Hillerton *et al.*, 1985).

Social facilitation

The main food-producing farm animals are species which live in social groups. If cattle, sheep or pigs are taken from their group and housed individually they eat less (Kidwell *et al.*, 1954; Cole *et al.*, 1976; Webster *et al.*, 1972; Foot and Russell, 1978). This could be a response to lack of companions in general or to lack of companions at feeding time. Even when food is continually available, farm animals usually synchronise their feeding. Hughes (1971) found that chickens in cages synchronised their feeding much more often than would be expected by chance. Sheep tend to graze at the same time and cattle usually do so but horses graze at different times (Arnold and Dudzinski, 1978) (Fig. 9.5). As a consequence of such effects, the duration of grazing is much more constant when animals graze in a herd than when they graze individually for both sheep (Arnold and Dudzinski, 1978, p. 19) and cattle (Hodgson and Wilkinson, 1967). Pigs also prefer to eat when other pigs do (Hsia and Wood-Gush, 1982) and piglets synchronise suckling (Stone *et al.*, 1974). Kilgour (1978) showed that weaned

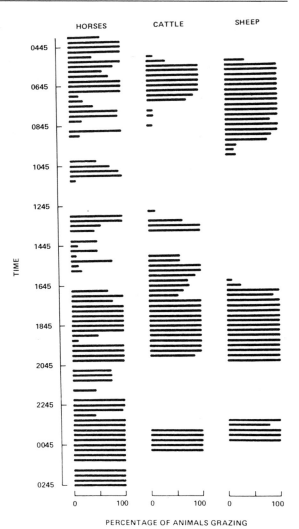

Fig. 9.5   The percentage of horses, Merino sheep and cattle grazing is shown at 15 min intervals during a day. Sheep graze together for concentrated periods but horses graze individually and for more of the day (after Arnold and Dudzinski, 1978).

piglets went to the feeder when they heard younger piglets suckling.

The rate of feeding is also affected by the presence of one or more companions. Chicks pecked more frequently and ingested more when a companion was present (Tolman and Wilson, 1965) and an apparently satiated hen took more food if a hungry hen was introduced to its cage (Katz and Revesz, 1921). A similar effect among calves has been demonstrated by Barton and Broom (1985). A calf fed on a milk replacer was given a feed alone early in the morning but its companion calf was not fed. If the companion was then reintroduced to the adjacent pen and given milk which it drank, the first calf which could see the second drinking, consumed more milk replacer. In a subsequent experiment the first calf was again fed alone, then the second calf was introduced to the same pen but was muzzled. When milk replacer was made available, the muzzled calf tried to drink and stimulated the first calf to take even more milk. The results are shown in Table 9.1. These results, together with observations of calves feeding when housed in groups of ten, showed that food intake by young calves can be increased when others can be seen and heard feeding. Hence, since competition is relatively unimportant in these calves (Barton, 1983a, b), the chances that any calf will receive too little milk replacer are reduced if several teats (about one per 2 calves) are provided close together (Barton and Broom, 1985).

Table 9.1
Social facilitation of milk feeding by calves

	Mean milk intake (litres)	Mean sucking rate (litres per min)	Mean sucking duration (seconds per day)
Calf alone	5.5	0.68	487
Calf with hungry calf in next pen	7.5	0.62	724
Calf with muzzled calf in same pen	9.2	0.64	864

Data from Barton and Broom (1985).

Competition and feeding behaviour

Individuals competing for food may be successful because of their fighting ability, or because of threats which provide some information about their fighting ability. This is not the only ability which might lead to success, however, for as Syme (1974) points out, competition for a food item is often resolved by the faster mover acquiring it. The hen which runs and pecks fastest is most likely to obtain a grain thrown to a group of hens. If a limited amount of food is available, the faster eater often gets more than slower eaters. This applies especially to pigs or cattle feeding from a trough. For many generations, trough feeding of a limited quantity of food has resulted in selection for animals which can ingest food at a high rate. Even at pasture, animals graze at faster rates when they know that the herbage available is limited. Benham (1982a) found that a herd of cows moved to a new strip of pasture every day showed most grazing immediately after introduction to the new strip. The biting rates and the incidence of aggression were highest at this time.

The effects of competition on food intake have been apparent from many farm animal studies. Wagnon (1965) found that heifers kept with older cows lost weight whilst those fed separately gained weight. The heifers were unable to feed adequately because the space available at the feed bunk or trough was inadequate for all of the animals and the older cows actively prevented the heifers from feeding on many occasions. In such competitive situations some breeds, e.g. Herefords, may be prevented from having access to food for as much time as other breeds, e.g. Aberdeen Angus (Wagnon et al., 1966). Observation of fights and other competitive encounters often makes it clear that individuals recognise one another and consistently defer to some and take precedence over others. The competitive order which can be described need not be linear and need not be the same in all situations or when assessed using different measures (Broom, 1981, p. 252), but the behaviour of animals at the top and bottom of the order are often very different when the animals are feeding. The frequency of disturbance whilst feeding and the consequent duration of feeding, are apparent when the paths of cows high and low in the competitive order are compared (Albright, 1969) (Fig. 37.3). Calves which did badly in competition were found to obtain less concentrate food and to gain weight less well when the trough length was insufficient for all animals to feed at once (Broom, 1982).

Competitive orders have been found to be positively correlated with food intake, growth rate, egg production or milk production in some studies but not in others (Syme and Syme, 1979). One reason for this is variation in the way that the food is provided. All situations where animals in a group are unable to feed at one time should be avoided whenever possible. Since most farm animals synchronise their feeding behaviour, any feeding situation which results in some individuals trying to feed but being excluded from the food source is a bad one. Feeding troughs should also be designed so as to minimise any fighting or threats at the time of communal feeding. Bouissou (1970) found that cattle would feed from a trough alongside other animals much higher in the competitive order if a barrier which extended over the trough was present, but they would not do so if there was no barrier or an inadequate barrier (Fig. 37.2). Where clearly demarcated feeding places with a place for each animal to put its head are provided, there should be enough of these places for each animal in the group. More space per animal is required if no barriers of any kind are provided.

Feeding by cattle

Cattle have to rely for food intake on the high mobility of the tongue, which is used to encircle a patch of grass and then to draw it into the mouth, where the lower teeth and the tongue are used to hold the bound grass while it is broken by a head movement. The nature of a cow's eating process is such that it is virtually impossible for the animal to graze less than one centimetre from the ground. After taking a series of bites, the cow manipulates the plant material, chewing only two or three times before swallowing. The head is swung and steps are taken so that the next bites can be taken from a new area. The bite size, rate of biting, number of head swings, and rate of stepping are affected by the pasture height. Some data from a study carried out on a rotationally grazed pasture at Shinfield, Reading, UK are shown in Table 9.2. When similar measurements were made by Broom and Penning at Hurley, Berkshire, UK on cows on two set-stocked pasture with two average pasture heights, bite rates were not proportional to average pasture height. The cows avoided longer, coarser grass and grazed at a constant rate on shorter grass with a higher proportion of leaf on both pastures. Chacon and Stobbs (1976) found that as *Setaria* pasture in Australia was eaten down, bite size declined markedly and bite rate increased to a maximum. This and other work by Stobbs (1973, 1974) emphasised that cows show clear selection for leaf. On day 1 of the study, 32% of the herbage dry matter available was leaf, the rest being stem and dead material, but 98% of the intake was leaf. The intake was assessed using fistula samples. By day 13, only 5% of available herbage was leaf but 50% of intake was still leaf.

Table 9.2
Grazing by Friesian cows on ryegrass pasture of two different heights

	Short grass	Long grass	
Mean length of longest shoot (cm)	13	30	$p < 0.01$
Time grazing in 24 h (h)	7.9	6.9	$p < 0.01$
Time walking in 24 h (min)	56	30	$p < 0.01$
Mean bite rate (bites/min)	51	47	$p < 0.02$
Mean chews per 100 bites	30	38	$p < 0.01$
Distance walked, head down (m/min)	2.5	1.9	$p < 0.01$

Data in part from Broom (1981).

When cattle on free range have grazed down an area they will move to another area. Decisions about whether or not to move will depend upon the average return from that area as compared with what the animals know to be the average return from the habitat as a whole. Cattle in fields also use their previous experience in deciding how much energy to invest in attempting to graze after pasture has been grazed down. If they know that they will be moved to a new paddock or strip each day they graze very fast at the beginning of the day, thus competing with one another for the available herbage, and do not graze much in the latter part of the period on the day's strip. When animals are moved on after a few days when the pasture has been grazed down they learn how to train farmers to move them at the appropriate time. The cue which they train the farmer to use is the sight and sound of a row of cows standing by the fence and bellowing.

For cattle, as for other ruminant grazers, the amount of energy obtained from the food is often limited by food-processing time. The maximum rate of processing is limited by the cross-sectional area of the gut. A consequence of this is that it is important for the grazer not to waste digestion time on poor quality food if good quality food is available (Westoby, 1974). This is the reason behind the active selection of leaf over stem. It is also a reason for choosing to eat some pasture plant species rather than others (Ruckesbusch and Bueno, 1978). Selectivity results in certain plants being eaten down in the pasture while others are left untouched. In addition to those of poor nutritional quality, plants may be avoided because they are hairy, or spiny, or poisonous. Cattle in loose-housing spend about 5 h per day eating. Their rumination time is also reduced. Although cattle in feedlots are in a very unnatural environment they still show diurnal rhythms similar to those evident in natural grazing, but their total eating time is much reduced. In place of natural grazing bouts, feedlot cattle have about 10–14 feeding periods, with approximately 75% of these occurring during daylight hours. If hay or silage is fed,

5 h per day may be spent on active eating, as in the loose-housing system. Eating time becomes reduced as roughage is reduced and the proportion of concentrate feed is increased.

Eating space is important in determining the number of cattle which may eat at one time, and this establishes the maximum amount of time a pen of animals may eat over a 24-h period. When eating space is restricted, feed intake of the group shows a compensatory increase in rate of consumption. Groups of feedlot beef cattle were fed experimentally in single stalls, with only one eating space provided for each pen of animals. The eating behaviour of the stall-fed groups was compared with that of trough-fed groups. The stall-fed cattle ate faster and differed in their diurnal eating pattern when compared with the cattle fed from troughs. The diurnal pattern of cattle waiting to eat from the single stalls did not differ from the diurnal eating pattern of trough-fed cattle. The ability of cattle to eat successfully from a single feeding space was related to the protection offered by the stall. Dominant cattle did not prevent subordinates from gaining access to the stall. Low ranking cattle replaced higher ranking cattle as frequently as they themselves were replaced by higher ranking cattle (Stricklin and Gonyou, 1981; Gonyou and Stricklin, 1981).

Cattle feeding indoors also modify their feeding behaviour according to the food supplied and show clear preferences. The time taken to consume food varies according to its volume, the concentrates which may be in it, whether it is wet or dry and the way it has been processed before being given to the animals. Alfalfa requires more chewing before ingestion than ground corn which, in its turn, requires more chewing than shelled corn. Given a choice between silage and hay, milking cows will spend more time at the silage, often two-thirds of the total eating time, while spending the remaining one-third at hay. In a study of food choice, it was found that green fodders and roots were preferred to protein while cereal chaff was preferred to straw.

Many studies of cattle in field situations show

that they graze mostly during the hours of daylight and cover, on average, about 4 km per day. The distance travelled increases if the weather is hot or wet or if there is an abundance of flies around. During the season of hot weather, more grazing may be done at night than during the day. In each 24-h period there are four main periods of high ingestive intake:

1. shortly prior to sunrise;
2. mid-morning;
3. early afternoon; and
4. near dusk.

Of these distinct periods, the hours prior to sunrise and around dusk appear to be the periods of longest and most continuous grazing. During other times of the day, cattle graze intermittently and idle, rest or ruminate. Selectivity of pasture and food plants increase, prior to the periods of high intake, becoming very marked during a high intake phase. After such a phase, grazing becomes intermittent again and the level of selectivity decreases.

The time cattle spend grazing during the 24 h period is 4–14 h. The periods of rumination may also total 4–9 h and the number of ruminating periods may be 15–20. The number of drinks taken per day is between one and four and the hours spent lying down are usually in the 9–12 h range. These figures may vary in different respects between beef cattle and dairy cattle and in tropical and in free-ranging herds, but behaviour in domestic cattle is usually fairly stable and the figures given are general norms (Stricklin *et al.*, 1976).

Grazing behaviour has been studied in the Chillingham herd of wild cattle in Northumberland, UK, which for centuries has been free from interference except during part of the winter when hay is given (Hall, 1983). The general pattern of grazing during summer has major grazing periods around dawn and dusk, and during mid-morning and early afternoon. During winter, little night-time grazing takes place.

Grazing bouts, defined as periods of uninterrupted grazing, can be up to 3 h in length. Grazing-bout length is significantly longer for females than for males in summer, but this difference is not evident in winter. Grazing-bout length is significantly correlated with time since the last grazing bout, and with time to the next. Daytime observations show that the amount of grazing during each hour is not correlated with time since sunrise, but is significantly greater for females than for males.

The males, which are not castrated, spend less time grazing (at least during the day), and show shorter grazing bouts (during summer) than do females. Males apparently make use of the time thus made available for elaborate social interactions.

Rumination

Following ingestion comes rumination, which allows cattle to regurgitate, masticate and then swallow food which they have previously ingested into the rumen. Thus animals can continue their digestive activities at leisure, when away from a preferred grazing area or sheltering during bad weather. Usually cattle prefer to lie down during rumination although in bad weather, e.g. heavy rain, they may prefer to stand or walk about slowly. Rumination does occur in young calves, but only takes up a proportion of daily time comparable to that in adults at about 6–8 months of age. During the 24-h cycle, rumination takes place about 15 to 20 times but the duration of each period may differ vastly; it may last only a few minutes or it may continue up to one hour or even more at one stretch. The peak period for rumination is shortly after nightfall; thereafter, it declines steadily until shortly before dawn when grazing begins. Times may differ, however, according to diet; cattle are able to regurgitate, remasticate and reswallow long hay more quickly than ground hay or concentrates. The relation between the time spent grazing and the time spent ruminating varies depending on the season and the abundance and quality of the herbage provided, together with the area available to the cattle and the size of the herd. The time spent ruminating amounts, on average, to three-quarters of the time spent grazing. Good quality herbage nearly always shortens the time spent ruminating, while herbage which is rough increases the number and length of ruminating periods. In the spring and autumn the time spent grazing almost totally eclipses the periods of rumination, but in the summer they are almost equal (Rickard *et al.*, 1975).

The factors which may disturb or cause the cessation of rumination are various. During oestrus ruminating nearly always falls away, but it does not stop altogether. Any incident which gives rise to pain, hunger, maternal anxiety or illness affects ruminating activities. The periods before and after parturition are not conducive to rumination and it may decline to a low level. Sometimes it is noted that the longer rumination is interrupted or delayed, the more difficult it becomes for the animal to resume this activity.

Drinking

This activity refers to the total consumption of water, including that water which is often contained in the animal feed. Cattle usually drink one to four times a day in temperate climates; they do so more often in hot weather and when there is a high proportion of concentrates in their food.

Cattle drink using their muzzles and the tongue plays little part in the process while the nostrils are kept above the surface of the water. Cattle usually drink in the forenoon, early afternoon or evening but rarely at night or at dawn. More drinking is done on old pastures than in nutritious grazing areas. Cattle given an abundance of feedstuff—a situation which may occur during housing—tend to consume more water than they would normally. In addition to hot weather and an abundance of various types of feedstuffs, milking also increases water intake. Thus after milking and especially after the evening milking, cattle drink water whenever possible.

Several other factors alter or discourage drinking activities. The water intake increases during later pregnancy and lactation, and the intake varies according to the ambient temperature, breed, age, body size, intake of pasture and the level of nutrient and salt in the food provided. European breeds of cattle drink more than tropical breeds. European cattle (*Bos taurus*) drink 30% more water per unit dry matter ingested at 28°C than Zebu cattle (*Bos indicus*) and 100% more at 38°C (Winchester and Morris, 1956). This is because Zebu cattle conserve water better. Cattle fed on foodstuffs with a high level of protein drink much more than those on a lower protein supplement. The amount of water consumed by pregnant heifers has been calculated to be 28–32 litres per day while the average daily intake of water by non-pregnant adults is about 14 litres.

Feeding by sheep

The general features of ingestive behaviour of sheep are those common to cattle. There are periods of movement and eating as well as of drinking, idling and lying down and ruminating, interspersed with periods of intensive ingestive activity. Some animals eat less than others, others spend more time lying down, but there are particular features of behaviour which typify the sheep.

Grazing activity is largely confined to the daytime, and the onset of grazing is closely correlated with sunrise. Grazing is concentrated during the whole daylight time available, but sheep do not graze continuously. They have specific phases during the 24-h cycle when ingestive intake is very high, and other phases when grazing is punctuated by ruminating, resting and idling. The ruminating behaviour of sheep varies from breed to breed. Some breeds prefer to split up into groups throughout the area, occupying particular spots.

The longest and also the most intensive periods of grazing take place in the early morning and from late afternoon to dusk. The number of grazing periods over each 24-h cycle averages four to seven and the total grazing time usually amounts to about 10 h. Although adult sheep usually eat more than lambs, the pattern of their ingestive intake is less uniform than in lambs.

The number of rumination periods may amount to 15 during the 24-h cycle. Although the total time of rumination may be from 8–10 h, the length of each period may differ vastly; from 1 min to anything up to 2 h. The adult intake of water is 3–6 litres and the number of urinations and defaecations total approximately 9–13 and 6–8, respectively. The average grazing intake of an individual sheep may differ greatly from that of the main flock and the amount ingested may also be affected by the presence of lambs. It is widely recognised that sheep prefer certain pasture plants (Arnold, 1964; Broom and Arnold, 1986). The fertility of the soil, the use or non-use of fertilisers, the geographical situation of the grazing land and the nature of the climate, all affect the grazing behaviour of the flock (Arnold, 1960, 1982).

In cases of restriction sheep nibble the grass very close to the ground and faeces are often deposited where there is good quality grazing. Sheep do not normally consume plants or grass which have been contaminated by faeces, but when circumstances dictate, the sheep do consume the good herbage in spite of such contamination.

Sheep are known to have well-developed senses of smell, taste and visual recognition of food, but their intake is almost unaffected when they are made to eat without the aid of vision. They do not often, however, eat plants which are hairy or greasy (Gibb, 1977).

It has been suggested that sheep are able to select what items of food they eat and thereby correct any nutritional deficiencies or excesses. Certainly sheep with definite nutritional deficiencies have been known to correct their nutritional balance by consuming plants and grains which will do so. Sheep generally accept food of a balanced quality rather than food of a more erratic composition. Findings in this field have not been uniform, however, and many sheep are found to persist in eating a particular crop or plant which further upsets an already unbalanced nutritional condition.

One evident aspect of the feeding activities of sheep is that they are fairly adaptable regarding the plants, grass and crops which are made available to them (Engels *et al.*, 1974). They do tend to develop particular likings for certain crops and may even prefer one type of food, which is exactly the same in content as another but prepared differently. They are able to adapt themselves to a particular species of grass or plant if there are no other nutrients to be found and, eventually, the disliked food plant apparently becomes palatable. The stage in its development and its body weight have an effect on a sheep's food intake, more so than adjustments to sensory faculties. On average, sheep consume food equivalent to 2–5% of their body weight per day.

Possibly as a result of allelomimetic behaviour, sheep often form specific paths to water sources and follow a recognised route rather than a direct one across grazing land, regardless of the time factor involved. They also generally tend to frequent a particular watering place. As with feeding, the amount of water consumed varies according to breed, quality of pasture and weather conditions, for seasonal changes greatly influence the amount of water consumed by drinking.

Rumination

Cud-chewing periods number about eight in 24 h and in this respect are not very different from the ruminating periods of cattle. Rumination in sheep, however, occurs at irregular intervals throughout the night and day and, although there may be a higher frequency of rumination early in the morning and the fairly regular rumination in mid-afternoon, these tendencies are not marked and cannot be said to be characteristic of all breeds of sheep. It has not yet been ascertained exactly what induces the onset and cessation of rumination. The consumption of chopped hay apparently invokes more frequent rumination than long hay. When sheep are fed small quantities of food at regular intervals instead of receiving one large feed, they show a marked increase in rumination and regurgitation.

Feeding by horses

Horses graze by cropping the pasture close to the roots with their incisors. Whilst grazing they cover large areas and seldom take more than two mouthfuls before moving at least one step further, avoiding grass patches covered in dung. They maintain some distance between each other when grazing in groups. The young foal does not graze very efficiently until it is several weeks old. By about the end of the first week of life, however, the foal has begun to nibble the herbage in association with its dam.

Horses do not drink very frequently in a 24-h period and many may only drink once a day. When they do drink they typically consume very large quantities of water, taking up to 15–20 swallows. The preference of horses for different plants and seeds mixtures have been studied. Horses were found to prefer grazing a clover-rich seeds-mixture pasture, with varieties of perennial ryegrass, timothy and cocksfoot to other species present (Archer, 1971, 1977). Less palatable pasture plants were red clover, brown top and red fescue. Observations on eliminative behaviour and grazing indicate that olfactory stimuli are important in directing feeding behaviour towards certain plants and away from contaminated areas of grass (Francis-Smith, 1979; Ödberg and Francis-Smith, 1976, 1977). This leads to differentiation of pastures into "lays" and "roughs" (Carson and Wood-Gush, 1983b). It has been shown that the greatest source of variability in grazing behaviour results from individual differences in animals. Different animal species select different plants or parts of plants while grazing. Most horses select the short young growth of plants, and often show a preference for the more fibrous grasses.

They also graze the higher-carbohydrate grasses in a mixed pasture.

Studies have been made on browsing in the ingestive behaviour of native Scottish ponies (Shetland and Highland) in various environments and geographical regions (Fraser and Brownlee, 1974). The ponies showed preferential selection of rough grazing including privet hedges, dead nettles, burdock and fallen leaves, in autumn and winter particularly. Ash leaves seemed to be particularly favoured. The bark of trees was often eaten; in restricted areas of grazing a number of trees could be debarked to a height of 2 m, the bark eating commencing at the lower levels of the tree trunk. The bark of some trees was apparently sought in preference to others; while poplar was a principal choice, ash, oak and rowan were also favoured. Ponies were observed to paw out thistles and eat them with their roots. Thistle and nettle eating were practised more noticeably in winter than at other seasons and were observed even in pastures where no scarcity of other herbage was notable.

Social facilitation strongly influences grazing in horses. Transmission of feeding habits from the mare is obtained by young foals. Group size and leadership may also influence grazing by dictating the timing of group activity.

Extremes of weather such as strong heat, wind or rain reduce the time that horses spend grazing. Season affects the grazing animal through seasonal changes in the weather and the state of the sward. Grazing at night is more common during the summer than the winter in ponies and the beginning and end of daily grazing periods are correlated with the times of sunrise and sunset (Pollock, 1980).

Feeding by pigs

Rooting is a salient feature of ingestive behaviour in pigs. Even when pigs are fed with finely ground foodstuffs they continue to show rooting activities. The snout of the pig is a highly developed sense organ and olfaction plays a large part in the determination of behaviour, not least in feeding activities. Pigs are omnivorous and, at free range, eat a variety of vegetable materials. They may also eat some animals such as earthworms. Under modern systems of husbandry, however, it is usual for pigs to be fed on compounded feedstuffs. Pigs consume a sufficient quantity of food of this type for 24 h, in as little as 15 min of each day. When provided with this food in feed-hoppers the time spent each day on feeding may be somewhat longer.

Self-feeding pigs randomly space their eating and drinking periods throughout the day. Of the two, eating is the preferred activity. Pigs quickly learn to drink from mechanical devices which supply water when some plate or button is pressed. Water drinking is influenced by both animal size and environmental conditions. Under normal conditions of management, full-grown pigs consume approximately 8 litres of water daily. Pregnant sows may drink in excess of 10 litres per day and lactating sows up to 30 litres.

The quantity of food that pigs consume is marginally affected by the palatability of the feedstuff. They appear to prefer feedstuffs with some sugar content. Preference is also shown for other constituents such as fishmeal, yeast, wheat and soya bean. Substances which reduce the intake of food include salt, fat, meatmeal and cellulose. As a general rule, pigs appear to eat wet foodstuffs more readily than dry ones, though much depends upon palatability. Under management conditions where pigs are hand-fed they typically show hunger when feeding time approaches and it is evident that the temporal arrangement of their feeding activities is very well defined. The speed of eating in the pig is found to increase as body weight increases.

Appetite can have a genetic basis in pigs. It has also been noted that certain families of pigs eat more than others and that pigs from these families are usually faster growing. The selection of highly productive pigs, in many cases, involves very little more than selecting those genes which promote eating.

Breeding sows must regain body weight after the end of lactation and, for this reason, they are very competitive at feeding time. The introduction of individual feeding stalls for sows has been a great help in dealing with this situation. The stalls operate best when sows are allowed access to a communal exercising area between feeds. Electronic sow feeders can also work well.

Social facilitation is an increase with synchrony in particular activities in the presence of others engaged in the same behaviour. The pig is a highly social animal and social facilitation is a common feature in its behaviour including its ingestive habits. When a group of pigs, unknown to each other, are mixed, aggression initially is the dominant behaviour but this soon becomes increasingly inhibited and, as it does so, social order results. As aggression is waning, feeding is waxing. In fact, feeding will be pushed beyond the level peculiar to any individual pig isolated from the group.

Community feeding has various effects on behaviour; feeding behaviour is evidently stimulated by the sight of other pigs feeding (Hsia and Wood-Gush, 1984). Pigs in groups are found to consume more food than pigs kept individually. Well-grown animals kept in pens in groups of six to eight should, therefore, be given enough feeding trough space to consume their own ration of food, without adjacent competitors being able to poach off them. It is estimated that pigs of approximately 90 kg live weight should have a minimum trough space of 35 cm each. There should be enough room for all pigs to feed at once. Even when the hoppers are well filled, if these are too few, the pigs will not be able to avoid competition in obtaining their full daily quota of food. Fighting among feeder-pigs in groups is significantly greater with single trough-space feeding than with long trough feeders. Competition can be minimised by giving groups of self-fed pigs access to several feeders at a time, and the incidence of behaviour such as tail-biting and ear-biting can be reduced considerably when these are provided (Hansen *et al.*, 1982). Barriers separating the heads of the pigs whilst feeding also reduce the incidence of fighting (M. R. Baxter, personal communication).

Growing pigs do not always show, in their watering behaviour, a direct response to systemic water requirements. Growing pigs have a daily water turnover of about 250 ml/kg when fed dry pellets at the rate of 4–5% of body weight daily. Water intake is unchallenged or slightly decreased when food intake is allowed to increase. Both reduction of food supply to half its usual amount, and fasting, significantly increase drinking and water turnover rate. Pigs, therefore, consume more water when food is restricted; a behaviour attributable to hunger (Yang *et al.*, 1981).

Some pig husbandry systems require food to be delivered at regular intervals at less than the ad libitum intake. Such a feeding routine can cause the water consumption of some pigs to increase by up to five to six times its normal level. It is now clear that polydipsia occurs as an aberration when pigs are kept under certain husbandry conditions. Behavioural observations and water turnover studies reveal that water for abdominal fill is often taken during the afternoon.

Feeding by poultry

In addition to pecking and swallowing, minor variations occur in the ingestive behaviour of the fowl. Free-range poultry, when they grasp a large food object in the bill, may run with it while calling. Again on free range the domestic hen typically makes two or three backward scratching movements with alternate feet before stepping back one pace to peck at the area of ground which has been disturbed. Poultry typically peck at their food with jerky head movements directed like small hammer blows. Sometimes poultry will sweep their bills in hoppers of soft feed, displacing it from side to side. In the typical food-pecking action the bird's eye are closed at the time of the strike. The pecked item such as grain is then grasped between the mandibles and, following this prehension, the head is jerked upwards and backwards as the food is swallowed.

Fowls usually eat most either at the start or at the end of the day, or both, but not in the middle of the day. Laying birds tend to eat more at the end of the day than non-layers, and non-layers more in the morning. Reproductive state appears to be the most important single factor causing variation in feeding patterns. Variation is also associated with the strain of fowl, age of bird and diet. The type of feeding pattern shown depends mainly on how much is stored in the crop at the end of the day and how hungry birds are in the morning. With non-laying birds, an increase in feeding at the end of the day depends on an ability to predict the onset of darkness, but with laying birds it can also be a direct consequence of the timing of oviposition or egg formation (Savory, 1980; Savory *et al.*, 1982).

Hens in large flocks show certain feeding characteristics. Their total feeding times and lengths of feeding bouts are greatest and the number of feeding bouts least when the feeding space is unpartitioned. Synchrony of feeding behaviour occurs in flocks when the distance between partitioned feeding space is 10 cm or greater. When feeding space is partitioned, the likelihood that the two birds would eat together at the same site increases with the distance between feeding space. Dominant birds exhibit the longest feeding bouts and greatest total feeding times but are less likely to feed in the same space as another bird. Birds high in the social hierarchy of the flock exhibit less synchrony of feeding behaviour than subordinates. The size of the flock in which the birds are raised has no clear effect on behaviour (Meunier-Salaun and Faure, 1984).

Evidently early husbandry conditions do not influence behaviour shown during feeding in later life. However, social attraction has a greater influence on the feeding behaviour of hens than is generally assumed. In view of this, in attempting to determine the requirements of laying hens for feeding space, attention must be paid to social attraction as well as to the competition at the feeders. Free access to long troughs creates optimum feeding conditions.

Poultry drink frequently each day and some

studies have shown that fowl will visit a drinking fountain in their pen 30–40 times daily. The drinking behaviour alters with growth. Marked changes occur in immersion angle, swallowing angle and distance from the waterer in growing broilers. Birds make progressively fewer trips to the waterer to take a large number of higher volume drinks as they develop (Ross and Hurnik, 1983).

The appetite of poultry has been subject to enormous study and is evidently complex. Birds do experience hunger behaviour after fasting, as shown in pecking rates, for example. Undoubtedly young chicks, in association with their hens, learn certain aspects of feeding behaviour from them. In the selection of food, visual stimulation evidently plays a part and food preferences are recognised. Certain cereal grains such as wheat are apparently preferred to others such as oats. Poultry have specific hungers and studies on the fowl indicate that this specificity is a means whereby feeding can be adjusted to special bodily needs. A need for calcium is a notable one, particularly in laying birds.

With free access to food, poultry concentrate their feeding in discrete meals, but there is evidence that hunger and satiety mechanisms have only loose control over initiation and termination of meals. Hunger and satiety are concerned with neural and humoral feedback processes which involve the brain, eyes, mouth, alimentary tract and liver.

10 Body care

Care of the body, through skin hygiene, evacuation and actions which regulate body temperature and other physical and chemical variables are important parts of the self-maintaining behavioural complex in farm animals. Indeed, the provision of appropriate environmental conditions so that animals can maintain themselves is very important for good welfare on farms (Sainsbury, 1986). Acts of body care, such as scratching, shaking and licking, are usually brief and there are several different forms of each; as a result they are not very conspicuous as a system. But these acts are important and numerous and their total occurrences, per day, constitute a significant proportion of the total activity. Another feature of this behaviour is the flexibility of its acts, allowing it to intrude into other major behaviours such as feeding and resting. Body care evidently has a comparatively high priority ranking among maintenance behaviours. Common behavioural acts subsumed under the heading "body care" include grooming or preening, defaecation and urination in a disciplined and selective way, sheltering from wind, shading from sunshine, bathing and wetting the body in heat.

Animals take care of their body surfaces in an organised, deliberate way and become involved in various activities in which areas of the body surface are treated in apparently satisfying ways. The interface between the body surface and the environment is perceived via the sense of touch. The attainment of comfort and the avoidance of discomfort depends greatly on touch perception. Animals seek and secure comfort as a matter of high priority at all times of normal function. Cattle may stand in the cool water of a pond or stream in high temperatures, turn their faces away from strong chill winds, or turn their backs into driving snow. The entire herd often adopts a similar orientation in the course of thermoregulatory tactics.

In high temperatures, pigs will bathe in water to head height and wallow in mud, giving their bodies muddy and moist surfaces suitable for heat loss and protection from the sun. Sheep will shelter under hillside ledges and alongside hedges when cooled after shearing or heated with full fleeces on hot days (Fig. 10.1). Animals in cold conditions will huddle to afford mutual shelter or to conserve the body heat of every individual engaged in the tactic. As an example of a group tactic, horses often generate herd gallops in snow, thus raising body temperature.

General

In principle, comfort is sought and discomfort is avoided. Open sunlit places are used freely and preferentially by cattle in mild temperatures (e.g. about 23°C) but shade from direct sunlight is sought in higher temperatures (e.g. over 28°C) by most European breeds of cattle. Shorn and

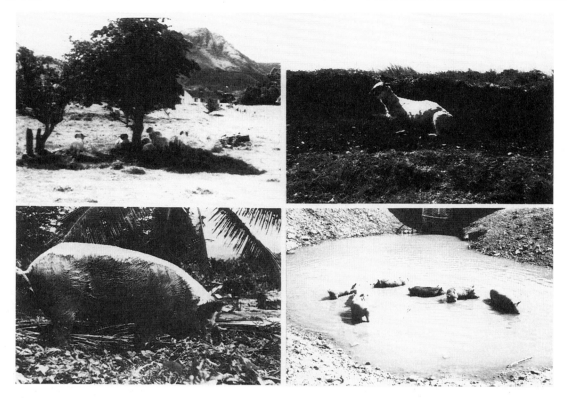

Fig. 10.1   Thermoregulatory tactics in sheep and swine in warm weather. Top left: rams sheltering from sunshine. Top right: shorn sheep sheltering from sun and wind. Bottom left: pig rooting and grazing in a tropical location with the protection of a mud coating from wallowing. Bottom right: swine bathing in a pond in summer.

unshorn sheep in early summer will seek shade from direct sunshine and shelter from wind according to fleece cover and ambient temperatures (Lynch and Alexander, 1977; Alexander *et al.*, 1979; Johnson, 1987). Sheltering and orientation from rain and snow, in cattle and horses, are particularly noticeable when the precipitation is wind-driven.

Shelter from flies is often difficult for grazing animals to achieve unless they can find an area receiving air currents, for example high ground. Cattle respond to flies which irritate or bite by agitating the head and ears, shaking folds of neck skin, other skin movements, tail switching, kicking and stamping. Hillerton *et al.* (1986)

and Harris *et al.* (1987) found that the frequency of ear flicks by cows was proportional to the numbers of the fly *Musca autumnalis* on the faces of the cows and that the numbers of kicks and stamps were proportional to the numbers of the biting fly *Stomoxys calcitrans* on the legs. If the cows had fenvalerate-impregnated ear tags, fly numbers were reduced and fly dislodging behaviour was reduced. Horses show similar behaviour when troubled by flies, often shaking manes and forelocks as an additional means of dislodging flies and creating air turbulance to deter settling. There may also be social responses to a fly problem; cattle and horses may gather closely together and with tail switching they can set up a fairly proficient fly screen for themselves. In the presence of very dense fly populations, cattle will be more likely to stand in close groups with their heads together (Schmidtmann and Valla, 1982). Occasionally they lie with their underparts—belly, brisket, neck and throat—on the ground. This ''grounding'' action seals off many sensitive skin areas from exposure to fly irritation. Such behavioural defences against flies may be very important since flies may carry disease. For example, the fly *Hydrotaea irritans* carries the pathogens which cause summer mastitis in cattle (Hillerton *et al.*, 1983).

Generalised comfort-seeking is directed towards extensive skin areas of the common integument as distinct from localised skin areas which receive attention in grooming. Animals often show clear preference for the tactile nature of the substrate on which they will more readily stand or lie, if given the opportunity of choice. Pigs prefer most to lie on straw as compared with other substrata, especially at night (van Rooijen, 1980). Horses prefer to stand on turf and further prefer to do so on a slope with the forefeet on a slightly lower level than the hind feet. The storage organs of rectum and bladder are normally emptied when they become distended and postures of defaecation and micturition or urination are adopted in ways which limit soiling of the hind limbs and tail.

Grazing or penned animals avoid soiling the sites which they have chosen for eating and sleeping by evacuating their urine and faeces at other selected locations. The ruminating species seem to have a comparatively low priority for orderly excretion but horses and pigs show very clear forms of eliminative behaviour which minimise the soiling of chosen eating and grazing sites (Ödberg and Francis-Smith, 1977; Petherick, 1983a). They avoid lying down where they have eliminated, when afforded space to do so. Horses often urinate at the edge of restricted grazing areas and will return regularly to defecate at a specific site chosen for this until, in some cases, large faecal piles are formed. The controlled eliminative behaviour of the pig is

remarkable and is evidently well organised in very young pigs, even under conditions of very restrictive penning in that they have clearly demarcated dunging areas. These are normally located in the coolest, dampest part of their pen.

The behaviour of grooming has certain characteristics common to most species. Scratching about the head parts with a hind foot is one; licking certain accessible parts is another. There are few body areas which are not scratched or groomed in this way by cattle, horses and pigs. Other grooming activities are peculiar to the species. Horned cattle frequently rub their horns and horn bases against accessible solid structures. Rolling in horses is one form of skin attention not seen in other farm animals, although dust-bathing in poultry is analogous. Chickens will dust-bathe if sand or other suitable material is available but will dust-bathe in dry food if there is no alternative. When prevented from dust-bathing they will show the behaviour with a lower latency and a higher frequency than if they have not previously been thus prevented (Vestergaard, 1980).

The eye, face, nose and nostrils of ungulate animals receive hygienic attention by the animal rubbing its face up and down the side of the appropriate foreleg, which may be held out in front of the other to be more accessible. In nasal cleaning, horses do not use their tongues to clean out their nostrils as do cattle, but they snort to do so. Nasal secretions in livestock can be considerable. In severely cold weather these secretions can freeze and become obvious on the muzzle. Abnormal nasal discharge in all livestock may accumulate in some illnesses. This is partly due to their excessive production and partly due to the fact that body care behaviour is suppressed in most illnesses so nasal cleaning may cease.

Organisation of body care

Some of the tactics employed in general body care are practised with remarkable precision with regard to location, position, posture (even awkward posturing), group density and duration. The timing of grooming behaviour is affected by various causal factors including hormone levels. Prolactin induces grooming and the dopamine system also supports grooming. Comfort behaviour may be opiate-related (Cools *et al.*, 1974). Prolactin may stimulate dopaminergic turnover in some brain areas, including the nigrostriatal system and striatal dopamine seems to be involved in ACTH-induced grooming (Drago *et al.*, 1980). Apparently the mechanism of prolactin-induced excessive grooming involves the dopaminergic system projecting into the nigrostriatal system. It is known that opiate-induced and sustained grooming behaviour is dependent on an intact catecholaminergic central system, and that dopaminergic terminals are indispensable for this effect (Perkins and Westfall, 1978).

The simple assumption can be reasonably made that scratching in animals mediates between a condition of itch and relief and that comfort is obtained by the activity. In ill-health generally, the body care activities become reduced or arrested. In many illnesses the coats of affected animals lose their normal clean and orderly appearance. Such coats, lacking the effects of friction from rubbing, moisturising from licking, removal of debris from scratching and brisk shaking, become "staring" or "harsh" in appearance. Sick animals, with reduced body care motivation, may not discriminate in choice of resting place or time and place of evacuation. Since they are probably also lying for longer periods than usual, their coats may become heavily soiled, particularly about the hindquarters. Similar deterioration in coat condition is also the result of chronic stall-housing or enclosure with inadequate bedding; circumstances which defy the operation of body care behaviour. For example, veal calves kept in crates cannot groom normally and there may be physical as well as psychological consequences.

The possibility of being thwarted by housing conditions may lead to normal body care becoming altered by circumstances. Excessive self-grooming occurs in young calves which are subject to acute restraint. This restraint may result in dopamine-mediated, excessive grooming either because normal grooming of the hindquarters is thwarted or because few other activities are possible. Anomalous self-licking is comparatively common in some systems of intensive calf rearing which involve isolation and extreme restraint of the animal.

Some comfort-seeking relates to the adoption of specific positions and postures of the body. These postures often change in "comfort-shifts" before and after episodes of sleep. In such "comfort-shifts", the anatomical–dispersive behaviour effects a change in a resting arrangement of the body to a fresh position or posture, while the general resting phase continues.

The term "position", in applied behavioural usage, means the relation of the animal's trunk (i.e. its chest, side, belly and back) to the ground, floor or walls of its immediate environment. "Position" therefore refers to states of standing, lying, sternal resting, leaning and lateral recumbency. The term "posture" signifies the distinctive relation of the extremities of the head, neck and limbs to the trunk of the animal's body. In various standing postures the extremities may be flexed or extended; in recumbent postures the limbs may be retained beneath the trunk or held alongside it.

With animals lying flat on their sides, the position of lateral recumbency, upper limbs may be held towards the body or away from it. Usually the upper limb is placed before the lower fore limb and behind the lower hind limb. Posture is also manifest in the disposition of the limbs in the standing position; in some cases the term stance can be used to include both position and posture. Mixtures of position and posture also occur in variations of the resting state. Frequent changes take the form of "comfort-shifts". Anomalies in positions and postures sometimes occur in states of behavioural disorganisation.

Comfort-shifts occur periodically in resting phases, including recumbency. Many of them are minor positional changes such as partial rotation of the trunk; most are small postural adjustments of the limbs, and tail movements. Their frequency is commonly several times per hour, but this is reduced during some illnesses. Their absence or reduction can lead to the development of oedema, necrosis, ulceration or abscesses over points of pressure, e.g. the tarsal joint. In other instances the occurrence of comfort-shifts in behaviour increases significantly and this is indicative of a state of discomfort. Such discomfort may be associated with pain, as in colic, or the first stage of parturition, for example. Frequent comfort-shifts can relate to less specific forms of discomfort associated with poor quality of husbandry accommodation. Comfort-shifts may become almost continuous in some circumstances leading to manifest restlessness affecting an individual or any number of animals simultaneously in a group. Comfort-shifts can become so frequent and intense as to constitute a state of agitation in conditions of extreme pain or discomfort.

Special and species features of body care

Grooming

Cattle lick and thereby clean every part of their bodies that they can reach. To groom inaccessible parts they often make use of trees and fences and by using their tails they keep off flies and brush their skins. The value of grooming is seen in that it helps to remove mud, faeces, urine and parasites and thus greatly reduces the risk of disease. It has been estimated that calves groom themselves on 152 occasions and scratch 28 times a day for a total time of almost one hour daily (Fig. 10.2).

When one animal grooms another, it is commonly found that the one engaged in cleaning is slightly below the other in the social order (though normally within three positions). In large mixed herds, adult males will groom each other more often than younger animals

or females. Their grooming is applied mostly around the area of the head and neck.

Grooming behaviour can be seen as auto-grooming (self-grooming) or allogrooming (of others). Autogrooming can be body-based such as in licking, scratching with a horn or foot, rubbing one part on another, such as head on leg. Some autogrooming is "environment-based" as, for example, when an animal rubs against a post, a tree, a stone, a wall or a fence. Sometimes autogrooming is done by rubbing on or against a cooperating association animal. Allogrooming is "body-based" and is shown by mutual licking; active licking of an inactive associate animal; nipping with the teeth. Massaging and nose-rubbing applied to others is common as allogrooming in swine.

Horses show notable "environment-based" autogrooming type when they rub and roll their bodies on the ground. When the horse is about to roll it sets itself down, with some care, on a selected spot of ground. This animal rolls onto its side and rubs its body onto the ground surface. The rubbing lasts a few moments and the horse rotates towards sternal recumbency, from which position it rolls once more onto its side to rub again. This process is usually repeated and in some of these rolls the horse usually rotates onto its back, holding this position long enough to twist its back once or twice, working the skin of the whole of its back onto the ground. From this position the horse usually rolls back to the starting position but occasionally the entire rolling episode may terminate with the horse rolling from the supine position on to its other side, thereby going through 180 degrees of rotation. At the conclusion of rolling the horse stands and carries out very vigorous shaking of the whole body. Each shake begins at the anterior end and passes down the body to the hind limbs. During this shaking the animal's entire hide ripples and dislodges debris, including dust picked up in rolling. This skin-rippling effect of shaking is a phenomenal feature of grooming. It cannot be appreciated by naked-eye observation, but the process is revealed by fast cinematography and slow-

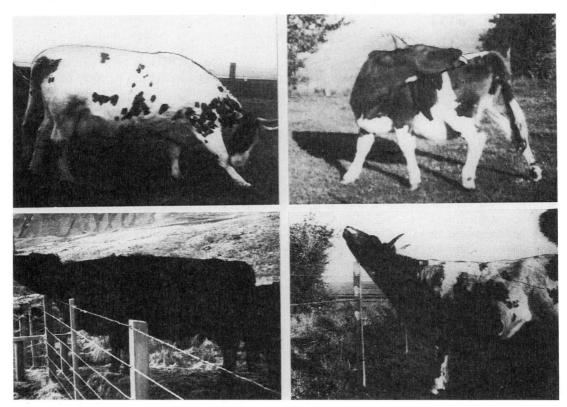

Fig. 10.2   Self-grooming activities in cattle. Most parts of the body surface can be reached by these acts. Inaccessible areas are groomed by friction against objects.

motion projection. The rippling creates a surprising looseness of skin. The shedding of debris is also quite remarkable as a result of such a simple, natural and brief session of body shaking. The explanation of the efficiency of this grooming lies, to some extent, in the vigour with which each of the steps is executed. The actual work involved in body care is well illustrated by this behaviour.

Another form of equine grooming is nipping of accessible body areas with sharp, repetitive biting actions. Mutual grooming between horses in pairs is common. The horses face towards each other and nip areas of the other's back not accessible to themselves, usually behind the withers. This behaviour can be sustained for many minutes during which each animal is continuously nipping actively at the same rate, though not necessarily in rhythm. Horses groom their crests by rubbing them to and fro beneath a manger, tree branch, etc. Manes can become damaged in this way under some circumstances.

Yet another form of equine grooming is scrubbing of the buttocks. This is another region which cannot be attended to by nipping or rolling. A swaying action of the rump is used against a convenient structure such as a post, tree, building, gate or fence. Special scrubbing places become adopted and fences can be broken down by such continual use. While this behaviour can be a sign of parasitism in the horse, it is also normal grooming and has no clinical relevance unless the incidence of the action becomes significant. The more normal effect of this grooming is two-fold. It scrubs the skin of the buttocks and the outer face of the tail head, removing scurf. It also causes the tail to be pressed into and across the skin of the dock, wiping this hairless region which can accumulate skin scales, salt from sweat, sebaceous grease and small faecal accumulations.

Preening and dust-bathing are notable forms of body care in poultry. In preening, which is body-based grooming, the bird cleans its plumage with its beak, uses brisk and repetitious head actions as feather vanes are "combed" and separated. Ducks "oil" their feathers by such action which has a waterproofing effect. Beak action goes down to the shaft calamus particularly on the primary and secondary remiges. The feather cover on the dorsal and ventral surfaces of the trunk are preened according to the bird's ability to flex and rotate its head and neck.

Through dust-bathing, which is environment-based, the bird is able to apply attention widely to the body, including plumage inaccessible to the beak, by friction against a suitable substratum. On a loose substratum the bird can excavate a shallow depression wide enough to contain its body. Within this the bird can use vigorous body movement and work the loose material into its feather cover, even scooping such material over itself while lying on its side. After such dust-bathing activity the bird will stand erect and forcefully shake out free debris from the general plumage to complete this modal action process in avian body care.

Thermoregulatory behaviour

This form of body care is employed when the enviromental temperature or other atmospheric factor, such as wind speed or precipitation, presents the animal with a challenge to its state of comfort, due to chill or wetness. In thermoregulation, animals such as cattle may stand broadside to the sun's rays on a cool day. They may seek the shade of trees, avoiding direct solar radiation at free range on a hot day (Gonyou *et al.*, 1979). In experimental and farm situations, farm animals can learn to operate switches which switch heaters on or off and hence control their environmental temperature (Baldwin, 1972; Curtis, 1983).

Much body care relates to thermoregulation, as has been stated previously. Some notable examples of this are included in the following illustrations. Swine running outdoors in hot climates have a predilection to wallow in mud. Sheep shelter below ledges in the terrains of highlands and moorlands in high wind, driving snow and hot summer days. Cattle shelter in close groups beneath shade trees during hot hours of the day in the tropics. Piglets huddle in tightly knit ranks in cool environments. Cattle have a predilection to stand with their feet and lower limbs in water for long spells on warm sunny days. Cattle turn their backs into driving rain or snow, closing their inguinal region by adducting their hind limbs closely below them. Horses turn their hindquarters into strong winds. Poultry seek shade from hot direct solar radiation and may crowd dangerously in such flocking if the shade area is restricted. Poultry take up roosting positions with their wings held out from the body when heated. Outwintering livestock make strategic use of tree clumps, woods, walls, buildings, etc. affording leeward protection from chilling winds.

In circumstances of communal sheltering the individual space normally maintained by the group members, as a fairly constant feature of their social organisation, usually is surrendered. This facilitates huddling, a behavioural arrangement which, in itself, is a proficient thermoregulatory tactic. It is important to the animal and of high priority in times of critical metabolic conservation.

The adaptive mechanisms of livestock, living under various climatic conditions, have been given detailed study by animal scientists over the last two decades, but it is only recently that the behavioural aspects have been closely examined (e.g. Mwanjali *et al.*, 1983). The differences in response to heat, solar radiation and the immediate environment are thus becoming better known and they are found to vary greatly between breeds and from one area to another. The level of temperature at which the so-called European breeds of cattle are able to maintain a normal body temperature (the thermo-neutral zone) is said to be about 0–20°C. Tropical breeds, on the other hand, are able to maintain a normal body temperature in ambient temperatures of about 22–37°C. There is evidence to suggest that some tropical breeds are even able to carry on normal activity and locomotion in temperatures in excess of 37°C. Both types are, however, found to use behavioural methods in attempting to control their temperatures.

Farm animals are capable of maintaining their body temperatures within very narrow limits using heat from within the body and are termed endothermic. The adaptive significance of this ability stems primarily from the marked effects of temperature upon the rate of chemical reactions in general and enzyme activity in particular. Endothermic animals are spared the slowdown of all bodily functions which occurs when the temperature falls. However, the advantages obtained by a relatively high body temperature impose a great need for precise regulatory mechanisms since even moderate elevations of temperature begin to cause nerve malfunction and protein denaturation leading to death. Convulsions occur at a body temperature of 41°C and 43°C is the limit for mammalian life. In contrast, most body tissues can withstand marked cooling to less than 8°C, which has found an important place in modern human surgery when the heart must be stopped since the physiologically dormant cold tissues require little nourishment.

Heat stroke, the development of a body temperature at which vital bodily functions are endangered, should be distinguished from heat exhaustion. The former is due to a breakdown in heat-regulating mechanisms, whereas the latter is not the result of failure of heat regulation but rather of the inability to meet the price of heat regulation. Heat exhaustion is a state of collapse due to hypotension brought on by depletion of plasma volume (secondary to sweating) and by extreme dilation of skin blood vessels, i.e. by decreases in both cardiac output and peripheral resistance. Thus, heat exhaustion occurs as a direct consequence of the activity of heat-loss mechanisms; because these mechanisms have been so active, the body temperature is only modestly elevated. In a sense, heat exhaustion is a safety valve which, by forcing cessation of work when heat-loss mechanisms are overtaxed, prevents the larger rise in body temperature which would precipitate the far more serious condition of heat stroke.

The first, most general, and most easily recognisable evidences of adaptive behaviour in cattle are the movements directed towards seeking shade, particularly when ambient heat greatly exceeds body heat. Though the behaviour of both Aberdeen Angus and Brahman cattle in cloudy, overcast conditions is much the same, differences become apparent when the two breeds are in conditions of direct solar radiation with little or no air movement. There is a definite change in the behaviour of Aberdeen Angus, which seeks out shade and consequently spends less time grazing than do Brahman cattle, which are less inclined to undertake adaptive behaviour under such conditions. On the other hand, adaptive behaviour of the Aberdeen Angus is much less marked if there is good air movement, regardless of the change in temperature. Cattle living in tropical rain forest and equatorial areas of the world show a greater need for shade than those living in sparse or semi-arid areas where rainfall is low and shade limited. It has been found that Dwarf Shorthorn cattle in Nigeria may spend as long as 4–5 h resting in the shade during the day and, to compensate, as long as 3–5 h grazing during the night. In this way their behaviour may be nearer that of the temperate breeds, such as Aberdeen Angus, Hereford and Holstein, than that of the Brahman breed.

The ability of newborn piglets to adapt to their environmental temperature is very limited as they are prone to lose body heat rapidly. The behavioural mechanism for dealing with this problem is huddling. From the time of birth, young piglets display huddling behaviour as an organised attitude for most of the day (Signoret *et al.*, 1975). During huddling they lie parallel to each other, often with head and tail ends alternating to some degree along the row. Whilst lying closely together side by side, they usually have their limbs tucked underneath them. When a group is large, some of the piglets in the middle may overlie others. Interruptions in huddling result from occasional "comfort-shifts" in individuals. The result of this huddling behaviour is that the quantity of heat lost by the piglets is much less than would otherwise occur. Although huddling behaviour is characteristically shown in the litter early in life, it is nevertheless a behavioural pattern which is retained by the pig into adult life as a means of conserving body heat and deriving tactile comfort.

In severe weather when a high wind is blowing horses cease to graze and direct the hindquarters into the wind. The tail is held close to its dock and this allows it to be blown between the hind legs. The tail hair then shields all of that hairless area of the perineum, the inguinal region and the inner thighs. By this means the horse spares itself the loss of heat and energy reserves. The combination of cold wind and precipitation can inflict great climatic stress upon a horse.

Thermoregulation in swine

The physical inadequacies of pigs in thermoregulation are various. Characteristic of the species in domestication is the thick layer of subcutaneous fat and also, partly as a consequence of that feature, an absence of loose skin. Sweat glands are very few and their distribution is almost entirely confined to the snout. These factors tend to cause a progressive accumulation of body heat in warm surroundings. The relatively poor body cover of hair makes the animal particularly vulnerable to the effects of direct solar radiation (Mount, 1968, 1979).

Pigs with limited experience of direct sunshine are evidently highly prone to heat stroke when suddenly exposed to it. In heat stroke the animal is hyperthermic, prostrate and respiring at its maximum rate while its associated circulatory responses fail increasingly to cope with the physiological emergency (Morrison *et al.*, 1969). The course of the prodromal state is short, possibly 1–2 h, and the duration of unrelieved heat stroke is probably about the same period before terminating in death. The circumstances associated with heat stroke are predictable and are those which expose the animal and force it to physical exercise in a high ambient temperature. Clinical cases are therefore most commonly found in association with inadequately shaded pens and with the effort of farrowing, breeding and being driven on foot.

In spite of its physical inadequacies the pig does possess efficient heat-regulating systems, but these, apart from respiratory responses, operate through cooling behaviour such as wallowing, moisture and shade seeking (Fig. 10.3). Wallowing in water is highly effective in alleviating hyperthermia (Ingram, 1965). A pig wallowing in mud quickly acquires a thick coating of mud over its lateral and ventral surfaces and its limbs. After the pig has left the wallow this coating adheres and dries out to form, over much of the animal's body, a protective insulation against the sun's rays. By absorbing heat from the pig, this superficial layer of caked mud can also assist in relieving hyperthermia. These factors permit pigs such as breeding sows to graze and forage actively in an environment which otherwise could not be economically utilised for extensive pig husbandry.

Sheep sheltering

Among free-ranging sheep, sheltered areas are constantly being identified and confirmed as a result of exploration. Mixed flocks of unshorn and recently shorn sheep show behavioural differences in location. During calm weather, in

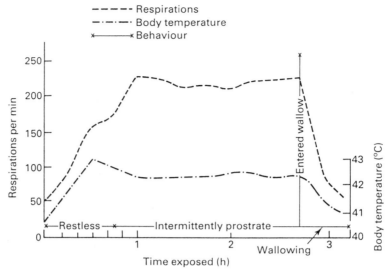

Fig. 10.3 Behaviour in relation to incipient heat stress in a pig. Wallowing is seen to control the syndrome after physiological responses have reached plateaux of limitation without relieving the condition.

daylight, sheep largely remain as one flock, but in windy weather, and at night, most shorn sheep congregate in a shelter while unshorn sheep remain away from shelter (Alexander *et al.*, 1979).

The inclusion of recently-shorn sheep in a flock of unshorn animals does not lead to an increase in the proportion of unshorn sheep likely to lamb in shelter. Unshorn sheep, in the presence of shorn sheep, appear to avoid sheltered areas and the colder or higher areas of grazing are preferred spots for them (Lynch and Alexander, 1977; Mottershead *et al.*, 1982).

In hot sunny conditions, sheep will often use the shade of a tree or other shelter. Sherwin and Johnson (1987) recorded a significant positive correlation between the proportion of the day spent shading and the daily maximum air temperature. Such behaviour is an important means of regulating body temperature since for newly shorn animals the heat load due to solar radiation can be similar in magnitude to the metabolic heat production of the animal (Stafford-Smith *et al.*, 1985). There is much individual variation in the strategies used by sheep which are being heated by direct sunlight, however, Johnson (1987) found that whilst some sheep in a group which he studied spent much time in shade during the hotter part of the day, others stayed in the sun and allowed their body temperatures to rise, but had lower respiratory rates and consumed no more oxygen than those which stayed in the shade.

Defecation

With few exceptions, such as rabbits, animals avoid the ingestion of their excrement and avoid grazing where there is faecal contamination. Horses and pigs feed in a different area from that in which they defecate and cattle refrain from grazing close to dung pats. Where slurry from a cowshed was spread on a field and left for seven weeks, cows preferentially ate clean herbage if it was available but grazed the tops of the herbage over the slurry if there was no alternative (Broom *et al.*, 1975.)

Horse defecation

While horses are defecating or urinating they usually cease other body activities. Stallions show careful and deliberate selection of the spot where defecation is to occur. Following defecation, a stallion usually turns and sniffs the spot where this has taken place. After defecation, in the case of both the stallion and the mare, the muscles of the perineum contract and the tail is lashed downwards several times.

While urinating, the stallion and the gelding adopt a characteristic stance, the hind legs being abducted and extended so that the back becomes hollowed. Urination takes place with the penis released from the prepuce. Following urination, the stallion again sniffs around the area before walking away.

The mare, when urinating, does not show the same marked straddling posture as is shown by the stallion; nevertheless, the posture is similar in that the hind legs are abducted from each other. Following urination by the mare, the vulvar muscles contract. More elaborate but similar patterns of urination are shown by brood mares with young foals and by mares in oestrus.

As already mentioned, horses typically show care in selecting areas for defecation. They return again and again to the same patch. These patches can accumulate large quantities of faeces during a grazing season. Adult animals defecate 6–12 times per day, depending on the nature of the feed eaten. Normally urination occurs less often during the day and horses have been noted to urinate as few as three times per day. Urine is passed commonly when the animal is freshly bedded and during rest periods in the hours of darkness.

Bovine defecation

Although the eliminative behaviour of cattle is neither notably regulated in the frequency of its occurrence nor specifically directed at a certain area, large amounts of faeces are often placed closely together. At night and during harsh weather cattle tend to bunch and this appears to be the main reason for the close deposition of faeces. The animals pay little attention to their faeces, often walking and lying amongst excreta but avoid grazing close to faeces. There is evidence that in some dairy cows allelomimetic behaviour engenders excretion; when one alarmed animal defecates or urinates others may commence to do likewise.

The normal defecation stance for both male and female animals is one in which the tail is extended away from the posterior region, the back arched and the hind legs placed forward and apart. The posture assumed is such that there is the least likelihood of incurring contamination. This attitude towards hygiene is also seen in calves which appear to take more care than adults to expel the faeces well away from the body. Unlike the female, the male bovine animal is able to walk while urinating and only displays a slight parting of the legs while doing so. The posture assumed by the female while urinating is very much the same as they employ while defecating and the urine is expelled more forcefully by the female than the male.

During the 24-h daily cycle cattle normally urinate about nine times and defaecate 12–18 times. The number of times cattle engage in eliminative behaviour and the volume that is expelled, however, varies with the nature and quantity of food ingested, the ambient temperature and the individual animal itself. High consumers such as Holstein cattle may expel 40 kg of faeces in the 24-h cycle while lower consumers such as Jerseys are found to defecate some 28 kg under the same husbandry conditions.

Pig defecation

Evacuation in piglets occurs on the day of birth using postures characteristic of older animals. As the piglets' neuromuscular coordination improves so they are able to hold these postures without falling over, falling asleep, trembling or sitting down. The posture for defecation is the same for males and females: the animal squats, curls its tail up over its back, flattens its ears and half closes or fully closes its eyes. This same posture is used by females when urinating. Males stand with the front legs slightly advanced, causing the back to depress; they urinate in a series of squirts, unlike the female which ejects a continuous stream. The characteristics of ear flattening and eye closure are less pronounced when urination is occurring. At defecation piglets do not regularly re-use the same site, so the place where any given piglet will eliminate cannot be accurately predicted. Elimination does not take place at random in the pen, however, for specific sites are chosen by pigs for defecation and urination (Fritschen, 1975; Whatson, 1978).

In spite of a reputation to the contrary, pigs are extremely clean in their habits if the system of husbandry imposed upon them gives them the opportunity to express their normal defecatory behaviour. Pig premises which are appropriately designed to create dunging areas are usually properly used by pigs. Even in the most limited quarters, pigs reserve an area for sleeping accommodation and an area for excretion. This sleeping area is kept as clean and dry as possible. Under conditions of crowding, it is sometimes difficult for groups of pigs to maintain organised eliminative behaviour as, for example, when growing pigs are allocated less than one square metre of floor area each. Organised, group eliminative behaviour is largely learned during infancy, perhaps from mature animals and if the defecatory characters are not acquired by learning at an early age they may not be properly acquired. Such pigs, in their turn, are unable to pass on organised behaviour of this type. These pigs are usually observed to be contaminated with their own faeces and their presence as a large proportion of a pig herd is a reflection on the system of management.

When penned pigs are exposed to high ambient temperatures and their normal behavioural methods of controlling hyperthermia cannot operate, it is commonly found that pigs defecate close to water. In farrowing pens, the piglets usually defecate near to a wall and particularly in the pen corners (Petherick, 1982). They avoid defecating in the area used for resting. Fattening pigs also tend to defaecate near to a pen wall and orientate parallel to, or with their hindquarters towards, the wall. This behaviour could be exploited to keep farrowing pens clean by having perforated floors around the pen perimeter and there are good economic and farm management reasons to exploit this tendency (Baxter, 1982).

11 Locomotion and other movements

The essence of behaviour is bodily movement. This includes action patterns and locomotion, displays, etc. giving the whole animal many of its ethological properties and qualities. All the functional systems such as body temperature regulation, feeding and reproduction incorporate various kinetic features. Descriptions of bodily motility refer to the bases of physiological activities such as breathing, anatomically localised actions such as blinking, specific goal-related acts such as drinking and gross activity of the whole animal such as locomotion, positional alteration or stretching (Brooks and Stoney, 1971). Gross activity is the category of behaviour considered here.

The original ecological niche of each species demanded different behavioural strategies and consequently species differ amongst one another in the amount and type of movement required to maximise use of their natural habitat. Movement is vital in pastoral living and the ungulate farm animals have a legacy of ingestive demands which they have met through their locomotion. Animals move to sustain life such as in the search for food and the avoidance of danger. The study by Low *et al.* (1981) on the many features of maintenance behaviour of cattle in Central Australia is a definitive account showing the central role of kinetic behaviour in maintenance. The three-part report by these workers is

a classical example of ethological macroanalysis which brings out general features of kinesis in grazing cows.

The topics discussed in the rest of this chapter are postures and movements at rest, gaits during locomotion, distances travelled and the need for exercise. Circumstantial subjective evidence suggests that freedom to move is a pleasure to animals. Observing calves at springtime turned out to grass or racehorses anticipating their morning gallop gives the impression that freedom to run is a pleasure in itself to the animal.

Postures and movements at rest

The complex neuromuscular system which controls body posture and movement is organised to limit fluctuations in the animal's centre of gravity in order to maintain stability and equilibrium. Adjustments of posture are additionally used to keep the animal in equilibrium when it is either stationary or moving (Massion and Gahery, 1979). Postural adjustment is also needed during rest, grooming, feeding and display and there is a minimum amount of space which is needed in order that such adjustments are possible. Descriptions of grooming behaviour often include reference to stretching movements but although some of these movements are involved in body surface maintenance, others serve a different function. Stretching enables an animal to keep its joints and muscles in a state such that they can be used effectively when required. Stretching is often performed after a period of rest or after a period when the limbs are folded.

Most stretching occurs as pendiculation in a series of actions as follows: flexion at the throat, arching of the neck, straightening of the back, elevation and movement of the tail and full extension of one and then the other hind limb (Fraser, 1989). Extension of the fore limbs or wings, singly or together, is a related exercise (Fig. 11.1). Animals which are prevented from stretching and subsequently provided with an opportunity to do so will spend a much longer

than normal period showing the behaviour. For example, hens confined in a battery cage so that they cannot stretch their wings will spend longer stretching their wings after a long period of confinement than after a short period (Nicol, 1987). Similarly, calves which have been closely confined show more vigorous activity when given space than calves reared with more space to move around (Dellmeier *et al.*, 1985; Friend and Dellmeier, 1988).

Other important movements which do not involve locomotion are those involved in standing up and lying down. Characteristic sequences of movements are involved, e.g. see Fig. 11.2, and the animal needs a certain amount of space for these. Petherick (1983a) calculated how much room a pig needs for lying on the sternum, and for lying with the legs stretched out. This

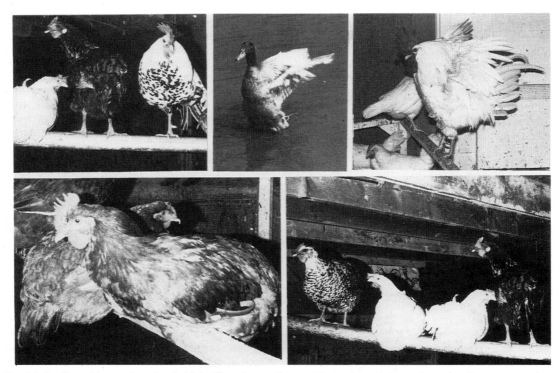

Fig. 11.1 Stretching and resting in birds. Top: forms of stretching — hen, drake and rooster. Bottom: roosting — poultry and guinea fowl.

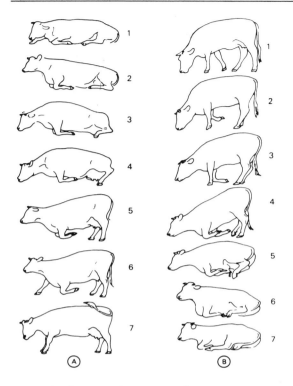

Fig. 11.2 The typical sequence of movements which occur when a cow stands up (A) and lies down (B).

space is shown for a range of body weights in Fig. 11.3. Baxter and Schwaller (1983) filmed the movement of pigs when standing up and lying down (Fig. 11.4 and 11.5) and were able to calculate the minimum space requirements of pigs from this.

Locomotion and gaits

In locomotion the limbs act synchronously in any one of a variety of given patterns, each of which is termed a gait. Two forms of gait pattern exist, symmetrical and asymmetrical. In symmetrical gaits the movements of limbs on one side repeat those of the other side, but half a stride later. In asymmetrical gaits the limbs from one side do not repeat those of the other. Symmetrical gaits include the walk, the pace and the trot. Asymmetrical gaits include the various forms of the canter and gallop, including the lope and the rotary gallop.

The full cycle of leg movement during the phases of support, propulsion and flight is termed a stride. A stride is a full cycle of movement of all limbs, while stride length is the distance covered between successive imprints of the same foot. The sound produced when a foot strikes the ground is the beat. If each foot strikes the ground separately the gait will be a four-beat gait. If diagonal pairs are placed down simultaneously, as in the trot, the gait is two-beat since only two beats will be heard for each stride. The canter is a three-beat gait in waltz time. A lead leg is that leg which leaves the ground last during the canter or gallop. The gallop, of course, resembles the canter, but since it has more propulsion it has an extra "floating phase" at the end of each stride.

Within each stride each limb for a time acts in a support phase and in a non-supportive or swing phase. In the walk the support phase is longer in duration than the swing phase and determines the stability of this gait. As the walk speed is increased the duration of the support phase decreases while that of the swing phase increases.

The gaits of the walk, the trot and the canter are the forms of quadruped motion fundamentally involved in all locomotor behaviour. These have been described in definitive terms for the horse, by Leach *et al.* (1984) and Waring (1983). As a kinetic law, the animal naturally changes from walking to trotting at a speed below which walking requires less energy than trotting and above which trotting requires less energy than walking. The same principle is true for changes between the other gaits and thus the natural gait at any speed incurs the least expenditure of energy. Within each gait there is a speed at which energy expenditure is minimal (Hoyt and Taylor, 1981).

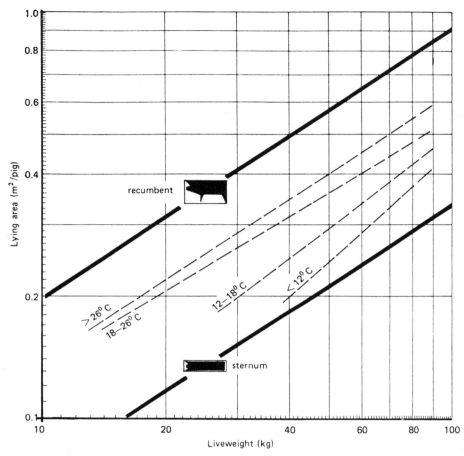

Fig. 11.3   Relationship between floor area occupied by resting pigs and air temperature (after Hauptmann *et al.*, 1972).

Walk

The walk is defined as a slow regular symmetrical gait in which the left legs perform the same movements as the right, but half a stride later and in which either two, three, or sometimes four legs support the animal at any one time. The support role is more important in the fore legs, which are nearer the centre of gravity, and the propulsive role is more important in the hind limbs (Wentink, 1978). Approximately 60% of the static weight is supported by the fore legs. The sequence of leg movement in quadrupedal walking is Left Front (LF), Right Hind (RH), Right Front (RF), Left Hind (LH) which always results in a triangle of support which includes the centre of gravity. Animal statues and models often show impossible leg positions.

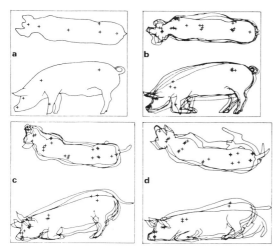

Fig. 11.4 Stages of movement in lying down by sows (from Baxter and Schwaller, 1983).

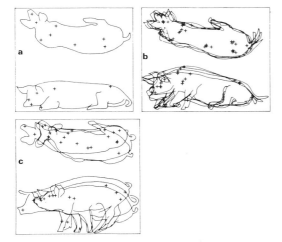

Fig. 11.5 Stages of movement in standing up by sows (from Baxter and Schwaller, 1983).

Trot

The trot is a symmetrical gait of medium speed in which the animal is supported by alternating diagonal pairs of limbs so the sequence is LF and RH then RF and LH. The fore limbs are free of the ground longer than the hind limbs to allow the front feet to clear the ground in advance of the placement of the hind feet, on the same side. If there is a period of suspension between the support phases, the gait is referred to as a flying trot. A slow, easy, relaxed trot is called a jog or dog trot. Sometimes the term dog trot is used to mean that the animal travels in a straight line with the hindquarters shifted to the left or right. The trot is occasionally classified also as ordinary trot, extended trot and collected trot. Standard bred horses use the extended trot in racing when the limbs reach out to increase stride length and speed. The hackney uses the collected trot which is characterised by flexion and high carriage of the knees and hocks—a gait suited for snow or marshland running.

Canter and gallop

The canter is essentially a slow gallop. It is a three-beat gait with one diagonal pair of limbs hitting the ground simultaneously. The hoof falls are typically as follows: (1) one hind foot, (2) the other hind foot and the fore foot diagonal to it simultaneously, (3) the remaining fore foot. Hence the sequence written in comparable form to those above is: LF and RH, RF, LH. The canter is a gait in which the horse can use its neck muscles to advantage by the accentuated upward swing of the head which helps to raise the forequarters and to advance the leading fore limb. As the horse tires in the canter it will bob its head more to utilise this minor auxiliary system.

The gallop is an asymmetrical gait of high speed in which the animal, during parts of the stride, is supported by one or more limbs, or is in suspension. If the limbs are placed down in a circular order with two close together in time, then a gap, then the other two, e.g. RF LF, LH RH, the gait is referred to as a rotary gallop. If the hind limb leads through to a fore limb of the opposite side, e.g. RF LF, RH LH, the gait is termed a transverse or diagonal gallop. Horses seem to prefer the transverse gallop whilst dogs use the rotary gallop. In the transverse gallop the placement of the limbs, and therefore the support pattern, is transferred from the initiating hind limb diagonally to the fore limb of the opposite side. As in the rotary gallop two forms of this gallop exist, dependent on the order of foot falls, e.g. LH RH, LF RF (a right lead transverse gallop) or RH LH, RF LF (a left lead transverse gallop).

The jump

As they prepare to jump, all horses strut with the forelimbs, thereby changing the momentum of forward movement into vertical impulse. In horizontal locomotion, the hind limbs hit the ground separately so as to maintain the rhythm and fluidity of stride. In jumping, however, these limbs hit the ground at a similar distance from the jump (approximately 2.00 m) and are spatially separated by only 0.09 m. This action of the hind limbs allows a more symmetrical and balanced upward propulsion. This synchronous and symmetrical action of the hind limbs at take-off allows these limbs to coordinate their movement in the air phase when the hind limbs are raised in unison following lift-off (Leach and Ormrod, 1984).

In the approach to a jump, if the fore limbs landed in a synchronous manner while the horse was moving at this speed, it is likely that a smooth transition from horizontal to vertical movement would not be possible. Disruptive changes would result in reduced overall speed and efficiency of the jump performance. The lightened weight of the fore limbs, and the recoil resulting from the elastic storage of energy in these limbs from strutting, probably help the fore limbs to clear the jump.

Distance travelled

Although horses are sometimes very active in cold weather, frequently galloping about their territories, other farm livestock limit their movements in cold or wet weather (Shreffler and Hohenboken, 1980). It is believed that this is done to conserve metabolic heat. Cattle and sheep periodically attempt to travel or roam away from their home range (Arnold and Dudzinski, 1978; Squires *et al.*, 1972; Wagnon, 1963). Given the opportunity, they will sometimes travel at the walk for considerable distances. One purpose in herding sheep traditionally is to return them periodically to their home grazings after roaming. Cattle and horses also roam, even leaving adequate grazing conditions to do so. One feature of note in this travelling behaviour is the "Indian file" order of following a lead animal which is frequent. The social aspects of being a leader in this situation are discussed further in Chapter 17. Animal routes are often seen, most clearly from the air, as pathways which criss-cross grazing ranges. They are even found in most paddocks. Animal walks are not, therefore, reserved for ambitious excursions but occur frequently, even regularly, in normal domestic conditions.

Daily distances that grazing herbivores travel are largely affected by the location of food and water. In paddocks where water is close to good quality food the distance walked by animals is small and occurs mainly as movement while grazing, but if water is some distance from food then walking to and from water contributes a greater part of daily distance travelled. The location of water and the quality of forage have a significantly greater influence on the distance travelled by cows than either forage quantity, stage of lactation of the cow, body condition of the cow, or time of year. Horses at range, for example, may travel up to 65–80 km (40–50 miles) daily to water. Sheep will also travel great distances regularly to water where vegetation and water are both scarce. While these travelling demands do not usually exist in conventional farming, this travelling ability is nevertheless shared, to some degree, by all grazing livestock. Even when environmental conditions are similar different breeds of sheep travel different characteristic daily distances, Border Leicester sheep travelling 14 km, Merinos 13 km and Dorset

Horns moving 9 km (Squires *et al.*, op. cit.). Daily distances travelled by cattle range from 0.9 km on a 0.1 ha paddock to 24 km under drought conditions on rangeland and of sheep travelling between 0.7 and 14 km daily depending on their environment. The size of home range and diurnal movements of New Forest ponies also depend on the location of food, water and shelter with ponies travelling further when these resources are more widely distributed (Tyler, 1972). In the study by Low and colleagues (op. cit.) it was recorded that some cows on the large paddocks on Tablelands in North Australia regularly walked 16 km daily to and from their foraging area. During a period when forage was scarce and dry the cattle walked 24 km daily to forage. This study indicated that paddock size has a definite influence on daily walking schedules, as do the palatability or availability and location of forage. To this must be added the walking ability of the individual cow. In one study it was noted that the distance walked and run by calves varied from 12 m per half hour in the first week of life to 80 m per half hour at 8 weeks of age.

Species-typical movements

Cattle

Cattle under free range on pastures in a wide variety of natural conditions in Australia, South Africa, New Guinea and the USA spend from 30–110 min per 24 h in locomotion. In addition to this, 500–600 min per 24-h day are spent in mobile grazing. All of this amounts to about 10 h per 24-h day of movement per grazing cow. The most influential factors of the environment affecting gross activity are those which make thermoregulatory demands on the animal, such as the necessity for sheltering. Cattle at pasture during the night are equally active in bright moonlit nights and in dark nights. Frequent changes of activity occur at night, such as changing from grazing to ruminating, to lying, to standing, to walking. As a result of these changes cattle are more restless at night. This relative restlessness occurs irrespective of nocturnal disturbances (Arnold and Dudzinski, 1978).

Differences between day and night behaviour are readily apparent in the data given by Low and colleagues in their Australian study (op. cit.). More time, in longer unbroken periods, is spent in active behavioural activities such as grazing and ruminating in the daytime, partly because more time is available in the daytime throughout the year, and more time spent lying down both resting (including sleep) and ruminating at night. This distinction remains in the data when standardised for unequal day length in different seasons. At night, despite less time being spent in the more active behaviours, there are more transitions, indicating that the cows are more restless then. However, cows in daytime change from resting to ruminating more frequently, indicating some restlessness during the warmer part of the day as well. The sequence of activities show that in the daytime, standing resting is the main pivotal activity, whereas grazing is the main pivotal activity at night. Restlessness is very evident in cattle after re-grouping (Tennessen *et al.*, 1985).

Horses

Locomotion in the horse has been described above in detail. During locomotion, horses are capable of effecting quite spectacular jumps, both in distance and height covered. Few horses, however, can jump off until they are taught to jump and, indeed, untaught horses may avoid obstacles only 60 cm high rather than clear them by jumping. Normally horses avoid jumping over ditches and show a reluctance to jump over horizontal obstacles in general.

It seems very likely that the wild ancestors of our horses travelled great distances during each year. They may have migrated in temperate countries, spending the summer months in the colder North and moving South for the winter.

Sheep

The distance travelled by sheep while grazing is affected both by the immediate environment of the flock and by genetic differences affecting the behaviour of different breeds in adapting to the particular habits in which they were reared. Thus Cheviot sheep travel further than Romney Marsh sheep when both breeds are kept in hilly country, but only a little further when both graze on flat areas. Ewes of Hampshire breed travel less than those of either Columbia or Rambouillet breeds. The distance covered by sheep, under temperate conditions, may be quite constant over long periods. The only major alteration to this behaviour occurs shortly before the breeding season when movement, particularly amongst the rams, becomes less regulated. Generally sheep travel about 7 km per day, although any increase in the duration of grazing times results in a corresponding increase in distance travelled. Likewise, any increase in available feeding space has a similar effect. These effects, however, are usually temporary and cause no major alterations to the overall behaviour of the flock.

Certain activity characteristics of sheep are of practical interest. Lamb activity declines after sunset, and throughout the hours of darkness the majority of lambs lie down and are then more easily collected. Experiments show the importance of moving sheep through yards along the same path and in the same direction for all handling procedures (Hutson, 1980). Alternative visual stimuli can be used successfully to attract sheep to move along races and facilitate husbandry practices. Sounds and odours have no such attractive effects (Franklin and Hutson, 1982).

Pigs

While young pigs are nimble and able to run about, the mature domestic pig, with its relatively massive trunk, is physically ill-equipped for movement at speed. Well-grown pigs there-fore run distances of only a few metres. They are, however, able to trot at a reasonable speed over longer distances.

Pigs have long periods of inactivity each day. During these periods they typically rest in huddled groups. Various studies have shown that pigs are fairly active during the night hours. This appears to be so particularly in the case of sows in oestrus. Distances travelled by wild pigs vary greatly according to terrain and food availability.

Poultry

Synchronised limb movements begin in the chick before hatching (Provine, 1980). Locomotion in the hen is by walking and running, but many hens are capable of flying distances of about 10–15 m. Much activity is invested in pecking for food but exercise activities are also common. Exercises include full extension of one wing after another. More usually when one wing is out-stretched in a backward direction the leg on the same side may also be extended backwards. Wing-flaps, while the head and body are held very erect, represent another form of exercise. Many forms of caging in current use virtually prevent these activities of basic motion.

Jungle fowl and feral domestic fowl do not travel large distances but stay in a small home range. Within this area, however, they are very active and frequently walk and fly from one place to another. They utilise trees and other vantage points for perching so need to fly at intervals to reach these.

The need for exercise

Agricultural livestock and probably other animals have an apparent need for movement and try to exercise frequently (Fraser, 1982b). The nucleus accumbens is apparently important in the control of locomotion. It is in the ventral forebrain region located above the olfactory tubercle and organises the continuity of locomotor limb movements (Brooks *et al.*, 1973).

Animals travel predictable distances during their daily activities on free range. Even when the need to travel has apparently been removed, as in the intensive farm environment, animals still try to do so. Maintaining a minimum level of activity keeps animals physically prepared for any necessary movement. The high incidence of lameness in intensively kept farm animals may be a result of the lack of exercise preventing proper activation of limb joints, muscles and pedal tissues. Even the productive farm animals require opportunities for exercise. Horses certainly need exercise on a daily basis. It is now clear that severe kinetic restrictions result in gross forms of anomalous behaviour.

The inherent nature of kinesis is apparent in the studies on fetal behaviour. Movement as a form of exercise is detectable in the mammalian fetus and in the chick embryo. Each normal equine and bovine fetus makes many thousands of movements during gestation, these movements having been likened to isometric exercises which promote good development of muscles and joints, and which prepare the fetus for postnatal life. The isometric exercises carried out in the uterus therefore prepare the fetus for the earliest activities, which are normally standing and searching for the dam's udder, necessary for survival in neonatal life (Fraser, op. cit.).

When severely limited in activity due to constraint, some animals perform, with high frequency, stereotyped activities of very specific and definitive forms. The causation of such activities is discussed in Chapter 32.

It must be assumed that a significant reduction of general activity will frequently be associated with husbandry systems which feature close restraint or confinement. Husbandry constraints which inhibit locomotor activity make the environmental circumstances of chronic restriction impose two main tangible deficiencies in the physiology of perception; viz. hypostimulation (reduced stimulus input) and hypokinaesthesia (diminished sensory receipt of body movement feedback). Although hypokinaesthesia can be a neurological impairment of endogenous origin in medicine, its origin is clearly exogenous in animal husbandry.

It is generally understood that exogenous stimuli are perceptible, external factors, whereas stimulation is the excitation process within the receiving sensorium of the perceiving animal. The quantity of stimuli can obviously affect the level of satiation in stimulation. Stimuli of the same type can lose their potential value for stimulation but a deficit in one type of stimulus can be compensated by an increase in another, alternative stimulus—that is to say, by variability. Through variability, stimuli can contribute to the quality of pooled stimulation in the animal's sensory system. Beneficial environmental quality, at least in this regard, can be assessed on the basis of its potential for stimulus variability.

Abnormally decreased motor function, or activity, is termed hypokinesia. Differing forms of this condition occur, but the critical effect of this state clearly must be a reduction in the animal's sensation of its own movement. The various forms of sense organs in the animal's moving parts, such as tendons, joints and muscles, respond to mechanical action, movement, position, touch and pressure, and obviously constitute a major share of the sensory input of animals. In addition, experience of gravity is obviously not the same in the static animal as in the mobile one. The sense of muscular effort that accompanies motion of the body is precisely the deficit of reduced sensory input which is at the foundation of some kinetic dysfunctions. Hence hypokinesia may lead through hypokinaesthesia to the production of self-stimulating, sometimes repetitive motor activities. The environmental inadequacy thus contributes to behavioural problems in intensive husbandry systems.

Episodes of wing-flapping in the red jungle fowl and the domestic chicken demonstrate that the frequency of wing-flapping in the chicken has not been altered by domestication even though some domestic hybrids are now physically unable to fly (Provine, 1984). Vigorous wing-flapping still occurs in heavy, flightless strains of chickens. These findings by Provine are relevant to the controversy concerning inherent behaviours in farm animals. They indicate that domesticated species continue to carry the neural basis for motor components of "natural" behaviour. Evidently neurobehavioural processes can be stable throughout domestication even though the motor performances of motion can become diminished, or eliminated.

12 Exploration

All farm animals are strongly motivated to explore and investigate when they encounter a new environment. Only when the environment has become very familiar to them does the exploratory behaviour subside, but it reappears in an animal's behaviour after any change in its environment. Hence animals appear to maintain a potential for generating activities which focus the senses upon additions, changes, salient features and novelties in its close environment. Habituation to familiar stimuli occurs although familiar areas may be revisited, presumably to check for changes. Exploratory behaviour equips the animal with a system of behavioural adjustability which can be brought readily into operation (Syme and Syme, 1979).

Exploratory system

The exploratory system in behaviour is evident through many animal activities. This system can be outlined most simply as causal factors and consequent activities as follows:

1. Need in the animal for perception of environmental characteristics.
2. The activation of the exploratory behaviour.
3. The receipt of sensory feedback from the environment and hence information which can be used.

4. Reduction in the causal factor level as a result of sensory input.
5. The return of the cycle to a basal level of readiness with the lodgement of the information in the memory.

Hence *exploration is any activity which has the potential for the individual to acquire new information about its environment or itself.*

The role of investigative behaviour in the facilitation of learning is considerable (Toates, 1982). When a new stimulus is perceived, a state of heightened awareness is induced, more information is gathered and an addition to the animal's experience occurs. Some activities involve interactions with the inanimate environment using species-specific procedures which involve environmental testing and investigations: horning of trees, bushes and turf; scraping earth and snow; nosing artifacts closely to sniff and to touch with the upper lip; rooting into soil and bedding; head-pressing on fenced perimeters for movability; leaning on upright structures for yield; licking hard surfaces; and overseeing from vantage points.

The functions of exploratory behaviour

Each of the functional systems of animals requires that some exploration and investigation occur before it can operate effectively. The efficient exploitation of food sources must be preceded by location of these and estimation of efficient routes to use when acquiring food. Water sources and places where water loss is minimal must be found. Physical hazards must be located if they are to be avoided successfully. Exploration of other individuals and of own ability must occur if adequate sexual and social behaviour is to occur. Most of all, exploration is necessary if effective anti-predator behaviour is to be shown. Animals which are cryptically coloured or which need to hide must find a good resting place. Those which flee or show other active responses to predators must investigate the characteristics of their surroundings and learn about them so that they can respond appropriately and effectively. If predator attack is imminent, animals must scan their surroundings and be ready to respond to environmental changes.

Given the obvious selective advantage of showing exploratory behaviour it is not surprising that animals give a very high priority to such behaviour. Barnett (1963) reported that rats explore a novel arena even if they have been deprived of food and are offered both food and the opportunity to explore. Cattle also show such investigation (Kilgour, 1975).

The kind of exploration shown varies considerably from species to species. All animals must explore their own abilities and must investigate the characteristics of their environment but active movement in a new area and responses to novel objects depend on sensory usage. A rat put in a novel arena walks around sniffing but a bird or ungulate may explore by looking around. Objects are manipulated by primates but may not be touched at all by animals which cannot gain information in this way. Investigation of various small novel objects by zoo animals was studied by Glickman and Sroges (1966). Obvious active investigation was highest amongst primates and carnivores, less for rodents and lowest for reptiles. Marsupials studied by Russell and Pearce (1971) investigated more if they were carnivores than if they were herbivores. It is likely that the objects were usually being treated as potential food items.

Wild animals are much more cautious in their responses to novel objects and rats (Shorten, 1954) and buntings (Andrew, 1956) avoid them for some time. Such behaviour is more likely to have an anti-predator function.

Exploration and fear

As Hinde (1970) points out, exploratory behaviour and fear responses are overlapping categories. Animals moving around their environment and examining various aspects of it may be said to be exploring, but those same movements may occur when the animal is anticipating predator attack. They may occur after an active predator has been detected. At some point the behaviour might be called a fear response but it is difficult to decide exactly how to distinguish between exploration and fear. As most behavioural changes which have been called fear responses are associated with adrenal activity, it is best to limit the term fear as follows (Broom, 1981, p. 168). *Fear responses* are taken to include only those activities which either (1) follow adrenal activity and are a preparation for danger, or (2) are a response to detectable danger. The diversity of uses of the word fear is discussed by Archer (1979).

Trial and error behaviour

Trial and error behaviour can be a form of exploration of the animal's own abilities. An action is attempted and, if the consequences are beneficial, it is repeated. Such actions are of particular value as the animal grows and matures. An example of improvement in the performance of behaviour is seen in the behaviour of the long-legged, short-sighted, newborn foal. The foal's rising attempts, which begin soon after birth, involve coordination, balance, effort and change. Several failures to stand up usually occur, with the foal falling back down, but with successive tries improvements occur. Soon the foal is able to rise to a fixed, partly upright posture. Thereafter the ability to rise and stand is achieved. The process of rising from a lying to a standing position is completed too fast for maturation to be much involved.

When the foal is ambulatory, its exploratory activity becomes engaged in "teat-seeking". By trial and error activities the foal locates and investigates the mare's limbs, the ventral region of the mare's inguinal region, and ultimately her mammary gland. The trial and error activities in the foal's teat-seeking behaviour are often extended over a substantial period. With highly successful foals it may be completed within 30 min. In others it may take several hours. In still other, rare instances, there may be total failure. When the trial and error activities terminate in success, they do not require to be reproduced in full on the next teat-seeking occasion.

Trial and error behaviour occurs during interactions between a young animal and other individuals so the opportunity for social exploration is important. Livestock confined separately from one another cannot show this behaviour and do not usually develop behaviourally in the same way as others of their own kind. In addition, exploratory behaviour becomes significantly suppressed during many illnesses in animals, particularly those which have depression as a component in the syndrome. Indeed, the opinion could be held that absence of all exploratory behaviour is strongly diagnostic of clinical states of depression in animal disease.

It will be evident that needs of animals are not merely elemental ones such as need for food or water; some are complex, such as the need for stimulus diversity. Other needs are compound in nature, such as the need to be able to maintain the body surface or the need to associate with other individuals. Animals need to be able to show various aspects of exploratory behaviour and if they cannot do so, adverse effects may ensue. They need to explore that part of their environment which they expect to be especially relevant to their survival. In other ways also they have to acquire their own terms of reference. They apparently need to determine their own characteristics, abilities, limitations, social status, etc., since they expend much activity investigating these factors. They do this through social exploration and constant empirical interactions with their animate and inanimate environments. Animals constantly test their powers of reach and prehension in feeding. They can determine their social tolerance in mutual grooming. They can learn of their strength through pushing. They can also learn, through play, their personal powers of flight, attack and defence. It is not possible to generalise about the importance to the animal of having the opportunity to explore in these various ways but there is no doubt that depriving animals of some sorts of exploratory behaviour is extremely aversive. Under circumstances of very close and chronic confinement attempts to explore often become redirected and produce alternative behaviour which is likely to be a simple but maladaptive activity. For example, the repetitions characteristic of stereotyped self-stimulating behaviour.

Factors affecting exploratory behaviour

Cattle and sheep explore any new field they are put in and pay most initial attention to the field boundaries. They are likely to follow the boundary before exploring the interior of their enclosure. In these initial activities they may be bunched in a closer intra-group spatial organisation than usual. In small pastures which permit overall vision, the group disperses quickly and adopts the extensive spacing characteristic of grazing. In large pastures several days or weeks may elapse before part of it has been explored by all the stock in it. In tall grass or land in which there are obstructions to view, sheep may explore far from their point of input. In such situations some breeds of sheep, such as Dorsets, show little exploration while others, such as Finnish Landrace, explore much more. Prior experience of similar terrain influences cattle, sheep and horses to explore extensively while poor exploration is likely to be shown if prior experience of a similar environment is lacking. Animals raised on mountainous land and on ranges explore differently in changed environments.

The efficiency of exploration is vital to the production of appropriate responses. Continual adjustments in behavioural response following exploratory behaviour are obviously of major importance to the free-ranging animal within its environment (Arnold and Dudzinski, 1978). The sensory information which the animal perceives as a result of its exploratory behaviour and its investigative activities form part of the animal's experience and is used to produce appropriate forms of behaviour (MacPhail, 1982). In systems of close confinement attempts to explore lack outlet and normal development of behavioural responses cannot occur.

A factor which is often associated with close confinement is the absence of possibilities to explore, investigate and interact with social companions. Livestock held in social isolation show a variety of abnormalities of behavioural development. It has been said, for example, that a horse confined on its own "is in bad company". Acts of anomalous behaviour, such as pathological "mouthing", occur relatively more often in animals confined alone than in others. These behavioural disorders might be other examples of anomalies resulting from a redirected exploratory behaviour.

The "flank touch" behaviour of isolate-reared lambs is a model of an abnormal response to environmental novelties shown by socially deprived young animals. When first exposed to the novel environment of the open-field arena at 14 days of age, isolate-reared lambs exhibit withdrawal behaviour. They are slow to initiate movement and display little ambulatory behaviour. They vocalise much less frequently than lambs raised with other sheep. It is observed that being reared in isolation influences the lambs' interaction with an inanimate stimulus (Zito *et al.*, 1977).

Unlike lambs from natural rearing groups, isolate-reared animals are slow to investigate

the stimulus and often turn to face away in an attempt to avoid the stimulus. Thus, it appears that the isolate-reared lambs tend to avoid the situation of a novel environment by withdrawing and avoiding interaction with the new environment. Such a study demonstrates that differential rearing will influence the behavioural response of lambs to a novel environment in such a way that socially-deprived lambs have deficits in exploratory capacity. A deficit of this nature would not provide the animal with good survival prospects in a natural environment. Similar observations have been made on foals. Naturally mothered foals in novel situations are more active and vocal than orphan foals (Houpt and Hintz, 1983).

When exploration is thwarted, acts of self-stimulation occur. Common to many abnormalities in the behaviour of confined animals, self-stimulatory activities apparently flourish in conditions of frustration or hypostimulation. These activities are often mouth-based and in many cases the tongue is used in the manner of tasting. Evidently, trigeminal orosensory reception, originating in the mouth region, is a major source of stimulation. Some acts of abnormal swallowing also appear to have self-stimulus value.

Self-stimulation is implicit in forms of self-directed behaviour. A most extreme form of self-directed behaviour is self-mutilation, a condition which will be described in Chapter 33. The "flank-touch" behaviour of lambs held in isolation has been given as a less dramatic form of self-directed behaviour but is of no less significance. It appears to be non-functional, stereotyped behaviour which occurs in lambs disturbed by isolation and diminished in exploratory activities. This behaviour is characterised by the lamb repeatedly reaching back and touching its flank with its muzzle. In test situations the "flank-touch" was seen significantly more often in isolate-reared lambs than in controls.

Housing effects may modify calf exploratory behaviour. It has been found experimentally that calves from restricted-housing in single pens show a higher incidence of rapid movement within a novel environment than calves from a loose-housing system in which they are able to move freely and to interact with their peers and mothers. When approaching a stimulus object, calves from a restricted-housing system adopt a hesitant ambivalent posture, suggesting a conflict between the tendencies to approach and to withdraw from the novel stimulus (MacKay and Wood-Gush, 1980). It has been observed that calves from a single pen system have a greater tendency to approach a novel stimulus than calves from a group-housing system. Calves from a group-housing system are equally likely: (1) to approach a novel stimulus, (2) to withdraw from it, or (3) to continue doing what they were doing at the time of stimulus presentation.

The completeness of exploration is an important distinction between normal and abnormal exploratory activities. Trigeminal denervated rats tested in novel situations showed initial exploratory sequences but they terminated these sooner than normal rats in the same situation. The time spent exploring was decreased and the resting time was increased following trigeminal orosensory denervation (Miller, 1981). The exploratory behaviour of socially deprived animals, regardless of how it may be initiated, is characteristically abbreviated. Incomplete exploration is a poor basis for adaptation and an animal with such a behavioural deficit must be at a biological disadvantage in many situations. Two relevant facts are clear: exploratory deficits will result in cognitive deficits, and associated fearfulness will probably create stress predisposition in various demanding husbandry situations.

Species-typical exploration

Cattle

One of the main features of exploratory behaviour in cattle is that it is effected by an animal only as long as the emotions of fear or apprehension are not present. The animal's curiosity is aroused when it sees an unfamiliar object or hears an unknown noise. What may induce exploratory behaviour in one animal may very often be ignored by another. Older animals, being more acquainted with the objects and sounds of their environment, are less curious and exploratory behaviour is therefore a more prominent characteristic of young animals. When curiosity is first aroused, the animal assumes a posture similar to that of surrender or submissiveness, but with nostrils quivering and sniffing. The size and nature of the object, in which the animal has become interested, determines the speed of approach. It sniffs the object and may lick it or even, if the object is malleable enough, chew and swallow it. This kind of exploratory behaviour is often induced by the sight of familiar objects in unfamiliar surroundings or vice versa. As mentioned above, however, the animal's curiosity is rarely followed through if it has any cause for fear or apprehension. It is a common finding that the most dominant cattle in herds are also the most exploratory (Kilgour, 1975). Isolation-rearing leads to inadequate social behaviour and subordinate positions in a rank order (Broom and Leaver, 1978), so it is not surprising that MacKay and Wood-Gush (1980) found such animals to be more fearful of novelty.

Sheep

In temperate conditions, a flock will set out into the pasture, moving together and then fanning out. However, although they may move some distance from each other, sheep will often form subgroups within the main flock and continue to exist as a concerted group, following a routine of movement around the grazing land. The rearing conditions influence the mode of behaviour lambs use to cope with a novel environment. Lambs raised in a social environment respond to novel situations by actively searching the area and interacting with the stimulus. In contrast, isolate-reared lambs reared in socially deprived environments attempt to avoid the stressful situation by showing withdrawal behaviour (Moberg and Wood, 1982).

Horses

A great deal of exploratory behaviour is shown by the newborn foal. This behaviour is directed towards the pasture, the ground, the premises and their boundaries and other objects in the environment within its touch. In the course of this exploratory activity the foal may nibble and mouth unfamiliar objects. Such keen exploratory behaviour is not shown to the same degree in adult horses, except between themselves. They nevertheless acquire familiarity with the area allocated to them. The home range becomes marked and mapped out by deposits of excreta. Preference for home range is very strong among horses and they typically show more willingness to be moved towards home than away from home.

Pigs

Much of the general activity of pigs appears to stem from their exploratory behaviour. They show very well developed exploratory behaviour, most of which is directed at objects at floor level which are investigated by sniffing, nibbling and rooting. Such actions may have a destructive effect on objects, where these are subject to continuous investigation by a group of pigs, which are severely restricted in their movements. This is apparently a contributing factor to the vice of tail-biting. The tendency to over-investigate specific items in their environment can be controlled to a degree by providing additional objects for investigation and some pig breeders, aware of this fact, provide growing pigs with objects to be used as toys. These include motor tyres and chains suspended from the ceiling. The provision of straw bedding also provides an alternative outlet for the investigatory activities of pigs.

Poultry

The domestic fowl in most modern systems of husbandry has no opportunity for exploratory activities, but birds at free range show a considerable amount of exploratory behaviour in the form of food-searching which may take them several hundred metres away from their home site in the course of each day in extreme cases. Birds also seek out suitable ground in which to settle and dust-bathe. Visual inspection of strange objects is carefully practised by the fowl. The fowl's vision is evidently good and it has been determined that the hen's colour vision is trichromatic and similar to human vision in the appraisal of colour. Under natural conditions hens will often seek out nesting sites in locations quite remote from the core area of their home range following territorial exploration.

13 Spacing behaviour

Spatial factors influence many activities of animals, especially when they are at pasture (Arnold and Dudzinski, 1978). The animal must maintain, use and negotiate space in order to fulfil basic physical and social requirements. Spacing of animals falls into two general types: (1) individual space which is defined in terms of the individual and hence moves with it, and (2) home range and territory which refer to a static area used by the animal. In order to appreciate why spacing behaviour occurs as it does the ecology of the animal must be considered (Dudzinski et al., 1978; Hediger, 1963). Spacing of social animals gives much information about social organisation and is subject to dynamic change as individuals adjust their relationships continually. Nevertheless, fixed social and individual distances give a group its characteristic nucleo-spatial architecture (McBride et al., 1969; Arnold et al., 1981; Hinch et al., 1982; Mankovich and Banks, 1982; McBride and Foenander, 1962). The spacing of the members of a social group at any moment depends upon the activities of the group members, as is clearly demonstrated by the work of Keeling and Duncan (1988) on domestic fowl.

Farm animals are "contact" species; they allow fairly close physical proximity between one another, except in special circumstances related to sexual, maternal and aggressive behaviour. The distance they maintain between themselves and other animals, especially poten-tial predators, is much greater. This latter *flight distance* is the radius of space within which the animal will not voluntarily permit the intrusion of man or other animals which might be dangerous. In domesticated animals the flight distance to man shrinks with appropriate husbandry and human socialisation (Done-Currie et al., 1983; Hutson, 1984). With good stockmanship involving careful contact it may disappear, but most farm animals retain some flight distance, or in other words they maintain an avoidance zone (Metz and Mekking, 1984). Sudden intrusion within this may cause an unexpected defensive reaction from the animal. Reactions to such intrusions include startle, alarm, fight-or-flight display and vocalisation (Craig et al., 1969; Syme et al., 1975).

When animals limit their movements to a home range this will include resources such as food. These resources will often be defended so that an area of land may become basically a substitute goal, representing the food, etc. it could provide. The farm animals function typically in herds or flocks whose group members possess varying values of social status permitting their integration into the group using common territory (O'Brien, 1984; Pamment et al., 1983; Salter and Hudson, 1982). Within the group there is usually a struggle for status in the social dominance order and this could be seen as a struggle for territorial property (Welsh, 1975). The term *agonistic behaviour* is often used for behaviour involving threat, attack or defence. However groups of farm animals like those liberated perenially into rural niches such as common grazings, ranges and ranches, devote little energy to fighting or threat. Through systems of social organisation, group harmony is a prominent feature of collective behaviour (Winfield *et al.*, 1981). Conspicuous features of group behaviour are social facilitation and synchrony of action so that the members of a group are often involved in the same activities.

Types of space

Home range

The home range is the area which the animal learns thoroughly and which it habitually uses. In some cases the home range may be the animal's total range. Within a home range, such as an extensive area of pasture, there may be a core area. This core is the area of heaviest regular use within the home range. The demarcation of a core area may not be too precise but generally includes resting areas.

Territory

A territory is an area which is defended by fighting, or by demarcation which other individuals detect so that the mark or other signal is a deterrent to entry. It need not be permanent, but in any relocation of an animal geographically, the new territory which the animal would require and seek would have to provide for requirements of nutrition, shelter, resting, watering, exercise, evacuation, periodic movement and defensive shifting. In many species, territories are used to attract a mate.

Individual space

Most animals actively preserve a minimum distance from themselves and attempt to prevent others from entering this space. This minimum distance, within which approach elicits attack or avoidance, was called the *individual distance* by Hediger (1941, 1955). It includes the physical space which the animal requires to occupy for its basic movements of lying, rising, standing, stretching and scratching. An example is seen whenever birds like gulls or swallows are standing in a line along a rail or wire. This space is somewhat expanded in the head region to accommodate the greater amount of movement of the head in the course of ingestion, grooming and gesturing.

The advantages of maintaining an individual space (Broom, 1981, p. 195) can include reductions in (1) damage to the body due to contact, (2) interference and competition whilst feeding, (3) impedance when starting to flee, (4) disease or parasite transmission, and (5) the chance of rape. Individual space can vary according to activity, for example Walther (1977) reported that male Thomson's gazelles walk 2 m apart, nest 3 m apart but graze 9 m apart. Walther considered that the high figure when grazing could be due to the similarity of the grazing posture to threat display, but problems of interference with grazing behaviour may also be a cause. The term social space is sometimes used for the individual space which is maintained by an active animal.

Association versus avoidance

Although farm animals maintain individual space and sometimes defend territories, they also actively remain close to certain other individuals. Some of such association is between mother and offspring (Chapter 24). Other association is between animals reared together or between animals which form a set attachment later in life. Calves reared together are much more likely to be recorded as associating than are those from different rearing groups (Broom and Leaver, 1978; Bouissou, personal communication). Pairs of cows which spend much time close together and often also mutually groom one another have been described by Benham (1984).

A special type of spacing behaviour results when individuals with close bonds arrange themselves so that they establish a "distance to nearest neighbour". Domestic herbivores, when grazing, maintain close contact with one and possibly other individuals but the distance to that nearest neighbour varies much less than distances to other individuals in the group. In 60–70% of animals an individual is the nearest neighbour of its nearest neighbour. This gives a spatial structure of pairs of individuals within a group, the spatial association with one other individual being stronger than any other type. In free-ranging situations the distance to second-nearest neighbour can vary considerably, whereas the nearest neighbour distance varies much less because of common pairings.

When farm animals of different species are kept in a field together they may utilise the area similarly for grazing so the nearest neighbour of a horse could sometimes be a cow. However, they normally rest in single species groups.

Spatial needs

Spatial needs in farm animals are both quantitative and qualitative (Box, 1973; Petherick, 1983a). Quantitative needs relate to space occupation, social distance, flight distance and actual territory. Qualitative needs relate to space-dependent activities such as eating, body care, exploration, kinetics and social behaviour. It is often necessary for animals to remove themselves from visual contact with others. Hence the quality of space includes the presence of barriers, places where the head can be put so that others are not seen, or dark places where concealment from an aggressor can occur.

The minimum spatial need is for that amount of room which physical size and basic movements require. Even the stalled animal, for example, needs distances of length, breadth and height in which to stand, lie and articulate its major parts, including head, neck and limbs. In the acts of raising and lowering the body, the animal is required to make forward and backward movements (Baxter and Schwaller, 1983). During these, the weight, or the centre of gravity, is shifted strategically to or from the forequarters or hindquarters. The animal uses the weight either as a counterbalance in rising or as a direct pull in lying. Another need for length is in stretching the head and neck forward and one or other hind limb backward. Lateral articulation of the head and neck is still another frequent and necessary form of movement. In lying the animal's need for space is increased through partial rolling of the body and the extension of hind limbs. The requirements for such movements are described in detail for cows by Cermak (1987).

As well as physical space, there is an extension of personal space into that invisible but recognisable room which the animal maintains in many social situations. This space is used to keep some separation between itself and others of its kind—its conspecifics. In ranging animals this space is continuously adjusted by changing physical relationships. It is preserved in many instances by gestures of threat or intention. Among the farm animals this space is often subject to compression, through enforced grouping. It appears that the last portion of this personal space to be surrendered under such circumstances is a "bubble" of space about the head. Destruction, or long-term loss, of this head space leads to futile negotiation of interpersonal spatial needs and increases the incidence of aggressive exchanges within an enclosed group. In cattle this head space appears to be about one metre in radius at its optimum. As with other spatial needs, individual space, including head space, can be surrendered without manifest aggression in a variety of circumstances such as short-term crowding and resting.

Corners are important features of enclosures and apparently increase the conceptual space of an enclosure. The square has more preferred space than the triangle and the triangle more than the circle. Group size, available area, stocking density and shape of the available area are all variables that influence spatial need. However, where aggression occurs, corners may be places of danger for weak, subordinate animals. This has been clearly demonstrated for poultry in group-housing systems where corners are best avoided. A curved barrier can be used to exclude access to corners.

Crowding

Groups of individuals whose movements are restricted by the physical presence of others are said to be *crowded*. A high density means more likelihood that one animal will come closer to another than its individual distance. As a consequence, the intrusion into individual space may result in an aggressive response or an avoidance reaction which, in turn, results in a further such intrusion. Crowding does not necessarily result in increased agonistic behaviour but it often does so. If a high social density causes adverse effects on the fitness of individuals then the term *over-crowding* is used. However, as Stokols (1972) points out, some animals can be crowded without being over-crowded. The distribution of resources is of great importance in determining whether or not individuals are adversely affected by high density. Crowding in the presence of many food sources, shelter sites, etc. can lead to no adverse effects whilst local crowding around a single food source can be harmful to some of the animals present. In all situations it is essential to consider the quality of living space (Box, 1973), as well as the social density.

Crowding has an effect on how much animals move about. As broiler chickens get older they fill the space in which they are kept. Newberry and Hall (1988) monitored the movements of chickens from 4–9 weeks old at the low stocking density of 0.134 m^2 per bird. The area occupied per week declined from 134 to 49 m^2 and the distance moved per hour declined from 4.5 to

2.3 m as the space available declined. If the stocking density was increased to a space allowance of only 0.067 or 0.041 m^2 per bird, the decline in movement was more rapid.

Very high densities of rodents can lead to adrenal hypertrophy, high blood pressure, kidney failure, impaired immune responses and reproductive failure (Christian, 1955, 1961; Calhoun, 1962a, b). The effects of crowding on production and welfare of farm animals have been reviewed by Syme and Syme (1979) and are discussed in Chapters 37–39. Crowding of cockerels results in reduced weight gain in cockerels (Craig and Polley, 1977). The optimum density for growth and egg production in poultry results in the average individual being healthy and not subject to serious attack by others in the group but the weakest individual in that group may be badly pecked or often unable to feed in the same conditions (Broom, 1981, p. 262). Crowding of pigs increases fighting (Ewbank and Bryant, 1972), lowers food consumption (Bryant and Ewbank, 1974) and reduces food conversion efficiency (Heitman *et al.*, 1961). Bryant (1972) recommends a minimum area per pig of 0.7 m^2 for pigs of 50 kg fed ad libitum in order to avoid overcrowding.

High social density is not the only factor in grouped livestock which can increase competitive behaviour and lead to adverse effects on individuals. A large number of individuals in the group can also have such effects. Al Rawi and Craig (1975), working with domestic hens, reported that for a constant cage floor space allocation of 0.4 m^2 per bird, the frequency of aggressive pecks was three times higher if group-size was 28 than if it was 8. Individual hens interacted with each other bird and at this density such interactions involved much pecking. When group-size is increased further, however, birds cannot move around to interact with each other individual. Craig and Guhl (1969) found that the frequency of competitive interactions did not increase when group size was increased from 100 to 400 at constant stocking density.

Spacing behaviour of farm animals

Cattle

Cattle show territorial aggressive acts by butting or threatening to butt. In defending their head space they "hook" with sharp oblique head swings. Bulls are prone to practise more spectacular territorial behaviour than cows. In small paddocks, bulls become strongly territorial, a behavioural feature which is age related. Strong territorial behaviour becomes a feature of bull behaviour at about four years of age. In the territorial display of the bull they dig the soil with their fore feet, scooping loose soil over their backs. They horn ruts into the soil, rubbing their heads along the ground. At the conclusion of the display they stand and bellow repeatedly. It is common for a specially selected site, or stand, which may be a prominence of land, to be used for this display.

Beef cattle under high crowding conditions in pens show clear preferences for certain locations with their pens. They tend to position themselves around the outer edges and corners of pens. The central areas of pens are less often occupied. The fact that the animals use the outside suggests that the ratio of perimeter to area of enclosure is important. The more crowded the animals, the greater the importance this relationship is likely to be in alleviating crowding. The amount of area needed per animal also depends on features of the enclosure. Beef animals on slatted floors require less area per individual than others on solid floors. In a sense, the area beneath the slats serves as extra space by reducing space otherwise occupied by excreta. Increasing the viewing area, across aisles for example, serves to meet some perceptual spatial need.

Distances between subgroups in cattle increase as forage conditions deteriorate but individual space is maintained even on rangeland and on intensive pasture. Bulls are often located on the margins of the herd. Bulls require a great social distance at relatively younger ages than steers, and the presence of heifers increases the distance between bulls, at the same time reducing herd scatter. Among housed dairy cows where a choice of stall is available, preferences may develop. Dominant cows prefer to occupy adjacent stalls while lower ranking cows avoid stalls previously occupied by dominant cows.

Spacing patterns in cattle are very similar to those in sheep. Dairy cows under intensive pasture conditions have a modal distance to nearest neighbour of 8.8 m. Free-moving cattle on extensive rangeland in Northern Australia have an average value of 9.2 m for nearest neighbour spacings. Again "pairing" tends to occur, especially on rangeland where the distance to second-nearest neighbour can be greatly increased.

Cows when lying mostly keep within 2–3 m of one another, compared with 4–10 m when grazing. In unlimited grazing space, bulls have a greater social distance than steers with individual space averaging a 25 m radius. Cows lower in social status tend to keep on the periphery of the group. Under crowded conditions, spatial arrangements may change and cows low in social dominance rank may then move about more than those in higher rank, apparently to avoid impinging on the individual space of dominant animals. In such crowded conditions the individual distance of high-ranking cows is greater than that of low-ranking cows. With a small idling area, frequency of urination increases, particularly amongst the low-ranking cows.

Horses

In territorial aggression, horses fight with their own typical offensive and defensive weapons (Arnold and Grassia, 1982.) They may bite, kick out with their hind feet and strike with their fore feet when the flight distance is violated. Both hind feet may be kicked out, for example, after backing up to the intruder. The double kick is delivered directly to the rear without aim. Kicking out defensively, with one hind limb, is sometimes called the mule kick, although it is used by horse-kind generally. The mule kick is a precisely directed kick with one hind foot. The farm species often share a common territory such as a grazing area, without interspecific aggression. Horses, however, may show aggression to cattle and sheep grazing with them by biting, kicking or chasing them.

Free-ranging horses spend much of their time grazing, about 12 h or more being common. In relatively arid areas, horses often travel very long distances daily to water. Their grazing range, under these conditions, is probably limited by the availability of water. When snow is on the ground horses can obtain fluid by eating it and are then independent of running water and can utilise different ranges. In free-ranging horses, trips to water and salt each day are a requirement. Horses will also show preference for certain areas of shade if there is a choice.

Ponies grazing on moorland areas have home ranges which are often shared or which overlap considerably. Summer and winter ranges may overlap or be separate but, in general, different areas have different intensities of use at different times of the year according to their ecological value to the animals.

Equine behaviour includes territorial rituals. Stallions pass faeces in specific sites where their dung may become heaped. All horses use certain territorial spots for defaecation. These areas are not grazed. A restricted grazing territory for horses soon becomes divided up into "lawns" and "roughs". The lawns are the areas closely cropped and the roughs are the dung areas which remain ungrazed, except in starvation conditions.

Sheep

Sheep threaten one another by means of head movements. If no submissive response occurs they may push, butt or tug at wool. Amongst animals which know one another well, however, a look suffices as a threat and leads to avoid-ance. In sheep, spacing among individuals varies considerably with breed and location. In extensive moorland and mountain country, sheep keep a greater distance apart than sheep on lowland ground. This may be a matter of adaptation or the result of the wider dispersion of suitable food. In situations of dispersion, e.g. mountainous areas, the modal distance to the second-nearest neighbour is three times that to the nearest neighbour on lowland grazing. This is the result of the persistence of "pairing" which is a feature of permanent hill flocks. If a flock is dispersed for any reason, pairs and small groups still go around together so social cohesiveness is preserved. Within each flock home range, there is a series of overlapping home ranges, each with its group of sheep.

In the main, sheep tend to form groups which remain in a particular area. In hilly country sheep "bed down" on hills themselves and move to the hillier areas, if possible, during winter. In hot weather they seek out the shade of bushes and trees and areas close to water. Although these home ranges are specific in the areas covered, neighbouring sheep may share common ground and small numbers of sheep often settle down along a boundary, or in a corner of a small grazing area common to another small group from an adjacent pasture. Although rams also have specific areas in which they tend to remain, their boundaries are less clearly defined than those of ewes, and they may change their locale just prior to their breeding season.

The associations formed between individual sheep in natural flocks of Dorset Horn, Merino and Southdown sheep were studied in Australia (Arnold *et al.*, 1981). When the Dorset Horns were grazing, the associations between individuals were within "feeding" home ranges. In the Southdown, the individuals associating together used widely dispersed areas of the paddock, rather than one general area. Merinos dispersed into subgroups only under extreme food shortage and then the sex and age groups segregated as in the other two breeds. Wide variations evidently occur between these breeds of sheep in their spatial organisation. In one

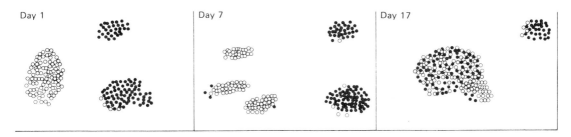

Day 1   Day 7   Day 17

Fig. 13.1   When two groups of 100 Merino ewes were put together at a density of 15/ha, they rested (camped) as shown on the first, seventh and seventeenth days. Complete flock integration took 20 days (from Broom, 1981, modified after McBride *et al.*, 1967).

critical study the inter-pair distances in two-breed combinations were measured in an open field at the beginning and end of a two week period. Sheep from a mixed-breed group showed no preference to be nearer sheep from any breed group, but those from separated groups developed a preference to be nearer members of their own group. Overall, these observations show that, irrespective of breed, flocks of sheep drawn from different sources do not readily integrate into a socially homogeneous group. Even when sheep of the same breed, but from different flocks, are mixed they may take a long time to integrate (McBride *et al.*, 1967). The effect is shown by Fig. 13.1.

In the Merino, in which subgroups rarely form, home ranges develop only when food shortage forces the group to disperse more widely. Otherwise, the Merino sheep does not develop home ranges even under the most extensive conditions. The difference is probably due to a varietal difference in flocking behaviour since Merino sheep form close flocks and remain as a single flock if they can maintain visual contact. They move around the environment as a single unit in most circumstances. Sheep of other breeds, e.g. Scottish Blackface, form subgroups under nearly all conditions, and all breeds of sheep that form home ranges have this characteristic.

Modal distances in metres between nearest neighbours in sheep of different breeds show a range from 4 to 8.6 on mountain and moorland

and from 3.4 to 4.4 on lowland grazing. These figures show that pairings are readily formed by sheep and they can be managed better in pairs. For example, the design of the transition zone from a pen to a race can be improved by allowing two sheep to enter the race in parallel.

Pigs

Pigs threaten to obtain or defend space by means of head movements which may be followed by barking, pushing with the nose and shoulder barges if no submissive response is given (Jensen, 1982, 1984). The stocking density in groups of pigs is known to have various effects upon their behaviour. Social encounters in penned pigs take place most often at or near the food source. These social encounters lead to clear-cut results when a hierarchical system has previously been well-established. When growing pigs are allocated only about 0.75 m^2 of pen each, there is a rise in severity of social encounters. When the stocking density is any higher than this it is found that individual pigs, which are low in the social hierarchy, are unable to avoid the consequences of aggressive encounters. The productivity of the unit is thus adversely affected.

Pigs, more than other farm animals, practise intense contact behaviour and show comparatively little territorialism except under feral or semi-feral conditions. The space in the region around the head, however, tends to be preserved by most animals. In addition, members of a group often observe a "social limit" which is the maximum distance any animal will move away from the group. They do require space, however, to employ avoidance tactics that mitigate aggression. The recognition, when managing pigs, of an "avoidance system" in the social behaviour of pigs is very important.

Avoidance is an inverse response in agonistic situations and it is the positive factor affecting agonistic control. The generally accepted belief that aggression establishes and operates the social system is inadequate. The avoidance behaviour, which often occurs in the absence of any aggressive act, is the vital component of the behavioural mechanism which generates social stabilisation. Of course, avoidance is an overall strategy which calls for specific behavioural tactics, and these tactics need space for their practical operation.

Poultry

Territorial behaviour which changes with season occurs in feral domestic fowl. In the breeding phase, well-defined territories are held by dominant males where they mate with the females which then raise a brood nearby in a home range. For the rest of the year each male has a harem, and the harems utilise overlapping home ranges (McBride *et al.*, 1969; Duncan *et al.*, 1978). Chickens even display home range behaviour under intensive conditions.

Site attachment has been observed in domestic fowl housed in flocks of 200–400 hens. The further a bird moves from the centre of its area, the fewer birds it pecks and the more birds it is pecked by. Thus, pecking pressure appeared to operate as a reinforcer, maintaining each bird within its site of attachment. Observations have been made of male spacing, mating and

agonistic behaviours in pens of mated domestic fowl and site attachment is found with cocks living close to the wall. High-ranking males appear to move over smaller areas than do low-ranking males. In small pens (1.85 m² per cock) the effects of fixed sites were negligible.

Cock crowing is considered to be a territorial pronouncement. With adequate territory, cock crowing is usually limited, notably to early morning. Where cockerels are crowded together and actual territory is nil, as in battery systems for artificial insemination purposes, excessive crowing is a remarkable and disturbing feature. Large flocks of hens do not have an even dispersal of their individuals, but their spatial distribution is evidently not random. A territorial arrangement of flock members seems dependent on facial alignment of nearby birds so that a preferred angle of between 90 degrees and 180 degrees is kept. Birds which may be generating additional stimuli through physical or behavioural characteristics are given great distance. Territorial organisation of flocks is evident in free-ranging birds and, when territories overlap, agonistic encounters will occur in that area. It has been found that hens in laying cages, given extra viewing area, show less behavioural evidence of stress.

Threats by dominant neighbours depend on the distance between the males and the orientation of the mating subordinate towards the dominant bird. Clear trends are not always evident in detailed spatial analyses of data on poultry activity, but studies confirm that there is differential use of areas by individuals. High-ranking birds are frequently in front of and beside the food dispenser but the perch is not monopolised by the high-ranking animals. It in fact is used heavily by the lowest ranked animal. The second-lowest ranking animal spends a great deal of time on the cage floor very near the perch. Thus the perch seems to serve as a sort of refuge rather than a controlling position.

14 Rest and sleep

Passive punctuation of behavioural sequences with less active periods interspersed among the most energy-consuming phases produces rhythms of living (Hartman, 1973; Ruckebusch, 1974). Inactive behaviours are functional as tactics of temporal organisation and self-conservation (Allison and Cichetti, 1976). In their simplest forms, self-conserving tactics include *ad hoc* resting and short-term inactivity (Horne, 1977; Petre-Quadens and Schlag, 1974).

In the examination of inactive behaviour, various forms are seen in practice (Balch, 1955; Bell, 1960; Blokhuis, 1983, 1984; Carson and Wood-Gush, 1983b; Faure and Jones, 1982a, b) (Table 14.1). In this variation, similarities are seen between species and some species-specific characteristics also occur (Howard, 1972; Klemm, 1966; Petherick, 1983b; Ruckebusch *et al.*, 1974). Inactivity is much more obvious in the intensive methods of animal agriculture. Most of these production systems provide an abundant supply of food and water, while in extensive animal husbandary, food requires time to be foraged. Concentrated compounded food can be consumed in much less time than roughage and, in the ruminants, less digestive time in rumination is required. All of this creates time, free from ingestive work, in which inactivity, such as idling, flourishes as an ethological phenomenon.

All healthy animals stand idling or lie down each day to rest. A significant proportion of life is spent at rest (Meddis, 1975). Resting and sleeping are governed by timing controls, more obviously than certain other cyclic activities (McGrath and Cohen, 1978; Yeates, 1963). The function of rest and sleep may originally have been to minimise the danger of predation when active behaviour was not necessary. An immobile individual in an inconspicuous position is less likely to be detected. However, sleep is shown by predators as well as prey. A second function must be energy conservation. For some kinds of animals and in some circumstances a function may be restorative, allowing metabolic recovery. Whatever the evolutionary origin, this system, requiring periods of passive behaviour, is of critical importance in the maintenance of the animal and receives high priority in environments to which the animal is adjusted (Mayes, 1983).

A biological clock evidently exists that measures time and issues temporal signals to the rest of the body (Allison and van Twyer, 1970; Aston-Jones, 1981). At the cellular level there appear to be cyclic variations in macromolecules within the cell (Merrick and Sharp, 1971). Rhythms of brain activity also occur (Table 14.2). Rhythmic activity is also a feature of the endocrine system. Of fundamental significance is the fact that levels of deoxyribonucleic acid (DNA) and ribonucleic acid (RNA) show rhythmical diurnal changes. A master clocking

Table 14.1
Common terms and forms of inactive behaviour

Term	Behavioural forms
Idling	Stationary standing for an extended period with some limited limb-shifting and positional changing. The animal may be using available time free of active maintenance requirements. Idling may simply take the form of passively waiting for the next phase of an established husbandry routine, such as milking.
	The term loafing is essentially similar in meaning but has been reserved mainly for ruminant inactivity in the standing position in which no rumination (as evidenced by "cudding") is taking place. Ruminant loafing is under strong social facilitation in herds and flocks. A specific pastoral locus is often used in this behaviour when it becomes established in habit.
Drowsing	A stable state of wakefulness in which there are signs of light sleep with head movement and eye closure. The animal is in an inactive state in one of certain variable postures. The animal may have a fully upright stance, such as is usual in the horse. Sitting on the sternum is a common postural form of drowsing in several other species, including cattle. In the latter case, no cudding would occur. Dogs will lie on the sternum with the fore legs flexed under, or extended with the head positioned between them. In poultry the neck is withdrawn and the tail held down.
Resting	Typically, rest is taken in a recumbent posture with evident wakefulness. In rest, the recumbency is seldom lateral. The fore legs are flexed beneath the thorax and the spinal column is held in a lateral arc in which the head may be carried round to the side of the body.
Sleeping	Sleep is seen as evident somnolence often in extended recumbency. The usual sleep position is flat on the side with legs extended. True sleep occurs in the form of both "brain sleep" with (electroencephalogram delta waves) and "paradoxical sleep". In the latter, rapid eye movements (REM) can be seen below the closed lids. Minor leg movements also occur, especially of the distal limb and the digits.

Table 14.2
Types of EEG waves in mammalian brains

Type	Rate	Site	Behaviour
Alpha rhythm	Medium	Neocortex	Relaxed wakefulness
Beta activity	Medium/fast	Neocortex	Alert wakefulness
Delta waves	Very slow	Neocortex	REM sleep; deep sleep
Theta activity	Slow	Hippocampal formation	Deliberate activity; orientation
Sleep spindles	Medium	Neocortex	Drowsing moderately; deep sleep
Olfactory rhythm	Fast	Olfactory bulb; pyriform cortex	Alert

system in the body seems to exist which adapts the rhythms of organs and cells to the environmental temporal cues such as photoperiod stimuli. Cells in the lateral hypothalamus show a diurnal rhythm of responsiveness to stimulation. The reticular formation may programme sleep and wakefulness but the suprachiasmatic nucleus in mammals and the pineal in birds are clearly of major importance in the control of rhythms.

Two forms of sleep exist: brain sleep (slow-wave sleep or quiet sleep), and the sleep of the body (paradoxical or rapid eye movement sleep, REM). Slow-wave sleep (SWS) is quiet sleep in which EEGs show a low level of electrical activity in the brain. Paradoxical sleep is so called because of the paradox of manifest sleep in association with electrical activity in the brain typical of wakefulness. Paradoxical sleep is also characterised by rapid eye movement (REM). The two types can best be differentiated from wakefulness and from each other by electroencephalograms. In slow-wave sleep, the EEG is characterised by synchronous electrical waves of high voltage and slow activity. In paradoxical sleep the EEG shows low voltage and fast activity similar to that seen in the wakeful state, but there is very little muscular activity and the animal is more difficult to arouse than when it is in SWS. During body sleep, or paradoxical sleep, the muscles of the eyes frequently contract, hence the term rapid eye movement (REM) sleep.

Light stimuli are transmitted via the optic nerve ultimately to the pineal gland which is evidently an intermediary unit in the synchronisation of diurnal rhythms of behaviour. Signals from the pineal body may travel to the medial forebrain and the reticular formation of the spinal cord, thus influencing the behavioural predisposition of the organism.

Sleep alters the distribution and the patterning of neuronal activity in the brain. Although the brain consumes energy, it does not perform physical work on the environment. Instead, it processes information and diverts neuronal metabolism largely to vital functions. The following sleep stages have been defined:

Awake: Normal responsiveness to stimuli. EEG either beta activity or alpha rhythm.

Drowsing: A transitional state in which the animal is sluggish. The EEG is irregular in rhythm and of variable low to medium voltage in amplitude.

Light sleep: EEG shows sleep spindles. Animal is readily awakened.

Moderately deep sleep: Sleep spindles interrupted by delta waves and there are rapid eye movements (REM).

Deep sleep: The EEG tracing consists entirely of delta waves. This stage, can include REM, paradoxical, activated or desynchronized sleep and is distinct from the other forms of sleep.

The depth of sleep is usually determined in terms of the intensity of stimulation, usually of a sound stimulus, required to awaken the sleeping animal and increases in the order given above.

REM sleep occurs in all mammals but not all the manifestations of REM sleep are exactly alike in all species. Animals are more difficult to arouse from REM than from other sleep states. Heart beat and breathing tend to be more irregular and on the average faster during REM

than during non-REM sleep. Even though phasic movements are common, postural muscle tone diminishes, especially in the muscles of the trunk, neck and shoulder. While the rate of cerebral metabolism is slightly lower in non-REM sleep than in the awake state, in REM sleep it is slightly higher.

These multiple changes in cerebral and somatic functions have suggested that REM sleep is in some fundamental way different from the other sleep stages. Thus pineal melatonin is present in higher quantities in plasma at night. Melatonin levels also appear to be the link between the photoperiod and annual cycles of sexual activity. Day length influences the relative amounts of body serotonin, a precursor of melatonin, and melatonin present in the pineal. These influence the organism's resting behaviour.

The build-up of serotonin may induce drowsiness and sleep. Experimentally, cerebrospinal fluid of sleep-deprived goats induced sleep in rats. Clinically, tryptophan, a precursor of serotonin, may be used to induce sleep. Acetylcholine has been implicated as the neurotransmitter responsible for wakefulness and noradrenaline that for REM sleep.

General rest and sleep

While it may be perfectly valid to count as secondary benefits of sleep the recovery of tired body systems, or the behavioural advantage of staying out of sight of enemies, there is evidence that processes occurring during sleep contribute to the health of the brain.

There are two possible ways in which sleep can serve cerebral functions:

1. It could be that during sleep, neural materials that were consumed during waking are recovered or resynthesised.
2. It may be that during sleep neural waste products that have accumulated are eliminated.

However, the sleeping brain is not inactive

but sensitive methods of estimating glucose metabolism in animal brains have shown that overall metabolic activity is reduced in two distinct states: slow-wave sleep (SWS) and REM state. Slow-wave sleep in this context includes all four sleep stages already defined. It has been suggested that in REM state the forebrain is aroused, although disconnected from the lower CNS. Disconnection implies that sensory stimuli are less readily registered and that motor commands are not reaching lower motor circuits as shown by decreased muscle tone. The brief movements frequently made in REM sleep are considered to originate from CNS structures other than the forebrain, such as the brain stem.

Young animals not only sleep more than older ones and adults, they also spend a large fraction of their time in REM sleep. The time spent in REM and total sleeping time varies among adults, but it is relatively stable for any one individual. Lost REM time disturbs animals and there is some reason to believe that REM sleep is important in some specific way. It has been suggested that brain tissue in the REM state performs some essential function for which it has little or no opportunity in either the waking or the SWS state. Perhaps in REM state the traces required for long-term storage of memory are being consolidated. Certainly learning can be hindered by depriving an animal of REM sleep.

The problem with this brain recuperation theory is that animals of some species sleep much less than others and some individual people are able to go for many months without sleeping. Perhaps the recuperative processes can occur during non-sleep states, even if they are normally best carried out during sleep.

Control of the sleep–wake cycle

A little more is known about the control of the sleep–wake cycle than about its biological function. Several theories have been proposed. The most conspicuous feature of sleeping is its regular alternation with waking. Consequently much study centres on the biological clock that drives the sleep–wake cycle. Best known is the theory that the forebrain is alerted by the excitation of the reticular formation of the mesencephalon and pons. In one series of experiments large electrolytic lesions were made in the brain stem. If such lesions destroyed the reticular formation of the upper midbrain on both sides, the animals did not wake up from general anaesthesia, but remained comatose with EEG dominated by sleep spindles and delta waves. Other animals had stimulating electrodes implanted in the midbrain reticular formation, but their brains remained otherwise intact. Low-intensity, high-frequency electrical stimulation through these electrodes easily woke these animals not only from natural sleep, but also, transiently, from light general anaesthesia.

The circuits believed to be involved in controlling the alert state of the animal became known as the ascending reticular activating (or arousal) system, sometimes abbreviated to ARAS. Excitation of this system puts the forebrain in the alerted state. The reticular formation of the upper brain stem is, in fact, the normal pacemaker of the sleep–wake cycle. Left to its own devices, the forebrain would lapse into sleep characterised by the spindle bursts and the delta waves of the cortex. Excitation in the ascending reticular system seemingly acts on thalamic nuclei, and through them on the cerebral cortex, causing the desynchronisation of the EEG, behavioural alerting and awakening of the animal.

Hippocampal theta rhythm occurs only when the neocortex is desynchronised. These hippocampal theta waves are related to one or more of the following behavioural states:

1. Orienting and exploring,
2. Active locomotion such as walking,
3. Any purposive voluntary movement,
4. High emotional arousal, with or without movement.

These are the main features of the alert condition which contrasts and alternates with sleep. It appears that some clock-like oscillator seems to engage and disengage the reticular activating system, allowing the forebrain sleep overnight and alerting it in the day.

In addition to electrical impulses involving the brain stem, sleep has neurochemical dependence. This concerns the serotonergic neuron system originating in the raphe nuclei of the brain stem. The ascending connections of some serotonergic neurons appear to induce sleep, especially slow-wave sleep.

A sleep-inducing serotonergic system is evident from experiments in which serotonin-deficient animals were shown to sleep little, or at least less than normally, and interventions that enhanced the activity of central serotonin systems caused increased sleep. It has been suggested that central noradrenergic circuits, with cells originating in the locus coeruleus, are also responsible for REM sleep. A hypothetical circadian clock would engage the serotonin system which initiates slow-wave sleep, and once slow-wave sleep is in progress, the noradrenergic system would begin a cycle of its own. Each time the noradrenaline cycle reached its high point it would interrupt slow-wave sleep and induce an REM period. The aminergic brain-stem relationship with the reticular formation may be the mechanism of a biological clock.

In keeping with the role of monoamines in regulating the overall level of alerting the forebrain, monoaminergic fibre terminals often do not form proper synapses with individual neurons, but end in a series of beads or varicosities apparently broadcasting transmitter substance among many cells. The varicosities of the axons may or may not have synaptic junctions. At non-junctional sites the monoamine becomes expressed into the extra-neuronal tissues where concentrations can build up and become diffuse to establish a permeated inter-neuronal chemical state. Such a situation would be entirely consistent with the neurobiology of sleep in all respects.

General idling

General observations on farm animal behaviour can hardly fail to take note of the fairly common occurrence of groups of stationary livestock in a somnolent state. Cattle and sheep take up stationary resting attitudes while ruminating. This may occupy about 5 h of each day, but there are periods of wakeful rest without rumination. Observers of such periods have referred to this behaviour as "loafing", or "idling". The terms are used to describe the circumstances when there is no active grazing and the animal remains standing at rest without ruminating. Such events are variable in time of occurrence and in duration.

Although the absence of ruminating highlights loafing behaviour in the ruminants, this type of inactivity can also be easily observed in the simple-stomached domesticated animals, notably the horse. Loafing is typical of ungulates, and such observations on this behaviour, as have been noted, refer exclusively to hoofed livestock. Perhaps the upright inactive stance is useful for rest (Rugh *et al.*, 1984) and is a basic use of the hoof. No other type of foot is as suitable as the hoof in stationary positions on surfaces of various types and conditions, ranging from mud to ice. The single hoof of the horse is better than the cloven hoof for high-speed locomotion, but the equine limb is also well-designed for stance. In the horse, support in standing is provided by arrangements of ligaments and tendons which form strong, flexible, elastic supports. This helps the animal maintain a standing position with very little muscular effort. Both fore and hind limbs have the "stay apparatus", which is mainly ligamentous, while the "check" and "reciprocal" apparatuses, in the fore and hind, respectively, are composed of structures which are either completely tendinous or are tendinous projections of certain leg muscles. Both stay and check apparatuses function mainly to support the fetlock joints, and bind and brace the sesamoid bones, and are clearly well-named. The suspensory ligaments of both fore and hind limbs assist in this.

The reciprocal apparatus is both muscular and tendinous, being made up of an extensor and a flexor muscle with the long tendinous insertion of each. These muscles (peronous tertius in front and superficial digital flexor behind) are in combination with the distal ends of both the femur and the tarsus to form a parallelogram, which causes the stifle and hock joints to articulate in unison. Thus, if the stifle is maintained in extension, the distal leg will bear the weight of the horse with little additional muscular effort. Horses are thus able to drowse, and even engage in slow-wave sleep, while standing.

Although they "idle" in stationary standing poses, cattle, unlike horses, are unable to rest satisfactorily in an upright stance for extended periods. They therefore become fatigued more severely when movements or husbandry disturbances prohibit recumbency. Sternal or lateral recumbency can be variants of ungulate idling; cattle certainly "sit" sternally at rest, without ruminating. Other animals, such as birds, have different postural tactics—in the forms of roosting, or squatting, for example.

Although it is unusual to see all the members of a group of horses lying down at one time, they idle simultaneously. The element of social facilitation, or group effect, is clearly one major factor which is operant in resting behaviour in most groups of animals. When animals lie down together, they appear to surrender readily their individual, portable space. Idling may be a form of active group behaviour, serving as a buffer against social stressors and serving as a behavioural mechanism for stress alleviation.

Drowsing

The condition of drowsing as a phenomenon is widely recognised in farm animals (Fraser, 1983); it has been studied by Ruckebusch (1972b). Drowsiness is a definite stable state of wakefulness, as opposed to alert wakefulness. The state of wakefulness occupies 85% of the 24-h period in the herbivorous species but only

67% in pigs. Cows spend the greater proportion of this wakeful period in the state of drowsiness than do horses. A considerable amount of the wakeful period of farm animals well-accustomed to their environments is spent in the drowsy state, when they are not asleep or actively ingesting or searching for food (Fig. 14.1). In drowsing the threshold to audio stimulation remains low. Cows and sheep frequently ruminate while drowsing.

Drowsing or somnolence may be defined as an intermediary state between wakefulness and slow-wave sleep characterised by a small decrease in muscular tone and respiratory rates. It is a stable, wakeful state which ends in an abrupt transition to either wakefulness or slow-wave sleep.

During their respective circadian cycles different species exhibit different amounts of drowsing. The ratio of drowsing to total wakefulness is smallest in the horse, both during the 24-h period (9.1%) and during the night (26.6%). The largest ratio of drowsing to wakefulness occurs in the cow, which is 96% drowsing at night. The pig has the greatest number of periods of drowsing with a total of 52 periods of brief duration and a total time of about 5 h per 24 h. Horses exhibit a large number of periods also and record the shortest duration, averaging approximately 3.7 min. Sheep and cows show approximately the same number of periods, but those in cows are of much longer duration (mean 18.8 min). Drowsing occurs in occasional daily periods in poultry (Hishikawa *et al.*, 1969). The hen drowses in a squatting position and drowsing phases are interspersed with true sleep when birds perch on roosting places at night (Ookawa, 1972; Ookawa and Gotoh, 1964).

Horses, cattle and sheep spend approximately 85% of the 24-h period in either wakefulness or drowsing. An equilibrium seems to exist between these two states. In the horse the shift is towards wakefulness, in the cow towards drowsing. This is possibly associated with the different temperaments of these two animals. The proportion of drowsing can be increased in a single individual when in a protected environment, as

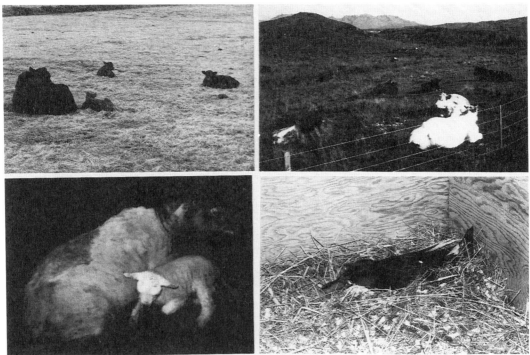

Fig. 14.1 Resting forms. Top left: "stayer" cow and lying-out calves. Top right: group-effected rumination in beef cows. Bottom left: resting in close contact — ewe and lamb. Bottom right: duck nesting/resting.

is the case in domesticated breeds. Drowsing is the most common feature of wakefulness in adult ruminants (cattle and sheep) and even in the sheep foetus near term electroencephalography (EEG) clearly shows brief phases of drowsing and sleep (Ruckebusch, 1972a). In adult sheep, spindling characterises the EEG pattern of drowsing. Cows reached a greater depth of drowsing than the other species which gives this species some of its ethos.

Data on farm animal sleep

General

In the definitive studies on sleep in farm animals by Ruckebusch, horses slept only during the night, cows and sheep mostly at night. With regard to position, horses spent the majority of this time standing, i.e. 80%, sheep 60%, while cows and pigs assumed a recumbent attitude, 87% and 89%, respectively. In addition, pigs spend a very high proportion of their daylight hours in recumbency (Table 14.3, Fig. 14.2).

Ruckebusch and Bell (1970) observed that sleep was generally distributed in two or three periods during the night, and during each of these periods transition from slow-wave sleep to paradoxical sleep was usually repeated three or four times. Paradoxical sleep occurred in horses, cows and sheep only during the night-time, but in pigs it was not restricted to this period and these animals had a higher incidence of sleep than the other species except when preoccupied with food.

Table 14.3
Hours per day spent awake, drowsing and sleeping in horses, cattle, sheep and pigs

Animal	Diurnal period	Awake	Drowsing	Sleeping
Horses	Day-time	12.9	0.9	0.6
	Night-time	5.3	1.5	2.8
	Total	18.2	2.4	3.4
Cattle	Day-time	10.6	1.2	0.2
	Night-time	1.9	6.3	3.8
	Total	12.5	7.5	4.0
Sheep	Day-time	10.0	1.6	0.6
	Night-time	5.9	2.7	3.2
	Total	15.9	4.3	3.8
Pigs	Day-time	7.4	2.5	2.0
	Night-time	4.4	2.5	5.2
	Total	11.8	5.0	7.2

After Ruckebusch (1972b).

Swine exhibited the greatest number of periods of paradoxical sleep both during the 24-h period (33) and during the night-time (25) and those of shortest mean duration, 3.2 min and 3.0 min respectively. The smallest number was recorded from sheep (7), and horses showed paradoxical sleep periods of longest duration (5.2 min). The ratio of paradoxical sleep to total sleep was highest in horses and lowest in sheep. Pigs also exhibited a high ratio of paradoxical sleep to total sleep.

Patterns of sleep, or hypnograms, can be used as an indication of stress in husbandry. Disinclination to lie at rest is seen in horses with orthopaedic conditions and in cattle with hardware disease. The normal sleep and resting characteristics of animals should be appreciated for purposes of assessing welfare so that abnormalities

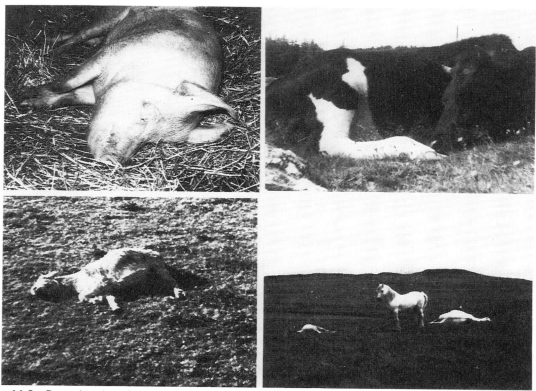

Fig. 14.2   Deep sleep in a pig, cow, donkey and two horses during day-time.

which may have symptomatic significance can be detected. A horse lying down at night in a normal posture is probably asleep. An adult horse that lies down during the day (unless in the company of its foal) or rests in sunshine may be abnormal and should be carefully observed for other evidence of illness. Although cattle do not sleep much, they may be difficult to arouse when they are asleep at night. Pigs lie and sleep a lot so that protracted resting and sleep are positive indices of normal function. Some clinical conditions cause disturbed patterns of resting and sleep in all animals. Significant clinical signs include sleeping fitfully and rising from resting postures frequently.

Management practices should interfere as little as possible with normal circadian patterns of maintenance behaviour. Interruption of activity cycles and loss of sleep may play an important role in the etiology of the stress-related diseases associated with newborn management, livestock transport, mixing of strange animals and introducing new animals into established groups.

Species-typical features

Cattle

Rest and sleep are important for cattle, as for other farm animals, and a free opportunity for such behaviour is a necessity. At pasture, cows have ample opportunity for resting. In a tied stall or a cubicle-house system where one lying place is allocated per animal, individual cows have ample opportunity for lying and resting. In a cubicle-house system when there are more cows than there are cubicles, this condition changes (Wierenga, 1983). Under these conditions the lying time of cows is reduced in proportion to the amount of over-occupation. The effect is reduced lying time among the low-ranked cattle due to a shortage of lying places during the night, when cows prefer to rest (Arave and Walters, 1980).

Even a few hours of lying deprivation raises the need for this behaviour since lying deprivation results in a significant increase in lying when this again becomes possible. Cows, well-accustomed to their environment, rarely indulge in non-REM sleep whilst standing. If recumbency is prevented they adapt without difficulty to non-REM but are not able to perform REM sleep. Cows under stall conditions sleep in non-REM and in REM phases in a recumbency position during the night-time. However, they are capable of indulging in non-REM, but not REM sleep whilst standing. By keeping them standing for 24 h selective REM sleep deprivation can occur (Webb, 1969). Preventing recumbency at night results in partial sleep deprivation since food intake during the day reduces available sleep time. In non-REM sleeping episodes cattle progressively exhibit irritability towards the presence of personnel and the time spent in drowsiness is halved.

Recumbency with the head fully supported on the ground is a well-known behavioural attitude of cattle when resting. When no restraint prevents its turning the head back along the flank, "the milk-fever position" is a characteristic attitude that occurs 6–10 times each night. These features, together with rapid eye movements (REM) and relaxed neck muscle tone, indicate periods corresponding to paradoxical or deep sleep identified by cortical low-voltage fast activity. These simple criteria can be used for the identification of the state of deep sleep in cattle.

The relaxed neck musculature is revealed by the animal when it adopts the "milk fever posture" in which the head is turned round to the flank and is supported on the ground or occasionally on a hind leg. Twitching of the ears and facial muscles also occurs in this deep sleep when rumen contractions become very slow.

During the day cattle usually rest in sternal recumbency while ruminating. About 5 h per day may be occupied in this fashion. They may also lie at rest without ruminating. While not actively grazing, cattle may also spend time standing at rest without ruminating. This idling time is variable but is short in healthy cattle. In daylight, a total time of less than one hour is likely to be spent in lateral recumbency and episodes of rest in this position are normally brief. These may be associated with periods of sleep.

The fore limbs are curled under the body and one hind leg is tucked forward underneath the body taking the bulk of weight on an area enclosed by the pelvis above, the stifle joint and the hock joint below. The other hind limb is stretched out to the side of the body with the stifle and hock joints partially flexed. They will occasionally lie with one or other fore leg stretched out in full extension for a short period. Cattle will also occasionally lie fully on their sides, but do so only for very short periods while holding their heads forward, presumably to facilitate regurgitation and expulsion of gases from the rumen. Adult cattle take up the sleeping position seen in calves with their heads extended inwards to their flanks. This is certainly a normal resting and sleeping position taken by adults periodically, although it is also a posture typically adopted in milk fever.

Most characteristic of ruminant rest are the extensive periods of drowsiness usually associated with rumination. At this time they usually lie on their sterna. Rumination and sleep are inversely related so that sleep time decreases with alimentary development. Sternal resting increases but sleep decreases as the percentage of roughage in the diet increases.

Since cows choose one side of an open building as a rest area, in designing free-stall housing for dry cow comfort, provision of a downhill slope to a cow's right as she faces the stall and access to a dry lot during warm weather would be ideal.

Horses

Horses are polyphasic animals as regards sleep or rest periods; 95% of horses have two or more such periods per day. The total length of time spent recumbent per day is approximately 2.5 h, with slight variations associated with age and management. Twice as much time is spent in sternal recumbency as is spent in lateral recumbency and normal adult horses rarely spend more than 30 min continuously in lateral recumbency; the mean time spent continuously in this position is 23 min.

Horses lie down and rise in a specific manner. In descent the forelegs are flexed first, then all four limbs. The head and neck are used for balance as the animal lowers itself. In sternal recumbency, horses do not lie symmetrically. Their hindquarters are rotated with the lateral surface of the bottom limb on the ground. In lateral recumbency the upper limb is invariably anterior to the lower fore limb, which is usually flexed. The hind limbs are usually extended with the upper limb slightly posterior to the lower limb. To rise the horse extends the upper fore leg. The forequarters are raised so that the lower fore leg can be extended. At the same time both hind limbs begin to extend, but the main thrust of rising comes from the hind limbs.

A sound horse seldom remains lying when it is approached, probably because a standing horse is better able to flee or to defend itself. It is interesting that a dominant stallion in a herd lies down first, before subordinate horses. Horses may be able to drowse and even engage in slow-wave sleep while standing by means of the unique stay apparatus of the equine limbs. REM sleep, however, occurs almost always whilst lying down.

Adult horses do not lie for very long periods. Mares with young foals tend to lie longer than usual when the foal is nearby and sleeping in full lateral recumbency. Mature horses are unable to lie in this flat-out posture for long periods of time before their respiratory functions become impaired. The full weight on the thorax of the horse, when laid flat, appears to be such that circulation to the lungs becomes inefficient after about 30 min. This is not the case among foals and young horses, however, and these subjects can be seen to spend many hours in the day sleeping on their sides at full stretch.

During the day the horse is awake and alert over 80% of the time. At night, the horse is awake 60% of the time, but drowses for 20% of the night in several separate periods. Stabled horses are recumbent for 2 h per day in four or five periods. Ponies are recumbent for 5 h per day and REM sleep occurs in about nine periods of 5 min average duration.

Management practices can affect equine sleep patterns. When moved from stable to pasture, they do not usually lie down during the first night and total sleep time remains low for a month. If horses are tied too short in a stall, so that they cannot lie, they do not have REM sleep. Horses stabled only at night may limit sleep until they are free during the day. Sleep deprivation may occur when they are transported long distances and must be tied short in stalls for support. Diet also affects sleep time in horses, as it does in ruminants. If oats are substituted for hay, total recumbency time increases; fasting has the same effect. Whenever possible horses rest on high slopes and ridges during the afternoon (Keiper and Berger, 1982).

Pigs

Of all farm animals, pigs spend most time resting and sleeping. Sleeping in groups simultaneously is usual and they may be recumbent in rest or sleep for as much as 19 h each day. Pigs also drowse and about 5 h are spent in this state daily. Of the total sleep time, slow-wave sleep occupies 6 h per day on average and REM sleep averages 1.75 h in about 33 periods.

Pigs are characterised by extreme muscle relaxation during sleep. While this is difficult to appraise in a mature sow, young piglets exhibit profound relaxation. When a sleeping piglet is picked up, it is found to be totally relaxed.

Sheep

Sheep are awake for about 16 h per day. They drowse for about 4.5 h per day, far less than cattle. Slow wave sleep occupies 3.5 h per day

and REM sleep occurs in seven periods of an average total of 43 min.

Poultry

The natural resting characteristics of poultry have a number of definite characteristics. According to physiological criteria, rest in poultry has been defined in several substates termed alert-rest, drowsiness, sleep and paradoxical sleep. In behavioural studies two substates are distinguished, namely drowsing and sleeping. These two resting postures of these states appear very similar, as follows:

Drowsing

This consists of two stages:

1. The neck is more or less withdrawn; the head is moved regularly and the eyes are open; the tail is slightly down.
2. The neck is withdrawn; the head is motionless and sometimes drooped; the eyes are closed or are slowly opened and closed; feathers are slightly fluffed; the wings may droop; the tail is down; and while standing, a slight crouching posture is adopted.

Drowsing can occur in either a sitting or a standing position.

Sleeping

The head is tucked into the feathers above the wingbase or behind the wing; feathers are slightly fluffed; sometimes the wings droop; while standing, a slight crouching posture is shown; and the tail is down. Sleeping can be performed either in a sitting or a standing position.

When perching for the night, they prefer special places. This results in competitive behaviour during the phase of initial perching. Resting is usually on perches at night but this is not the case during the daytime. In litter, birds do not create a resting site; they simply stop whatever they are doing and assume a resting posture in a convenient spot. Drowsing postures gradually develop throughout the flock from one to the other. When the hen assumes the sleeping posture, it moves its head slightly forward, turned at 180%. It puts the beak at the proximal end of the wing and pushes the head between the wing and the body while making a vibrating movement with the head. This movement also occurs in ducks. While sleeping, occasionally jerky movements of the head and neck occur and sometimes there is a soft peeping noise. External disturbances during drowsing cause an alert posture; arousal from sleeping is more difficult than from drowsing.

Resting postures are very uniform among birds. In the sleeping posture, the head is above the centre of gravity, and this may give stability to the bird in situations of muscular relaxation during physiological sleep. The sleeping posture could be a behavioural adaptation, reducing head loss via comb and wattles and closing in the vent. Although all poultry rest in a sitting as well as a standing position, sitting is most common. Sitting is a very stable position, as poultry possess a mechanism by which the feet close around the perch when the animal sits. Sitting is advantageous from the point of view of energy conservation, as metabolism is 40% less and heat loss decreases 20% as compared with standing.

Resting shows rhythmic organisation in poultry, starting with perching activity before sunset changing to activity before sunrise. Light is evidently the main cue for this organisation. During the day, resting was shown mainly in perching or squatting by about two-thirds of the flock in the alert resting posture. The deeper resting states are mainly shown at night. This shows the influence of environmental circumstances on sleep type and quantity which may be relevant in determining poultry welfare. External factors such as lighting, temperature, length of the dark period and external disturbances influence resting. While most maintenance behaviours are concentrated in the light period, preening occurs during the night, probably because this is the only behaviour that can be performed adequately and efficiently on a perch in the dark.

During the night, all poultry normally rest on perches. Perching during the day is associated with a short resting or preening bout and the lower perches are preferred for this. About one hour before sunset, birds start perching for the night. Usually it takes 30–60 min for the whole flock to take their places. Much flying on and off the perches is seen during this period. Fowl prefer to use the higher perches, but some individuals also use the lower ones. Poultry resting and sleeping on perches draw the head and neck close to the body and grasp the perch firmly with their feet, maintaining this position for several hours. In roosting, preference is shown for locations high from the floor area but such perching is not possible in a battery cage system. In cages with sloping floors there is a preference to sleep on the highest available place on the slope. Though this is apparently a poor substitute for a perch, which is preferred whenever present, fowls evidently adapt to such facilities, probably at some physical expense.

In poultry, the genetic strain is an important factor affecting perching behaviour. Some strains almost completely fail to use high perches but Appleby (1985) has shown that early experiences affect later perch use. These strain differences are not due to weight disparity or to social pressure. Some birds perch whereas others are non-perchers. A perching facility increases the time spent on the perch by perchers but does not convert non-perchers into perchers. The type of material, such as wood or wire, from which the perches are constructed has little effect on behaviour, but perch shape and size do have an effect. In some strains there are no significant preferences for wire or litter, but some birds avoid wire. The welfare implications of perching from these results are interesting. The type of perch most commonly used in semi-intensive housing may well be inadequate, so more appropriate perches could be designed.

15 General social behaviour

A most pronounced feature in farm animal behaviour is the active way in which individuals associate with each other (Syme and Syme, 1979). Such behaviour serves many purposes, including species cohesion and ecological integration. Social affiliations are basic to systems of passive transmission of learning. The group effect, inherent in social facilitation, influences communal activities. The intimate association of individuals permits the organisation of numbers of animals into family units, breeding groups, herds, and flocks. The discipline which the social force brings to the component individuals of animal assemblies ensures the common pursuit of tactics required for living. Social motives are manifestly related to survival and the behavioural phenomena dependent upon them, therefore, are found to be pursued with vigour.

Animal relationship with man, when it has been successful, ranges from the near familial to the habituated, but in all events the domestication of various species has depended on this capacity for social affinity. Domesticability ensures its own type of survival, different from natural survival perhaps, but no less biologically real in a final analysis. Social compatibility with man was evidently a prototypic feature of the domesticated animals. It is certainly essential to their efficient manipulation in husbandry. In the farming of animals, their readiness to form their own social groups allows them to be organised easily into close groups, even to be crowded (Metz, 1981; Metz and Mekking, 1984).

In many social species of animals, normal behaviour depends upon being in a social group. Through the phenomenon of social facilitation, time budget allocation of the majority of individuals in a group dominates and prevails generally. The increased likelihood of showing certain activities is a further development in grouped animals. For example, many animals in total isolation do not show the same degrees of maintenance activity, such as ingestion, as shown within groups. It would almost appear that optimum group size aids productivity. The one feature of farming which receives most notice today is the collective management of animals as groups rather than as individuals (Tsuyoshi *et al.*, 1981).

The useful description of social behaviour depends upon an appreciation of the complexity of the subject. The terms listed below are those of Broom (1981).

Social organisation. This term includes:
Physical structure—the size of the group and its composition in respect of age, sex and degrees of relatedness of group members;
Social structure—all of the relationships among individuals in the group and their consequences for spatial distribution and behavioural interactions;
Group cohesion—the duration of association

of the members of the group and the frequency of fission in which one or more members leave the group.

Some terms used in the description of social structure concern the roles of individuals in the group.

Leader: the individual which is in front during an orderly group progression. Other colloquial uses of this word are best replaced by different terms in order that the descriptions used in behaviour research should be as precise as possible.

Initiator: the individual which is the first to react in a way which elicits a new group activity. This new activity may be similar to that of the initiator but need not be. For example, a movement to a new feeding place may elicit the same movement by others but an alarm call may elicit freezing behaviour.

Controller: the individual who determines whether or not a new group activity occurs, when it happens and which activity it is. The controller can also reduce the likelihood that certain activities by individuals occur. The control may sometimes be exerted by force or threat but the more common situation is that in which members of a group look to the controller before changing activity or moving as a group. Examples include the old mare in a group of New Forest ponies, or the hind in a group of red deer, or the male in a group of gorillas or baboons who determines when the group will move to a new area (Schaller, 1963; Kummer, 1968; Tyler, 1972). Initiators may try to start such group movements but be unsuccessful unless the controller decides to move.

Competition: the situation where individuals seek to obtain the same resource. This need not involve any physical confrontation between rivals, for as Syme (1974) points out, the fastest mover may often succeed in obtaining a food item. In other circumstances, the cleverest rather than the strongest or the fastest may be successful.

Hierarchy: a sequence of individuals or groups of individuals in a social group which is based upon some ability or characteristic. The term is most frequently used where the ability assessed is that of winning fights or displacing other individuals. The hierarchy might involve just two levels, as in the case of a *despot* who wins against a set of equal individuals (Carpenter, 1971). Usually hierarchy refers to a series of levels like a *linear peck-order* (Schjelderup-Ebbe, 1922) or a linear series with some triangular relationships in it. Such an order might reflect an ability to dominate other individuals, the subordinates, restricting their movements and access to resources. However the term dominance order is seldom appropriate as orders are usually based on specific measurements such as winning fights or displacement from a feeder rather than an assessment of real dominance. Various matters explaining these concepts further are discussed later in this chapter.

General features

Numerous behavioural phenomena are seen in domesticated animals in the course of social interactions. Pair bonds are notable associations. Social relationships between and within sexes and age groups are also prominent in each species and are aided by communication (Ploog, 1970). Among enclosed animals, modified social behaviours are seen. The domesticated animal's social interaction with people varies considerably from species to species, dependent on the system of husbandry and whether the animal has experienced unpleasant human actions. This form of special relationship involving the positive association of the animal with man is termed socialisation. Inter-species affiliations can occur in remarkable forms.

Farm livestock associate together in groups. Even under free-range farming systems voluntary grouping is very evident (Tyler, 1972; Wagnon, 1963; Wagnon *et al.*, 1959, 1966). Sheep, cattle and horses maintain visual contact. Swine show more body contact and keep in auditory communication. When disturbed suddenly, most sheep and horses first bunch together and then run in a group from the source of disturbance. Pigs and cattle move in looser groups. During the bunching of animal groups in natural or high-density situations, individuals may be forced to violate the personal space of others. Social interactions at such close quarters depend on the position of the animals in the dominance order. Dominant and subordinate postures and responses are appropriately adopted. This stability of social relationship requires:

1. Recognition between individual animals;
2. Established social positions; and
3. Memory of social encounters which establish social status.

Commonly given estimations of the total number of group members that can be recognised or remembered by each individual are 50–70 in cattle and 20–30 in pigs.

Piglets show some competitive fighting within a few hours of birth for the preferred anterior nipples of the sow. Lambs and kids do not develop a stable social order until some time after weaning. In semi-wild cattle, bull calves stay in cow herds, dominating the females up to about two years of age and then move into "bachelor" bull groups.

Social dominance effects can be very important in cases of high stocking densities or poor farm design. Inadequate trough space, narrow races, inadequate space in indoor housing or lack of feeders can mean that dominant animals command resources at the expense of subordinate animals. The latter will suffer and health and general production can be affected. Documented examples include the higher internal parasite load of subordinate grazing stock during droughts when scarce food is commandeered by dominant stock.

Leadership

In their affiliative movements, animals often respond to the initiative of a lead animal by following (Sato, 1982; Squires and Daws, 1975). The common "follow" responses of pigs are not as marked as in sheep, in which the follow reaction is part of the strategy of flock cohesion. All herding and flocking animals show "follow reactions" in various social circumstances involving movements (Rathore, 1978, 1982). Leadership exemplifies the follow reaction so evident among sheep in which it is often provided by an old ewe. Older animals are more likely to effect leadership and the status of the animal in the social hierarchy may not be a determinant factor. In cattle the lead role is often taken by animals out of the middle of the dominance system. In the movements of cattle during their husbandry routines, the order of following remains very consistent. Leadership may be shared but the follow order tends to be organised and to persist from event to event.

Several observers have reported that the voluntary order of cows going for milking at each milking session is fairly consistent (Reinhardt, 1973). Dairy cows organise themselves into a specific order for entering the milking shed according to their milk yield, with high yielding cows taking an advanced position in the order. The movement order to milking is quite consistent though the rear animals have more fixed positions than the "leaders". Evidently the follow reaction in an order system can be influenced by the "reward" of milking. Types of leadership in cattle have been subdivided into three categories as follows:

1. Leadership during movement to and from locations of eating, drinking and sleeping. This establishes movement order.
2. Leadership in the initiation of grazing and resting which is the basis of an initiative order.
3. Leadership in direction during grazing activity which is a more obscure form of lead-and-follow behaviour.

In the suckler herd studied by Benham (1982b) some individual cows always moved at the front of the herd and ran around to the front if the herd changed direction. It was clear that they were leaders but not controllers of movement. Acceptable explanations of the overall system are given by Sato (1982), who points out seasonal factors as follows: summer temperatures may inhibit the development of grazing while association will be increased to avoid the attacks of biting flies. Sato observed that the summertime lowering of grazing and the development of association frequently caused heifers to react as follows. With seasonal reduction in associative behaviour the increased grazing drive in cooler temperature caused heifers to behave less as followers and to show dispersive grazing formations. Since grazing essentially involves dispersive movement, "follow reactivity" is readily obscured. Aggregative movement, on the other

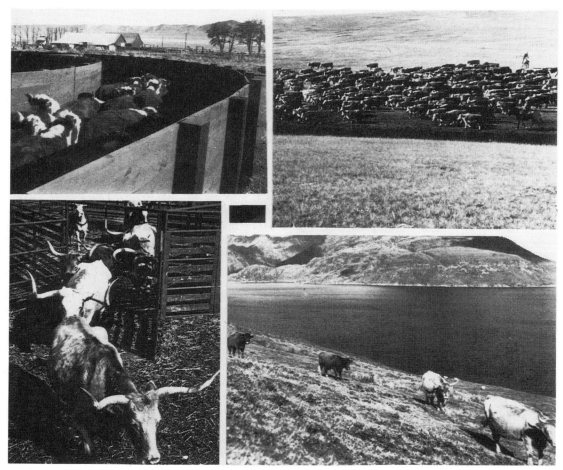

Fig. 15.1   Forms of followership in cattle. Top left: following in a curved, solid-sided passageway guiding stock to a lairage. Top right: herd following on a range. Bottom left: single file following through a race. Bottom right: separated-out line of following on Highland grazing.

hand, may have amplified follow-behaviour through social support of initiative switching (Fig. 15.1).

Changes from grazing to resting or from resting to grazing take place as follows. When an individual cow initiates activities different from the remainder, it returns to the activities of the rest of the herd if the remainder do not follow. Drifting occurs when a neighbour begins to follow, until the behavioural policy of the whole group is changed. Each animal is dependent on the herd influence and leadership ranking is not simply a measure of individual preference in effecting reactivity. Apparently the follow reactions of cattle largely result from reciprocal action between the salient maintenance need of the individual and the group effect of the herd. This general rule is modified by the fact that freely active movement of high-ranking animals

and negatively-derived, independent movement of low-ranking animals can both have an effect on the determination of order systems among cattle. The milking order may not be the same as the order when travelling; the travel order may differ from the order going through gates, doors or out of yards, into races or other linear controls.

Some use is made in animal management of the "Judas" animal to lead groups in to slaughter premises. Using the natural movement pattern of the species concerned, sheep, cattle and horses can all be trained to lead. Under free-range conditions the older grazing stock can transfer to their offspring information about seasonal pathways, areas of good pasture and watering places if this familial bond is not disrupted before weaning. In this way, home range areas can be established efficiently. Sheep in

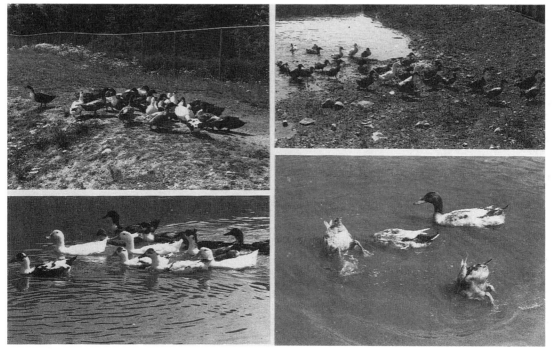

Fig. 15.2 Some "group effects" in ducks. Top: group feeding and following on land. Bottom: formation following and feeding on water.

extensive pastures may establish separate home range areas on the basis of familial leadership and its social cohesion. Such cohesion contributes to social facilitation.

Social facilitation

Within groups, the activity of the majority seems to prevail so as to direct behavioural policy for all. This group effect serves as a basis for the holistic strategies of group behaviour. Social facilitation in flocks (Fig. 15.2) and herds

(Figs 15.3 and 15.4) are involved in daily movements, and in stampedes, marches and migrations which persist as outstanding behavioural phenomena in animals. Social facilitation is more likely where there is adequate association, ability to communicate and react, a potential for mimicking activities, similarity of motivational state and suppression of intra-species aggression.

One example of social facilitation is the increased likelihood of pecking by a chick where another chick is seen or heard pecking. Another example is that of cows in a field which are more

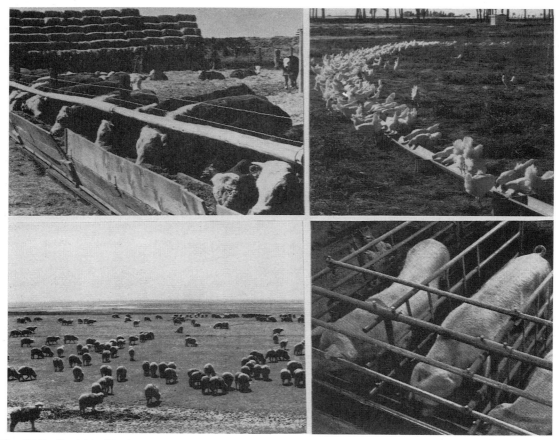

Fig. 15.3 Social facilitation effected by a variety of husbandry systems potentiates various forms of behaviour, notably feeding.

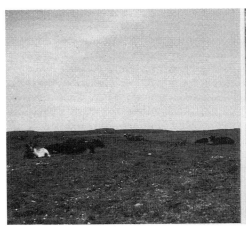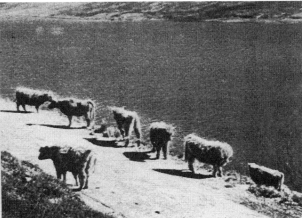

Fig. 15.4   Social facilitation as evidenced by group behaviour in a common activity. Left: day-time ruminating in cattle at pasture. Right: idling in cattle.

likely to start grazing or lying if others in the herd do so (Benham, 1982a). The amount consumed may also be affected by social facilitation. In studies where pigs ate to satiation (Hsia and Wood-Gush, 1984) or calves drank milk to satiation (Barton and Broom, 1985), the presence of a second hungry animal resulted in the first animal consuming more.

Social order

In groups of animals which have been together for some time there is often a clearly established hierarchy. This can result in maximal group-bonding and minimal aggression, creating the social stability which is a vital requirement in good animal husbandry (Schein and Fohrman, 1955). A social hierarchy is not an inviolable structure, however, it is merely the state of settled-out relationships between individuals. Of greater importance are other relationships which need not involve any aspect of competition. Friendship pairs are formed and these involve mutual tolerance. The function and durability of the hierarchy is dependent upon component relationships and upon on-going, operative avoidance tactics. "Dominance

hierarchy'' may be a misconception for a social relationship based in a mixture of social arrangements. It seems that animals use organised tactics of stable social living which may well prove to be their own pacts and systems of pacts. Such relationships may lead to bachelor grouping and association in which there is matriarchal dominance.

Formerly it was thought that social order was the result of social dominance through aggression and for that reason it was commonly termed the "aggression order". This view is not now tenable. Beilharz and Zeeb (1982) have drawn attention to a need for proper appreciation of the term dominance in the context of social systems. The use of dominance should be restricted to the phenomenon that can occur in every pair of animals in which one member can inhibit the behaviour of the other (Sato, 1984). The order of the group is therefore the sum of all such inhibitory relationships. Dominant animals probably have been aggressive in the past to obtain their dominant positions, but a dominant animal need not be aggressive subsequently (Reinhardt and Reinhardt, 1982). Measures of the dominance position of animals in a herd should be based on observations in the particular herd, contain sufficient observations to be reliable and reflect the actual magnitude of differences among animals.

Dominance relationships are the result of learning, with many different factors being involved in the formation of a relationship. Once learned, dominance relationships persist for a long time (Syme and Syme, 1979). Although unsettled dominance relationships are found in young animals, mature animals of all species of domestic livestock generally have clear unidirectional dominance relationships. The dominance order of the group may be no more than the sum of the individual relationships within the herd.

Social dominance is not usually exerted when sheep or cattle are grazing or are resting. In horses, however, subordinate animals deliberately avoid moving too close to dominant animals and dominant animals frequently threaten subordinates while eating. Social dominance is exhibited in competition for supplementary feed given in a restrictive place, or at water troughs in cattle, sheep and horses.

Dominance in flocks of sheep of similar age when feeding at troughs is not related to weight. In flocks of mixed ages the youngest and oldest are the least competitive. Under severe competition the poorer competitors cease trying to feed. The same general pattern has been observed in horses and goats.

In one study it was observed that a definite "rank order" existed among five goats penned together on a permanent litter of straw and provided with a ration of oats and hay, fed from the floor. The mature animals dominated the younger ones. Within the younger group, one goat dominated the other; these two subordinates were not permitted access to the feed by the dominants until it had become spread out on the bedding in the course of which it became contaminated. After about six months of confinement, the two goats at the bottom of the rank order showed signs of unthriftiness, anaemia and diarrhoea. Faecal samples showed gastro-intestinal parasites only in the subordinates. Treatment for parasitism was carried out, but the subordinate pair died (Campbell and Fraser, 1961).

Much behavioural observation on "aggression orders" in farm animals, and in pigs particularly, is now unfortunately suspect since the subtle behaviours of avoidance–submission, such as "head-tilting" in swine, went unrecognised. Similar head-tilting is seen in sheep and may occur in other animals. The range of significant social behaviours among swine have been outlined by Jensen (1984). To this list must be added the very aggressive gesture of "aiming" observed as an upward lift of the head in the direction of a threatened conspecific at a distance of 2–3 m.

These behaviours provided all the social exchange involved in maintaining social stability in a permanent herd of free-ranging sows. In a study of the social system of this herd as compared with commercially kept herds it was concluded that the dominance order, measured as "avoidance order", seemed to be maintained mainly through the behaviour of the subordinates. They performed the most social acts, mainly submissive and flight behaviour. These were mainly received by the dominant animals. The view is expressed that these facts support the use of the term "avoidance order" as a measurement of social dominance, instead of the "aggression order". Jensen observed that confinement and semi-confinement decreases the social activity, measured as number of observed interactions per time unit, and leads to unsettled dominance relationships combined with high aggression levels. Semi-confinement systems do not provide sufficient space for a stable social system and the frequencies of aggressive behaviours were actually highest in semi-confinement. Systems in which animals are in small groups having individual feeding stalls and an area of secondary space, provide enough area for the sow to settle dominance relationships and to keep the aggression level fairly low.

It is clear that housing methods of animals which provide more space of appropriate quality will become increasingly used in intensive farming in order to keep energy-wasting and stress-inducing aggression within groups under control. Within systems which provide security of position at feeding and secondary space for resting it is possible for a constantly settled avoidance order to exist.

The avoidance system

An avoidance order emerges in loose-housed dry sow groups and this order actually regulates the aggression level in the group. Both "retreat" and "head-tilt" are behaviours used significantly in determining the "avoidance order". They are usually preceded by nose-to-nose or head-to-head threats and are usually followed by "no reaction". This means that avoidance behaviour seems to diminish aggressive outcome in social interactions. An avoidance order has important effects of the regulation of aggression in sow groups.

In some situations of spatial restraint an avoidance order becomes unstable. The reason for the unstable avoidance order in the higher restraint system is not clear, but possibly if the available area is too small to permit the animals to perform subordination behaviour this will cause settled pair-relations to break down in frustration.

The recognition of an avoidance system in social behaviour of pigs is apparently a change in fundamental comprehension. The phenomenon of an avoidance system, at once so obvious and so subtly obscured, has been overlooked by many ethologists studying aggression.

Avoidance is an inverse response in agonistic situations and it is the positive factor effecting agonistic control. Evidently the generally accepted belief that dominance, by itself, established and operated social hierarchy, is inadequate. The avoidance system in behaviour, which operates within the dominance system, is the vital component of the behavioural mechanism which generates social stabilisation. Of course, avoidance is an overall strategy which calls for specific behavioural tactics, and these tactics need space for their practical operation. In social stabilisation, one suspects that the behavioural system components which make the underlying avoidance system work have to be prompt behavioural responses which are minute, discrete, speedily learned and imperatively unambiguous. Avoidance serves to reduce contests between individual animals, but if the contest develops, various types of tactic can be adopted. This gives scope for a variety of courses in games of conflict among animals.

16 Association

Associative arrangements in which one animal spends more time closer to another than the mean group inter-individual distance develop within groups of animals (Arnold and Dudzinski, 1978; Fraser, 1981, 1982a). Pair bonds are a notable feature of associative behaviour; these pair bonds are not by any means confined to the relationship between the mother and its offspring. Within herds, it is often found that discrete pairing through mutual selection of each other's company is a common social strategy which operates to the advantage of both, particularly in agonistic situations involving other dominant animals. The associative characteristics of animals are now recognised as a clear manifestation of their conscious choice for company which must represent a basic biological need.

Many different sorts of behavioural associations are featured in animal groups (Dickson *et al.*, 1967). Any hierarchical organisation of behaviour manifests itself through social association and utilisation of private space (Dietrich *et al.*, 1965). Association with man is a special form of affiliation (Chapter 17).

The social organisation of a flock or herd depends basically on recognition by the individual of its status in relation to other individuals. Sheep of a single breed put together into a pasture quickly develop a flock or group identity so that if other sheep are put into the pasture it takes several weeks for the two groups to become integrated (McBride *et al.*, 1967; Fig. 13.1). Social order, once established, is very stable. Introducing strangers into a herd does not alter the rank relations between any pairs of cows. Existing rank structure is not changed fundamentally by oestrous cycles, even though social activity increases during oestrus.

In free-living sheep and goats the females and the juveniles use certain fixed areas, which may change with season, with the males associating in bachelor groups in other areas but joining the females during the breeding season. The basic social unit in these groups is the female with her most recent offspring. Associated with this unit are likely to be related animals, for example a yearling and the female's mother. The stable unit is made up of numbers of subgroups of related individuals. In large bachelor male groups the associations between individuals are looser and the composition of the groups may change frequently, but in small bachelor groups there is much cohesion (Fig. 16.1). This group identity is due in part to group odour because anosmic sheep mix freely with strange sheep. Sheep and cattle prefer to associate with others of the same kind.

The sense of smell is used by cows to recognise other cows even in pair-competitive situations. The vomero-nasal organ (VNO) may be responsible for this. It has been found that social hierarchy, determined by conventional interindividual aggression contests, is distinctly

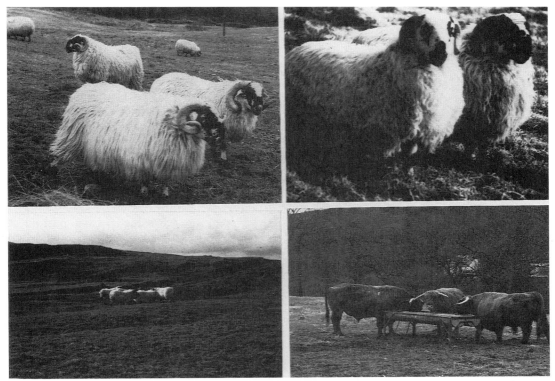

Fig. 16.1 Bachelor groups in sheep and cattle featuring close social bonds and harmonious behaviour. In rams bachelor grouping becomes broken up when the breeding season commences. Bachelor groupings appear to suppress libido.

changed by experimental inactivation of the VNO. Steers which were higher ranking pre-treatment generally lost rank and lower ranking steers gained rank over controls. This has led to the postulate that the VNO has a role in social aggressive behaviour that contributes to social hierarchy in cattle.

Association in farm animal species

Cattle

Domestic cattle in a free-range situation move from place to place in groups in which indivi-

duals maintain close proximity to one another. Dairy and beef cattle often lie in groups and grazing animals often stand within a few metres of one another, seldom moving out of view of the rest of the herd. Associations during movement, other active periods and resting periods are not random. A study of young dairy heifers by Broom and Leaver (1978) showed that associations were much more likely among some heifers than among others. In this study, animals which were reared together as calves were more likely to associate when adult and Bouissou and Hövels (1976) obtained the same result. However, other associations also formed and the occurrence of such associations in a suckler herd of mixed ages is described in detail by Benham (1982b, 1984). The animals in the suckler herd often allogroomed (licked one another) and spent most of their waking time together. It is likely that social licking has effects on the psychological stability of the animals concerned as well as cleaning the skin and hair.

Sheep

The development of social organisation has been followed in sheep (Arnold, 1977). The first social bond a sheep develops is with its dam. Once the bond is established it remains in females unless broken by separation. Ewes and lambs during the first four weeks of the lamb's life are found to stay within 10 m of each other for over half the time. The formation of "weaner" flocks breaks the dominant social bond in the lamb's life and a new social organisation has to be developed with the formation of small groups in which inter-animal distances are low. Gradually, these groups become larger until a flock is eventually formed. A flock identity creates a unitary force for adult sheep. Any groups of small numbers within contact distance immediately run together when disturbed.

Lambs after weaning tend to form numbers of subgroups before a flock tendency is shown. The size of subgroups increases with age from weaning up to four months old. This is unrelated to the size of the paddock or space available to the animals. Even as late as 11 months of age subgroups may be formed. Normal adult flocking behaviour appears to be established by 15 months of age. Three characteristic flock structures have been described as follows:

1. A tightly knit flock,
2. A flock widely dispersed, but with uniform spacing between individuals.
3. A flock split up into subgroups but which remains a social entity with membership of subgroups continually changing.

Pairing is common in sheep and such pairing is not related to twinning. In most cases twin lambs do not develop a lasting paired arrangement. Some pairings may only last for a few weeks or months, when fresh pairings may form. Pairings of twins are seen in cattle, however, and such pairings are evidently of a lasting nature. The association between twins observed in cattle is probably stronger because twin cattle are more rare and the pairs studied are reared as pairs and do not know other individuals from birth, as occurs usually in the case of twin lambs.

An important feature of behaviour in sheep is their marked synchronisation of activity and well-developed practice of social coexistence. In a comparative study of two separated flocks of sheep kept on the same grazing pasture for several days and nights, there was found to be no difference in the start or finish of the major grazing periods. Likewise, it was noticeable that no single animal was the instigator of any grazing or resting period. Although individual sheep rested or grazed at different times from the main flocks, the presence of any dominating animal, which influenced the pattern of behaviour of the combined flocks, was not noted.

When resting, social distance is greatly reduced and an analysis of 72 flocks showed that when resting, sheep occupied an area of 10 m² per sheep. Distance to nearest neighbour is one attribute of social arrangement; the cohesion of all members of a flock is another. This cohesion varies with environmental factors. The average distance between neighbouring sheep when grazing varies from 4 m to more than 19 m. The greatest distances are for hill breeds of sheep and the smallest for Merinos. The average distances of the nearest neighbours among sheep in all breeds is within 5 m but breeds differ on this basis and fall into four classes of dispersion. Merinos are the closest, lowland breeds are next, hill breeds are further apart, with the mountain breeds being the furthest apart.

The orientation of individuals to one another is an important factor in maintaining social contact. Sheep in flat paddocks are orientated when grazing, but not when engaged in other activities. Sheep align themselves to each other with angles of 110 degrees which coincides with the angle between the optical axes of the sheep, i.e. "line of sight". This allows them to have their nearest neighbours in full view. Since young sheep associate in close knit bunches this angular arrangement is not seen in them to the same extent as in adults.

Horses

Whilst being a typical herd species, horses also show a marked preference for certain individuals of their own species. Two horses encountering each other for the first time show much more mutual exploratory behaviour than is seen in the other farm animal species. Exploratory behaviour at introduction involves an investigation of the other's head, body and hindquarters using the olfactory sense.

As with the other farm animals, horses show a form of social order when they live in groups and a social hierarchy becomes established within these groups. The older and larger animals are usually found to be high in the dominance order. Stallions do not necessarily dominate geldings or mares. A dominant individual often dictates the movement of the herd through the grazing area and will sometimes break up exchanges between other horses. Socially dominant horses are sometimes found to have more aggressive temperaments than the others. Horses running at pasture show special features of behaviour if the group contains a stallion and breeding mares. Stallions usually drive younger male animals to the perimeter of their groups, but will not show any aggressive attitudes towards them if they remain there. The stallion attempts to herd a group of brood mares together. The normal size of a 'harem' amongst horses is about seven to eight mares. The colts tend to form a bachelor group after splitting off from the herd at the age of about one to two years. Fillies may or may not join this group.

Mares that have been kept together will continue to associate closely and consistently when put with other mares. In mares from different studs, such close associations are not formed, although most individual mares are found to associate closely with certain individuals. In herds of both sexes, colts and fillies tend to separate from the mares and stallions. The stallion usually attacks members of the younger group if they approach too closely. The stallion will round up the mares on the periphery of his herd or "harem" but will ignore or repel fillies.

In free-living ponies close groups are formed. Most groups are family groups with fillies remaining with their mothers for two or more years. When they leave their mothers young mares frequently change groups, often joining older mares with foals. Stallions in winter form bachelor groups. Groups of young males have a loose social organisation with members leaving to form other groups for a period and then rejoining the original. Stallions without mares often live as solitary individuals.

The formation of close social bonds in horses is essential for group stability and is important to plan for these in the management of domestic horses.

Pigs

The social organisation of groups of pigs is known to include the establishment of a social hierarchy (Fraser, 1974; Jensen, 1980; Jensen and Wood-Gush, 1984). For the social hierarchy to function properly, the size of a group and the space allocated to it are important (Jensen, 1982). It is also necessary for the members of the group to be capable of prompt recognition of each other. In pigs, it is still uncertain how the mechanics of recognition operate, though it is evident that different types of recognition exist. A form of face-to-face recognition appears to operate during an initial introductory period in the formation of a hierarchy. Sensory clues such as olfactory stimuli are probably involved in the maintenance of the social structure. It is also evident that pigs in an established group are quickly able to recognise an alien in the group.

Visual and olfactory cues seem to be the principal differentiating features of pigs for each other.

Poultry

The chick shows early social responses to adult calls and to clicks from other embryos (Vince, 1973) while still in the shell and it may give low-pitched distress calls if cooled or rapid twitterings of contentment if warmed. Chicks which are hatched at slightly subnormal temperatures give distress calls as their moist down dries and they lose contact with the egg shell. Contact with a broody hen or other warm object prevents these calls. Newly hatched chicks are attracted to the hen by warmth, contact, clucking and body movements. This attraction is greatest on the day of hatching. They develop the behaviours of maintenance, in particular to eat, roost, drink and avoid enemies, in the company of their mother. In chicks the most sensitive period for learning the characteristics of the mother is normally between 9 and 20 h after hatching. The attachment to the mother is further strengthened as her voice and appearance are recognised. As the down starts to disappear from their heads, the hen rejects the chicks by pecking at them and the clutch becomes dispersed. The clutch is the basis of flock organisation and even after it has dispersed chickens need company. A chick

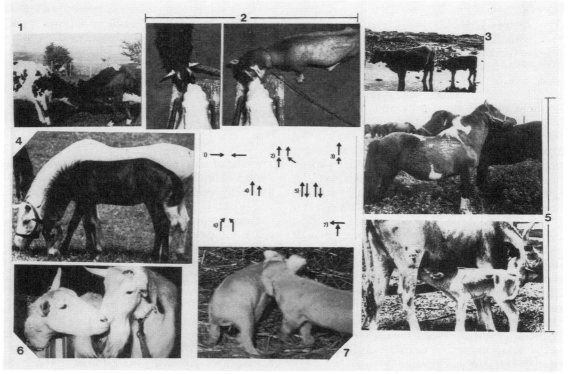

Fig. 16.2   Examples of two-animal formations. 1, typical head to head positioning; 2, perineal nosing at breeding; 3, progeny following mother; 4, mother and young grazing together; 5, "parallel-and-opposite" position commonly recognised in situations of nursing and mutual grooming; 6, nose to nose, nose to mouth; 7, agonistic lateral approach.

reared in isolation tends to stay apart from the flock. Flock birds eat more than single birds due to social facilitation.

Adult flock formation depends on tolerant association. Strange birds are initially attacked and are only gradually integrated into the flock. Newcomers are relegated to positions near the bottom of the peck order and only active fighting will change this. Hens and cocks have separate peck orders as males in the breeding season do not peck hens.

The geometry of association

In flocks and herds it is common for animals to have as nearest neighbour an individual with whom they have a relationship. It is common for the angle of alignment between the animal and its nearest neighbour to coincide with the central axis of the orbit. The angle of relation is therefore an oblique one. In pairs of animals the geometric alignment between the two individuals has been found to conform to several distinct patterns having a geometric basis. The seven forms of these which have been noted are shown in Fig. 16.2. In these formations animals typically align themselves head to head, head to tail or head to side. In some of these the angle of alignment is parallel and opposite, parallel and similar, and opposite in direction at 180 or 90 degrees. These are not necessarily fixed relationships, but are nevertheless frequent.

17 Social interaction

Amongst socially living animals, a high proportion of all behaviour takes the form of social interactions and affiliations (Hafez, 1975; Wilson, 1975; Broom, 1981; Craig, 1981; Barash, 1982). Among closely confined animals social behaviour is seen to be dependent upon the system of husbandry. The social interaction between man and animal is an important ethological feature (Kilgour and Dalton, 1984).

Social relations between man and animal

The removal of the young animal from its own dam to be raised by a human leads to social attachment to humans. The optimum time for such relationships and developmental processes to be formed varies with the species. With precocial species which are behaviourally competent at birth, like cattle and sheep, the optimum time is from birth to four to six days. A leader–follower relationship may occur in which the animal follows the human for food or companionship. If the attachment to humans has been very exclusive, such hand-raised animals may later relate sexually to humans. In species that develop a dominance–subordination type of social structure it is important that the human caretaker be dominant, particularly when the animals may be dangerous as adults. The dairy bull asserts increased dominance with maturation and growth. For such an animal, domi-

nance is best established at the appropriate time for the species, usually early in life when no punishment may be needed. Since the social dominance interactions are fairly specific for individuals, the fact that one particular person dominates an animal is no guarantee that another will be able to do so with the same animal (Schafer, 1975).

The hand-rearing of animals can be very beneficial to animal and owner in that individuals survive and thrive which would not otherwise have done so. However the problems which can arise as a consequence of bonding socially with man at the sensitive period in development must be considered in later management of the animals. Animals which are handled more by man may change their social responses to members of their own species as well as to man. Waterhouse (1979) handled regularly some young dairy calves in a row of hurdle pens and found that these calves showed less social interaction with their neighbours. There were no long-term adverse effects on social interactions in this study but there are reports of regularly petted animals and of entirely hand-reared animals, not adjusting well to social conditions. It would seem inadvisable to handle some young animals in a group much more than others (Broom, 1982). The other problem which can arise is of misdirected sexual behaviour, playful behaviour towards a person by an animal which has grown large enough to be dangerous, or of aggression towards people by an animal which has little fear of man because of its early social experience with man. This problem is soluble by taking care to socialise the animal with its own species at an appropriate time, rather than keeping it with only human company.

Having pointed out that farm animals can form social attachments to people, it should be emphasised that lack of contact with man is a much more important problem on farms. The most common relationship between a farm animal and the people whom it sees is that the animal is afraid of the people. This fear is extreme in poultry and may be extreme in sheep, pigs and other animals. If the stockman (a term which refers equally to woman or man) treats animals roughly or inconsistently then there are effects on welfare and there may be effects on production. Milk production by dairy cows is much affected by the behaviour of the stockman towards the animals (Seabrook, 1984, 1987).

The work of Hemsworth, Barnett and collaborators has shown that early handling of all the members of a group of pigs can have effects on the later responses of the pigs to man, the ease with which the pigs can be handled when older and the reproductive performance of the animals (Hemsworth *et al.*, 1981a, b, 1986a, b; Hemsworth and Barnett, 1987; Gonyar *et al.*, 1986). Using a standard test of latency of and amount of approach to a person, it was found that sows on different farms varied greatly in their responses to man. The average level of fear of human beings was negatively correlated with the reproductive performance of the pigs on the farm. In several experimental studies, pigs were either minimally handled, or stroked and patted when they approached (pleasant handling), or slapped or prodded with an electric goad when they approached (adverse handling). The pleasant handling resulted in the smallest behavioural and adrenal cortex response to man, highest growth ratio, highest pregnancy rate in gilts and earliest mating responses in boars (Table 17.1). It is clear from these results that the welfare and production of pigs is substantially affected by the extent of controlled

Table 17.1

The effects of handling treatments on the level of fear of humans and performance of pigs in four experiments. After Hemsworth and Barnett (1987)

Experiment and parameters	Mean for handling treatment		
	Pleasant	Minimal[a]	Aversive
Time to interact with experimenter (s)[b]	119	—	157
Growth rate from 11–22 weeks (g/day)	709	—	669
Free corticosteroid concentrations (ng/ml)[c]	2.1	—	3.1
Time to interact with experimenter (s)[b]	73	81	147
Growth rate from 8–18 weeks (g/day)	897	888	837
Time to interact with experimenter (s)[b]	10	92	160
Growth rate from 7–13 weeks (g/day)	455	458	404
Free corticosteroid concentrations (ng/ml)[c]	1.6	1.7	2.5
Time to interact with experimenter (s)[b]	48	96	120
Pregnancy rate of gilts (%)	88	57	33
Age of a fully coordinated mating response by boars (days)	161	176	193
Free corticosteroid concentrations (ng/ml)[c]	1.7	1.8	2.4

[a] A treatment involving minimal human contact.
[b] Standard test to assess level of fear of humans by pigs.
[c] Blood samples remotely collected at hourly intervals from 0800 to 1700 hours.

human contact with the animals. The same must be true of all farm animals.

A study of the effects of handling by farm staff on the later responses of dairy heifers was carried out by Bouissou and Boissy (1988). Animals which had been handled on three days per week during months 0–3 or 6–9 showed some improvement in ease of handling at 15 months when compared with unhandled controls. A substantial improvement in ease of handling and reduced heart-rate and plasma cortisol responses to novel situations were shown if the heifers had been handled for three days per week each month during months 0–9.

Among agricultural animals overcrowding and poor management may lead to upsets in normal behaviour and abnormal behaviour, injury or unthriftiness may result (Arave and Albright, 1976). While most basic behavioural traits of each species do not alter appreciably as a result of domestication, the normal social behaviour is modifiable by human caretaking (Stephens, 1974).

Animal interactions

Social interactions between animals are affected by the number of animals associated together in a common group (Arnold and Pahl, 1974; Dickson *et al.*, 1967). Social interactions in such circumstances are affected by the position of the interacting animals in the "peck order" of the group. The ranks of the animals encountering each other in a social situation determine how dominant or subordinate responses may be exhibited (Dietrich *et al.*, 1965).

During the bunching of animal groups in such natural or even high-density situations, individuals may be forced to violate the individual space of others. Social interactions at such close quarters depend on the position of the animal in the dominance order. Dominant and subordinate postures and responses are appropriately adopted. The same responses tend to be very consistently shown in all encounters between the same animals. Consistency of social interaction requires that the individuals are able to recognise one another and that their social positions have not been altered as a result of confusion in large groups, illness or temporary removal (Stricklin, 1976). Stability of association requires the following circumstances:

1. Recognition between individual animals,
2. Established social positions,
3. Memory of social encounters which establish social status.

Aggressive encounters between animals within a fresh group are frequent while the group is developing its own "peck order" (Syme and Syme, 1979). With the development of the order there is stability and aggressive encounters become reduced. Aggressive social interactions in the development of a "peck order" usually involve aggressive acts such as biting, butting or pushing. The introduction of a new individual is disturbing and even hazardous due to the sheer mass of separate aggressive encounters which the newly introduced animal will receive from most members of the group in turn, or sometimes in concert (Signoret *et al.*, 1975).

Pair bonds are a notable feature of social behaviour and bonds of this type are not limited to the interaction between the mother and progeny. It is often found that symbiotic pairing, through mutual selection of each other's company, is a common social strategy which operates to the advantage of both animals, particularly in agonistic situations involving dominant "third-party" animals. The social interactions of animals are now recognised as manifestations of their conscious choice and need of company. Learning is not necessarily involved, but the early bonds formed between parent and young may be generalised to include other species members (Fig. 17.1).

Since aggressive behaviour is most seen when groups of pigs, cattle or horses are first formed, the frequent changing of group members should be avoided. Production of milk and other physiological responses can be affected for several days while aggressive social interactions

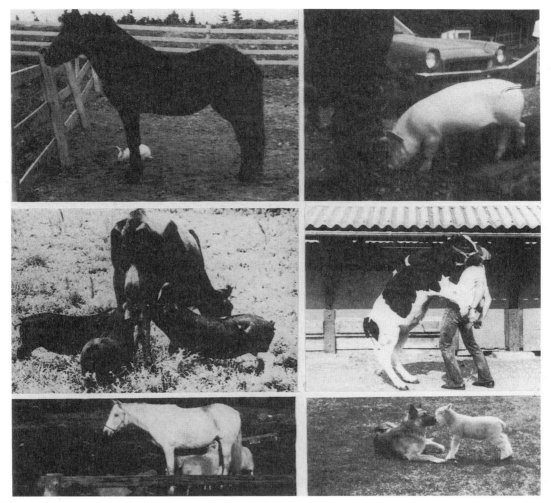

Fig. 17.1 Inter-species relationships can result in striking bonds. Top left: horse and rabbit in a strong companion bond. Top right: a friendship bond between a horse and pig (photograph by G. Thorne). Mid-left: a nursing bond between a cow and pigs. Mid-right: A bull with a social bonding to a human (photograph by H.H. Sambraus). Bottom left: maternal bond between a mare and sheep (photograph by G. Thorne). Bottom right: a close social bond between a bitch and a lamb.

are taking place. Sometimes tranquilisers have been used to aid social tolerance when strange pigs have to be penned together or when wild horses have to be collected.

Although young sheep seldom show overt social dominance (Morgan and Arnold, 1974), rams compete at the start of each breeding season and sheep may show aggressive butting if intensive husbandry conditions increase competition over food or bedding areas. Butting in cattle and sheep, biting of the mane or withers in the horse, and pushing, biting and side-ripping with the tusks in boars, are the common form of agonistic behaviour. Piglets show some competitive fighting within a few days of birth for preferred nipples of the sow. Other farm species do not develop a stable social order until some time after weaning.

In semi-wild cattle, bull calves stay in the cow herd and dominate the females by about two and one half years of age and then move into the bull group. Social-dominance effects can be very important in the case of high livestock densities or poorly designed farms. Dominant animals can command resources at the expense of subordinate animals due to inadequate trough space, narrow races, inadequate space in indoor housing or lack of feeders. Subordinate animals can suffer poor health and general production can be affected. Documented examples include the higher internal parasite load carried in some subordinate goats and high death rates during droughts when scarce food becomes commandeered by dominant stock.

Social behaviour of chickens

Newly hatched chicks are attracted to the hen by warmth, contact, clucking and body movements. This attraction is greatest on the day of hatching. They learn to eat, roost, drink and avoid enemies in the company of their mother (Fölsch and Vestergaard, 1981). Chicks rapidly learn the characteristics of their environment on the first day of life (Bateson, 1964; Broom, 1969a). Thereafter they are more likely to approach the familiar and avoid the unfamiliar but this rapid learning period can be extended if no appropriate stimuli, such as mother or siblings, are detected. The attachment to the mother is further strengthened as her voice and detailed appearance are recognised. The period spent with the mother is terminated when she rejects the chicks by pecking at them when the down starts to disappear from their heads. Soon after this the brood is dispersed.

Hens and cocks have separate peck orders as males in the breeding season do not peck hens.

The male order is less stable than the female owing to greater aggressiveness. The peck order is most clearly seen in competition for food or mates, and subordinate hens may obtain so little food that they lay fewer eggs. Dominant hens mate less frequently than subordinate hens but dominant males mate more often than subordinate males. Birds in a flock kept in a state of social disorganisation by the removal and replacement of birds eat less, may lose weight or grow poorly, and tend to lay fewer eggs than do birds in stable flocks. Additional feed and water troughs distributed about the pen enable subordinate hens to feed unmolested, and an adequate number of nesting boxes gives these birds the continuous opportunity to lay. If space permits, flocks of over 80 birds tend to separate into two distinct groups and at least two separate peck orders may then be established. Large, dense flocks are subject to hysteria (Hansen, 1976).

The clutch or brood is the basis of flock organisation and even after it has dispersed, chickens need company. A chick reared in isolation tends to stay apart from the flock. Flock birds eat more than birds which have been kept singly. Adult flock formation depends on mutual tolerance. Strangers are attacked and are only gradually integrated into the flock. Newcomers are relegated to positions near the bottom.

Social behaviour of domestic turkeys

Domestic and wild turkeys have similar flocking patterns and social organisation, but management practices, of course, determine the size and composition of domestic groups. Flock groups are self-organised according to a social dominance order that is less stable than that of chickens. Among males penned together some changes in rank may occur every few days. Certain varieties of turkeys tend to dominate others; e.g. Black over Bronze over Grey and in mixed sex groups, males dominate females.

The most common social interaction is a

simple threat. One bird may submit to the other, otherwise both birds warily circle each other with wing feathers spread, tails fanned, and each emits a high-pitched trill. One or both turkeys may then leap into the air and attempt to claw the other. The one that can push, pull or press down the head of the other will usually win the encounter. Such bouts usually last a few minutes. Haemorrhages may occur during a tugging battle since richly vascularised skin areas may be torn, but actual physical damage is usually slight and birds do not fight to the death. An injured lower ranking bird must be separated from the group, however, until its wounds heal, as other birds will tend to peck and aggravate the wound with fatal results.

Turkey incubation takes 28 days and the poults move freely shortly after hatching. They become socially attached to the mother during the first day or two though occasionally they become attached to siblings, humans or other objects. Normally imprinted poults form tightly knit groups which may initially cluster for warmth but are cohesive even in fairly warm environments. Birds tend to "tidbit", feed or wander as a group, and if they are with the mother, she is the focus of activity, providing leadership and defence against intruders. Vocal and visual signals are used by both parents and young to stay in contact until the poults are at least eight weeks old. Fighting is rare prior to three months of age, but increases to a peak at five months, when social orders are formed. Males fight more vigorously among themselves than do females.

Social behaviour of ducks

Most domestic ducks are promiscuous breeders. The drake will attack sexually any female he may meet and he plays no part in the selection of the nest, incubation or care of the young. Muscovy adult males are solitary and aggressive towards other males. Their displays are primitive and their calls are simple. The female, when alarmed, utters a weak quack. A hissing noise with tail-shaking, crest-raising and swinging of the head in the males is both a threat to other males and a sexual display towards females. As female ducks generally avoid displaying to males they tend to be chased extensively before mating is possible. Following fertilisation the female retires to her nest site and commences daily egg-laying. The nest is not continuously occupied, however, until incubation begins with the final egg.

Domestic ducks artificially incubated and kept in a man-made, man-controlled environment, adapt immediately to a natural environment. They take to swimming and diving for food, no matter what age, after getting their feathers, without the influence of a mother duck or other ducks. They automatically start feeding on grass and weeds found in run-off areas from a pond and also dive for any substance found on the bottom of a water-filled area. Usually one or several ducks watch over the flock while feeding on land or on water. A mother will protect her ducklings while they are feeding.

In more natural surroundings ducks will take to water together as a way of avoiding human or threatening presence. They are fast moving and very agile on water but exactly the opposite on land, especially if it is rocky or rugged terrain. Ducks can easily inflict bruises and cuts on their bodies trying to avoid capture because their bodies are so low to the ground. Ducks of different flocks do not fight but they do not readily accept each other until they have shared the same space for several months. Mingling is gradual and at times each original flock may still swim in the formation of original group. This formation is a triangle shape with a leader, usually a drake, at the head.

18 Reproductive abilitation

Reproductive activities are not ever-present features of behaviour. Their induction requires processes of maturation and stimulation which enable the animal to produce efficient reproductive activities and responses. Most reproductive behaviour depends upon hormonal state and also upon sensory stimuli. The process of acquiring reproductive capability has been termed here abilitation.

The abilitation of reproductive behaviour is dependent on a wide range of factors including neural mechanisms, hormones, pheromones and the sensory reception of a variety of stimuli. This brings the animal into a state of reproductive capability which then often overshadows other classes of behaviour by its high priority in motivation (Schein and Hale, 1965).

Sensory factors

Olfaction

The sense of olfaction is of critical importance in the stimulation of a wide variety of responses in animals. Reproductive responses, for example, are quite evidently under the control of the olfactory senses to a very large extent (Whitten, 1956; Whitten and Champlin, 1972). Odour can be seen to have a stimulatory value in arousing the male sex drive. Odorous substances produced by one animal which convey information to another animal are termed pheromones (see Chapter 7). The importance of the role of pheromones in the breeding behaviour of animals is becoming much more widely acknowledged (Izard et al., 1978). These pheromones have various sites of production and routes of elimination. For example, they are produced in the submaxillary salivary glands and excreted via preputial fluids in the boar (Melrose et al., 1971; Patterson, 1968; Perry et al., 1972; Signoret, 1970). A variety of male animal odours are detectable even to man, for example the smell of the billy goat which has its principal effect on female members of the same species.

The production and the reception of odour are clearly important in influencing behaviour. Odour plays a large part in the establishment of the strong bonds between a mother and the newborn animal. These bonds are dependent firstly on mutual recognition through odour (Alexander et al., 1974; Fraser, 1968).

Visual stimuli and photoperiodism

Although odour is the principal means by which early recognition occurs between mother and young, visual recognition soon takes over as the secondary means of mutual identification.

It has been known for some time that relative length of the light period of each day is a factor in determining breeding behaviour in farm animals. Seasonal breeding, for instance, is largely determined by the changes in the daily photoperiod. Photoperiodism operates in two principal ways:

1. Some animals exhibit their reproductive activities during that portion of the year during which the daily light period is long. It is widely known that for horses the normal breeding season commences in the spring—that period of the year when light is becoming stronger and the number of daylight hours greater—and continues through summer (Berliner, 1959).

2. Some animal species confine their breeding behaviour to that portion of the year characterised by the minimum amount of daily light; sheep and goats are examples of this. Most breeds of sheep and goats commence their breeding seasons in the autumn, when the daily photoperiod is less than the dark period and the light period is diminishing further day after day (Fraser, 1968).

Clearly, the natural light stimulus for those farm animals that show seasonal breeding is a complex one involving the absolute quantities of light and dark as well as relative quantities of light each day which are changing dynamically. Although it is generally believed that daily fluctuations in the photoperiod emphasise the change taking place in daily light rations, it is also clear that the fixed nature of the photoperiod is important, i.e. seasonal breeding animals maintain their breeding activities as long as an adequate quantity of light (or of dark) is delivered. When the photoperiod fails to provide adequate stimulation for the animal a refractory period develops during which the breeding performance is arrested.

Visual stimuli are often combined with olfactory stimuli in eliciting reproductive behaviour. The stationary form in oestrous females is the "key stimulus" for the male to initiate copulatory behaviour. In the case of the newborn, attempts at suckling are released and directed to the mammary region and the teat after being orientated firstly to the darkened underside, thereafter to the angular area of this underside and a vertical limb, to the prominent mammary region and finally to the lactiferous sinus and the protruding teat. The young animal soon learns the direct route to the mammary gland.

In the male, mounting is apparently released by a form presenting a dorsal surface and supports. Bulls will mount dummy cows or "phantom cows" which are of very simple form having only metal frame and a covered body. Most bulls tested with a "phantom cow" mount the dummy. Similarly, boars will normally readily mount a dummy sow consisting of a tubular frame with a padded covering. The simple form of the mounting releaser helps to explain why some bulls and other male animals with inadequate mating experience will attempt to mount from the side or even the front of the female subject.

Auditory stimuli

Vocal expression by animals results in auditory stimuli being exchanged. Auditory stimulation has been studied in horses and pigs. In the latter species most study has probably been devoted to the effect of auditory stimulation on breeding. There is abundant evidence that auditory stimulation plays a large part in maintaining the close bond between the dam and the newborn animal. Clearly animals react to auditory stimulation of a great variety of types. They show certain reproductive responses to certain sounds.

Hormonal and pheromonal facilitation

Reproductive behaviour is based upon the sexual differentiation in the brain which occurs at an early age. Processes of sexual behaviour depend on stimulation by oestrogen in the female and testosterone in the male. Reproductive behaviour in any species is the species-typical repertoire associated with courtship, mounting and coital action in males, and courtship, soliciting and coital acceptance in females. During epigenesis, critical periods exist for the determination of sexual behaviour. A common critical period for sexual differentiation does not appear to exist but the sheep has this critical period in the fetal phase of life.

The neuromuscular mechanisms for most of the components of sexual behaviour are present in both sexes. Given appropriate stimulation, typical heterosexual behaviour can develop. The type of sexual behaviour displayed is the result of the degree of hormonal or other stimulation applied to elicit it (Hurnick, King and Robertson, 1975). In female sheep and goats male-like behaviour induced by testosterone includes most of the distinguishable male components including mounting and pelvic thrusting. In the intact ewe the difference between male and female behaviour appears to be one of length of hormonal stimulation (Lindsay and Robinson, 1964). Thus a dose of either oestrogen or testosterone can induce female oestrous behaviour in ewes within 24 h. Continuous stimulation by either of these hormones can result in a progressive change from female to male behaviour. Ewes treated in this way are effective as males in inducing the ''male effect'' in anoestrous ewes (Signoret *et al.*, 1982).

Sex pheromones act through the olfactory system which includes the vomeronasal organ and the olfactory bulbs. The pheromones may be produced in secretions of the genital organs, the skin glands or occur in the urine, faeces or saliva. The steroid compound produced in the boar and transmitted by saliva foam to the female to produce the immobilisation reflex is a notable example of a pheromone facilitating behaviour. The steroid is released in the saliva when the boar courts the sow and results in the characteristic immobile stance. A sow in oestrus will give a standing response when this steroid in an aerosol is directed towards her snout. With domestic sheep also, it has been suggested that rams stimulate oestrous activity in non-cycling ewes through olfactory receptors in the ewe (Fletcher and Lindsay, 1968).

Seasonal and climatic breeding responses

Sheep characteristically limit their breeding activities to specific seasons. Whether ''breeding'' is taken to mean mating or parturition, it is plain that when seasonal breeding occurs the newborn is provided with environmental circumstances favouring its survival to puberty. In cases where the young are born at an inclement period it is found, as a rule, that the rate of maturation is relatively slower in such species and considerable time is needed for the maturation of the young before they are subjected to the stresses of their first full winter. The periodicity of breeding is governed by the necessities of the young. For the most part, however, seasonal breeding is reflected in mating behaviour.

In a seasonally breeding species, for example the horse and goat, the reproductive activity by both sexes is intensive in the breeding season and subdued, reduced, or absent during the remainder of the seasons. The duration and intensity of oestrus have been observed to alter with seasons. In the mare, oestrus is normally longer in duration during the season of full breeding than at other times. In some breeds of cattle it has been variously noted that significant differences in the duration of oestrus occur with season. In breeds of sheep which breed throughout most of the year, the intensity and duration of oestrus have significant seasonal variations. When the breeding season is a very limited one the intensification of mating drive is evident in the male animals.

Temperature effects

Even with constant breeders temperature changes associated with climate seem to be able to affect reproductive behaviour. It is a frequent observation in cattle breeding organisations that a sudden spell of cold weather is associated with a drop in the numbers of cows in oestrus. Some other species such as goats, indigenous to areas which have equable climates but with marked periods of rainfall, show degrees of seasonal breeding in relation to rainy seasons. It is often observed in indigenous cattle that breeding becomes intensified with precipitation and the associated rapid growth of herbage. Some native breeds of cattle in West Africa are reported to show increased reproductive activity in relation to rainy seasons. Cold daily temperatures are considered to have some slightly beneficial effect on reproductive behaviour in sheep.

The effect of low environmental temperatures on the intiation of the breeding season in sheep is real though slight. Cold days apparently hasten slightly the onset of reproductive activity. It is universally observed in the practice of artificial insemination of cattle that a sudden spell of cold weather is associated for a short while with a drop in the number of reported oestrous cases. In a study of 46 000 inseminations in cattle in central Europe, weather conditions and occurrence of oestrus were correlated. Good weather led to more cows coming on heat but poor, deteriorating weather led to a reduction in the incidence of oestrus.

In other cases, daily peaks of mating activity are apparently associated with fluctuations in male sex drive. Bulls and boars exposed to high temperatures during the summer in hot climates show marked reductions in libido. Libido is inhibited in bulls, in air temperatures of 40–50°C. These effects are transient, however; if affected animals are cooled by wetting, libido quickly returns to normal. It is common in South Africa to find boars extremely inactive during the hot hours of the day, sometimes totally ignoring the presence of oestrous sows. Liberal wetting with cold water is usually effective in improving the sexual activity of such boars. The conclusion can be drawn that excess body heat specifically inhibits libido but is only temporary in effect.

The heat of summer days in central and southern Europe can adversely affect reproduc-tive functions in dairy cattle. This may also be true of many other animals. In general, it can be concluded that temperature changes, e.g. high temperatures, seem more likely to affect the behaviour of continous breeders than others and that isolation apparently inhibits male sexual activity during day-time in the tropics and in warm climates.

At some point, an increasing ambient temperature will make it difficult for an animal to dissipate heat and hyperthermia will tend to develop. Discomfort due to climatic heat can be aggravated by heat increments within the animal as a result of physical activities. Clearly, it is physiologically appropriate that there be limitations on behaviour during hyperthermia, even at a subacute level. The decline in male sexual activity with increasing environmental temperatures therefore has homeostatic significance. It is most likely that the control of this homeostatic mechanism is placed in the hypothalamus.

Inherent rhythm

As stated earlier, breeding rhythm is not just a response to variation in the environment; environmental factors only create the capacity for a rhythm which is endogenous, the environment acting as a zeitgeber or time-giver. This particularly applies to yearly periodicity. The better the endogenous factor (or inherent rhythm) is developed, the more will the time-giver function merely as a synchroniser of events. Breeding periodicity results from the interaction of the two agencies of environmental and internal rhythm together, although the goat and the sheep both tend to maintain internal rhythm for about a year when transferred across the Equator. Among ewes sent from England to South Africa, some immediately change to the Southern Hemisphere breeding season while others change slowly. Within two years, all such ewes switch to breeding during the autumn months of the Southern Hemisphere.

Evidently, the nature of internal rhythm has

not yet been made clear. An animal, of course, does not possess just a rhythm but has a multitude of rhythms in its physiological organisation, with each behavioural element having its own relationship with the environment.

Daily patterns

Breeding in several species tends to occur at particular periods of the 24-h day. Sheep, for example, are observed to mate mostly around the hours of sunset and sunrise, particularly the latter. In Welsh mountain sheep most mountings by rams occur in the early morning, about the time of sunrise. This is mainly due to the fact that about 75% of oestrous periods start during the night. The commencement of mating ewes occurs commonly about the hour of sunrise and also at sunset. This tendency is most evident in the early part of the breeding season. The onset of mating activity appears to become more uniformly distributed in time as the breeding season progresses.

Although first signs of oestrus are at dawn, evening twilight exists as a secondary peak period of initial oestrous behaviour. The rams are active throughout most of the 24-h period, going around the paddock investigating ewes every 20–40 min. It seems unlikely that the significant diurnal incidences of mating in sheep reflect fluctuations in libido, since such rams are usually found to have satisfactory libido when hand matings are carried out in the hours of the day when matings seldom are seen to occur under natural conditions. This points further to the role of the female rather than the male in the crepuscular mating character of the sheep.

In the Red Sindhi breed of cattle in Pakistan the onset of oestrus in 60% of cases occurs most often at night. A preference for mating during the night is evident in Brahman cattle and in various breeds of *Bos indicus*, but this by no means precludes day-time breeding. However, nocturnal mating is the rule in the swamp race of Asiatic buffalo (*Bos bubalis bubalis*). By contrast, the river race of Asiatic buffalo practise day-time mating.

In general there are long-day breeding seasons and short-day ones. Among domesticated species, examples of long-day breeders include the horse and donkey and short-day breeders include sheep and goats. The domesticated horse breeds in the spring and early summer but the Przewalski horse, the closest remaining link with the prehistoric horse, breeds in the summer. Mares do not have an absolute anoestrous season in winter and it has been estimated that only about 50% of mares go into true anoestrous at this period. Many breeds of sheep at tropical and near tropical latitudes breed at all seasons. It seems as something of a general rule that, among those species which manifest seasonal reproduction, long-day breeders are those which have long gestation periods (9–11 months) and short-day breeders have short gestation periods (5–7 months).

In most species, the breeding season appears to be controlled not by a single factor, such as periodicity, but by a combination of external stimuli, including behavioural ones. These vary in different species but nevertheless act through sense organs and mediate the internal rhythms of the individual through the hypothalamus and pituitary.

Illumination

Much more is known of the role of external factors in seasonal reproduction, with photoperiodicity well recognised as the principal agent.

The nature of photoperiodicity has been quite well elucidated in relation to female sheep in which the natural stimulus to seasonal breeding is understood to be shortening daylight. Experimental attention to this phenomenon has been principally directed at bringing sheep into heat outside their normal breeding season by exposing them to schemes of diminishing periods of light per day. Sometimes this has been done with controlled nutrition and temperature. Such treatments have been found to be very effective but involve a considerable latency of response, often 13 to 16 weeks. The picture is very similar in the goat. Extra-seasonal breeding can be induced in the goats treated with artificially controlled light: dark ratio. Gradual light reduction can induce heat periods in goats. Conversely, increasing light results in the cessation of oestrous cycling in the goat.

In addition to the gradual light reduction, one important element of the seasonal phenomenon appears to be a breed-specific sensitivity to some absolute quantity of darkness per day. The natural stimulus is undoubtedly composite but this single aspect of it may be of no less importance than daily reductions in light quotas.

In the goat there seems to be a natural need for daily light and dark, in a ratio of approximately 1:1 or more, for full breeding function in this animal. This approximate ratio is available virtually all the year round in the tropics and between the autumnal and vernal equinoxes in the high latitudes. In the tropical location no season is encountered in which reproductive reduction amounts to impotence. However, it is noteworthy that in wet weather in the tropics the general behaviour of goats is of an inactive character. Even when no seasonal behaviour changes are noted, the exiguous variation attributable to weather changes can create a demarcated breeding season in tropical regions where weather changes such as precipitation frequency are very closely linked with season.

Photoperiodism is the outstanding environmental clue for facilitating those reproductive responses of a seasonal nature. The study of photoperiodic responses, in general, has revealed that some developmental processes are controlled by the length of day. Day-length can control the annual cycle of reproduction or the beginning of breeding rest periods. Photoperiodic responses are due to the length of day (or of night) more than to light quality. Breeding responses induced by photoperiodism can be produced when the length of natural day is extended by artificial lighting of very low intensity. Experiments of this nature have shown that the duration of the photoperiod is more important than the intensity of light. Proximate factors in the environment evidently facilitate the endogenous rhythm.

The influence of constant daily periods of darkness has been studied in Scotland in ewes of Suffolk and Cheviot breeds. During two consecutive anoestrous seasons ewes were provided with simple treatments of 17 h and 16 h dark-housing per day for four-week and two-week periods. Compared with controls, significant results were obtained after one month of treatment but not with two weeks. Oestrus was induced in all ewes treated with 17 h of darkness and in 93% of Cheviot ewes treated with 16 h of darkness. There was a latency of response of 38 days from the commencement of treatment in Suffolks. A latent period of 50 days was observed in Cheviots in both anoestrous seasons. Induced heats continued to recur regularly into the natural breeding seasons of the two breeds. A gradual decrease in the proportion of light is therefore not necessary to stimulate breeding. A fixed and suitable light: dark rhythm is sufficient to hasten the onset of the breeding season in the sheep (Fraser, 1968).

Fixed day-length of a given quantity has already been found in Japanese goats to be as effective as graduated shortening of light hours in the induction of oestrus. The natural stimulus for seasonal oestrus in sheep and goats has components which are both absolute and relative in nature and these components can function independently in operating a breeding rhythm.

The breeding seasons of the sheep and goat are determined in most instances by the times when the majority of females come into oestrus. It is generally supposed that the males will have their reproductive efficiency seasonally influenced in a manner which will coincide with the female's breeding season. Rams have been found to be lacking in libido during the anoestrous period, but rams penned and subjected to controlled light breed out of season. The sexual behaviour in male goats also demonstrates seasonal variation. In the autumn, sex drive is strong and in the period from spring to autumn sex drive is relatively weaker. The period of full breeding function in male goats corresponds very closely with the breeding season of female goats in the same locality. In breeding behaviour of the male goat, reduction in qualitative performance rather than a total inhibition in the reproductive drive is found.

Responses to artificial photoperiodism have been observed in the horse but since this animal is a "long-day breeder" it is found, as expected, that increased light is the positive stimulus. Mares of the Shetland breed—a breed with a very restricted breeding season—can be made to undergo sexual rhythm by irradiation with strong artificial light. It is found in the northern latitudes of Japan that an additional five hours of artificial light after sunset during the month of November improves sex drive in the stallion.

Courtship

Courtship involves male and female behaviour but males are often more active. Many pre-coital components of behaviour tend to be species-specific. These include nosing of the female's perineum, nudging, flehmen, flicking out of the tongue, striking out with a fore limb and low-pitched bleating. Butting of the female's hindquarters is also occasionally seen in both of these species. Mounting intention movements are sometimes shown by males as in all livestock.

The behaviour of courtship will receive later description but attention should first be focused here on three of its salient components, viz. female-seeking, nudging and tending. The seeking by males of females in oestrus goes on almost continuously, under free-breeding conditions. Nosing the perineum and the hindquarters of females is a common male activity. The male may drive the female forward in differing ways. Many male animals, such as rams and boars, will actively pursue females in pro-oestrus.

Nudging in some form or other can be seen in the pre-coital behaviour of all the farm animals and is prominent in courtship behaviour. Nudging behaviour prompts the female to move forwards. In oestrus, the female responds with a stationary stance. This facilitates mating and provides reciprocal stimulation for the male. Rams nudge by pushing with their shoulders and striking the hind limbs of the ewes with their fore feet. Butting is another form of nudging shown by all the ruminants including bulls, rams and goats. Boars root sows.

Tending behaviour is displayed by the farm animals when environmental opportunities permit. The male maintains close bodily contact and association with the female. Both sexes contribute to this temporary alliance. In the tending-bonding there are often phases when the male animal rests his chin over the hindquarters of the female. This chinning behaviour is notable in cattle and represents male testing of the female's receptivity by tactile sense.

19 Female sexual behaviour

Three characteristics of female mammals are of particular importance in their effect on the likelihood of successful mating behaviour: attractiveness, proceptivity and receptivity (Beach, 1976). Attractiveness, or attractivity, is measured by the extent to which a female evokes sexual responses from males. This will depend upon odours which she produces, visual qualities, etc. and on her proceptivity, the extent of invitation or soliciting behaviour. Receptivity is the willingness of the female to accept courtship and copulatory attempts by the male. Variations occur in the degree of attractiveness, proceptivity and receptivity in oestrus female animals (Holmes, 1980; Tilbrook, 1987). Some studies, for example, have shown that many ewes permit about six matings during each heat period. When competition between ewes exists for a limited number of rams, it appears that older ewes are usually more successful than maiden ones in obtaining repeated matings (Fraser, 1968).

A number of reports show that natural matings have the effect of shortening the duration of oestrus in cattle. It is reported that the period of receptivity in cattle is shortened by as much as 8 h when natural circumstances are provided and repeated matings take place. These studies also show that when some female animals are "teased" with vasectomised males, the duration of oestrus is slightly shorter than otherwise. This substantiates the recognition that oestrus is not under endogenous control alone and that its manifestation is subject, in part, to environmental factors including biostimulation (Bailie, 1982; Esslemont and Bryant, 1976; Esslement et al., 1980).

Oestrus is the state during which the female seeks and accepts the male. The behavioural features are synchronised with various physiological changes of the entire genital system essential for mating and fertilisation. The signs of oestrus are characterised for each species but variations occur between individuals. Seasonal and diurnal variations also occur in oestrous manifestations (Bellinger and Mendel, 1974; Foote et al., 1970) (Table 19.1).

Behaviour in general is altered when the mating drive in the female subject is evoked. The usual routines of behaviour are disturbed during overt oestrus and typically there is a reduction in ingestive and resting behaviour, while locomotor, investigative and vocal behaviour are increased. All of this is secondary to the essential character of oestrus, namely receptivity to mating (Lagerlof, 1951).

The influence of environmental factors on overt oestrus is very real and was not adequately appreciated formerly. Apart from those environmental factors which ensure health, such as nutrition and housing, others, of a biological nature, are also influential on oestrus. Recognition of these biological factors improves the modern concept of oestrus occurrence and

Table 19.1
Behavioural characteristics of heat in farm animals

Animal	Typical oestrous behaviour
Horse	Urinating stance repeatedly assumed; tail frequently erected; urine spilled in small amounts; clitoris exposed by prolonged rhythmical contractions of vulva; relaxation of lips of vulva. Company of other horses sought; turns hindquarters to stallion and stands stationary.
Cow	Restless behaviour; raises and twitches tail; arches back and stretches; roams bellowing; mounts or stands to be mounted; vulva sniffed by other cows.
Pig	Some restlessness may occur, particularly at night from pro-oestrus into oestrus. Sow stands for "riding test" (the animal assumes an immobile stance in response to haunch pressure). Sow may be ridden by others. Some breeds show "pricking" of ears.
Sheep	May be a short early period of restlessness and courting ram. In oestrus proper ewe seeks out ram and associates closely with it; may withdraw from flock. Remains with ram when flock "driven".
Goat	Restless in pro-oestrus. In heat most striking behaviour includes repeated bleating and vigorous, rapid tail waving; poor appetite for one day.

affords improvement in the detection and management of this critically important phenomenon.

The term oestrus applies principally to behaviour but it must be acknowledged that it also describes some internal physiological processes. Although the two facets of oestrus can occur separately, this is rare, and it is normal for them to exist simultaneously. When oestrus is shown, behaviour in general changes and many of the animal's usual behavioural routines become disturbed. There are often alterations, and reductions, in feeding and resting, for example. These are secondary to the essential characteristic of oestrous behaviour which is the coital drive.

Features of oestrous intensity

Quiescent oestrus

The dichotomy of the discrete physiological and the overt behavioural characteristics of oestrus is evident in the condition known as silent oestrus. Oestrus in cattle can sometimes be so subdued as to be virtually undetectable, this state being referred to as "silent heat" or "silent ovulation". It constitutes a problem in swine, cattle and horse breeding (Cronin, 1982; Dyck, 1971; Hemsworth *et al.*, 1978a).

While sub-oestrus indicates a very low intensity of oestrus, "silent heat" is a term which has been used to describe the condition in which oestrous behaviour is apparently absent in an animal which is nevertheless undergoing the ovarian changes typical of oestrus. The term "silent heat" is unsatisfactory since "heat" implies intense oestrous behaviour; silent oestrus, sub-oestrus and silent ovulation are more suitable terms for the condition.

In cows and mares, silent ovulation and sub-oestrus can be detected by repeated manual palpation of ovaries per rectum so as to ascertain progressive cyclical changes in the ovary of the anoestrous subject. It is important to differentiate between sub-oestrus and anoestrus, the latter having quite different causes and implications. Paradoxically, the animal in sub-oestrus is potentially fertile although mating capacity is absent.

Silent ovulations occur in other farm animals. Normally they precede the overt heats of the breeding season in the sheep. Silent ovulations are also reported in sows and quiet oestrus occurs in horses, particularly among thoroughbreds under controlled mating methods.

Aberrances of oestrus

Anoestrus is the condition in which a female animal fails to show cyclic recurrence of oestrus. Anoestrus normally occurs, of course, when the animal is pregnant or when it is in its non-breeding season. Some animals such as sheep will occasionally show oestrus in the non-breeding season, as will some pregnant animals. As many as 2% of pregnant cattle show oestrus during pregnancy.

Onset of oestrus

The onset of oestrus in cattle seems to occur at random at any hour of the day or night, although more mutual riding behaviour is shown at night. There is a suggestion that among cattle indigenous to tropical climates, that a much higher frequency of oestrus occurs during the night. Similar observations have been reported in sheep in warm climates where it has been noted that approximately 75% of them commence oestrus during the night. Even in northern latitudes the commencement of oestrus in sheep is during the night in the majority of cases.

Vocalisation in oestrus

Cattle and goats in general employ vocalisations in oestrus, presumably to summon and maintain the attendance of the male. In addition, the vocalisations of many males appear to have considerable effect on the manifestation of oestrus in the female.

Cattle and goats bellow and bleat while in oestrus and the ewe also can occasionally be heard to bleat during heat. The sow is reported to make grunting sounds in heat and it is this species particularly that the effect of male vocalisation on the manifestation of oestrus in the female has been most closely studied. Although the influence of boar odour on heat manifestation appears to be considerable, the "chant de coeur" of the boar is a more effective stimulus than odour in the induction of sexual receptivity in the sow.

Duration of oestrus

Few animals have a normal oestrous cycle which is so notoriously irregular in duration as the horse. This irregularity is found in the horse at all latitudes. Although the mare usually remains in heat for fully a week, it can last much longer. A common range in the duration of oestrus in the mare is four to ten days. Shorter heats more often occur as the breeding season progresses (Table 19.2).

Although it is considered that the true oestrous period of cattle lasts 18–24 h, some variation is reported in them also. A significant seasonal difference occurs in the average duration of bovine oestrus. Oestrus has an average duration of 15 h in the spring as compared with 20 h in the autumn. The oestrous period has been considered to be shortened by mating. Heifers when mated to vasectomised bulls tend to ovulate earlier than those not mated. The period of receptivity is shortened in many cows after natural service.

The heat duration in the sheep appears to be under influences very similar to those in the cow. No seasonal difference in duration of oestrus apparently occurs in Merino ewes but Merinos have shorter oestrous periods than some other breeds. Mating appears to reduce the heat period in the sheep (Table 19.3).

The determination of the duration of oestrus in the ewe has been based on the period throughout which the male will mate with the ewe. Several experiments have shown, however, that a decline in the ram's libido, specifically for the individual stimulus ewe, occurs after a number of matings and when a fresh stimulus ewe is presented there is restoration of libido. This suggests the possibility that duration of oestrus in the sheep, as estimated by the course of mating with a given ram, may be frequently underestimated. Heat periods of three days' duration have been noted in Suffolk and Cheviot ewes.

The length of the period of oestrus in the goat is sometimes longer than the usual estimates in sheep. The limits of the goat's heat period are

Table 19.2
Temporal features of oestrus in the mare

Feature	Occurrence		Remarks
	Average	Range	
Age at first oestrus	18 months	10–24 months	Breed variations occur
Length of oestrous cycle	21 days	19–26 days	Length of cycle is largely dependent on length of oestrus, e.g. 5 days oestrus has 21 days average cycle; 10 days oestrus has a proportionally longer cycle (26 days).
Duration of oestrus	6 days	2–10 days	Heat periods early in breeding season are usually long (10 days) and tend to get shorter as breeding season advances.
First oestrus post-partum	4–9 days	4–13 days	Ninth day after foaling is common time.
Breeding life-span	18 years	16–22 years	Breed variations occur
Breeding cycle and season	Seasonally polyoestrous. Natural breeding season is spring and summer (i.e. seasons of increasing light) in either Northern or Southern Hemispheres. Extended breeding time in tropics. Nearer the Poles the breeding seasons are very restricted, also a feature characteristic of northern breeds, e.g. Shetland pony.		

more easily determined because of the clearer signs of heat in this species. The period of oestrus is one to three days (average 34 h) in most goats.

Post-partum oestrus

Since complete involution of the uterus requires several weeks following parturition in all animals, there are no physical grounds to expect oestrus to occur soon after parturition. But this is true only for some species; several show normal heats very soon after parturition.

The mare is the best known example of a species showing early oestrus after parturition. This early heat is called the "foal heat" and occurs on the average about nine days after the birth of the foal. The foal heat is often short and is of low fertility but is otherwise apparently normal. It has been observed that 65–69% of mares of most breeds show oestrus not later than the twentieth day after parturition.

Heat is not rare in sows about three days after farrowing (Benjaminsen and Karlberg, 1981). Cattle show a much more delayed heat after calving and this heat is further delayed if the subject is nursing a calf or is being milked frequently each day. In Red Sindhi cows after calving, cows whose calves were weaned at birth returned to oestrus in 110 days as compared with 157 days for cows whose calves were not weaned. In most European breeds of cattle the first oestrus occurs at an average of 31.7 days after normal calvings. The wide variation in the heat interval in dairy cattle is commonly taken to be associated with the rate of milk production, with high producing cows taking longer to show the first post-partum heat. Cows running with a bull after calving show heat about 27 days earlier than similar cows without exposure to a bull. The heat interval is commonly about six months after calving among dairy cattle which nurse their calves.

A number of sheep of various breeds, which have seasonal breeding rhythms, show heat

Table 19.3
Temporal features of oestrus in sheep and goats

Feature	Occurrence		Remarks
	Average	Range	
Sheep			
Age at first oestrus	9 months	7–12 months	Usually occurs in first autumn when well grown.
Length of oestrous cycle	16.5 days	14–20 days	Very long intervals usually indicate intervening silent heat
Duration of oestrus	26 h	24–48 h	
First oestrus post-partum	Spring or autumn		Some ewes show oestrus while lactating
Cycle type	Seasonally polyoestrous		7–13 heats per season according to breed. "Silent heat" commonly precedes overt oestrus.
Breeding life-span	6 years	5–8 years	Short breeding life for hill ewes
Breeding season	Precedes shortest day of year but varying in extent according to breed.		Northern breeds (e.g. Blackface) have shorter season than southern breeds) e.g. Suffolk, Merino. Latter can breed bi-annually.
Goat			
Age at first oestrus	5 months	4–8 months	Kids born in spring show oestrus in autumn of same year.
Length of oestrous cycle	19 days	18–21 days	Short infertile cycles (e.g. 4 days not uncommon. Short cycles in tropics.
Duration of oestrus	28 h	1–3 days	Seldom less than 24 h.
First oestrus post-partum	Autumn		Tropical breeds can sometimes be bred while lactating.
Cycle type	Seasonally polyoestrous		8–10 heat periods.
Breeding life-span	7 years	6–10 years	Shortest in tropical breeds.
Breeding season	Commences about autumnal equinox		September to January in Northern Hemisphere. Extensive season in tropics.

quite soon after lambing, before the onset of their anoestrous season.

Species-typical oestrous behaviour

Sheep

Relatively quiet heat is the rule in sheep rather than the exception. Oestrus in the ewe is extremely difficult to detect if there is no ram in the flock. But, with a ram in the immediate environment, it is usual for the ewe in oestrus to associate closely with it for most of a 24-h period. Ewes frequently initiate the first sexual contact by seeking out the ram and thereafter following the ram while heat persists. Some-times the ewe will rub herself against the ram. Further behavioural evidence of oestrus sometimes appears as tail shaking but this only occurs at mating. Different grades of intensity occur in the sex drive of ewes, although the general mating pattern is similar in all. Many ewes in oestrus actively seek out the male and, when a choice of ram is possible, it is the most active ram which is generally chosen. Although the normal period is recognised as being just over 24 h, oestrus can last for up to three days in some ewes. Mutual riding among ewes, one of which is in oestrus, has not been reported.

Goats

In very sharp contrast to the sheep is the manifestation of oestrus in the goat which has very marked behavioural signs. Goats of any breed probably show more conspicuous oestrous behaviour than any other farm animal. For the one to two days of oestrus the female demonstrates a rapid tail waving; the upright tail quivers vigorously from side to side in frequent bursts of flagging. There is repeated bleating throughout oestrus; the animal eats less than usual and has a tendency to roam.

Cattle

It is uncommon for very intense manifestations of oestrus (for which the term ''heat'' should perhaps be reserved) to be observed in cattle. Signs of such oestrus include general restlessness, raising and switching the tail, arching or stretching of the back, roaming and bellowing. The most noticeable element of behaviour, however, is the mutual riding which takes place between the oestrous subject and conspecifics. These are often the closest social associates of the subject. Ultimately it is the cow in oestrus which stands to be ridden but this does not wholly preclude the subject, in its turn, riding others, male or female. (see Table 19.4).

The behavioural signs of oestrus in cattle include the following points:

1. There may be an increase in general activity in ways that could be generally termed restlessness.
2. The oestrous cow bellows more than usual.
3. Grooming activities, in the form of licking other animals, are increased.
4. Typically, the oestrous cow frequently makes mounting attempts on cattle. When several cattle in a group have been prompted to mount each other, through the initial activity of the oestrous cow, it may become difficult for an observer to identify the cow in the group which is in true oestrus, but when one animal in particular is standing to be mounted by others it is usually the animal in oestrus.
5. Oestrus lasts for a period of 12–24 h and it is commonly observed to be of shortest duration in young cattle.

Table 19.4
Behavioural signs of bovine oestrus

Behavioural signs	Intensities of display		
	Intense	Intermediate	Weak
1. Restlessness	++++	+	−
2. Bellowing	+++	++	+
3. Licking other animals	++	++	+
4. Mounting other animals	+++	++	+
5. Standing to be mounted	++++	+++	+++
6. Jerky movement of lumbosacral region	++	++	+
7. Arching and stretching the back	++	++	+
8. Appetite reduction	+	−	−

Considerable variation occurs both in the intensity of oestrus shown and also in the degree of notice taken of an oestrous subject by other cattle in the group. Only a small proportion of the group participate in mounting the oestrous animal. When two or more heifers are in heat they are not of equal interest to other heifers. Even with the same animal no great similarity in mounting attraction at successive heats is shown. The stage within the oestrous period does not appear to influence the mounting behaviour of others. The repeatability of degrees of expression of oestrus in individual cattle is low. Selection against weak oestrus is therefore of little value but some consistent individual differences are observed between cows in the intensity of their heats, indicating a genetic basis to intensity.

Ovarian dysfunction in cattle

Ovarian dysfunction alters the nature of reproductive behaviour. Typically it manifests itself either by anoestrus or by abnormal oestrus. Follicular cysts are the most common cause of both types of syndrome. Most other forms of ovarian dysfunction suppress oestrus. With oestrus suppression, two types of syndrome occur, namely sub-oestrus and anoestrus. The two syndromes are sometimes confused but have very different significance.

In sub-oestrus, the ovary of the animal exhibits the normal cyclical changes without overt oestrus occurring. Some cases with histories of anoestrus can reveal evidence of full ovarian function on rectal palpation by the presence of either an active corpus luteum or a graafian follicle. These cases properly are diagnosed clinically as sub-oestrus. Sub-oestrus is of common occurrence in the early post-partum period. Again, sub-oestrus may only reflect poor or inadequate observation by attendants, for example, oestrus may be short and may occur at night. ("Silent heat" is a stockman's term used synonymously with sub-oestrus.)

Anoestrus is only a symptom and is not in itself an independent disorder. It must always be remembered that pregnancy is a principal cause of anoestrus. Anoestrus under other circumstances requires special consideration as a symptom of several types of ovarian dysfunction.

Arrested ovarian function without a responsible lesion is not infrequently associated with anoestrus. In such cases no gross physical abnormality may be present in the ovaries but these are found to be smooth-surfaced, being free of corpora lutea and graafian follicles. The condition may be a consequence of high production pressure or other environmental adversity. Since it often has the status of a herd problem, in very large dairy herds, it must represent a widespread problem.

Horses

The mounting behaviour between females so typical of oestrus in cattle is not observed in mares. Oestrous behaviour in mares shows a range of characteristics peculiar to this species (Fraser, 1970b). The intensity of oestrous behaviour varies probably more than in any of the other farm species. A mare in oestrus frequently adopts a urinating stance. During these periods of straddling, mucoid urine is ejected in small quantities which may splash at the animal's heels. Following this, the animal maintains the straddling stance for a time with the hind limbs abducted and extended. The tail is elevated so as to be arched away from the perineum. The heels of one or other hind hoof are commonly seen to be tilted up off the ground so that only the toe of that hoof remains touching the ground. While this stance is maintained the animal shows flashing of the clitoris by repeated rhythmic eversions of the ventral commissure of the vulva (Fig. 19.1). The duration of equine oestrus is four to six days on average but varies, some lasting only one day and others lasting up to 20 days.

The company of other horses is sought and particular interest is shown towards the male. In the presence of the stallion, the mare in typical heat will direct her hindquarters towards him and adopt a stationary stance. It is found, however, that some mares of fractious temperament, though in heat, may kick forcefully on being mounted by the stallion.

Abnormal oestrus

Five types of irregularity in equine oestrus are recognised.

Sub-oestrus.   In the mare, as in the cow, a form of ovarian dysfunction can be clinically recognised in which there is follicular development in the ovary without an associated behavioural oestrus being detected. This condition, commonly referred to as "silent heat" is featured in many cases of anoestrus in mares during

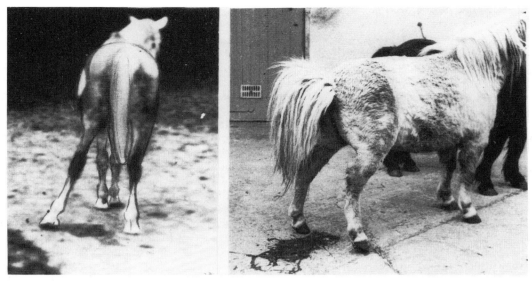

Fig. 19.1   Oestrous display in the mare showing tail-arching, hind limb abduction, toeing the ground, etc.

their natural breeding season. Normal ovulations usually occur in these cases.

Nymphomania. There is no doubt that excessive displays of oestrus or "nymphomania" are encountered in mares but this condition is not associated with true cystic ovarian disease. Nymphomania seems to be a condition of "transient persistence" of one or more follicles which eventually regress or ovulate spontaneously. The term nymphomania may also be used by horse breeders to describe excessive oestrus manifestations within a normal oestrous period. Normal oestrus periods can recur in infertile mares so regularly and frequently that a history of excessive oestrus is given and encourages an incorrect speculative diagnosis of "nymphomania". A mare with normally recurring oestrous cycles could be in heat 22% of the time. Sexual maturity may be more variable in mares than has been generally recognised. There is no doubt that there is great variation in the age at which young mares attain normal ovarian activity as evidenced by polyoestrus.

Protracted oestrus. The average duration of oestrus in the mare is commonly given as six days but wide variations in duration are common. Some workers in equine infertility have suggested that estrus exceeding ten days in duration is abnormally protracted. Certainly, infertility is common in protracted oestruses of this nature due to the inevitable delay in ovulation. It is thought that many cases of this type are more common at the onset of the breeding season and are also more common in young maiden mares.

Seasonal anoestrus. This is not uncommon in the winter in northern countries. European countries often report an incidence of about 50% of winter anoestrus in mares. The incidence in North America is at least as high as this and in Canada it is considered normal for most mares to be in seasonal anoestrus during the winter.

Simulated oestrus. Oestrus in the mare can in some cases be shown without associated follicular development on either ovary. In some of these cases, the behavioural signs of oestrus can be quite intense. At the present time, no satisfactory explanation for this condition can be given but exogenous oestrogens in the animal's diet might be responsible in some cases. Again, in some cases, there may be small follicles present in the substance of the ovary which may not be palpable but might have endocrine function.

Whatever the neuro-humeral background might be, the behaviour takes on the appearance of simulation. Simulated conditions (such as lameness) appear in states of learned helplessness in animals. The question remains unanswered, however, concerning the possibility that mares may simulate oestrus in certain circumstances.

Pigs

A salient feature of oestrous behaviour in the sow is the adoption of an immobile stance in response to pressure on the back. In pig-breeding practice this is often supplied by the animal attendant pressing the lumbar region of the sow or sitting astride the animal. The onset and the termination are gradual and of low intensity but the "standing" period is well defined and lasts less than a day on the average. The oestrous sow is sometimes restless when enclosed, this being rather more noticeable during the hours of night. Some breeds, particularly those with erect ears, show a conspicuous pricking of the ears in full heat. The ears are laid close to the head, turned up and backwards and held stiffly. "Ear pricking" is often shown when some movement is taking place behind the animal. Mutual riding is very much less common than in cattle but the subject in heat is often ridden by other females. Occasionally, among groups of sows, one particular sow will perform most of the riding.

While the level of oestrous behaviour expressed by the gilt influences her fertility, factors exist in the environment which are capable of affecting the expression of oestrus. The level of oestrus expressed can be determined by the back-pressure test in the presence of a boar, based on the willingness of the gilt to stand, and on the duration of this standing response.

Oestrous stimuli

It is now recognised that for oestrous responses to be shown in complete form, in many farm animals, it is necessary for some form of extero-stimulation or "biostimulation" to be provided. Male attendance which supplies prompting, as for example, in the form of nudging, is now appreciated to be an important contributor to oestrous displays in females. This male influence on oestrous behaviour, now termed "biostimulation", has been noted by some stockbreeders for many years, but was not accepted as a fact by animal scientists until the so-called "Whitten Effect" was reported. The Whitten phenomenon is one in which oestrus in mice can be synchronised and induced by the introduction of a male mouse into a colony of females. Carefully detailed experimental work on this phenomenon has established that the majority of the females come into oestrus as a result of being exposed to a specific odour from the male animal. There is evidence that this type of phenomenon may also occur among the various farm animals (Fig. 19.2).

It is known that the introduction of a ram to a flock of ewes can influence the commencement of the breeding season in that flock (Fraser and Laing, 1968). This effect can even be achieved without the ram having physical contact with the female members of the flock. Ram influence, being provided under practical conditions by "teaser" rams, undoubtedly brings on seasonal breeding activities in ewes more rapidly than occurs when they are left in an all-female group. The masculine stimulus may be provided visually by the sight or by the sound or odour of the ram. It would seem, however, that whatever the stimulus, it can influence the breeding behaviour of ewes over some distance.

Boars provide a range of stimulating factors

in the form of elaborate nudging and highly specific vocalisation, together with the production of pheromones, in order to induce maximum oestrous responses in sows. While other examples of biostimulation in farm animals show a latency in responses, this has not been noted in the pig to date. Indeed, in a sow which is already in oestrus, the standing response can be obtained almost immediately when some of the specific stimuli are provided, e.g. a recording of boar sounds or the dropping of small quantities of seminal fluid on the snout of the sow.

Evidence of biostimulation has also been obtained in cattle. It has been reported that, in several experiments in which teaser bulls are run with groups of newly calved cows, the so-called teased animals show signs of oestrus much earlier than similar cows in control groups. Breeding behaviour may be shown four weeks earlier in the teased group than among controls. The phenomenon of biostimulation and its significance must now be more fully appreciated.

It is clear that induction of oestrus in the farm animals is not only due to internal, endogenous factors, but also to external, exogenous stimulation. The latter stimulation is complex involving odour, sound, sight and touch. Earlier it was supposed that oestrus was entirely under endogenous control, but it is clear now that exogenous factors are of considerable importance. The problem of anoestrus—the failure to show oestrus during the periods of the breeding season or life-cycle when it should be shown — in farm animals might be attributed, in many cases, to the absence of exogenous factors through faulty husbandry as well as faulty observation and detection.

Genital stimulation

Oestrus can be prompted or induced to some degree by genital stimulation in ways which resemble phenomena of the "Whitten" type. Genital stimulation is evidenced by nuzzling, nudging and licking about the perineal region in the pre-coital behaviour of cattle, sheep and goats.

Synchronisation of stimulated oestrus

As might be anticipated, biostimulation afforded by the presence of the male in a group of females, in addition to inducing oestrus, has the added result of affecting most of the female population, simultaneously. In consequence, oestrus which has been prompted by biostimulation shows varying degrees of synchronisation (Fig. 19.2).

When the ram is turned out with a flock there is a high incidence of oestrus 18–20 days later. The introduction of a ram serves as a stimulus to terminate the anoestrous season and results in a degree of synchronisation of heats. Vasectomised teaser males in goats and sheep prompt the manifestation of oestrus in 91% and 97% of the females of the two species, respectively, after a latent period of one month. Biostimulation by the ram is especially effective during the transition from the non-breeding season to the breeding season of the given breed and also at the end of the breeding season.

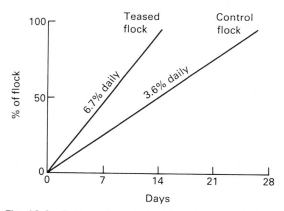

Fig. 19.2 Daily rate of lambing in teased (biostimulated) and control (non-teased) ewes. Following biostimulation both flocks were joined and one ram was introduced; this achieved close synchronisation of pregnancy.

20 Male sexual behaviour

The propensity to show sexual behaviour of male farm animals is referred to as libido (Wodzicka-Tomaszewska *et al.*, 1981). This develops at puberty and, after maturation, persists at a fairly constant level for the remainder of the animal's lifespan. Male libido is primarily dependent on the production of testosterone by the testis, but there is genetic variation amongst animals in its extent.

Some variations in libido can have quite considerable consequences in farm economics (Blockey, 1978, 1981). In the bull, libido varies in degree between age groups and between breed types (Chenoweth and Osborne, 1975; Couttie and Hunter, 1956; Foote *et al.*, 1976). In general, a lower level of libido is found in beef than in dairy breeds. Comparing the species, the highest levels of libido are generally noted among the seasonally breeding animals, for example rams (Banks, 1964). Clearly those species which concentrate their breeding season into relatively short periods require high levels of libido for effective reproduction during that time. The level of libido may change as a consequence of various factors. Young rams usually show low libido after introduction to a new group (Holmes, 1980). Also there are physical changes that occur in ageing bulls which are known to reduce their sex drive. Quite clearly, an animal which is experiencing discomfort or even pain during movement in mounting will, in time, have his breeding behaviour impaired. It is

also strongly suspected that temperamental factors can cause sexual inhibitions in stud animals (Fraser, 1957, 1960b).

While low libido in free-living animals can substantially reduce the number of offspring produced, in domestication unwise selection can permit its propagation and there is evidence that this has occurred in some of the beef breeds of cattle. It is recognised by practical flock-masters that, in some breeds of sheep, the rams have higher levels of libido than in others. There is also growing suspicion that certain breeds of pigs produce boars with inferior libido. Impaired or inferior libido is not always inherited. Obesity in stud animals often contributes to low libido. Some skeletal defects such as arthritis are also a common cause of poor motivation in breeding behaviour.

An interesting phenomenon of libido is one which is associated with its total absence. When entire male animals experience complete loss of their sex drive for some reason or other, they seek out the company of other male animals of the same species. The bachelor groupings which result when such male animals gather together are a phenomenon which has been observed in many species of free-living animals. Bachelor groupings can be noted when large numbers of bulls run together. They are also seen among rams during the long non-breeding season of the year. The purpose of bachelor groups is to suppress further any libido that individual males might have and such close male groupings quite clearly show successful adaptation amongst their members.

Male manifestations

One of the behavioural components of male sexual display in all hoofed stock except the pig is the "olfactory reflex" known as flehmen. In this the animal fully extends the head and neck, contracts the nares and raises the upper lip while taking shallow respirations. It occurs most usually subsequent to smelling urine and nosing the female perineum and is a form of odour testing. Schneider first reported the reflex in 1930 and descriptively termed it flehmen. He observed it in a variety of artiodactyls in a zoological collection. He found that the "expression" could be evoked by a variety of volatile substances.

The sheep and the goat have a great number of components in their courtship activities which are extremely similar (Clegg *et al.*, 1969; Lindsay, 1965; Price *et al.*, 1984c). They include the following acts: nosing the perineum, nudging, olfactory reflex, flicking of the tongue, striking out with a forelimb, low-pitched bleats. The male goat apparently has the largest repertoire of such acts, including some others such as:

(a) urine-spilling on to the fore legs which resembles urine-spilling on to the hind feet in reindeer;

(b) butting the female's hindquarters which resembles a component of bull behaviour; and

(c) false mounting attempts such as occur in some other species, particularly the horse.

Some components of male sexual behaviour are fairly characteristic of the given species. Bulls, for example, often pump their tail heads and pass small amounts of faeces in the precoitus. Certain major activities develop male sex drive. These are linked and are virtually common to all hoofed stock. These behavioural activities tend to flow into each other but can be separately described as follows:

1. Threatening and displaying.
2. Challenging and contesting.
3. Signposting and marking.
4. Searching and driving.
5. Nudging and tending.

Although these activities tend to flow into each other, they are best discussed individually.

1. Threatening and displaying is usually effected with the subject in a stationary position. The threat display of the bull occurs as a physiological state of fight-or-flight. In this state the animal arches his neck, shows protrusion of the eyeballs and erection of hair along the back. During the threat display the bull turns his shoulder to the threatened subject.

The threat display of the stallion involves rearing on his hind legs and laying back the ears (Collery, 1969, 1974). Threat displays are rarely shown by rams towards humans but, nevertheless, forms of threat are exhibited in the presence of other potential aggressors and in these circumstances the threat display usually involves vigorous stamping of a fore foot.

The readiness with which threat in any form is displayed varies and is logically thought to reveal something of the subject's disposition (disposition being a manifestation of temperament). Male temperament is found to vary a great deal in bulls although it is fairly consistent in many given individuals. The range of temperaments has been noted and described variously as "placid", "stable", "lethargic", "likely", "excitable", "aggressive", "apprehensive" and "timid". Some of these terms are anthropomorphic and without meaning to those with no knowledge of this animal but the terms are descriptive and serve to show the spectrum of male temperament.

2. Challenging and contesting apparently occurs to some degree among sexually adult males of all ungulate species. Challenging behaviour among male animals is typically seen where there is an opportunity for males to form pairs. When the challenges are taken up the outcome of the challenge eventually determines the "peck-order" or hierarchy. The peck-order also affects sexual status in free-breeding groups of animals. The male at the top of the peck-order may perform most of the breeding with the available females. Under domestication this type of circumstance is not usually permitted to develop. Nevertheless, breeders are not unfamiliar with "boss bulls" and "boss rams". The challenging behaviour of the bull has three main components which appear to run closely together and to occur in variable arrangements.

(a) The bull paws vigorously at the ground with a fore foot, with the head lowered. This pawing or scraping breaks up soil which is scooped over the animal's withers where it may gather as an earthy mantle.

(b) The animal rubs the side of its face and its horns into the area bared by pawing. This is done with the animal kneeling and with some vigour.

(c) The bull stands stationary, repeatedly bellowing with a broken voice (Fraser, 1968; Fraser and Sane, 1982).

3. Signposting and marking to indicate sexual territory. Domesticated male animals engage in behaviour which can be described as territorial. Pawing and horning behaviour by bulls creates bare patches of earth and these patches located throughout his territory are clearly a claim to possession of a given area ("stamping ground"). Stallions also claim territory; they do this at pasture where they urinate and defaecate at selected spots. Given suitable territory they mark it in this fashion, returning from time to time to defaecate and urinate again in the same places. These activities apparently serve the dual purpose of marking male territory and priming female sexual responses by pheromones.

4. Searching and driving. Searching for breeding females and then driving them before him is an activity of the male animal which now appears to be an important component of biostimulation, a system which is becoming better appreciated. The tending bond links male and female closely during the period of oestrus.

Many male animals, notably rams, engage in pursuit of females in the pre-oestrous phase. Bulls spend much of their breeding time searching through the herd, examining females.

Male seeking behaviour of females in oestrus goes on continuously under free-breeding conditions. Nosing the perineum and the hindquarters of females is a fairly continuous male activity (Wierzbowski, 1966). The experienced male animal is capable of detecting the pre-oestrus phase in the female and after locating a female in this state he will consort with her and will engage in "driving" behaviour. The male may drive the female forward in differing ways. Stallions force mares to move forward by nipping their hindquarters and often by biting them in the regions of the hocks.

5. Nudging and tending of some type are often shown by the male while consorting with the female before and during oestrus (Fig. 20.1).

"Nudging" in some form or other can be seen in the precoital behaviour of all the farm animals and is prominent in courtship behaviour. Nudging behaviour prompts the female to move forwards. Firm standing is the positive response to nudging (pushing the female with, for example, the nose or poll) by the male subject and provides reciprocal stimulation. Nudging is represented by the pre-coital behaviour of the bull and male goat, but other forms of nudging or promoting are also used. Nudging by the horse with the shoulder and with the chin can both be observed. Another form is seen in the stallion which he tests oestrus in the mare not only by sniffing her but also by biting and pinching her over areas of the body, working from the hindquarters towards the neck.

Once mating has occurred, freely associating partners of several species exhibit the so-called tending bond. Both sexes contribute to the temporary alliance, thereby facilitating repeated mating and ensuring optimum conditions for fertilisation to occur (Hemsworth *et at.*, 1978a).

"Tending" behaviour is displayed by farm animals when opportunities permit. The male maintains close bodily contact and association with the female whilst grazing near her. In the

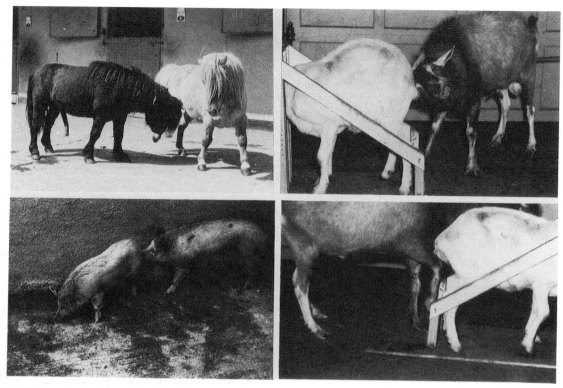

Fig. 20.1   Forms of ''nudging'' in the horse, pig and goat. Top left: stallion nipping the hind leg of an oestrous mare. Top right: buck goat butting perineum of female ''teaser'' goat. Bottom left: boar pushing sow with the snout. Bottom right: buck striking female with a fore leg.

tending-bonds of most farm animals there are phases when the animal rests his chin over the hindquarters of the female. This ''chinning'' behaviour is best seen in cattle but it also occurs in other species.

Motivational modifications

In domesticated animals it has been observed that the beef breeds of bulls which gain considerably in weight with maturity show reduction in libido with obesity. Many bulls of some beef breeds are found to be virtually asexual. Obesity in all animals generally affects libido as evi-denced by reduction in the reaction time. In the boar reduced libido occurs in subjects which have acquired skeletal defects, e.g. arthritic lesions. On post-mortem examinations of impotent boars, pronounced changes are often found in the skeleton, particularly in the larger joints of both fore and hind legs. The most constant finding is deformity of the hip joint. Impotent boars often suffer lesions of the hip joint although the level of libido is constant for most bulls throughout their working lives. Beef bulls sometimes show reductions in libido with ageing. In cattle the voluntary separation of bulls from cows during the hot months in tropical Australia has been attributed to the long-term stress of adaptation and under-nutrition. Such animals show the absolute loss of libido which is typically revealed by spontaneous male segregation. In many different circumstances spontaneous male segregation is shown by individual animals such as old Chillingham bulls. At other times such segregation is shown collectively by masculine groupings during the non-breeding season as, for example, in the bachelor parties of rams.

The level of nutrition can apparently exert some slight influence on libido (Wierzbowski, 1975). High planes of nutrition inhibit testosterone secretion in young bulls, while gross underfeeding impairs libido in some boars.

There is much variation amongst genetic strains in the libido of male animals, although a variety of factors can modify sexual desire in bulls and other stud animals. Uniformly poor libido, for example, was found in a set of monozygous triplet bulls.

Seasonal fluctuation in libido can occur but dominant males of certain breeds successfully retain their status from one season to another. Even in seasonally breeding species, there is some persistence in the strength of libido from one breeding period to another.

Some of the domesticated species showing seasonal breeding have been studied critically in respect to their libidos over periods of time, but none of them shows seasonal breeding in a form as dramatic as the rut and they do not show a complete absence of libido during the non-breeding season (Hafez, 1962). Seasonal fluctuations are widely observed in the libidos of the male goat and sheep. During each breeding season a level of libido is reached which is fairly characteristic for the individual. In tropical locations, seasonal waxing and waning of libido may not occur in some sheep. In Africa the mean libido is consistent throughout the year in the breeding activities of rams and goats. Rams and male goats are found to show seasonal reductions in libido which occur in the summer season (Fig. 20.2).

In considering the strength of sex drive as an indication of infertility in the male, it is important to stress the fact that there is no significant correlation between sexual behaviour and semen production or quality. For example, semen has been found similar in rams with normal libido and those with poor libido. In any assessment of the breeding ability of a sire, an adequate examination must therefore take cognisance of the efficiency of sexual behaviour, quite apart from semen characteristics.

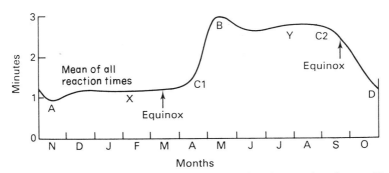

Fig. 20.2 Annual mean reaction (ejaculation) times in a group of 12 male goats in twice-weekly semen collections under controlled, experimental conditions. The breeding and non-breeding seasons are marked by plateaux (X and Y) in responsiveness. Changes (C1 and C2) in libido are closely linked to the two equinoxes showing that a photoperiod with a greater quantity of dark than light per diem was stimulatory in these animals. Highest and lowest responsiveness (B and A) are brief phases commencing and terminating the breeding season in this species in Northern latitudes.

Measurement of male libido

Measurements of sex drives in male animals have been determined such as:

(a) number of ejaculations in an exhaustion test;
(b) the reaction time (delay before ejaculation);
(c) proportion of failures to mount; and
(d) proportion of failures to ejaculate.

The importance of establishing a constant stimulus in any attempt at measuring sex drive has long been emphasised (Hale and Almquist, 1960; Fowler, 1975; Fowler and Langford, 1976). The reaction time and number of ejaculations per unit of time are valuable as basic measures of male sexual function.

Even highly objective measures, however, can be misapplied, by prior stimulation, for example, or by varying the stimulus conditions from time to time. Bulls in the presence of a constant stimulus animal show a gradual decrease in the number of ejaculations per unit of time until no further responses occur. The loss of response to a given stimulus animal may not interfere with the degree of response to other animals but the recovery of sexual response to the same stimulus animal ranges from poor to complete after an interval of a week.

These naturalistic methods may have their value but they may not reliably indicate small differences in libido between animals or between times. The negative aspect of ejaculation number is, of course, ejaculation failure and this criterion can be used in assessing libido in bulls or other stud animals over an extended period of breeding time. Failure to mount and ejaculate in a group of similar subjects in a standard schedule, provides a reliable assessment of libido if continued over a sufficiently long period.

Although sexual reaction times in male animals can be influenced by a variety of somatic and psychological factors, estimation of the reaction time provides a simple and, ordinarily, reliable measurement of libido. In a study of reaction times in 102 bulls of different ages and breeds it was found that subjects over four years of age had longer reaction times than others (Table 20.1). For bulls of four years of age and over, the reaction times of beef breeds were significantly greater than in dairy breeds. Under four years of age the difference was not significant. The dispositions of all bulls was observed in order to determine temperaments and these fell into three main groups, viz. stable, aggressive and apprehensive (Table 20.1). Reaction times of bulls with ''apprehensive'' dispositions were significantly greater than others. There is now general acceptance of the belief that apprehensive traits have a particularly inhibiting effect on copulatory activities. Further observations on reaction times in bulls confirm that reaction times are fairly consistent in the individual but have a skewed distribution in the population. Two very different averages have therefore been observed—a mean of 12 min and a mode of 2 min.

Reaction times of bulls, rams and stallions remain almost constant over intervals ranging from one to 20 days. After the first ejaculation, reaction time increases with successive copulations as repeated breeding progresses. It has been found that the mean reaction time of four random observations spaced well apart gives an extremely reliable indication of the long-term sexual responses of the animal.

Table 20.1
Average reaction (ejaculation) times (min) according to age, breed type and temperament for 102 bulls

A. Breed and age group

Age group	Beef bulls	Dairy bulls
4 years and over	24	12
Under 4 years	6	5

B. Temperament

Stable	Aggressive	Apprehensive
12	9	44

After Fraser (1957).

Male responsiveness

The key stimulus required to elicit sexual behaviour in the male is simple in the case of the bull. Bulls will mount and attempt copulation with a dummy consisting of a covered frame. The basic releaser for mounting in the bull is in the form of an arch or bridge of appropriate dimensions.

A simple dummy or "phantom" cow is used in some programmes of bull testing. Of 2500 bulls tested as many as 90% mounted the dummy. When given a choice, however, bulls preferred a live cow. The visual stimulus is considered to be of paramount importance in the bull. Bulls which are blindfolded will still serve, however, and clearly other stimuli operate. Olfactory cues were of great importance in the bull but individual stimuli are additive in nature and the simulus provided by the sight of a sexual object may be enhanced by the olfactory stimuli released by an oestrous female in her urine. The internal and external stimuli, involving conditioning and all the senses, are temporarily cumulative and the threshold may be exceeded by one, some or many stimuli according to the responsiveness of the subject. It is a general law of ethology that constant stimuli do not evoke a constant response. Responses fatigue, and such fatigue clearly occurs when the same stimulus is repeatedly offered.

In practice it is found that changing the stimulus animal or the setting results in a greater number of ejaculations per unit time in the bull and sheep. Sexual responsiveness in the male sheep can be readily restored, after exhaustion with one ewe, by presenting a fresh unmated ewe. Substantial changes of stimulus can have an adverse effect; for example, the responses of jackasses is poorer to mares than to jennies. Young boars with experience of natural mating take longer to respond to the dummy sow than do similar young boars without experience of natural service. In certain circumstances the male animal can be abnormally stimulated. Restriction and homosexual groupings of intensively confined animals are liable to produce abnormal intra-specific sexual behaviour.

Some breeds of domestic sheep and goats have such an intense breeding period that there are resemblances to rutting. The fighting which occurs between black-face rams at the outset of their breeding season closely resembles a rut. Head-on charges between rams can be so forceful that ruptures sometimes result from the impact. The abdominal viscera force open the inguinal canal and allow the passage of large portions of omentum into the scrotum. It is clear that fighting between breeding males can be merely mock battles from which no serious injuries result; but, on the other hand, such contests can be very real, vigorous and potentially harmful to the participants. Among domestic stock it would be extremely unwise to allow adult breeding males to fight on the assumption that the contest will be a mock, ritual event. Fatal trauma too often results in such circumstances.

21 Copulation

Coitus in farm mammals has its timing so arranged that most spermatozoa are introduced into the female genital tract before the ovum is liberated from the ovary—a requirement of fertility. Initial copulations are centred mainly in the earlier part of oestrus, with repetitions of mating occurring in the later part. The frequency of repetition varies. Differences in frequency are evidently greater between individual pairs than between species (Blockey, 1979). Coital repetition diminishes in the middle period of the day and in late oestrus. This contributes to the conservation of breeding resource in the male.

Mating results from the emergence of oestrous behaviour in the female and the activation of male sexual behaviour. Both sexes make equivalent contributions. The female contribution is now recognised (Hemsworth *et al.*, 1978a; Lindsay, 1978). Oestrous ewes, for example, studied in an extensive enclosure containing a tethered ram, approached the ram sufficiently closely to allow mating to occur. It has been noted that a ram tethered to a tree, while ewes were driven away daily, marked 66% of his flock in 52 days. In the same time, in a similar flock, a free ram marked 84%. The ewe's part in mating is emphasised by the finding that many ewes will breed with only one ram under natural conditions, even though there may be several available. Even with rams immobilised by tether, over 50% of ewes chose to breed with only one ram and less than 10% bred with all the available rams.

In cattle it is well known that the cow will actively seek out the bull, even mounting him herself if mating is delayed (Fraser, 1968, 1978a). Such behaviour supports the generalisation that both sexes exert considerable influence on mating activities as a whole (Holmes, 1980; Lindsay, 1965; Perry *et al.*, 1980; Rushen, 1983; Signoret, 1975).

The male contribution to mating stems from the male sex drive which, if fully functional, only requires minor environmental stimulation to be activated. Details of such activation have been considered in earlier chapters. The behaviour of pre-coital "courtship" activities merges into that of coitus to integrate with it (Table 21.1; Fig. 21.1).

Pre-coitus

In the immediate pre-coitus the basic response of the male is orientation towards the female. The male typically aligns himself behind the female, in the same long axis, until mounting occurs. Deviated stances occur in close association with impotence characterised by diminished drive. In the deviated pre-coital stance the male animal, while keeping his head at the hindquarters of the female, turns his body away from her alignment. Such disalignment sometimes precedes

Table 21.1
Coitus in farm livestock

Male reaction time	Pre-coital behaviour of male	Manner of intromission
Stallion Averages about 5 min	Noses genital region Genital olfactory reflex Bites croup region Penis erects fully	One to four mounts Several pelvic oscillations Terminal inactive phase
Bull Mode 2 min Mean 12 min Mean of beef breeds 20 min	Noses vulva Genital olfactory reflex Alignment Licks hindquarters	Single pelvic thrust coordinated with clasp reflex
Boar 1–10 min	Approaches sow giving series of grunts Noses vulva vigorously Champs jaw and froths at mouth	Short pro-trusions of spiral penis repeated till intromission occurs Pelvic oscil-lations followed by somnolent phase
Ram 30 s to 5 min	Noses vulva Genital olfactory reflex Paws with fore foot	Very quick single pelvic thrust with fore limb clasping
Goat 12–60 s	Bleating, stamping with fore foot, rapid licking Genital olfactory reflex	Very quick pelvic thrust

impotence, thereby allowing the latter to be forecast under conditions of controlled mating. Deviated position is held characteristically for lengthy periods of several minutes and the angle of disalignment appears to be greater with more complete forms of impotence. The implications of the phenomenon in the bull, ram and goat are that orientation becomes impaired with reduced sex drive but becomes re-established when sex drive is restored (Fraser, 1964).

Mounting

The salient component in mating behaviour is mounting. The neuroethological mechanism for the activity of mounting differs from that mediating intromission. Mounting by both sexes is seen in some species; it is particularly common in cattle. Female cattle will mount each other even when there is a male present in the group. The pig is another animal which exhibits mount-ing by females when one of their number is in oestrus. Mounting by females on other females in oestrus is a very rare event in the horse. As a rule, it does not occur in sheep.

The stimulus required to initiate male sexual behaviour is essentially simple in the case of the stallion, the bull, the ram and the boar (Sambraus, 1979). These animals will usually mount and attempt copulation with a dummy consisting of a covered frame. The mounting of "dummies" can be the result of a learning pro-cess in the boar.

As has already been pointed out, the male mating pattern is not sex-specific within the species. Temporary inversion in sexual beha-viour in individuals of both sexes is uncommon but does occur. The basic neurophysiological mechanisms of mating behaviour are vested in both sexes, so that two potential features of sexual behaviour are present in each individual.

Male animals seldom mount the females of species other than their own but stallions will mount female donkeys and jackasses will, likewise, mount mares. Such inter-species coitus allows mules to be bred. Occasionally sheep and goats will inter-mate but normal pregnancies do not result. Isolated instances of abnormal sexual behaviour have been reported in which the male of one species mounts females of a different species. Examples include bulls mounting mares, stallions mounting heifers. In each of

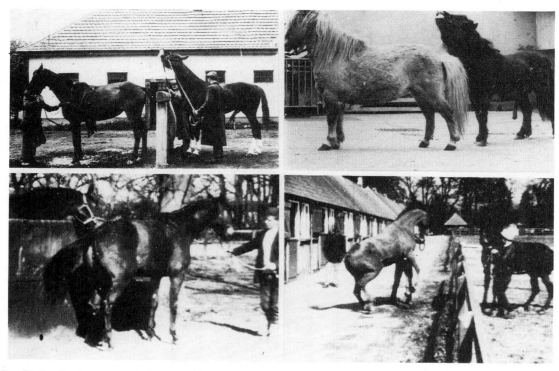

Fig. 21.1   Oestrous mares being tested for receptivity. Top left and right: positive responses in both sexes. Bottom left: stallion nips mare which responds with oestrous display. Bottom right: mare (on left) reacts negatively to stallion approach and contact.

these cases the animals involved were stated to have been in each other's company from early life and this suggests that the abnormal behaviour was a consequence of imprinting.

"False mounting" attempts by the male animal are commonly seen in courtship. In these instances dismounting subsequently follows quickly without any fore limb clasping or pelvic thrusting movements. False mounts show that the mechanics of mounting and of intromission are separately controlled. False mountings are to be seen in the mating patterns of the stallions, the sheep and the goat. In the stallion it is believed that some two or three false mounts are normal before effective mating is achieved.

In a detailed study of mounting behaviour in the stallion it was found that older animals mounted more quickly than younger ones, that blindfolded subjects mounted more quickly than others and that about two false mounts seemed to be usual before intromission and ejaculation were effected. In the stallions which were blindfolded it was observed that mounting was undertaken after the male had "shouldered" the female. The mounting behaviour of the stallion when presented with a dummy mare was also studied and it was noted that young inexperienced stallions mounted the dummy more readily when they were blindfolded than when they could see, but still more mounted the dummy when it was visible and sprinkled over with urine from an oestrous mare. All of this points to the positive stimulus of odour and the weak effect which visible features may have on mounting behaviour in this animal. Bulls, which have a significantly protracted reaction time, and which appear to have their mounting responses inhibited by environmental factors when presented with oestrous cows, sometimes respond to blindfolding by mounting promptly.

Intromission

Following normal mounting, penile intromission is effected, but this is dependent on prior penile erection. Erection in the stallion is much less rapid than in the ruminants. It may be for this reason that "false mounts" are customarily shown by stallions before mating takes place. In the bull, goat and ram there is a more rapid erection and protrusion. In the ruminant species intromission consists only of a single pelvic thrust which is followed by dismounting. In the stallion intromission is maintained for a period of a minute or more during which there is repeated pelvic thrusting and subsequently the adoption of a fairly static posture, after which dismounting occurs.

Clasping by the male during intromission and mounting is an important component of coital behaviour. The stallion and the bull effect tight clasping of the respective female with their fore legs adducted into her flanks. In the case of the bull, this clasping increases in intensity at the moment of penetration and ejaculation. Vigorous clasping also takes place in mating between sheep, but when the male and female are heavily covered by wool, clasping is inevitably impaired to some degree. Recent studies suggest that more effective mating takes place in sheep when the female has been shorn before mating activities commence; if this is true the explanation is likely to lie in improved clasping by rams which in turn improves mating action.

The manner of intromission in the pig is also unique. In this species, the male mounts and makes thrusting actions with the penis, which repeatedly makes semi-rotatory actions. Only

when the spiral glans penis of the boar becomes lodged tightly in the firm folds of the cervix does this action stop and ejaculation commences. It is clear, in fact, that the locking of the penis in the cervix acts as the essential stimulus to ejaculation in the boar. Although clasping is not easily shown by the boar, this animal employs a "treading" action with his fore feet on the back of the sow while mating. Large boars on small sows or gilts will clasp but in these cases it is common for the female to collapse and effective intromission or mating does not occur.

Treading is of course the important mechanical feature of mating in poultry. In the mating behaviour of poultry "waltzing" by the cock is the main pre-copulatory behaviour. In waltzing the cocks adopt a stilted walk around the female bird, tilting the body to one side. In freely mating poultry a high frequency of treading occurs in social relationships where the male chases the female frequently, or where the male waltzes to the female frequently. Treadings most often result from crouchings by the females, chasing the female, and previous treadings by other males. Sexual preference between particular pairs of birds are noted. In ducks, mating may take place on water or land and sometimes the mating drake will be assisted by another male pressing the female's neck onto the ground when the mating drake is mounting.

The erect penis on intromission has increased sensitivity to tactile stimuli and these, in their turn, effect ejaculation. Spinal reflexes are also involved in ejaculation. The release of oxytocin, on intromission, contributes to the ejaculatory process in the bull. Significant amounts of oxytocin are present in the bull's bloodstream immediately before and after service. Bulls which were not sexually stimulated or had served more than five times previously were found to have no detectable amounts of oxytocin in their bloodstream. At the time of bovine ejaculation there occurs also a peak record of the psychogalvanic skin reflex which is indicative of a neural–emotional event.

Repeat mating

Following ejaculation, male animals show a refractory period which is a state of sexual exhaustion. The state of sexual exhaustion is not principally a physical one, however, and refers mainly to the loss of stimulus quality by the female. A quick return to mating behaviour is shown by male animals when they are given an opportunity to mate a new oestrous subject.

It is the normal procedure among farm animals for repeated matings to occur with any given female. Stallions probably re-serve oestrous mares five to ten times in each heat period and most rams are noted to re-mate with ewes three or four times. Bulls are seen to re-mate with oestrous cows repeatedly perhaps on five or six occasions. Boars normally serve sows several times over a period of 24–48 h. Among poultry repeated matings are frequent (Craig and Bhagwat, 1974).

The boar is capable of a great number of services before exhaustion occurs. Boars can serve oestrous sows up to eleven times in one heat period. It was observed in a test that each of three boars ejaculated eight times during a 2–25 h test period in which nine oestrous females were available. In a test of mating ability in the bull, however, it was reported that 75 ejaculates were collected from one particular bull in a 5 h period of testing (Almquist and Hale, 1956). Some animals with less spectacular mating scores are nevertheless able to carry out large numbers of matings over longer periods of time. The sheep is the best example of this. It is estimated that the average ram mates 45 times per week in a large flock.

Variations occur in the degree of receptivity in oestrous female animals. Some studies have shown that many ewes permit about six matings during each heat period. When competition between ewes exists for a limited number of rams, older ewes are usually more successful than maiden ones in obtaining repeated matings.

Natural matings have the effect of shortening the duration of oestrus in cattle. The period of receptivity in cattle may be shortened by as much as 8 h when natural circumstances are provided and repeated matings take place. When some female animals are "teased" with vasectomised males, the duration of oestrus is slightly shorter than otherwise. This substantiates the earlier statement that oestrus is not under endogenous control alone and that its manifestation is subject, in part, to environmental factors including biostimulation.

Pairing

Among outdoor livestock, pairing is most conspicuous in the species which maintain sexual segregation for most of the year, forming intersexual arrangements only during the breeding season. This is notable in sheep living in free-range conditions.

In the much briefer pairing periods of other livestock a close tending bond is usually evident. A special positional arrangement has been noted in breeding cattle. Under field conditions cattle frequently adopt a "parallel and opposite" position during the period when they pair for mating. The parallel and opposite positioning of the male and the female clearly allows a most intimate bond between the individuals of opposite sexes when mating activities are in abeyance.

The mating and pairing arrangements in horses have been studied and described by Zeeb (1959, 1961). He noted that before pairing is established mares present their hindquarters to stallions and urinate. After biting by the stallion and kicking by the mare, pairing is often established by nose to nose contact between stallion and mare. During these activities, however, the stallion is constantly providing protection to his entire herd, circling it and examining other females, especially when they respond to his whinnies. Although the qualitative reproductive behaviour of stallions is very similar, there is a great difference between them quantitatively.

Impotence

Impotence is inability to mate. It has been fairly well studied in domesticated species because it is a factor which adversely affects the economics of animal breeding and because of its fairly common occurrence (Fraser and Penman, 1971; Fraser, 1973). Impotence, in the form of disinclination to serve, is the most common impairment of breeding function. Inability to copulate has been reported to be the most common cause of the disposal of bulls. Sexual inhibition appears to be a major factor in many cases of impotence. This includes the "somnolent condition" in the bull in which there is a tendency of the bull to appear somnolent, with its eyes shut, during chin-resting on the cow. Normally, of course, if chin-resting elicits a static response in the cow, the bull shows an increase in sexual activity.

The boar is also found to suffer commonly from impotence. The majority of boar infertility cases are not truly infertile, but are impotent due to defects in mating. Numerous studies show that peculiarities of mating behaviour are of prime importance in the etiology of infertility in swine. Many mating dysfunctions in boars seem to be associated with inability to achieve sufficient penile penetration for effective locking of the spiral glans penis in the sow's cervix.

Abnormal sexual reflexes occur in the stallion and these may be due to heredity, inhibitory reflexes or faulty management (Waring *et al.*, 1975; Waring, 1983). Undoubtedly genetic factors play a part in some forms of impotence. The effect of inbreeding in mating soundness in bulls has been widely studied. There seem to be more service deficiencies among inbred bulls than in cross-bred bulls. Inbreeding has an adverse effect on the mating activity of rams also. As a result of inbreeding, rams may lack the ability to recognise the olfactory signs of oestrus in ewes.

Many different factors can, of course, be responsible for states of impotence and in a variety of forms of impotence in bulls two major divisions exist:

1. Impotentia generandi, which is synonymous with the more common term infertility; and
2. Impotentia coeundi, which is equivalent to the term impotence.

Varieties of impotentia coeundi (or impotence) exist in bulls. These are categorised as follows:

(a) bulls with lowered sex drive;
(b) bulls with insufficient erection;
(c) bulls with faulty ejaculation.

Clearly the variety of physical, physiological, hormonal and genetic conditions which can be the basic causes of these forms of impotence can be very great.

Certain common physical disorders, whether distal or local to the genitalia, such as arthritis and posthitis, will readily impair an animal's mating actions, but a surprising number of impotence states are attributed, by experienced observers, to psychological factors in the subject. In some instances psychological factors have been alluded to in general terms but other reports implicate more specific psychological factors such as exaggerated apprehension. There seems little doubt that psychological factors, whether specific or non-specific are a common cause of impotence, or copulation failure, in farm animal reproduction (Fraser, 1960b).

22 Fetal behaviour

Features of behaviour emerge and change during the development of the animal. The courses by which these changes occur have now become recognised as an important branch of ethology. This special area of behavioural ontogeny not only reveals crucial patterns of infant behaviour in farmed animals but also shows the phenomenon of a time dimension in the programming of behaviour. A full appreciation of the behavioural as well as the physical development in young livestock is of critical importance in their optimal management.

Behaviour in the nascent animal reveals phenoma of neural programs relevant to neonatal survival (Cowan, 1979). An appreciation of such phenomena is important to optimal conditions in the perinatal period. Mortality rates in these newborn animals are great and cannot be controlled without progressive management, taking account of their specific behavioural needs. Development of behaviour in the fetus, the neonate and other young farm animals has received some keen study in recent years. The sheep fetus has been an excellent model for different aspects of this study. The major features of behaviour in the nascent subject are kinetic, postural, taxic and tropic.

In recent years there has been keen interest in the effect of the pre-natal environment on post-natal behaviour. Precocial neonates, such as foals, calves, lambs and piglets, have already been exposed to sensory stimulation of some kind before birth and it is therefore likely that sensations of position, gravity, touch, smell and taste occur within the uterus. It is known that sheep fetuses can hear some extra-uterine sounds (Vince and Armitage, 1980; Vince et al., 1982). The fetal ear of ungulates is completely formed and functional before birth (Humphrey, 1970). The quantity of amniotic fluid in fetal nostrils at birth is usually considerable, indicating that the olfactory mucous membrane has been in close intimate contact with the material which will later be expelled at the birth site.

In the embryonic domestic chick movements of the head, body, wing and limb begin as jerky actions at four days of incubated age. These continue as uncoordinated movements in irregular sequences, reaching a peak at the middle of the incubation period and continuing until a few days before hatching when smooth and coordinated movements develop. The embryonic movements have been shown to be under spinal control. Wing movements are evidently driven by a spontaneous neuromotor process. Similar spontaneous nerual activity probably underlies most mammalian fetal activity. By the time the chick is ready to hatch, synchronised limb movements resembling walking and wing movements that resemble flapping are present (Provine, 1984).

Fetal behaviour in farm animals has been the

subject of reported study for several years. The concept of fetal behaviour as an entity is not new. In regard to the human fetus, Hooker (1954) pointed out that "the skeletal muscle reflexes of the fetus are one manifestation of function and constitute its overt behaviour". Researchers have noted that although many kinetic reflexes in the fetus appear through reflex activity, spontaneous fetal movements also occur—in fact, they predominate. Much fetal behaviour develops in the organism by the reaction and integration of local reflexes which create complex functional activity. The concept of progressive behavioural development in the fetus recognises that given behavioural actions occur in given stages of development, in either an active or passive manner.

Features of kinetic behaviour in the human fetus have mostly been concerned with the living aborted fetus subjected to probe stimulation during a brief extra-uterine life while suspended in isotonic saline solution (Hooker, 1954; Hooker and Humphrey, 1954). On the other hand, fetal behaviour in farm animals has been studied by palpation, surgery, ultrasound, radiography and recently by fluoroscopy (Fraser *et al.*, 1975; Fraser, 1976, 1977; Fraser and Terhune, 1977a, b; Fraser and Herchen, 1978). While surgery and palpation in horses and cattle have provided information on fetal posture, the dynamic aspects of fetal kinetic behaviour have been found most amenable to study in sheep by the use of video-taped fluoroscopy.

As the major form of fetal behaviour, fetal kinesis occurs throughout the greater part of pregnancy and with gestational progress its different features become recognisable. In both medical and veterinary studies two forms of fetal movement have been recognised. In the human subject these have been called local reflexes and total pattern reflexes. In animal studies the terms used for analogous behaviours are simple fetal movements and complex fetal movements. Since some fetal kinetics in the large animals may be either spontaneous or reflex, the term fetal movement is considered preferable.

Human fetal reflexes have also been classified as negative and positive, depending on response to local stimulation. In the animal subject "positive" movements are those which show posture, position and adaptation for birth; since these positive postures and positions are sometimes temporarily abandoned—in a return to a supine condition—such returns might be termed "negative" movements, in accord with a medical perspective.

Action patterns and movement sequences in the fetus

In addition to singular movement and multiplicity of movement, episodes of great fetal activity occur. Behavioural units are desirable in detailed behavioural study. During the study of naturally occurring behaviour in a fetus the concept of the "action pattern" (Broom, 1981) is useful. When gross fetal activity occurs, this is the result of groups of complex fetal movements quickly following one another. It is therefore appropriate, in all types of fetal activities, to recognise the functional units of these as simple and complex movements. Simple and complex fetal movements are finite units, the study of which calls for periods of continuous scrutiny which include occurrences of action patterns such as rotation and pronation in the mature fetus. Fetal monitoring by video-taped fluoroscopy allows this to be done for comprehensive appreciation of fetal movements.

The action patterns of the fetus in rotation, extension and pronation, seem to be non-signal in nature. Rotation and pronation are the two notable action patterns of the fetus which must be described in terms of their structure. Other important aspects of the movements are the taxic, their relation to maternal anatomy, and the temporal, their timing during gestation. In addition, it is hoped that identification of the action patterns will lead to the search for their counterparts in the central nervous system.

Simple fetal movements

Radiography has been used in sheep to observe certain qualitative aspects of fetal activity during days 80 to 120 of the 150-day gestation in this animal. Simple fetal movements observed by this method are generally similar in form and of characteristic occurrence in each of the major mobile anatomical parts. The neck, fore limbs and hind limbs show most movement. These movements occur independently of fetal position. They are not subject to influence by the number of co-fetuses. Radiographic study has shown that simple fetal movements usually consist of exercise movements of major parts. These exercises are common and apparently autonomous. They take the form of extension and flexion, principally of the limbs and neck. Movements of the trunk were noted but were less striking. The main reason for this apparent disparity between trunk movement and movement of other parts may be the close coupling of the vertebrae of the trunk.

A number of specific features of this type of fetal kinesis were observed. These included the following:

1. The frequency of simple fetal movement was similar in both fore and hind limbs in the total population of 124 fetuses studied. This is consistent with the movements being general exercise.
2. The greatest degree of kinetic variation was seen in the neck. The most common movement of this part was lateral flexion. Extension of the neck was a notable feature only in pre-partum "engagement" of the fetus in the maternal pelvis.
3. Neutral positions of articulating parts outnumbered any other single position but did not outnumber flexions and extension combined. Evidently exercise is a prominent activity.
4. Fore limbs were rarely in opposing disposal, while hind limbs were usually in similar disposal. Symmetry of motion further suggests fetal control of these actions.

In any animal, repetitive muscular activity inevitably has the effect of establishing improved muscular development and muscle "tone". In pathological conditions of the fetus associated with reduced fetal energy, such as thyroid deficiency in the fetal sheep, muscular underdevelopment is a prominent finding. In thyrodectomised fetuses, a marked reduction was noted in the development of the appendicular skeleton, compared with controls. Simple fetal movement is evidently a phenomenon directly related to physical maturation generally, to muscular development in particular, and to kinetic competence most specifically. The application of this information probably lies in better recognition of the need for fetal activity with the nutritional management implications inherent in this.

Jaw movement

Periodic mouth opening and closing has been reported in the human fetus as a local reflex—the equivalent of a simple fetal movement. Continuous fluoroscopy on the sheep fetus has shown that jaw movements, which are of high frequency in nature, constitute a notable item of terminal fetal activity as an item of specialised simple fetal movement. Slow and rapid jaw movements can be distinguished, the former as early as 40 days pre-partum.

Rapid jaw movement is seen in the mature fetus in the form of rapid rhythmic mouth opening and closure. Most of these exceed ten in number per brief episode of oral activity. This rapid, rhythmic jaw movement is carried out with the lower jaw moving in the vertical axis in relation to the skull. This form of rapid rhythmic jaw movement represents vigorous sucking activity by the fetus (Fig. 22.1). Such episodes occur frequently in very late gestation. Involved with these are minor actions of head extension with the mouth open and ventral head flexion with the mouth closed. It has been determined that such actions represent swallowing. In addition, some rapid jaw movements are

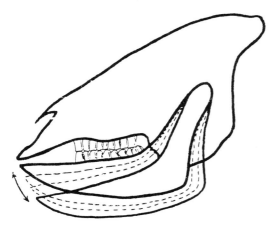

Fig. 22.1 Drawing of rapid jaw movement as seen by fluoroscopy in the sheep fetus during the two weeks before birth. This activity represents sucking which is therefore not simply a post-natal development. (Courtesy of R. Bowen.)

seen in the last week in which the lower jaw moves at right angles with the upper jaw, with the mouth evidently closed. This has been assumed to represent "chewing" mouth movement. It is clear, therefore, that the mature fetus engages in a considerable amount of oral behaviour including sucking and swallowing.

These observations dispel the notion that the "suck reflex" is a phenomenon which comes into existence for the first time post-natally. The first sucking activity (in the form of rapid jaw movements) is seen in the sheep fetus on average ten days before full term and occasionally as early as 16 days before birth. Fetal sucking has been observed at some point during the week preceding birth in all of the fetal lambs recently studied for this phenomenon (Fig. 22.2).

Complex fetal movement

While simple fetal movements, with the exception of rapid jaw movement, are common and evenly distributed throughout the second half of gestation, fetal movements of greater complexity become more numerous as full term is approached. Complex movements consist of close accumulations of physical actions occurring in series. Typically, complex fetal movements contain three to five individual component actions. In the terminal phase of gestation complex fetal movements in cattle, horses and sheep increase in frequency. Some episodes follow closely on each other, giving lengthy spells of fetal activity. Extremely intense fetal activity is frequently followed by an extended period of fetal quiescence. In the radiographic study using fluoroscopy, complex fetal movements are seen to have quality in addition to quantity in that they contribute to processes of action. Coordination of complex fetal move-

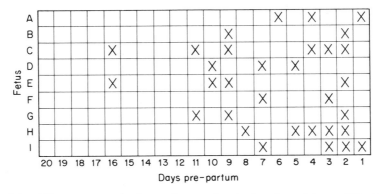

Fig. 22.2 Sequential rapid jaw movements observed pre-partum in nine sheep fetuses. (Courtesy of L. Husa.)

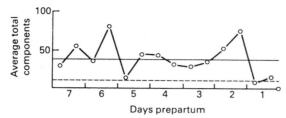

Fig. 22.3 The course of kinetic activity, determined by ultrasound, in a group of 12 bovine fetuses in heifers pregnant to the same bull in the last week of synchronised pregnancies.

ments develops and leads to their grouping into phases. Mass fetal activity occurs in lengthy phases in the pre-partum stage of gestation. The peak of fetal activity occurs three days prior to parturition in horses and about two to three days pre-partum in sheep and cattle; shortly before parturition, activity declines (Fig. 22.3).

Righting

The effects of complex fetal movements in subjects close to full term involve change in fetal postures and position. Much of this relates to so-called "righting behaviour" in the fetus which, in the case of sheep, is otherwise held in a supine position, the fetal spinal column resting on the maternal abdominal floor. The principal items in righting behaviour are:

1. General activity.
2. Extension of the carpal joints and digits of the fore feet towards the maternal pelvis.
3. Elevation of the head and neck.
4. Rotation of the head and its extension towards the maternal pelvis.
5. Rotation of the anterior trunk from the supine position through 180 degrees.
6. Attainment of a position of pronation (Fig. 22.4).

Essentially, these righting reflexes dictate a conversion from general flexion to strategic extension of certain parts; they evidently occur

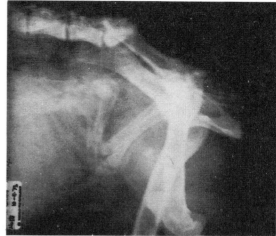

Fig. 22.4 Fetal pronation and engagement in the maternal pelvis.

during the two days before birth in the sheep, one day pre-partum in the bovine fetus and in first-stage labour in the equine subject. Further specific postural features of note during birth include the flexion and retraction of the elbows against the thorax and simultaneous flexion of the stifle joint before terminal conversion of the hind limbs from full flexion to full extension. Episodes of massive fetal kinesis precede the alerted phase when fetal postural extension first occurs, usually a few days before pelvic engagement and birth. Mass kinesis, involving approximately 3500 movements, coincides with these fetal "righting" actions. Typically this ceases before birth, when a phase of quiescent fetal behaviour prevails. Evidently the muscular competence necessary for such a scale of fetal activity is acquired by intra-gestational fetal exercising. Attainment of the birth posture by the fetus is the apparent function of terminal fetal kinesis.

The posture of alerted behaviour has been found to be most proficiently secured by the heavier, more muscular, fetus. This finding indicates the need for adequate muscular development if the fetus is to respond properly to terminal arousal, as yet an undefined phenomenon.

The quantity and quality of complex movements during the righting, or rotating, reflexes can probably only be carried out efficiently if the fetus is in a satisfactory muscular condition. If all of the essential righting reflexes are not accomplished, the fetal posture may be abnormal. The common abnormalities are: (a) the result of failure of one or both fore limbs to be extended into the maternal pelvis before birth commences; and (b) the result in deflection of the head to one side—a position which is exaggerated when the second, or expulsive, stage of birth forces the fetus into the birth canal. That these circumstances are conducive to the most common forms of fetal malposture encountered in dystocia in sheep, and other farm livestock, is too obvious to ignore. Absolute inertia of the fetus on the last day is likely to result in fetal malposture and birth difficulty. Inertia follows abnormally high spikes of fetal activity and is apparently a form of fatigue in the fetus.

The primary etiology of fetal malposture becomes opened for reconsideration given these findings. Already there are known correlations between pathologically reduced neonatal vigour in animals and certain conditions such as prenatal nutrition and placental insufficiency. Research is required to ascertain whether these and other conditions operate via fetal health which, in spite of decades of intensive study of fetal diseases in domesticated animals, has been a singularly neglected aspect of the subject of fetology.

These behavioural items listed in righting do not necessarily occur in the order given. This order is not always precisely followed in the course of "righting" behaviour—which can be more properly termed rotation. Both partial and total rotation is frequently undertaken, abandoned and restored by the sheep fetus in the terminal days of gestation. While this may also be true of the bovine fetus it is by no means true of the equine subject.

When rotation has been completely enacted by the sheep fetus and the posture of upright extension attained, and if the position of orientation to the pelvic inlet holds good, the fetus appears to squat to the pelvic lodge. This squatting may be sustained for variable periods of time such as 10–60 min. However, it frequently becomes abandoned and the fetus then usually returns to a supine position. In doing so the fore limb extension may still be preserved.

Pronation

As a result of periodic rotations, the fetus terminally adopts the prone and squatting posture appropriate for birth. This occurs several times before the birth processes become imposed upon the fetus. Eventually there is extreme extension of the head at the atlanto-occipital joint and this ensures "engagement" of the extended skull and fore limbs within the maternal pelvis. The atlanto-occipital and atlanto-axial joints in the anterior neck region are subject to considerable articulation. These seem to be the most active articular sites in the entire vertebral column. Their articulations relate to modifications in cranial or vertex presentation and the degree of extension of the head at key points in the birth process. Even then, partial engagement may be lost in a temporary regression in postural behaviour. Such regression is not uncommon. When phases of postural regression occur they modify fetal rotation, pronation and terminal extension, either partially or radically.

Fetal rotation leads to the "pandiculated" fetal attitude as a result of fully extended pronation. The fetal head, including the occipital poll, eventually becomes contained within the maternal pelvis so that a point-of-no-return is reached in the fetal position and final "engagement" is evidently complete.

The primary "righting" act of carpal joint extension has the effect of directing the fore feet into the maternal pelvis. The elevated and extended head follows, having changed from a cranial presentation to a facial one. When the head and fore feet are fully engaged in the birth canal, ewes began to show the behavioural signs indicative of pain in the first stage of labour. Fetal posture at this stage is also characterised by full flexion and closure of the elbow and other joints. In addition, although the distal fore limb joints are extended, the elbows are typically retracted against the lower antero-lateral region of the rib cage on each side. In this position the elbow joints are opposite to the intrathoracic location of the fetal heart. At this point, the fetal posture is one of extended pronation. Fetal posture and engagement at the pelvic inlet become fully organised on the last day of gestation, sometimes only in the last hours in cattle and sheep.

Attitude in expulsion

In the fluoroscopic study of lamb births it was noticed that, as the head progressed through the birth canal, the carpal joints, in a number of cases, remained momentarily fixed and hinged over the maternal pelvic inlet. This had combined effects, including:

(a) advancing the shoulders into the birth canal;
(b) apparently levering the head and neck forward: and
(c) retaining, and over-exaggerating, the fully flexed and retracted elbow-joint posture.

With the advance of the shoulder joints into the maternal pelvis, the fetal scapulae became laid in parallel position over the dorsum of the fetal thorax. These arrangements of the upper fore limb joints gave a bilateral Z-shaped bony support to the fetal thorax throughout the expulsive stage of labour.

When the terminal postural changes are effected, the fetus is wedge-like in overall attitude and the typical "birth posture" becomes attained. The X-ray studies have shown that the fetus, in natural birth, holds the elbows in this retracted position during the expulsive stage of

the birth process until the subject has been almost totally extruded. Ultrasonic records of heart action during sheep births show that fetal heart rates drop very suddenly and quite dramatically when the dam is exerting her full expulsive forces on the fetus during the second stage of parturition. It would appear that thoracic reinforcement with the flexed elbow may be of value to support heart action in the fetus at this time of considerable external pressure.

As birth of the anterior parts of the fetus progress, all the hind limb joints are flexed. These remain in this posture until the fetal abdomen is in the birth canal. At this time, the hind limbs convert to parallel posterior extension. Fetal expulsion is complete soon thereafter.

Final fetal postures in cattle

The postures of 1255 bovine fetuses were determined using a direct surgical examination in a caesarean survey. Incidences of variable features, including fetal presentation, head posture and the arrangement of limbs, were determined. The fetuses had incidences of 86.8% with anterior presentation, 90.2% with head extension, 96.1% with extended fore limbs and 56.5% with extended hind limbs in posterior presentation. Pronation, with extension of the digits and carpal joints of the fore limbs, was dominant. Reduced responsiveness was recognised in varying degrees from the minor one of one flexed fore limb, to the major one of deflected head with both fore limbs flexed.

Certain consequential features of kinetics emerged clearly from this caesarean study. The "alerted" behavioural state of the fetus, evident in maximal extension of the head, also involves fore limb extension, of the digital and carpal joints in particular. Fetuses showing postural arousal in the form of head extension, show equivalent responsiveness in fore limb extension as part of the engagement process of the fetal head in the maternal pelvis. Few cases of double fore limb flexion (only 0.6%) were found in association with head extension, while a comparatively high number (5.1%) showed double fore limb flexion in association with failure of head extension. When fore limb extension did fail, in the "alerted" or "aroused" fetus with full head extension, it occurred in one limb only. This is indicative of a reduction in arousal of a lesser order than in subjects with double fore limb flexion plus failure of the head extension. In the latter case an "aroused" state had evidently not been behaviourally established. To present the picture another way, it can be stated that fetuses showing head deflexion are apparently not adequately "aroused" and in these cases, therefore, flexion of both fore limbs is relatively common while single fore limb flexion is rare. This picture fits the concept held by many veterinarians that the bovine fetus at term makes "efforts to stand up *in utero*".

Fetal arousal, as evidenced by fore limb extension, was more commonly deficient in older cows. The posture of alerted behaviour tended to be most proficiently exhibited by the heavy male fetus in the younger cow. This finding may be an indication of the need for adequate muscling of the fetus in order to respond properly to terminal arousal, as yet an undefined phenomenon. Postural defects, chiefly head deflexion and fore limb flexion, appear to be associated with relative fetal inertia (Fraser, 1977) at full term when "alerted" fetal behaviour should occur.

The application of these data mainly relate to the etiology of fetal malposture and the recognition of dysfunction of posture as causes of bovine dystocia. Fetal postural function can evidently be better appreciated through the behavioural processes of fetal motoricity and kinesis.

Fetal "bunting"

In the pre-partum stages of gestation the monitoring of fetal activity in the sheep by fluoroscopy has shown that acts of bunting occur

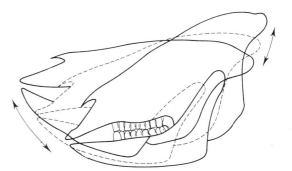

Fig. 22.5 Drawing of sharp, upward "bunting" movements of the sheep fetus as observed by fluoroscopic monitoring.

occasionally (Fig. 22.5). In this activity the fetus jerks the anterior pole sharply upwards by extension at the junction of the head and neck. This is done with the mouth closed. The behaviour very closely resembles the bunting acts of lambs at nursing in which they thrust the nose vigorously upwards at the ewe's udder when nursing is being initiated and before milk letdown has occurred. With the recognition of prenatal sucking it is to be expected that pre-natal "bunting" should also be evident in fetal behaviour. The sharp upward head movements of the fetus, while resembling udder bunting characteristic of nursing, appear to have no clear biological purpose in determining appropriate position or posture, although it might serve to orientate the fetus towards the pelvic roof.

Fetal play

Fagen (1981) in his definitive work on play asks the pertinent question "Is there play before birth?" His discussion on this question answers it in the affirmative. He points out that two functionally and ethologically distinct forms of pre-natal motor activity are known in some species of mammals.

1. Just before birth the fetus actively changes

its orientation *in utero* and attains the position in which it is born.

2. Long before this change in orientation, the fetus exhibits whole-body movements and movements of its body parts.

The phenomenon of pre-natal exercise raises the central question of the evolution and possible adaptive significance of phenotypic modifiability. Why should pre-natal exercise be the mechanism of choice to increase pre-natal work? Perhaps pre-natal modifiability is natural selection's way of ensuring that only those fetuses capable of performing the necessary movements will survive through birth. A fetus that did not exercise would become increasingly weak as a result of detraining and might not survive gestation or the parturient process.

Modifiability through self-generated movement ensures that organisms which are developing well will continue to do so, whereas organisms that genuinely fail to thrive will self-destruct at a rate proportional to their neuromotor inadequacy.

It is conceivable that much intra-gestational fetal movement is analogous to post-natal play. It might subserve one of the principal physiological functions of play, namely periodic increase in vascularity to the musculo-skeletal system. During the rapid epigenesis of that system, escalating nutritional demands on these tissues might be met by intense episodes of regional hypervascularisation.

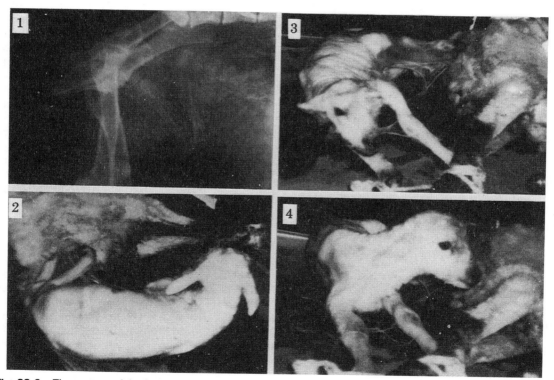

Fig. 22.6 The posture of the fetus during expulsion at birth showing the rapid emergence of the anti-gravity acts of head and neck elevation.

Conclusion

An understanding of fetal activity will result in appreciation of eutocia, of optimal circumstances of birth. A wide variety of neonatal disorders are related to perinatal misadventures but conventional obstetrical concepts have tended to be superficial regarding the role of the fetus in its acquisition of birth posture. It has often been the opinion that fetal posture and position are principally the result of maternal compressive forces. It may be that maternal compression will ensure that fetal "engagement" occurs and persists, but action processes are recognisable in terminal fetal behaviour are largely autonomous entities.

It is apparent that much fetal behaviour relates to the postural needs of the birth processes and it is now clear that some ante-natal activity relates to some post-natal practices. This is most obvious in fetal sucking. Admixed with some episodes of righting and rotation were instances when the fetus made vigorous attempts to raise the head and neck against gravity—rather than towards the maternal pelvis. Repeated examination of video-taped records of this show that this is another fetal movement which relates to post-natal practice since the first postural action of the expelled fetus is anti-gravity head elevation (Fig. 22.6).

The studies on fetal behaviour have drawn attention to the manifold role of kinesis. Attention is especially drawn to the quantity of kinetic work contained in the pre-partum period when righting behaviour is creating the birth posture. The work required in this consumes energy, and demands continuing fetal activity. The biological function of fetal kinesis is apparently two-fold: firstly to establish muscular competence, and secondly to create the characteristic birth posture. Together, these functions facilitate intra-partum survival which is doubtless the ultimate objective in fetal kinesis.

23 Parturient behaviour

Many free-living species seek out remote or concealed sites for giving birth and there are also strong indications that many domesticated animals deliberately try to avoid the hours of supervision when allowing the birth process to take place. However, because they can be kept under close supervision, the behaviour of farm animals during parturition is relatively well explored (Fraser, 1968).

Maternal behaviour occupies a central position in the life of the mother, the survival of her offspring, and in the social shaping of the individual animal. For the newborn the behaviour of the mother is critical, not only immediately for life, but for on-going adjustment to the finite environment into which it is born. Since the mother is the initial source of learning her response to the various activities of the young can shape the behavioural characteristics of the latter (Rheingold, 1963).

The process of birth passes through three very definite stages; this is particularly the case with species in which single births occur. The first stage refers to the dilation of the cervix and the associated behaviour of the animal. The second stage is the expulsion of the fetus itself. The third stage is the passage of the afterbirth or fetal membranes. These phases extend into the broader, more general behavioural periods of pre-partum, birth and post-partum (Table 23.1).

Pre-parturient period

The pre-parturient period extends from late gestation (the carrying of the fetus by the mother) to the beginning of the first stage of labour. Apart from certain changes in attitude towards any previous offspring still being nursed, there is generally little of significance in the animal's behaviour until parturition itself is very close. Once parturition is imminent, many animals separate themselves from the main group and select a site for the birth. Many species at free range choose inaccessible areas where the birth may occur unhindered. The domesticated ruminants often appear to withdraw from the grazing group when birth is only an hour or two away but, in some cases, the parturient animal has simply failed to keep up with the grazing drift of the main herd or flock.

Under intensive housing conditions natural pre-parturient behaviour is not possible. For instance, the feral sow builds a nest of grass in a shallow pit (Jensen, 1986) but in farrowing crates most sows show no change in behaviour until they are within 24 h of parturition. With sows in bedded farrowing pens of the traditional type it is observed in the pre-parturient phase that, while most of the time during the three days before the onset of labour is spent sleeping and feeding, an increasing amount of nest-building behaviour is also shown. This is usually evident in the form of chopping up bedding. The first

Table 23.1
Principal events in parturient behaviour

Animal	Immediate pre-partum period	Parturition	Post-partum period
Mare	May be shy of interruption. Anorexia only evident immediately before foaling. Whisking of tail is shown as parturition commences. No ''bed'' prepared.	At first: restlessness and aimless walking. Tail swishing, kicking, and pawing at bedding. Later: crouching and straddling, kneeling. Finally: mare lies down to strain power fully and regularly to expel fetus. Latter must rotate from a supine position through 180° for delivery.	Frequently remains lying on side for a period of about 20 min. Does not eat fetal membranes. Usually oestrus shown by 9th day (''foal heat'').
Cow	May separate from herd. Seek screened locality. Anorexia develops (1 day). Restlessness begins (several hours). No ''bed'' prepared.	Pain and discomfort expressed in very restless behaviour (alternately lying and rising). Animal more usually lies during expulsion of fetus. Expulsion of fetus slower than in mare.	Will eat fetal membranes if fresh, occasionally before uterine separation is complete. Maternal responses such as licking calf usually initiated promptly.
Sow	Gathers bedding material and attempts to make a nest. Becomes restless. Lies on side in full extension to farrow.	Shows signs of pain. Strains when fetuses are in pelvis. Tail actions signal each birth. The final expulsion of each piglet is usually done with one wave of abdominal straining.	Eats fetal membranes and fetal cadavers or parts of them. Lies extended on side for long spells accommodating frequent suckling by litter.
Ewe	Interest in other lambs; may separate from flock (66%). Most breeds seek some shelter. Restless, paws ground.	Repeated rising, lying. When straining, usually stands; lies during early expulsion.	Grooms lamb attentively, licking fluids, nibbling any membranes on lamb. Remains at birth site usually.
Doe goat	Sluggish walking. Becomes restless, agitated.	Shows clear signs of pain. Repeated straining, occasional bleating.	Variable attention to kid. Grooms by licking and nibbling. If a ''leaver'' may seem to have weak maternal drive.

changes in pre-partum behaviour are restlessness, with the sow frequently altering her position, either from side to side when lying down, or from lying to standing. This activity gradually increases until the sow changes position every few minutes. Intermittent grunting, champing of the jaws and increased respiratory rate are also prominent features. During this period the sow may attempt to make a nest, using its fore legs vigorously in attempts to accumulate bedding into a heap.

In the immediate pre-partum phase of all livestock, which is the 24 h before parturition, indicative behavioural features begin to emerge. The animal becomes increasingly restless and fre-quently alters her position and possibly also her disposition. Phantom nest-building may occur and sows provided with cloth strips manipulate them extensively at this time (Taylor *et al.*, 1986). Gradually, still greater restlessness becomes evident until a stage is reached where the animal changes her position every few minutes. Recognition of this pre-parturient behaviour in the pregnant animal allows the time of birth to be predicted accurately in the great majority of cases. Forewarning such as this allows the corrective husbandry of parturient animals and their neonates.

Similar behaviour to that in the parturient sow is seen in the cow. In beef cows changes in behaviour appear from a few days to a few hours before parturition. Sometimes restlessness is accompanied by the cow licking its flanks and/or swishing its tail. In dairy cows, some aspects of behaviour change as early as six weeks pre-parturition when the cow avoids social exchanges of butting or being butted. Such changes may relate to the physical burden of pregnancy as a result of which the cow becomes less agile in advanced pregnancy and so is less able to sustain social rank through agonistic behaviour. Two weeks before calving pushing at a crowded feed trough is no longer seen. The cow tends then to feed and drink when few other cows are at the trough. She also stays on the periphery of the herd when grazing and lying. Non-specific restlessness can begin in pregnant dairy cows as much as 14 days before parturition, with intensification 24–36 h before the cow calves (Johnston *et al.*, 1979).

Shortly before parturition some females show interest in recently born young of other females in the group. This behaviour indicates the early onset of the maternal drive under new hormonal influences. It is seen most frequently in ewes since there is a high probability in large flocks that ewes with newborn lambs will be mixed with pre-partum ewes. Pre-lambing maternal interest has been observed as much as two weeks before lambing, but it usually occurs in the 12 h preceding birth. Welch and Kilgour (1970) reported that there could be a high incidence of mismothering and poaching of alien lambs, especially at high stocking densities. The incidence may be up to 20% with some breeds of ewe and is less in primiparous ewes. In Merino flocks pre-lambing maternal interest often occurs within two hours of lambing. Interest varies from a brief inspection to cleaning, suckling and on some occasions to attempted adoption. Such ewes normally lose interest in other ewes' lambs at the commencement of parturition. "Stealing" of other young in this way occurs in mares and cows and may pose serious problems in group housing conditions (Edwards, 1983).

Immediately before parturition there are moments of restlessness culminating in almost

continuously restless and erratic behaviour. Sometimes, during the pre-parturient period, muscular contractions of the kind that herald the onset of labour itself may even take place so that one is given the impression that the actual birth is about to occur. There is strong behavioural evidence of the build-up of pain in the parturient animal during the late pre-partum phase. The biological evidence of this pain in mares, cows and ewes has been considered extensively, and it seems that the pain serves to signal the forthcoming events to the animal. This pain secures the entire attention of the parturient animal and its total participation in the birth process. Increasing restlessness and other evidence of a build-up of evident pain constitute the predominant indications of the late pre-partum period and the phase associated with the first stage of labour. Restlessness in mares is seen several hours before parturition, and both thoroughbreds and ponies typically start to sweat before foaling commences.

Increases in restlessness and withdrawal from group activity are characteristic of pre-partum behaviour in sheep, cattle and horse. Active separation from the group sometimes occurs but in a study of dairy cows, many did not isolate themselves before parturition (Edwards and Broom, 1982; Edwards, 1983). In sheep and cattle pawing and sniffing the ground may also occur. Pre-partum pawing is most notable in sheep. The length of time prior to parturition during which these changes in behaviour occur varies with the species. In sheep they occur quite close to parturition. Many ewes display uneasiness for the first time within an hour of birth, while virtually all will lamb normally within two and a half hours of such signs.

About two-thirds of all ewes display behavioural signs before parturition, the most common of which are walking in circles, pawing the ground, rising and lying, as in "comfort shifts". The physical correlate of pre-partum behaviour indicating discomfort and pain is dilation of the cervix resulting from advanced fetal engagement within the maternal pelvis. With the effacement of the cervix on completion of the first stage, the contents of the uterus can move through the open birth canal and invade the vagina. After the uterine contents have passed through the fully opened cervix the next phase of the part-urient process can begin.

The timing of parturition

Parturition does not occur randomly through-out the 24 h in most species which have been studied in detail. A higher incidence of birth at night has been reported for various mammals, including man, horses (Zwolinski and Sindinski, 1965; Rossdale and Short, 1967; Campitelli *et al.*, 1982) and pigs (Deakin and Frazer, 1935; Friend *et al.*, 1962). Conflicting results have been obtained for sheep and cattle. Wallace (1949) and Arnold and Morgan (1975) found no significant pattern of lambing time. Lindahl (1964), Handscombe (1974) and Younis and El-Gaboory (1978) recorded more lambing during the day but George (1969) found that whilst more Dorset Horn ewes lambed during the day, more Merino ewes lambed at night. Two studies on cattle (Arthur, 1961; Dufty 1971) have reported more calving at night and three studies (Richter, 1933; Ewbank, 1963; George and Barger, 1974) have obtained no such result. However these studies involved small numbers or imprecise timing so the results are not very convincing. Edwards (1979) studied 522 Friesian cows and reported no peak of calving at night or during the daytime (Fig. 23.1). Work by Yarney *et al.* (1979) has shown that Hereford cows calved at night more often if they were fed regu-larly in mid-morning and mid-afternoon rather than in late morning and late evening. Others, however, failed to repeat this result (Tucker *et al.*, 1985).

It was of particular interest in Edwards' study that whilst heifers calved evenly throughout the day, older cows were less likely to calve at milk-ing times (Fig. 23.1). This avoidance of milking time could be due to extra disturbance at this time but heifers showed no such avoidance, despite being subject to the same disturbance. It

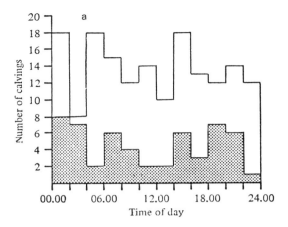

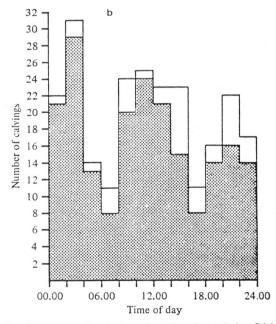

Fig. 23.1 The distribution of calving times during 24 h according to the parity of the cow. (a) First calvers; (b) third-eleventh calvers (median 5th). □ Unassisted calvings; □ assisted calvings (after Edwards, 1979).

is possible that some internal rhythm created during the lactation period is affecting behaviour. Whatever the cause, it is clear that the cows were able to avoid milking time, presumably by actively delaying the onset of the final stage of parturition.

Birth

Pain is most evident during the phase which corresponds with the second stage of labour, i.e. birth. As has been noted, the activities of the single-bearing (monotocous) dam are separable into three phases. In the multiple-bearing (polytocous) species, the parturient process is such that the activities of the second and third stages are interrelated, the two stages being interchanged at fairly regular intervals. It would be more accurate, therefore, to talk of only two stages, namely, the pre-parturient period and the period of fetus and fetal membrane expulsion.

The outer fetal membrane remains adherent to the uterine wall and, during the course of physical straining, becomes rent with pressure. This allows the amniotic bladder containing the fetus to bulge into the vagina—which is lined with secretions of cervical mucus and chorionic fluid—and effects further dilation so that the fetus enters the pelvic canal. At this stage of labour the contractions of the uterus are regular. Even at the end of this stage, they can be very strong and frequent. These events terminate the second stage with an acceleration in the expulsive efforts of the dam. Provided there is no impediment to its delivery, the fetus is then expelled by a combination of voluntary and involuntary muscular contractions in the abdomen and uterus. Repeated straining, particularly abdominal straining, is therefore the principal feature of maternal behaviour in birth. The straining efforts increase in number and recur more regularly when the second stage of labour has begun. At this time the strong reflex abdominal and diaphragmatic contractions are synchronised with those of the uterus. The

straining sessions are punctuated by resting intervals each lasting a few minutes. Further extrusion of the fetus is not necessarily achieved with each straining bout. The course of extrusion is subject to arrest and even retraction of the fetus back into the dam. One of the main obstacles to single birth is the passage of the fetal forehead through the tight rim of the dam's vulvar opening. Once the head is born the rate of passage of the fetus is greatly accelerated. The shoulders follow the head within a few minutes and, immediately after this, the remainder of the neonate very quickly slips out of the birth passage. The mother's vigorous straining usually ceases when the fetal trunk has been born. Often there is a short resting period at this point while the hind limbs of the neonate are still in the recumbent mother's pelvis (an event commonly occurring in unassisted horse births). Immediately on being born, ungulate neonates exhibit typical struggling movements and upward tilting of the face before they make efforts to stand.

During birth, the posture of the dam varies a great deal. Some remain recumbent throughout birth; in others there is alternate lying, standing and crouching. The ewe usually lies down during labour, but may stand occasionally, particularly if the final stage of expulsion is protracted. Labour is generally short and may only be about 30 min duration. Most lambs are born within an hour of first showing at the vulva. Some ewes have prolonged labour lasting over two hours; this is due, usually, to dystocia. With twins, labour is much shorter for second-born lambs than first-born lambs.

The posture of the cow during birth varies considerably. Throughout the first stage of labour the cow repeatedly alternates between standing and lying. For the first part of the second stage of labour the cow usually stands up, but for the birth of the head and fore limbs she lies down, generally on one side for final expulsion efforts with the two upper legs clear of the ground. Delivery is often completed in lateral recumbency, but the cow may be in the sternal position, or occasionally may remain standing. The duration of the second stage of labour is usually much shorter than the first stage.

Post-parturient period

In the immediate post-partum period, the dam is engaged in the third stage of labour which concerns, behaviourally, the expulsion of the placenta and the grooming of the neonate. Fetal membranes are usually passed fairly effortlessly by the dam during the first few hours following the birth. Many cows occupy themselves by eating the afterbirth after its final expulsion (placentophagia). Not all animals are placentophagic; cows and sows are, while mares are not. It seems that the two groups do have certain general behavioural characteristics which differ. The species that are placentophagic usually keep their newborn close to the birth site for several days at least, whilst those that are not placentophagic lead their young away from the birth site very early on in the post-parturient period. It has been noted that in natural circumstances mares foal at night and in the open so that, by daybreak, the foals can trot and have been led away by their mothers. Maternal behaviour is therefore related to the neonatal characteristics of following or hiding. Neonatal behaviour of the latter type is sometimes described as lying-out. This behavioural feature is widely recognised in many species, including cattle, sheep and goats (Kilgour and Dalton, 1984).

Parturient sites and lying-out areas are of necessity in the same vicinity. The birth and lying out sites of goats are concentrated in areas of intensive use by the goat herd, particularly the herd's night-camp. Birth sites chosen usually have some overhead cover which dims light and some elevated feature affording wind shelter.

In lying-out species, parturition is followed by variably long periods of isolation of the neonate from its mother. Follower species, such as the horse, maintain close and frequent contact between mother and offspring after parturition. Both strategies of post-partum behaviour have been interpreted as different means of minimising predation on neonates. Follower species characteristically have rapidly developing, highly mobile neonates and are able to provide some form of efficient defence of their young. Lying-out species give birth where cover is available for the vulnerable, non-mobile neonate which employs hiding as a tactic against predation (O'Brien, 1983).

Although the parturient animal of a lying-out species tends to choose a good birth site affording shelter and security, the mother may or may not remain close to the neonate (Hudson and Mullord, 1977). Depending on their use of one or other tactic such mothers may be "leavers" or "stayers". Such maternal behavioural variations can be seen again in cattle and sheep and has been given special study in goats (O'Brien, 1984a).

Following parturition individual female goats may either remain in the vicinity of their neonate during lying-out or leave the neonate alone while they forage with the herd. The individuals exhibiting these strategies are characterised as stayers and leavers. Stayer females tend to be older than leaver females. Female goats with twins are more likely to be stayers than the mothers of singletons. Staying and leaving are apparently maternal, age-related strategies.

Species-typical parturient behaviour

The mare

Free-ranging pony mares vary in seeking isolation but ponies sometimes move to a quiet sheltered area beyond the normal home ranges to foal (Tyler, 1972). Some pony mares simply stay behind when the group moves off grazing, while some stay with the group up to foaling time. The first sign of labour occurs when the mare becomes increasingly restless. She may perform circling movements, look around at her flanks, get up and lie down spasmodically and generally show signs of anxiety. At the onset of parturition feeding ceases abruptly. The mare rises and lies down again more frequently than before, rolls on the ground and slaps her tail against her perineum from time to time. Subsequently she adopts a characteristic straddling position and crouching posture, frequently urinating at the same time. The mare may also show flehmen, especially after the allantoic fluid has escaped with the rupture of the allantochorion about the end of the first stage of labour when extremely vigorous straining—typical of the mare alone—occurs for the first time.

Just before straining starts, an unusually high raising of the head is sometimes observed. But when straining begins the mare soon goes down flat on her side and the expulsive efforts become intensified. From the first signs of sweating it may be deduced that the first stage of labour, which may last up to four hours, has begun, but false starts are not uncommon. After some straining the waterbag (amniotic sac) becomes extruded; within it one fetal foot usually precedes the other. The bouts of straining become more and more vigorous until the muzzle of the fetus appears above the fetlocks. Although the straining bouts at this period are very vigorous the amniotic sac does not rupture. Most of the delivery time is normally taken up with the birth of the foal's head. Soon after this the remainder of the foal, except its hind feet, is expelled from the vagina. The reflex head movements of the almost wholly born foal finally burst the amniotic sac; the foal begins to breathe and its further reflex limb actions may extract the remainder of its hind legs from the dam. Although 98% of mares give birth in the lying position; final expulsion of the legs may be caused by the mare rising.

The duration of this second stage of labour is, on average, about 17 min although in normal circumstances it may vary from 10–70 min (Rossdale, 1968). Following the completion of birth mares often lie, in apparent exhaustion, for 20–30 min. As has previously been stated, mares do not eat their afterbirths although they do groom their foals. The usual length of time for the extrusion of the fetal membranes is about one hour. The foal attempts sucking within an hour of birth and begins to trot after about four hours. About 80% of mares foal at night and in the open if possible (Rossdale and Short, 1967).

Parturition is also usual at night in stabled horses, perhaps because this is when there is least human disturbance. The peak foaling hour in stabled mares is prior to midnight. In free-ranging mares birth is often in the dark hours of early morning. This gives the mare and foal all day to establish a bond and allows the myopic foal to travel in daylight.

Parturient synchronisation points to a form of maternal protection which may be either conscious or unconscious. For example, it has been found that many mares foal during the early summer when nutrition is at its height. Mares mated early on in the breeding season will often foal at the same time as those which mate later on in the season. Apart from this broad synchronising effect on gestation, it has been found that seasonal factors may also affect the time of birth. Comparing two groups of mares, it was found that the average length of time of gestation was eight days longer in those which foaled in the spring than those which foaled in the autumn.

Cows

Until the first stage of labour has begun physical changes rather than behavioural ones are apparent in the pre-parturient cow. Ingestive behaviour is, however, reduced at the time that labour is about to start. It is also at this time that the animal begins to show regular periods of restlessness; feeding sometimes recommences between these periods. Eventually the restlessness gives way to behaviour which is very similar to that encountered in conditions of colic. The cow appears apprehensive, looking all round her sides and turning her ears in various directions. At this period the cow will also perambulate excessively if she is at all able. She will also occasionally examine patches of ground and sometimes even paw loose litter or bedding as though gathering it into one spot.

The first stage of labour becomes apparent

when the cow shows intensive comfort shifting. She repeatedly goes through the motions of lying down and getting up again. She may also kick at her abdomen, repeatedly tread with her hind feet, look around to her flanks and shift her position frequently. About this time, also, the cow begins to pass small amounts of faeces and urine at intervals while arching her back and straining slightly. Cows tend to show these bouts of slight straining earlier in parturition than the other farm species. With time, the spasms of evident pain become better defined and more frequent. Finally they begin to appear regularly about every 15 min and each spasm lasts about 20 s. The spasms are manifested by several straining actions in quick succession. After some bouts of straining, the allantochorion or "first waterbag" is rent and a straw-coloured urine-like fluid escapes. After this there is usually a short pause in the straining and muscular con- tractions. This pause terminates the first stage of labour which may vary in duration from three hours to two days, though a period of four hours is a more common (modal) average time.

About one hour later the more powerful straining of the second stage of labour becomes evident and the amnion appears at the vulva. This time, straining occurs about every three minutes and lasts for about half a minute; it grows more powerful and more frequent when portions of the calf, such as its fore feet, become extruded at the vulva. At this stage the cow either adopts the normal resting position or lies on her side. In a study of calving in 82 Friesian cows by Edwards and Broom (1982) all were recumbent when calving unless there was human assistance. Her upper legs may even swing clear of the ground if she strains while lying flat on her side. Straining is virtually continuous until the head and trunk of the calf are extruded. Most cows which give birth easily and unaided remain recumbent until calving is completed. In a study by Metz and Metz (1987) 92% of such cows were still lying at the expulsion of the fetus, but when calving was difficult, 64% were standing by this time. The birth is completed with the breakage of the umbilical cord. Occasionally a cow rising after the main period of extrusion will do so with the pelvis of the fetus still lodged inside her own, and the retained fetus may swing from her for a period of time before dropping to the ground. Second stage labour, i.e. birth, is usually com- pleted within an hour.

The cow often licks up her uterine discharges before the birth is completed. Once the calf is born, she rests for a variable length of time and then rises and licks the fetal membranes and fluids from the calf. She usually eats the placenta and sometimes the bedding contami- nated by fetal and placental fluids as well (George and Barger, 1974).

Ewes and goats

Two phenomena widely reported to occur in lambing ewes are isolation-seeking and shelter- seeking. The fact that a ewe, when first seen with a newborn lamb, is often separated from the flock does not necessarily indicate that the ewe actively sought isolation from the flock prior to parturition. While 60% or more of most ewes lamb in isolation from the flock the remainder lamb in the area where the flock is grazing or camping. The majority of isolaters seek isolation actively, whilst the rest are passively isolated as they are left behind by the flock. Most ewes lamb on the site where the birth fluids spill, and most do not move away from the site where they commence labour. Many of those come back to the site to complete the birth process. Fewer Merino sheep seek isolation, and 90% lamb at the area where the flock is grazing or lying at the time labour starts. Fine-wool Merinos rejoin the flock as soon as they can after lambing and show poorer maternal behaviour than other types of Merinos (Stevens *et al.*, 1982) and most other breeds are better mothers than Merinos. Active isolation is strong in some other breeds. Evidently sheep of different breeds behave quite differently in seeking isolation at lambing. Lickliter (1985) reports that most (76%) parturient goats separate themselves from herd mates several hours prior to birth.

The biological advantages of parturition in isolation are two-fold:

1. The risk of interference by other ewes that are in the pre-parturient state is reduced.
2. The best opportunity for developing a close bond with the young is provided since the newborn lamb orientates itself towards the nearest object, preferably a moving one, which is most likely to be the maternal ewe if she has isolated herself.

Isolation-seeking is a behavioural tactic in sheep which, in the process of domestication, has apparently persisted in most breeds. Shelter-seeking by ewes, which may be associated with isolation-seeking, depends on weather conditions and the availability of shelter. Welsh mountain ewes, for example, seek shelter at lambing time in wind speeds greater than 11 km/h. At higher wind speeds where there is also a cooling chill factor, they choose progressively more sheltered sites for birth. In Soay sheep marked isolating and sheltering behaviour occurs about four hours before parturition with the ewe laying down in a sheltered position independent of what the other ewes are doing. Similar effects, of wind speed and chill, influence shelter-seeking by parturient ewes of other breeds but the Merino is a notable exception, showing flock cohesion (Alexander, 1960). Isolation and sheltering are evidently varietal tactics in the parturient behaviour of sheep (Stevens *et al.*, 1981). The motivation to seek shelter, when it occurs, must reflect a continuing effect of natural selection for survival.

Most lambing ewes display signs of nervous and restless behaviour: lying down and getting up again, paddling with the hind feet and other classic signs of discomfort. In 17% of ewes no initial signs of parturition were evident in one study although the sheep were kept under close supervision and almost constant observation at the appropriate times during two lambing seasons. Scraping the ground with a fore foot is common immediately before and after lambing.

Although there may be frequent lying down and rising before birth, most ewes remain recumbent until the fetus is partially or completely expelled. In cases of twin and multiple births the neonates usually follow each other within a matter of minutes (Arnold and Morgan, 1975).

The mean joint duration of the first and second stages of labour is 80 min. The process of parturition in ewes would therefore normally seem to be a fairly swift one. The standard deviation in time of lamb delivery is about 50 min and the lambing times would follow the normal distribution were it not for cases of parturition of over two hours due to difficulty in birth (dystocia). There is no apparent difference in duration between breeds or ages. Although ewes lamb at all time during the 24-h period, it has been observed over a period of time covering several lambing seasons that a disproportionately large number of ewes lamb during the four-hour period lasting from 7 p.m. until 11 p.m. and also during the early morning hours from 5 a.m. until 9 a.m. (Fig. 23.2). The distribution of births over the 24 hours appears to vary slightly with the breed of sheep. Merinos have a small peak between 17:00 and 21:00 hours; Suffolk ewes show a peak between 08:00 and 12:00 hours. Ewes may chew and eat parts of the fetal membranes but they do not consume the entire afterbirth (George, 1969).

The birth times of lambs and kids are synchronised to a degree; this is most evident in hill breeds of sheep. It has also been found in a herd of Angora does that, during one season, two-thirds of the kids were born within a four-day period. Immediately before birth a doe often appears fretful and nervous. The doe will paw bedding and will repeatedly lie down and stand up with signs of straining. Birth is usually complete within about one hour of first behavioural signs of first stage labour. Afterbirths are normally passed from about 20 min to 4 h after birth. Does often eat fetal membranes.

The development of parturition in does and ewes is fairly similar. Immediately after birth, the maternal orientation of the neonate allows the doe to administer further, more intensive, grooming of the young but maternal attention is

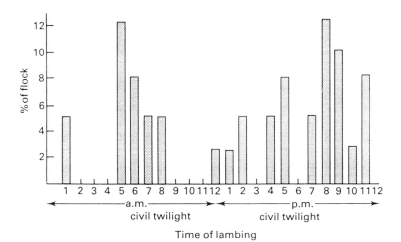

Fig. 23.2 Histogram of lambing times in flocks of Cheviot and Suffolk ewes observed experimentally over a three-year period. The bimodal distribution points to two peaks before and after morning and evening twilight. Parturition in the ewe appears to be loosely related to dark side of the crepuscular period.

variable. This may be related to the fact that many does are natural "leavers" of kids. Mutual recognition by the dam and the neonate is important (Gubernick, 1981). A doe will often reject her kid if it is taken away immediately after birth and returned after a lapse of time. In some cases it has been known for does to reject the young kid after only one hour of absence following parturition.

Sows

Prominent features in the pre-parturient sow include intermittent grunting, champing of the jaws and rapid breathing. During the 24-h period before parturition nest-building also takes place. The activity may start up to three days before parturition. The nature of these nest-building activities may, however, largely depend on the material with which the sow is provided. The sow will attempt to clean and dry her selected birth site and will chew long grass or straw to provide bedding, carrying it a considerable distance if necessary.

The location of the prospective birth site may be changed more than once. Pawing activities are evident where the sow uses her fore legs to move the bedding about. In general sows adopt and maintain a lying posture at rest before birth. It has been observed that free-living sows choose a wooded area to build a den with dry vegetation. The dens are lined with chewed-up undergrowth and leaves and the site of birth place is made dry and sheltered. In a concrete pen the sow will still pursue her nesting tendencies using any material that is provided for her use as bedding. She will often resist human attempts to disturb or relocate her nest. The amount of time taken over the building of a nest varies from one sow to another but they nearly all make use of straw, hay and any other dry material that is provided.

When farrowing is only a few hours away the sow alternately utters soft grunting noises and shrill whining sounds. As parturition approaches she begins to grunt more intensely and emits loud squeals. Farrowing more often occurs during the night than at any other time.

During the process of delivery the sow is normally recumbent and lies on her side, although there are occasions when some sows adopt a position of ventral recumbency (lying on the sternum). Vigorous movements of the sow's tail herald each birth and the piglets are expelled without a great deal of evident difficulty. Although, as has been stated, polytocous species more accurately exhibit only two stages of parturition, relatively little afterbirth is passed until all the piglets are born.

During farrowing, the recumbent sow may occasionally try to stretch out and kick with the upper hind leg or turn over on to her other side. These movements force out fluids and a fetus may be expelled at this time. Sometimes during the birth of a piglet, the sow's body trembles and if she is of nervous temperament she may emit grunting and squealing sounds.

Piglets are expelled at an average rate of one every 15 min. Nervous sows often stand up after the birth of each piglet; this may be associated with temporary reduction in pressure in the reproductive tract. The entire farrowing process normally lasts about three hours. The sow pays little attention to her young until the last one is born and, when finally she rises, she sometimes voids quantities of urine (Jones, 1966a, b).

The fetal membranes are expelled in batches of two to four after all the piglets have been born, although some small portion is often passed during the process. Many sows will eat all or part of the expelled afterbirth unless it is removed promptly.

Following the parturition she will often call her litter to suck by emitting repeated short grunts and may emit loud barking grunts if an intruder disturbs the nest. The sow rarely licks or grooms her young but sometimes appears to try to position the piglet near her udder or draw them towards her teats using her fore legs in scooping actions.

It is important to provide close observation over a particularly nervous sow for it is in such an animal that cannibalism is most likely to occur. With such a sow also, the young are sometimes crushed by sudden and erratic movements. The piglets can be removed immediately after birth if the sow shows signs of dystocia. After the process is over and her piglets are returned she will usually display normal responses towards them.

24 Maternal behaviour

With the birth of the newborn the vital relationship between the dam and neonate develops. This is established by the soliciting behaviour of the young animal and the acceptance of this by the mother. The maternal behaviour develops quickly perinatally and is in general characterised by collaborative behaviour unmatched in any other phase of the animal's existence. Commonly, the commencement of maternal behaviour is in the pre-partum period. In the sow, attempts at nest-making are usually shown at least 24 h before parturition and in some cases this nest-building is evident three days before farrowing. With the other farm species there is not the same biological need to "nest" since the neonates are more fully developed, and better coated, at birth.

Following parturition the maternal animal acquires a novel repertoire of behaviours orientated towards acceptance and maintenance of the newborn. As in some other "new role" situations the parturient animal has been behaviourally primed by an increased and special hormonal output. It appears that both the concentration of the reproductive hormones and their relative proportions to each other create the state of maternal behaviour. Most animals which normally are units of a flock or herd seek some degree of separation from their group when birth occurs. This arrangement allows the immediate association between a mother and her newborn animal to develop during their own

sensitive periods which persist for several hours following parturition. The pair, in comparative isolation, bond very quickly and efficiently together. The phenomena of sensitive periods and bonding have already been discussed. With an established bond the mother acts largely in the interests of the neonate as it develops.

Mother mammals often produce specific vocalisations post-partum. During grooming, both dam and offspring vocalise and this is important to the development of the maternal–neonatal bond. Three distinct sounds are made by cows; loud open-mouthed bellows are made during licking; soft throaty grunts are made later with the mouth closed; a similar but louder sound is made when the calf wanders away. When nursing their offspring, ewes have a low pitched gurgling call and goats give a series of low pitched, short bleats. Sows give characteristic grunts in a rhythmic series while nursing their litters as a prelude to milk let-down (see below).

Initiation of maternal behaviour

After giving birth the majority of mother mammals lick the neonate. The exceptions include the camel, pig and seal families. The new mother removes the amniotic fluids covering the neonate by thorough licking. Neonatal heat loss by conduction through thick amniotic fluid is reduced. Much grooming activity becomes progressively directed from the dorsum of the neonate and its head to ventral areas and limbs. These maternal attentions arouse the neonate and draw its primary interests towards its mother. In the course of grooming the mother inevitably lays considerable quantities of her saliva over the surface of her offspring. This soon dries out but it is distinctly possible that the dried saliva may impart a familiar pheromonal identity to the newborn. It is now clear that oral pheromones in the vehicle of saliva are important in the social exchanges of animals and most notably between young and mature individuals in recognisant situations. It is likely that the role of grooming is compound; it is certainly well motivated behaviour under the influence of prolactin, the hormone which evidently mediates much maternal behaviour, including grooming.

The changes in calf-licking by the mother

during the first six hours are shown in Fig. 24.1 (Edwards and Broom, 1982). This decline in licking over 5 h was shown when calves were licked by alien cows (Edwards, 1983), so the decline in licking is a consequence of the change in the stimulus characteristics of the calf rather than being due to a hormonal or other change in the cow.

While grooming is maintained until the newborn has been well-attended, it soon ceases. In the cases of animals with twins or triplets, maternal grooming behaviour may not be extended beyond the first born, especially in Merino sheep. Maternal experience plays a part here since ewes inexperienced with twins are more likely to neglect grooming the second born than would experienced ewes (Alexander *et al.*, 1983, Shillito-Walser *et al.*, 1983). The total time which ewes spend licking lambs is greater if twins are born but the second lamb is, on average, licked less than the first (O'Connor, personal communication).

Once the young animal stands the mother may act in a way which helps it to remain close to the mother and find the milk supply or she may show behaviour which is not helpful to the young. In studies of the responses of dairy cows to their calves Broom and Leaver (1977) and Edwards and Broom (1982) described aggressive behaviour and inappropriate maternal behaviour as being shown by some heifers. In the first study, such behaviour was more frequent if the heifers had themselves been reared in isolation for eight months whilst they were calves and corresponded with inadequate social responses to animals of their own age. In the second study, heifers were found to be more likely than were older mothers to butt or kick the calf as it approached. Some heifers repeatedly turned to face the calf thus making teat-seeking difficult. Heifers were also more likely to make movements which interrupted suckling.

When the animal has been born, dried and has gained its feet, almost all of its activities are initially concerned with teat-seeking. While the newborn is exploring its immediate environment in the course of teat-seeking, the dam does not

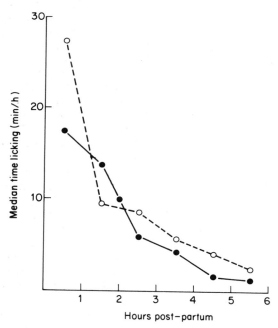

Fig. 24.1 The median time spent licking their calves by dairy cows during the first 6 h post-partum. Filled circles, heifers; open circles, second-plus calvers (after Edwards and Broom, 1982).

simply receive the soliciting approaches passively but shows positive orientation in accommodating them. The manner in which this is done is not always obvious at first, principally because the dam's behaviour is, superficially, one of inactivity. Typically, the dam will take a stationary position immediately adjacent to the newborn and will hold this position, permitting the progressive exploratory approaches of the young animal. Occasionally the dam may make an alteration in position or stance to correct the young animal's orientation. Inexperienced mothers tend to overcorrect at first. With the exception of swine, and occasionally of sheep, all farm animals give birth to singles or twins and, if they do so lying down, they rise to their feet very quickly and are therefore in the appropriate posture when nursing attempts begin. In the case of the sow, however, since large numbers are born in each litter, fetal expulsion occurs over an extended period.

Often several hours elapse between the first and the last piglets in a litter and the sow lies during the delivery of all of them. Her lateral recumbency is also the nursing position and by this means newborn piglets have access to the mammary region whenever they rise—usually only a matter of minutes after birth. All of this precludes grooming in its imperative form, characteristic of the other farm animals. Sows do nose their piglets, however, when the births are all over.

Following the grooming the mother has learned much of the identity of her young. Olfactory, gustatory, visual and auditory recognition has become established and will be reinforced progressively thereafter. From this time on, the maternal subject will give care to the young animal and defend it with much intensity. The maternal attitude towards the young resembles recognition of the latter, effectively, as an extension of herself. The young animal facilitates this by maintaining an intimate association with its mother, by vocalising for assistance or support, by numerous suckling attempts and by physical contact. Such reciprocity is rewarding for the mother.

Ewes separated from their lambs immediately after birth usually accept them on their return after absences of up to eight hours. Even when lamb interchanges are made ewes can accept lambs earlier put to them, after a lapse of some time without them. It appears that the ewe will lick the first recently born lamb or lambs presented to her within a period of several hours post-partum and that licking for a period of 20–30 min establishes an attachment and a basis for recognition.

Removal of a kid or lamb at the instant of birth and then returning it to the mother after variable periods of absence (two to four and a half hours) results in most of the young being totally rejected by their mothers. When goat dams are separated from their young for one hour immediately after parturition they subsequently fail to show the normal "individual specific" maternal care.

It is a common observation that sheep and goats will generally allow only their own young to suckle and will drive away alien young, suggesting that acceptance of young depends on the early sensitive period which is restricted to the first few hours post-partum. Modern opinion dismisses the legend that "handling" young animals will sometimes lead to their rejection by their mothers and points out that it is temporary removal from the dam and not "handling" *per se* which can lead to maternal rejection.

Some modifiability in the sensitive period in sheep and goats has been shown experimentally. Sheep and goat mothers, between 2 and 12 hours post-partum, in close proximity to alien neonates, were restrained until they permitted the alien young to suckle freely (average 10 days). All adoptions were successful although some sheep were given kids and some goats given lambs. These results showed that enforced contact between dam and young, after the normal critical period of the first hours post-partum had elapsed, can prolong the critical period effectively, although the enforced critical period requires to be very protracted.

Immediate separation of kids from their

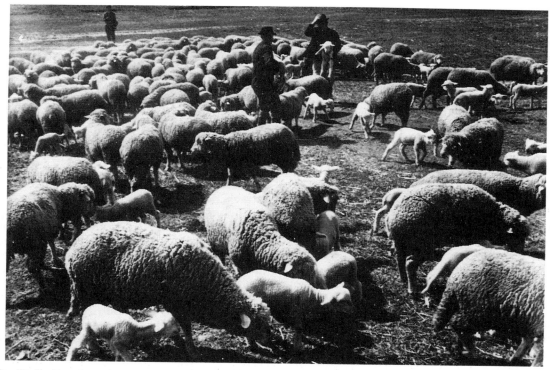

Fig. 24.2   Experienced ewes after short separation from their young actively seek out their own in a group by the sense of smell.

mothers at parturition, for periods as short as one hour, led to the later rejection of the kids by the mother goats. With only five minutes of contact, however, between doe goat and young immediately following the kidding, the rejection after separation (of up to three hours) could be prevented. It is considered that vision is not the principal factor involved in the maternal response. A form of olfactory priming seems implicated in the process as it affects the phenomenon of the maternal critical period in goats. Sheep and goat herders would agree that the odour of the young is the dam's prime criterion of acceptability (Fig. 24.2).

A marked difference is observed in the responses of experienced and non-experienced goat mothers on occasions of kid separation. Previous maternal experience may serve to increase the likelihood of activation and maintenance of maternal responsiveness in domestic goats. The use of washing coupled with close confinement appears to be an effective aid to the fostering lambs onto ewes, especially within the first day or two after birth (Alexander *et al.*, 1983). Fifty-five per cent of ewes one to three days after lambing failed to accept their own unwashed lamb after being separated from it for only 40–48 h, indicating that the ewe's memory for lamb odour is transient and/or that the odour changes with time (see Chapter 25 for further information on fostering).

Maternal motivation

If the mother does not become bonded the

maternal motivation does not fully develop but terminates fairly quickly. In dairy cattle, from which the newborn calves are usually removed without an opportunity for grooming, little or no evidence of a maternal motivation is shown one to two days post-partum. With some contact between cow and calf, however, the maternal motivation becomes strong and enduring. If a cow is left with her own calf for a 24-h period and the calf is then removed, the cow will still possess strong maternal motivation five days later at which time fostering alien calves onto the cow is still a practical possibility. This, in fact, is the basis of one calf fostering method which has been found to be a suitable one for multiple calf rearing on cows under commercial circumstances. It has been found that this fostering procedure serves to strengthen the bond between the cow and her adopted calves. A relationship can thus be made between the development of maternal responsiveness and maternal bonding in dairy cattle. In cattle, mother–offspring bonds are weaker with twins than with singles (Price *et al.*, 1985).

In sheep, the success of fostering appears to be positively related to the persistence of sucking attempts by the lamb, and negatively related to the aggressiveness of the ewe. Tranquilisation can thus be an efficient technique for fostering single alien lambs on post-partum ewes that have lost their own lambs; however, it does not facilitate fostering on ewes with their own young present.

Maternal motivation can modify the normal reactivity of the mother, causing her to show changes in reaction towards man. After a period of successful association by the mother with her young, maternal motivation may persist for months. Towards its termination, reduction in maternal behaviour becomes apparent. The mother shows increasing indifference to care-seeking behaviour from her young. This is the onset of the period of parent–offspring conflict (Trivers, 1974) when the reproductive potential of the mother is maximised by reducing or terminating parental behaviour but that of the offspring is maximised by encouraging the parent to continue parental care. This topic is discussed in detail by Broom (1981, p. 225). Parental behaviour can be manipulated by the offspring and is not just a matter of the parent deciding how much care to give.

In domestication some maternal behaviour appears to become pathologically altered by the duress of some forms of husbandry. Extreme aggression can be shown by newly farrowed sows towards attendants. This warrants cautious approach to such animals at this time, particularly if their piglets are to be handled. In some instances pathological behaviour in sows takes the form of cannibalism of their own litters. Immediate sedation of such cases is required; many of these will show normal maternal behaviour on recovery from sedation. Abnormal maternal behaviour is shown by a small proportion of individuals in all the domestic species. Much of this leads to rejection of the newborn animal and depriving the newborn animal of intake of colostrum which, for optimum passive immunity, should be ingested promptly after birth under calm conditions (Broom, 1983a). It is believed that the aetiology of several neonatal diseases is complicated by such perinatal, behavioural malfunction.

One feature of maternal behaviour observed in some ruminants is the concealment of the newborn (Lickliter, 1982, 1984). Free-ranging animals which have well-covered terrain in their habitat usually give birth to their young in some area with dense cover. After the first successful nursing, the female frequently leaves the young animal near the birth site and goes off at a considerable distance to graze. Periodically the dam will return to nurse the young animal but it may be some days before the dam is prepared to allow the neonate to remain with her constantly. These young animals also require this hiding, or lying-out, time to become developed sufficiently to be competent to associate actively with their mothers. Many of the species which show this characteristic of concealment of young also demonstrate synchronised parturitions. They also tend to have specific territories reserved for parturition. As a result of large numbers of females giving birth about the same time to their young in specific sites, pools of newborn animals are formed.

The domestic cow, for example, calving out of doors, will often do so in some concealed position and, having nursed the calf once, she will move away some distance while the satiated newborn animal remains lying in the lair. Stockmen occasionally have difficulty in finding the newborn calves of these "leaver" cows. Not infrequently the calf is found more than 100 m from the spot where the cow is observed. The link to the dam is initiated at the time of first nursing and improved on subsequent occasions when she returns to the calf in order to feed it.

The mare shows quite the opposite relationship with the newborn (which is a follower), refusing to leave it from the moment of birth. The sow is another example of an animal which does not readily allow itself to be separated from its newborn.

With any species, after the first few days postpartum, the dam aims at continuous close association with the young animal. In all species the nursing pattern at this time is determined by the young and by the mother, the dam making herself available for nursing almost continuously. As a parallel development the maternal behaviour becomes primed for the defence of the young. This defensive disposition causes some mothering animals to be singularly aggressive towards all other animals, including man.

The tactic of hiding the neonate is a notable feature in the goat (O'Brien, 1983). Newborn kids move away from their mothers and birth site 15 to 26 hours after parturition, and seclude themselves from conspecifics for four to seven days following birth. Goat mothers participate in the process by being "leavers", i.e. by not attempting to induce following, by rejoining the group and maintaining considerable distance from their young. Mothers are primarily responsible for determining the daily activity pattern and suckling frequency of their kids.

Milk "let-down"

All nursing and suckling behaviour is directed at the transference of milk from the mammary gland of the dam to the stomach of the young animal. The removal of milk from the mammary gland, however, is not by simply mechanical withdrawal alone; it requires also a positive milk-ejection process in the dam. Milk ejection occurs as a reflex and is an active unconscious process. This milk-ejection reflex is commonly termed the "milk let-down". The reflex is manifested by a sudden rise in milk pressure after stimulation which usually includes that of sensory nerve endings in the teat. The entire reflex path is a neuroendocrine arc which usually commences with udder stimulation and passes via peripheral and central nervous systems to the hypothalamus and the posterior pituitary where the arc is continued with the output of oxytocin. Oxytocin travels in the bloodstream to the udder where a sudden rise in milk pressure then occurs. With the establishment of this pressure, passive withdrawal of milk by the sucking animal is facilitated.

The mechanism clearly requires activation, e.g. by vigorous nosing of the udder by the young, and also requires time for oxytocin to circulate. The latter explains the slight delay in milk let-down which is commonly noted, e.g. in the suckled cow. Evidence of milk let-down is shown when the young remain stationary, rapidly gulping the milk released as a result of the rise in milk pressure. A circulation time after oxytocin is administered by intramuscular injection is required before let-down occurs. Latency periods (time of administration of oxytocin to time of milk let-down) in certain species have been recorded as follows: goat, 14 s; sow, 21 s; cow, 50 s.

Although the principal stimulus to milk let-down is undoubtedly local physical stimulation of the mammary gland, there may be other factors, such as odour, sounds, or visual stimuli contributing to it. Conditioning occurs in the stimulation of milk let-down; for example cows respond to many sounds and sights in the milking parlour by milk let-down. The let-down of milk can be prevented by factors leading to adrenaline (epinephrine) release. The complexity of the mechanisms involved in milk secretion makes it difficult to determine the details of the physiological derangement but the inhibition of milk ejection, resulting from loud noises or other disturbing stimuli, is caused by the resulting circulation of adrenaline (epinephrine) acting directly on the mammary gland. Electric shocks given to cows experimentally inhibit milk ejection if the shocks are administered one minute before milking commences but they have little effect if given after milk flow has begun. Practical experience supports the finding that milk let-down can be easily prevented but not so easily arrested.

The pig has complex nursing and suckling behaviour, consisting of several distinct phases of suckling by the piglets and a characteristic pattern of grunting by the sow. Experimental findings suggests cause-and-effect relationships between the different elements of sow and piglet behaviour, and the relationship of the behaviour of milk ejection. Synchronous features of pig nursing and suckling behaviour promote an even distribution of milk among all litter-mates (McBride, 1963; Hemsworth *et al.*, 1976).

Nursing and suckling

Nursing refers to the behaviour of the dam while the young are suckling and this behaviour is fairly characteristic of species and groups of species. As a general rule, the postures are typically those of open, upright stance in monotocous species and of recumbent extension in polytocous species. The sow lies on her side and in the first hours of life colostrum is available continuously. The first born piglets may go from teat to teat taking colostrum (Bourne, 1969; Hartsock and Graves, 1976). Later born piglets are less likely to obtain sufficient colostrum for a variety of reasons (Broom, 1983a). After about

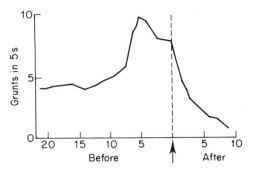

Fig. 24.3 Mean number of grunts per 5 s by six sows whilst nursing four or five times. The number of 5 s intervals before and after the onset of rapid sucking by piglets is indicated (redrawn after Whittemore and Fraser, 1974).

10 h, milk let-down becomes synchronised and periodic (Lewis and Hurnik, 1985). The sow gives a characteristic grunting call (Fig. 24.3) (McBride, 1963; Whittemore and Fraser, 1974) and milk is let down simultaneously from each teat. The piglets learn the call and the periodicity so they are ready on the teats. The milk let-down lasts only 10–25 s and occurs every 50–60 min. This system ensures that, provided there are not too many piglets for the teats (normally 14) all can suckle satisfactorily.

The nursing position of the sows is full lateral recumbency. Some sows lie on either side while others favour one particular side. A small number of sows stand at most sucklings. There may be some adverse consequences of these postures. Some sows which habitually lie on one side to nurse have a reduced milk supply on that side. Sows which nurse while standing often have lower milk yields than those which lie. It may be that lactogenic udder massage by piglets is restricted in abnormal postures and that this results in reduced lactation. This seems a probable explanation, for milk flow can be quantitatively stimulated by udder massage (Fraser, 1980a; Algers, 1989). Frequent episodes of udder massaging may delude an observer into thinking that suckling is more frequent than it really is. As many as one-fifth of apparent suckling episodes may involve no milk let-down.

In other farm species, on the first day of nursing activities the mother may feed the neonate hourly throughout the day and night. As the young animal reaches some weeks of age, the mother's nursings may become less frequent. At this time, although most mothers will have accommodated their young on demand until then, the maternal–offspring association may undergo some equalisation in which the mother may not permit suckling on every instance. Suckling attempts are not only responses to a need for milk but may reflect instead a need for comfort. When lambs are alarmed, for example, they rush to suck their mothers and the ewe tends to stand her ground and accommodates the lamb until her own flight distance is significantly encroached upon.

Maternal behaviour is an exceedingly complex phenomenon. A high degree of variability exists both among mothers of different species and among mothers of the same species. Certain aspects of maternal care show improvement with successive parturitions. It was observed by Alexander *et al.* (1984) that maternal behaviour, in the ewe, can change in the same subject as a result of learning from one lactation to another. Maternal behaviour as shown by sheep, for example, involves multisensory control and sophisticated learning ability (Alexander and Shillito, 1977; Morgan and Arnold, 1974; Morgan *et al.*, 1975). The "maternal care complex" is capable of progressive alteration as a consequence of the interaction of genetic, physiological and experiential factors (Wolski *et al.*, 1980).

The status of the mother in a social hierarchy also influences her maternal abilities. Those females which occupy lower positions in the social hierarchy may have poorer access to the food supply and hence produce less milk. In sheep, the poorest mothers are usually those which are poorly self-maintained.

25 Neonatal behaviour

The behavioural processes which unfold in the newborn animal in characteristic and predictable ways serve to show the quantity and detail of behaviour organisation which develops as a result of interaction between the genetic code and the environmental variables which are normally encountered in very early development. The control mechanisms for much of this early behaviour are located in the brain (Cowan, 1979). Neonatal behaviour is of vital importance since it is very closely correlated with survival prospects (Naaktgeboren and Slijper, 1970). Clearly it is essential for the mammalian newborn animal to establish a bonded relationship with the mother and to suckle from her quickly and successfully (Kuo, 1967). Norms of newborn activity are established and this allows appraisals to be made concerning satisfactory behavioural development.

Parturition exposes the newborn animal to a greater quantity and range of stimuli than it has previously experienced. Exploratory behaviour involves response to fresh environmental features including the feel of a solid substratum and sounds, sights and smell. Behaviour of the neonate is a mixture of patterns and processes by which the animal adapts to post-natal conditions and preparation for later life. Almost everything in its environment is unfamiliar except, perhaps, for some maternal features such as voice and the smell of the amniotic fluid. Exploration and orientation feature in the newborn animal's behaviour in the way in which it responds to changes in the surroundings using its senses (Wolski *et al.*, 1980).

Neonatal survival requires great adaptive success and is dependent upon prior fetal competence, together with a satisfactory puerperal history. The neonatal link with the mother is a major ethological phenomenon. The latter is essentially the bonding of the newborn individual with its dam. The initial work by the newborn to establish itself in a bond formation falls into several categories. Four primary stages can be recognised in neonatal behaviour during the formation of the neonatal–maternal bond. These are: coordinating recumbency; elevation; ambulation; and orientation and responding to stimuli.

Neonatal kinetic stages

Coordinating recumbency

Immediately after its birth, the neonate lies in extension. It soon raises the head and neck, flexes the fore legs, completes rotation of its sternum and flexes its hind limbs to rest on its sternum and one haunch. The head is shaken side-to-side, following which the limp ears become mobile and may become erect. The latter is a common localised behaviour which precedes rising and seems to indicate a state of increasing coordination and full awareness. The elevated head is positioned to the inside of a long arc of the neck and trunk vertebrae. This is a position from which the recumbent animal can attempt to rise for the first time. The initial post-natal recumbency facilitates grooming attentions by the dam which are directed at first over dorsal areas of the newborn.

Elevation

In the second stage of post-natal behavioural development the newborn animal attempts to rise to a full upright stance in a series of movements typical of rising in that species. Lambs and calves raise their hindquarters before their forequarters. Foals begin to rise by extending the fore legs and raising the forequarters before the hindquarters. The labyrinthine neck reflex initiates this rising process and the anti-gravity function of the inner ear system is functional in this behaviour. More than one attempt is usually made to rise before the newborn establishes upright equilibrium. A few falls occur and it is common for a "half-up" posture to be attained and held momentarily as a first measure of successful rising. Calves and lambs may have their hindquarters fully erected while they are still stabilised on their knees. Foals hold themselves partially up for a while on one fully extended fore leg. In the foal, extension and muscular tension of the fore limbs and neck are pronounced features of the early upright stance before competent upright mobility is established. When an upright posture is established, in these several species, the limbs are usually splayed to some degree before fine adjustment of stance is acquired (Fig. 25.1).

Ambulation

When the stance has been secured, attempts at walking are quickly initiated. First tentative walking steps occur as the typical four-step form of slow ambulation. In neonatal ambulation,

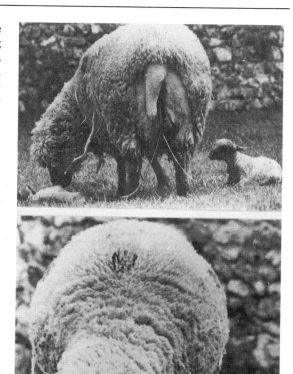

Fig. 25.1   Initial neonatal behaviour shown by twin lambs. Top: the first-born shows head elevation. Bottom: both lambs enter the second phase of neonatal behaviour simultaneously by their first rising attempt (photographs by E. Shillito-Walser).

unsteadiness is a prominent feature. This is apparently exaggerated by the presence of the eponychia, or collagenous pads over the sole of the fetal hoof. These pads have a protective role during fetal kinesis and are still present on the plantar hoof surfaces during the first walking activities. This soft eponychial tissue rapidly becomes shredded and removed from the soles by wear during early ambulation. The unsteady form of locomotion may further secure maternal attention. Neonatal motility in general appears to stimulate maternal concern and may promote the formation of the maternal bond.

Orientation

Myopia is a notable neonatal condition. This high degree of close visual competence is at the expense of long-range vision and visual accommodation; it varies in degree between species. Exploratory activities towards the dam typically take the form of close examination by "nosing" with the head and neck fully extended on the same level as the trunk. During these inspective activities the neonate may be intercepted by minor, but strategic, positional changes of the dam. The mother is normally quickly encountered in these exercises and then becomes the principal focus of neonatal attention and orientation. Such circumstances facilitate the learning of maternal and hence species characteristics. There is variation amongst species in the details of their responsiveness (see later in the chapter) but close visual examination, the use of tactile hairs or vibrissae on the neonate muzzle, and olfaction evidently function in this context. Undirected sucking towards the mammary gland may be facilitated by discrete maternal adjustments such as hind limb abduction and static posture. Once a teat-like protrusion is encountered, grasping and sucking occur.

These neonatal activities are the components of teat-seeking. Teat-seeking persists for two or more hours in the absence of reward. However these attempts will wane in time and the orientation of the newborn towards the mother will then diminish and terminate. Once terminated it will not naturally return but, by "shaping" the nursing behaviour through directive neonatal care, orientation can be re-established if the ability to suck remains in the disorientated neonate. After successful suckling, teat-seeking

becomes reinforced and learning occurs. Subsequent suckling is often aided by udder presentation, e.g. through horizontal rotation of the body in the recumbent sow and pelvic tilting in the mare. This presentation frequently takes place as a maternal postural adjustment prior to milk let-down. Given satisfactory stimulation, the lactiferous reflex, or milk let-down, occurs in the mother and complements the sucking actions of the neonate to implement ingestion. Sucking milk is self-reinforcing and, if undisturbed, continues until a meal has been taken. Fully-fed neonates sleep so readily as to suggest that sleepiness indicates successful milk intake.

Comparative aspects of neonatal behaviour

Foals

On average, foals need about 30–50 min to attain an upright stance after birth and they usually fall about three or four times in standing attempts before they have a secured stance. The time taken to stand is variable, especially in the Thoroughbred, in which breed neonatal activity may be influenced by genetics and management (Rossdale, 1970). While some very active and viable foals can stand in 15 min others, which could be considered abnormal in this respect, require more than two hours. In one study of over 400 foals (Fraser, 1980a, b) equine neonatal activity data were obtained under six headings as follows:

Stance

After their birth normal foals quickly attempt to secure an upright stance. In early standing attempts they usually fall about three or four times. The time taken to stand is variable within a common range of 20–50 min. Pony foals take an average time of 32 min. A stance within 40 min in the Thoroughbred is considered quick, while a stance after 90 min is considered slow. Some foals require two hours or more before they can stand unaided, but these are often very

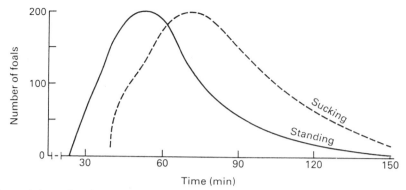

Fig. 25.2 Estimated time taken for newborn foals to stand and suck. Data taken from initial suckings observed in 435 foals mostly of Thoroughbred breeding.

large foals (over 70 kg in Thoroughbreds) and neonatal vitality is suspect with such a delay (Fig. 25.2).

Exploration

A great deal of exploratory behaviour is shown by the newborn foal. Much attention is directed towards the pasture, the ground, the premises and their boundaries and other objects in the environment within touching distances. In the course of this exploratory activity the foal nibbles and mouths unfamiliar object. Through such keen exploratory behaviour they acquire familiarity with allocated space and familiar territory is quickly adopted as the home range for which they then have affinity.

Rest

During the first week foals spend most of the day resting. In the next two or three weeks they rest about half of the time. They typically rest in a flat-out recumbent posture. Over six months, physical and physiological maturity of the chest and lungs do not allow them to lie flat so often and they then lie in sternal recumbency more frequently. Groups of foals tend to lie down together and this group effect of resting behaviour is very noticeable in larger breeding herds.

Play

Play in foals serves mainly as a kinetic function (Carson and Wood-Gush, 1983a). It begins by nibbling at the legs and mane of the mother. The very young foal remains close to its mother, often maintaining physical contact with her, even when they are walking together. Sometimes active play causes the very young foal, which is typically myopic, to collide with environmental obstacles.

Ingestion

Following stance, the foal suckles after an average interval of 21 min. Foals which stand quickly have a shorter than average interval (15 min), while those with delayed stance have an average interval of 32 min between stance and suck. In the following few days it seldom goes more than one hour between sucklings. By six months of age the foal's suckling episodes are reduced to about 10 per day. Further details of suckling and its role in the behaviour of the developing foal are described by Houpt and Hintz (1983) and Waring (1983).

From one week onwards foals gradually begin to eat grass. At first the young foal spreads and flexes its fore legs to reach grass and for a week or two, until its neck has grown, it is unable to walk and graze simultaneously. Foals graze about 15 min per hour by about three months of age.

Sequential events

The course of development of neonatal activities in the first critical three hours is indicated by the order and time of events in Table 25.1. One common behaviour which precedes rising and seems to indicate a state of full consciousness is erection and mobility of the ears.

Calves

This description of early calf behaviour is based on accounts by Broom (1981, p. 227) and Edwards and Broom (1982). The newborn calf is licked vigorously by its mother, often being lifted partially from the ground by the mother's tongue, and may be encouraged to stand by this stimulation. First standing usually occurs between 30 and 60 min after parturition except where birth has been difficult (Fig. 25.3; Edwards, 1982). The calf adopts a crouched stance with legs partly spread, shoulders lowered and the head and neck fully extended. It soon approaches a vertical surface like the leg of the mother or a wall and nuzzles against it. The nuzzling is concentrated at nose height and occurs more vigorously if a horizontal surface joins the vertical surface at about this height. This behaviour results in exploration of the

Table 25.1
Sequence of equine neonatal activities

Activity	Time post-partum (min)
Head lifting	1–5
Sternal recumbency	3–5
First rising attempt	10–20
Upright stance	25–55
First suckling attempt	30–55
First successful suckling	40–60
First defaecation	60
First urination	90
First sleep	90–120

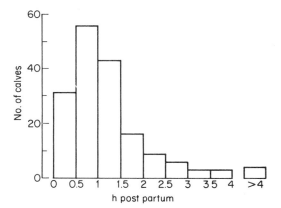

Fig. 25.3 The time to first standing for 171 dairy calves (after Edwards, 1982).

under-belly of the mother or of the underside of a table 75 cm high. The point where the leg meets the horizontal surface elicits the most attention. Selman *et al.* (1970a, b) emphasised that the shaded under-belly of the cow is attractive to the calf during its exploratory nuzzling. If the calf starts nuzzling at a fore leg it may spend some time exploring the axilla and if the exploration is by the hind leg, the inguinal region may receive close attention. Calves lick and suck at any protuberance which they encounter during their exploration. If a teat is found, the calf will take it in its mouth and suckling will begin. The exploratory nuzzling behaviour is usually referred to as teat-seeking as it is terminated by finding a teat, but it may be prolonged if no teat is found. Many calves fail to find a teat during their first search and some fail after several attempts. Edwards and Broom (1979) and Edwards (1982) found that half of all calves of cows in their third or later parities failed to find a teat within 6 h of birth (Fig. 25.4). This is because the pendulous udder and fat teats of older cows make teat-finding difficult. The calf's searching results in success in more than 80% of heifers' calves but often fails if the searching is directed at body underside level but the teats are much lower down. A variety of other factors affect the length of the delay before successful suckling

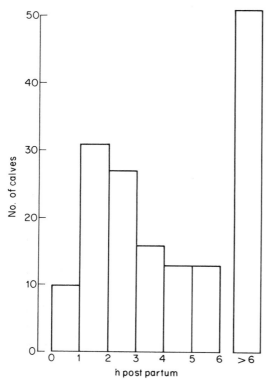

Fig. 25.4 The time to first suckling for 161 dairy calves (after Edwards, 1982).

and colostrum ingestion (Fig. 25.5; Edwards, 1982; Edwards *et al.*, 1982; Broom, 1983a). For example twin calves are often weaker than single calves and require two to three times as long to begin suckling (Owens *et al.*, 1985).

Many newborn calves lie-out; outdoors they may spend the first few days of life lying alone or with other newborn calves hidden in deep grass or rough vegetation. Lying-out animals are less precocious than "followers"; because of this they may have a slower sensory development which may be partially the consequence of a slower exposure to new stimuli. The calf benefits by being licked by the dam in order to stimulate physiological functions such as urination, defaecation and general awareness.

Newborn calves normally suckle five to ten times a day, with each nursing session lasting up to 10 min. The number of suckling bouts usually decreases with age, but this may vary depending on the rate of growth of the calf and the milk yield of the cow. Calves at six months of age suckle about three to six times per day. Dawn is a common nursing time. Other nursing bouts are centred around mid-morning, late afternoon and about midnight. Calves fed artificially with nippled milk hoppers show similar suckling habits. While sucking such feeders they often stand with their hindquarters deviated from the direction of their necks and prefer to touch a wall with their bodies in the course of sucking. This behaviour resembles the characteristic stance of the suckling calf with its mother in which it turns the side of its body and its hindquarters to be in contact with the side of the cow.

Mutual sucking is a common problem among bucket-fed calves raised together in crowded groups. Such inter-sucking can occur very frequently and can cause skin inflammation. Prolonged sucking of the ears, the umbilical region or the prepuce is typical. Calves that indulge in intersucking are often unthrifty, especially if urine drinking occurs. Calves with wet ears from sucking by others may have them frozen in extremely cold weather. The provision of a teat supplying water can substantially reduce intersucking in group-housed calves (Vermeer *et al.*, 1988). The persistence of inter-sucking behaviour in adult stock is not uncommon, especially in dairy herds. In a problem dairy herd, as many as one-third of the calves and one-tenth of the cows may be affected. Social facilitation by other milking cows may increase the incidence of the behaviour. Since the condition is difficult to control, culling of offending animals is usually necessary and it therefore represents a serious economic problem. Some dairy farmers prevent the problem by penning young calves individually but this is a drastic measure for a problem which is absent in many herds.

Increasing attention is now being given to numbers of calves being fostered on nurse cows to feed naturally. When cross-fostering is

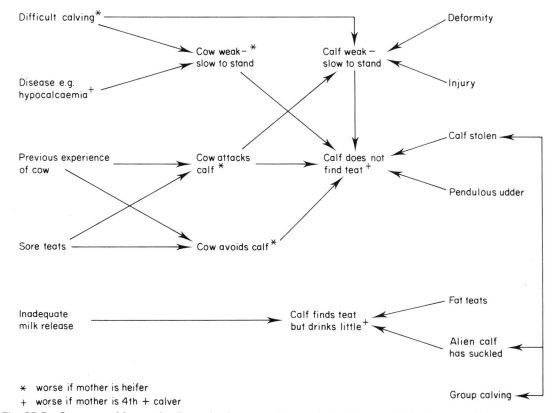

Difficult calving *

Cow weak – *
slow to stand

Calf weak –
slow to stand

Deformity

Injury

Disease e.g.
hypocalcaemia +

Previous experience
of cow

Cow attacks
calf *

Calf does not
find teat +

Calf stolen

Pendulous udder

Sore teats

Cow avoids calf *

Inadequate
milk release

Calf finds teat
but drinks little +

Fat teats

Alien calf
has suckled

Group calving

* worse if mother is heifer
+ worse if mother is 4th + calver

Fig. 25.5 Summary of factors leading to inadequate colostrum intake by calves (after Broom, 1983a).

attempted the normal procedure has been to present a cow, already in milk, with several young calves, perhaps newly born. Recent research on fostering has shown a much higher degree of success when the young calves to be fostered are presented to the nurse cow immediately following her parturition, before she has adopted her natural calf but while she is still in the sensitive period of maternal awareness. At this time such cows readily adopt numbers of fostered calves and continue to facilitate their suckling subsequently so that these calves grow better. In selecting calves for fostering it is necessary to realise that calves which have not suckled naturally at all in the first six days of life are unable to suckle later on a lactating cow. Cows

do sometimes allow alien calves to suckle (Kilgour, 1972) and although applying birth fluids from the cow to alien calves facilitates acceptance by the cow it is sometimes possible to foster successfully without this and at a late age. Kent (1984) penned three or four calves with a cow several days post-partum and found that calves were often accepted, especially if the stockman actively tried to prevent rejection.

Kids

It is observed that the initial response of the kid is to seek a rounded ventral surface without hair. When a hairless area is reached the newborn kid starts sucking movements. Under experimental conditions, when an udder was surgically transposed to the neck of a doe, kids quickly found it and used it.

Kids quickly establish themselves on a preferred teat and there is very little non-nutritive sucking, i.e. sucking without a need for milk. During the active suckling periods it is observed that the movements of the kid's tail corresponded exactly with the frequency of sucks during the major peak of milk let-down.

In the hiding or "lying-out" behaviour of newborn goats, kids move away from their mother and birth site towards the end of the first day post-partum (Lickliter, 1984, 1985). They then seclude themselves for four to seven days. The maternal doe goat participates in the process of kid seclusion by keeping a considerable distance from her young and by rejoining the adult goat herd (O'Brien, 1984a).

At the termination of the hiding phase mothers are responsible for determining the daily activity pattern and suckling frequency of their young. Kids choose their hiding sites and establish physical proximity to their dams at mother–infant reunions. These circumstances demonstrate the importance of the active role of the domestic goat kid to the development of the mother–infant relationship (Lickliter and Heron, 1984) and explain the common misunderstanding that doe goats often leave their newborn due to poor maternal motivation. The tendency to leave is a maternal tactic of this species.

Within 48 h of birth newborn goats have the perceptual and locomotor abilities to recognise their mothers and achieve close physical proximity to them. This represents a considerable achievement for a newborn animal. It involves the ability to store identifying characteristics of the mother very soon after birth and to match sensory input with this stored information on subsequent encounters.

Lambs

Lambs are born in an advanced stage of physical and behavioural development. With all sense organs ready to function from birth, this facilitates rapid learning so that the young animal can respond and adjust to the novel environment of the mother. They can stand, walk and suckle within the first hour, although many of lighter birth weight (e.g. under 3 kg) may require two hours. After the first successful suckling they become recumbent and sleep as in the other farm species. Their senses of sight and hearing, however, are evidently better developed than those of some other neonates, such as the foal.

The most noticeable behavioural aspects of sheep after lambing is the strong maternal relationship with the newborn which develops (Shillito-Walser, 1980). A ewe nearly always vigorously rejects any attempts by other lambs to suckle and will look after her own young exclusively.

Vision is important in the sensory development of young lambs since they are "followers" and characteristically move with their mothers throughout the post-natal period (Winfield and Kilgour, 1976). In following the ewe very closely, the lamb often puts its head down close to the dam's head while she grazes. Young lambs seem to recognise their own mothers very rapidly and sometimes will not respond to strange ewes when still only one day old. Since this recognition and following response occurs at a distance from the ewe, vision must be involved (Morgan and Arnold, 1974). Lambs reared outside recognise their dam in 95% of cases, versus 72% in lambs reared indoors. It is evident that the environmental conditions in which ewes and lambs are maintained can influence their ability to select their partners at a distance with the help of auditory and visual cues (Poindron and Schmidt, 1985). Sensory affiliation extends to twin lambs; twins or multiple lambs develop a strong bond between each other and learn to recognise each other by sight and sound. By response to voice and appearance they stay nearer to each other than to any alien lambs (Shillito-Walser, 1985a).

The earliest sensory experiences received by lambs are tactile and olfactory, followed by auditory and visual signals, all of which the lamb learns very rapidly. The odour of the inguinal region is used by the lamb when seeking the udder and the temperature and tactile characteristics of the udder result in the lamb spending some time exploring its immediate vicinity (Vince, 1983, 1984). Sound and vocalisations influence lamb behaviour very strongly. It has been shown experimentally that lambs can hear maternal bleating and throat rumbling sounds before they are born (Vince and Armitage, 1980). The sounds *in utero* are attenuated particularly in the higher frequencies. Since the rumbles have no high frequencies they may be familiar sounds when the lamb is born, particularly since different ewes have different rumbles. After birth the lamb first hears a low rumbling sound made by the ewe as she licks the lamb dry. The structure of rumble sound is very different from that of bleats. These rumblings made by ewes seem to help the lamb orientate to the ewe. This sound also keeps the newborn lamb near to the ewe, particularly in the dark. On other occasions ewes rumble to their lambs as "comfort sound" after separation, and also to keep their lambs near when mixing with other ewes and lambs (Shillito, 1975).

When a ewe is separated from her young she and the lamb will "baa" until they are brought together. Even adult members of the flock, which become disengaged from the others will "baa". They increase in vocalisation and become more animated in attempts to locate the main flock. Increased vocalisation has been shown to be accompanied by increased mobility. Vocalisation in a young lamb separated from its dam, or an adult sheep separated from the main flock, tends to be fairly intense initially. It declines, however, after about four hours of continuous separation.

Most newborn lambs are able to stand within the first half-hour following birth and nearly all are able to stand within the first two hours. The lamb's first attempts to suck are usually unsuccessful; it often seeks out the teat by nosing between the fore legs of the dam or any nearby object which the lamb may feel has maternal properties. If, at this point, the newborn fails to find the teat or is prevented from doing so by the behaviour of the mother, it may cease its attempts to suck.

Within about one hour of birth approximately 60% of newborn lambs have begun to suck and, in normal cases, nearly all lambs have sought out the udder within the first two hours. Once the newborn lamb is able to stand, it sucks and nibbles at any object which is at hand; this is usually the coat of the dam. While the dam is removing the placenta from the lamb, the latter finds its way to the region of the teats and udder. Sometimes the lamb is prevented from sucking by the diligent efforts of the mother to remove the placenta. Again, if the udder is too large, the newborn may find the teat difficult to grasp. However, once the newborn can facilitate milk let-down by pushing the teat cystern upwards into the udder with its mouth, progress in locating the teat again and sucking becomes very rapid. In the first week following birth, lambs suckle very frequently, sometimes on 60 to 70 occasions during the 24-h period. The duration of suckling at this time is usually from one to three minutes, but later on the young are seldom allowed by the dam to suckle for periods of over 20 s.

Single lambs do not usually favour one teat over another. In the case of twins, though, each lamb does develop a preference for one particular teat, but this may change where the other twin obstructs the arrangement. In cases where one of the twins is removed after a period, the remaining lamb begins to suck from both teats. Sometimes the dam facilitates suckling by lifting her hind leg on the side at which the newborn is attempting to suck. One aspect of behaviour characteristic of the newborn lamb is the vigorous wagging of its tail when involved in nursing. It has been postulated that this is a mechanism which entices the dam to smell the anal region and so recognise her young, for some ewes do not discourage the approach of another newborn if it is similar in appearance to her own.

Attempts to foster different or extra lambs on to a ewe often involve the application of birth fluids, for example on a cloth jacket which is put on to the alien lamb (Price *et al.*, 1984b; Alexander and Stevens, 1985a, b). Birth fluids still elicit a positive response from the ewe after they have been frozen and thawed (Levy *et al.*, 1983), so it should be possible to freeze such jackets for future use (Gonyou and Stookey, 1987). Other actions which promote alien lamb acceptance are stretching the ewe's cervix prior to introducing the young (Keverne *et al.*, 1983), using a masking odour, restraining ewe and lamb together (Alexander and Bradley, 1985; Price *et al.*, 1984a), and tranquilising the ewe (Tomlinson *et al.*, 1982).

Piglets

Piglets stand very quickly and move around the sow soon after birth, following the edge of her body. Their first response is to any nearby object, which is then investigated by the nose. Piglets have an extensive innervation in their snouts, the senses of touch and smell being very important in piglets. The smell and taste of the piglet's amniotic fluid expelled post-partum by the sow may help to keep the piglet near the sow. As with lambs, pre-natal sound could be an influence on piglet post-natal behaviour. Sows are generally vocal and the piglets are likely to have heard the sow's voice before birth. Newborn piglets learn to run to the sow's vocalisations, especially the grunts produced before milk let-down (McBride, 1963; Whittemore and Fraser, 1974), and they learn to communicate by vocalising themselves. Pig vocalisations have been well identified. Calls asking for contact are made by piglets exploring a new area and consist of closed mouth grunts which are distinctive. When a piglet has escaped from its home pen these characteristic grunts are made. The latter

may be the early development of the adult greeting call.

Piglet vision is good and rapidly improves in the post-partum period. Recognition of its "own teat" on the sow and its place in the teat order may be dependent on vision. The formation of the social organisation within the litter, which takes the form of the "teat order", is a notable behavioural phenomenon. Unproductive teats are avoided when there are enough teats for all (Jeppesen, 1981, 1982). The high degree of organisation inherent in the teat order is an important means of litter survival. It also facilitates proficient synchronous nursing which is important in the prevention of piglet inanition —a common cause of piglet mortality.

Although piglets can walk, see and hear within a few minutes of birth, certain physiological mechanisms, such as temperature regulation, are not fully developed at this time and temperature conservation by huddling is therefore a prominent feature of neonatal behaviour in the pig. Orientation is an important factor in piglet behaviour and disorientation is maladaptive. Newborn piglet mortality is high, commonly about 15%. Most of this mortality is due to crushing by the mother on commercial pig units. Normal healthy and well-fed piglets show positive orientation to their litter-mates and the sow's mammary region. Disorientated piglets and those which are weak are very liable to become crushed or chilled. Many young piglets fail to obtain sufficient colostrum and hence are weakened or more susceptible to disease (Fig. 25.6; Broom, 1983a).

Fostering of extra piglets on to sows is relatively easy in the first few days after parturition because sows generally accept piglets coming from their own nest. Hence the alien piglets can be placed in the litter group and are usually accepted. However some often show aggression to piglets fostered at more than four days of age and piglets fostered at more than seven days old do not gain weight at the normal rate (Horrell and Bennett, 1981; Horrell, 1982; Horrell and Hodgson, 1985). Piglets of up to 15 days of age can be successfully fostered if introduced to the

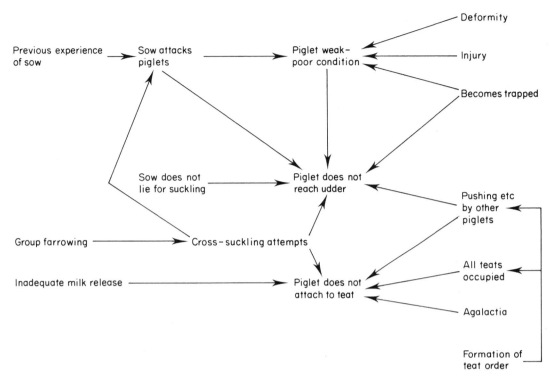

Fig. 25.6   Summary of factors leading to inadequate colostrum intake by piglets (after Broom, 1983a).

sow on the first day post-partum (Hartsock, 1985). One consequence of the acceptance of alien piglets by sows is that group farrowing can lead to the strongest piglets from several litters getting much milk and the weakest being ousted from their own mother's udder by aliens. In group farrowing situations incomplete nursings are more frequent (Bryant *et al.*, 1983).

Piglet ''teat order''

Much study on suckling behaviour in swine has been focused on the preference of young piglets for specific teats (Fraser D., *et al.*, 1979; Hemsworth *et al.*, 1976; McBride, 1963). A clearly defined social order prevails among litters in their suckling activities. Piglets generally suck the same teats forming a ''teat order''.

This order develops among piglets within their first day of life, often within an hour or so of birth. The order is altered when the sow first rolls over to feed the litter from the other side. Many observers have noted the singular preference piglets show for the anterior (pectoral) teats but the real preference is for a productive teat wherever it is on the udder (McBride, 1963; Jeppesen, 1982). Piglet birth weights alone do not determine the outcome of these teat competitions but very light piglets are at risk in their competitive world, especially if functional teat places are fewer than or equal to the total number of piglets.

Each suckling by piglets begins with a massaging operation in which the piglets rub their snouts forcefully in upward and circular directions into the mammary region of the sow.

The area massaged by an individual piglet is equivalent to a single segment of the mammary gland. The massaging process lasts approximately one minute. This is followed by milk ejection from the dam, a process which lasts an average of 14–20 s, during which the piglets suck vigorously. A final massaging operation follows which occupies variable periods of time, being frequently protracted. Replete piglets quickly assume recumbency.

Sometimes extended association occurs between the sow and her litter and another feature of piglet nursing can be observed then. After feeding, somnolent recumbent piglets may retain attachment to teats. As a result, adherence can persist between litter and dam from one feeding period to another. When this occurs it will tend to ensure that the "teat order" is preserved and that the entire litter feeds at each let-down of milk. Such adhesive behaviour would appear to have great survival significance by reducing agonistic behaviour and by operating against inanition.

Undue aggressive behaviour within the litter eliminates an increasing number of piglets from the established "teat order". Disturbing factors, such as frequent movements by the sow, can lead to increased agonistic behaviour in the litter, as a result of which places in the "teat order" are lost and mortalities increase. The initial sign of loss of teat position is disorientation in the piglet's suckling behaviour and such disorientated piglets are prone to be crushed beneath the sow as is the case also in disorientation due to inanition. In litters larger than 14 —where disturbing factors are great because 14 is the average number of teats on a sow—there is a significant increase in the numbers of piglets fatally crushed by the sow.

Various workers have studied and emphasised the relationship between piglet growth and anterior or posterior suckling position in the teat order. The usual interpretation is that the anterior teats are the most productive, that the piglets, therefore, compete for the anterior teats soon after birth, that the heavier piglets usually win their possession, and that these piglets show particularly large weight gain because of their anterior positions in the teat order. This interpretation began with a very few sows studied and the belief has become widely accepted. Research findings are not all in accord with this concept, however, since correlations between birth weight and teat order position are variable. Although in many circumstances the heaviest piglets at birth occupy anterior positions at the mammary gland, this is not always so. In many cases piglets nursing on anterior teats grow better than others during the first three weeks but this is by no means a constant finding. The anterior teats may be preferred because they are nearer to the source of grunts (Jeppesen, 1982) or safer from kicks (English *et al.*, 1977). As an explanation of teat order in piglets the following hypothesis has been offered by D. Fraser (1984):

During the first hours after birth, the piglets are attracted to the more anterior teats for reasons yet to be confirmed. The piglets may compete for specific teats based on aspects of teat quality, and may compete for anterior placs, but with tendency for the heavier piglets to obtain the anterior positions. During lactation, variations in milk yield and piglet performance are probably due to variations in teat quality and the vigour of the piglets, with a small statistical tendency for piglets on anterior teats to grow faster once the effect of birth weight is taken into account.

26 Juvenile behaviour

The post-natal bond to the mother is a major ethological phenomenon (Fig. 26.1), but newborn animals in groups pass from a phase when they are principally aware of their mothers to a phase in which they spend much of the time associating in peer groups. As the need for self-maintenance increases, so the peer group activities change. Play and rest, which initially dominate peer group activity, are augmented and eventually replaced by grazing groups. The young move between their peer group and their mothers in sundry activities. As a result, their primary social bonding is in kinship groups at weaning. Further changes depend on the social organisations characteristic of the species but social grouping remains the chief behavioural characteristic.

During the first week of life lambs, calves and foals form peer groups. In Merino lambs at four weeks of age 80% of lying, 60% of grazing and 100% of playing is done in peer groups. From 6 to 12 weeks of age Merino lambs when grazing keep nearer to each other than to their dams. However, lambs retain ewe contact, their dam usually being the nearest ewe. At a later stage the association with peers seems to become less important. From this mother–offspring relationship the matrilinear groupings form in home range groups when weaning by forced separation does not occur.

Juvenile characteristics

Calves

Newborn calves do not graze until they are several days old and their first attempts are usually inefficient. As the periods of suckling are reduced, grazing becomes more regular and calves become highly selective in their grazing intake. Calves at pasture with their mothers and others in a suckler herd form complex social relationships (Kiley-Worthington and de la Plain, 1983; Benham, 1984).

When calves are weaned they begin to show the clearly defined maintenance activities characteristic of adults. Maintenance activities, through lack of play opportunity, are modified in older calves penned individually. These calves kept in isolation may spend more time in standing at rest than calves in groups, which appear to spend more resting time in recumbency. These adolescent cattle have the behaviour of their maintenance activities apportioned as follows: feeding 22%; drinking 2%; rumination 28%; grooming 5%; resting 40%; and exploration 3%. Adolescent calves which have acquired behavioural schedules learn to anticipate feeding times and show restlessness as these times approach.

It seems that more frequent "nearest-neighbour" associations occur in groups formed of calves reared in a group, than for calves

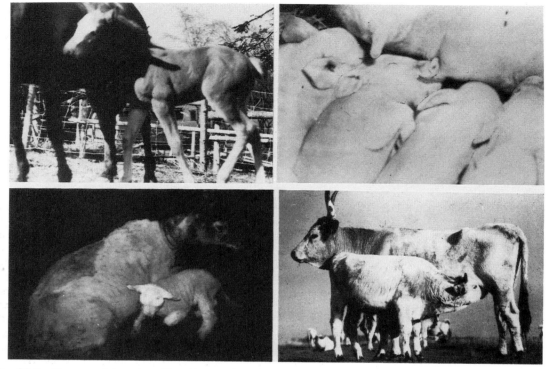

Fig. 26.1   The neonatal–maternal bond is one of continuous intimate association, often involving physical contact.

reared in isolation. When they are grouped together for only a few days of contact, calves in pairs create a bond, and consequently contribute toward the stability of any group into which they are put. Calves grouped in a lot with no previous social contact form an affiliate group within a week (Kondo *et al.*, 1983).

Lambs

Experimental studies have been made on following behaviour in young lambs by using a model of a ewe which circled in an enclosure (Winfield and Kilgour, 1976). The lambs' strongest following response occurred between 4 and 10 days of age. A weak response in animals less than four days old was explained to be the result of a lack of maternal reinforcement of the following response. In contrast, lambs older than 10 days recognise their dams very quickly and do not follow strange models. In fact, lambs will select ewes of their own breed when their dams are not present in a mixed flock of different breeds (Shillito-Walser, 1980).

For the first few weeks of life lambs stay quite close to their own ewes (Key and MacIver, 1980). By one month of age young lambs spend two-thirds of their time in the company of other lambs. By this age play is well developed. The gambolling form of play in this species is very typical. The play involves upward leaps, little dances and group chasing. Play is reduced as lambs grow and is becoming rare by four months. In general it appears that lambs are born in an advanced stage of development, both physical and behavioural. For example they can stand, walk and suckle within the first hour. Their senses of sight and hearing are evidently better developed than those of some other neonates, such as the foal. The course of their behavioural development is therefore fairly rapid throughout the nursing phase but can be affected by rearing methods (Moberg and Wood, 1982).

Lambs reared in isolation do not respond to other lambs or ewes. Exploratory behaviour in isolated lambs is adversely affected. Such lambs will not inspect a new object or run and chase other lambs. They withdraw from novel environments, vocalise less and are slow to initiate movement and investigate any new object or run and chase other lambs (Zito *et al.*, 1977). Lambs reared in peer groups without mothers, behave similarly to lambs reared with their ewes. The main effect on isolated lambs is not therefore the result of maternal deprivation but of social deprivation. Twin lambs develop a strong bond between each other and learn to recognise each other's voices and appearance and they stay nearer to each other than to an alien lamb when given a choice.

The distance of the lamb from its dam depends on her activity. If the ewe is lying or walking the lamb is usually within a metre of her. If the ewe is grazing the lamb has greater freedom of distance and activity. The distance between ewe and lamb when both are grazing increases rapidly over the first 10 days of life, reaching a final average distance of 20 m which is the average social distance between dam and offspring when grazing on pastures of abundant feed.

Lambs are strongly influenced by the food the ewes eat and this affects their own choice of food later. The pattern of grazing in lambs of six months of age has been determined by the breed of ewe that reared the lamb. When Welsh Mountain lambs were cross-fostered onto Clun Forest ewes they grazed restrictively as Clun Forest sheep, whereas Clun lambs reared by Welsh Mountain ewes grazed in a wide area over the hills, as did the breed which had reared them.

Lambs reared by mothers which ate grain whilst the lambs were very young and taking only milk were more likely to eat grain when older than were lambs whose mothers ate no grain (Keogh and Lynch *et al.*, 1982).

Foals

The maturing foal gradually undertakes sorties of increasing distance from its mother and progressively spends more time playing with other foals as it grows. The equine bond, however, persists over one to three years and can remain strong even when later siblings are born. As the foal matures it suckles less frequently, perhaps only about 8 to 10 times per day at six months. From one week onwards foals gradually begin to eat grass. They graze about 15 min per daylight hour by about three to four months of age. By one year of age foals spend about 45 min per daylight hour in grazing activity. At first the young foal must spread and flex its fore legs to reach grass and, for a week or two, it is unable to walk and graze simultaneously. Foals spend most of the day resting during the first week. In the next two or three weeks they rest about half of the time. Foals typically rest in lateral recumbency until they are over six months, when physical and physiological maturity requires them to lie flat less often and to lie in sternal recumbency more frequently. Groups of foals may lie down together and social facilitation of resting behaviour is very evident. In a herd of 15 mares and their foals, the foals, of 7 to 16 weeks of age, were found to associate in fairly fixed groups of two or three.

Piglets

The formation of the social organisation within the litter, which takes the form of the "teat order", is a notable behavioural phenomenon which has received previous description in which two important features were mentioned, viz. (a) the high degree of organisation inherent in the teat order as an important means of litter survival, and (b) proficient synchronous nursing, which is important in the prevention of piglet inanition.

Piglets suckle frequently when they are young. As piglets mature the number and duration of suckling bouts gradually decreases from about one every 20–30 min in the first few hours of life to about six per day at two months of age (Fraser, 1974). Piglets attempt to eat solid food by 7 to 10 days of age. They are particularly attracted to solid food which is sweetened and formed into small pellets. Solid food intake, however, does not become substantial until about three weeks of age unless the piglets are milk-deprived. Young piglets quickly learn to eat the same solid food as their mothers and often attempt to share the sow's food with her.

Many piglets are raised under conditions of isolation in specific pig production enterprises. Their behaviour, in isolation from sows, is significantly affected (Fraser, 1975a, b). For example, those reared in artificial circumstances of isolation from their sows suck one another and snout-rub excessively. They may defaecate frequently in the nesting area, in marked contrast to their normal discipline of defaecation which develops rapidly over the first few days of life. Normal piglet defaecatory behaviour by four days of age shows clear preferential use of a communal and restricted dunging area which is usually the corner of the premises furthest removed from the sleeping area.

Isolated piglets give distress calls frequently when being handled, while conventionally raised pigs only give such calls when hurt. Even when separated from the sow for a few hours, piglets exhibit considerable distress by vocalisation with either squeals or grunts. Vocalisations of distress increase with the length of isolation and, if isolation is imposed on piglets individually, distress vocalisation is greater than if the entire litter is isolated from the sow as one group.

Early weaning of piglets at three to four weeks of age is often practised to increase the number of litters which a sow might have over a given period. These early-weaned pigs massage and nibble one another, particularly over their bellies. They spend less exploratory time rooting or nibbling inanimate objects. Early-weaned pigs in cages rest by sitting on their haunches much more frequently than do piglets on straw bedding and show a disinclination to rest in the normal lying position.

The development of sleep has been studied in piglets during the first five weeks. The daily amount of sleeping does not change during this time and neither does the duration of sleeping episodes. Piglets sleep for about 26 min per hour and for the first five weeks of life this factor remains fairly constant. Cycles of sleep are not apparent in young piglets but on the average they sleep for about 10½ hours per day. This contrasts with pigs of three to four months of age which sleep about eight hours per day. The duration of one type of sleep (paradoxical or REM sleep) does decrease significantly as piglets develop. Young piglets commonly sleep in a crouched position, with all four legs folded under the body.

Chicks

The chick is active while standing in its shell. Before hatching it attains an upright position with the head and neck elevated. It gives various calls within the shell; calls of distress and satisfaction have been identified. When the chick breaks through the shell it quickly seeks a source of heat, making characteristic calls as it does so. The natural heat source is the broody hen with which the chick makes very close physical contact after hatching. Thereafter close company with the hen is maintained as the chick matures and this provides opportunities for learning to refine the behaviour of maintenance. The clutch of chicks with a hen maintains a close association with her and readily recognises her physical characteristics and calls. When the process of physical development of the chick causes the down to be lost from the head, the hen rejects it. The clutch then becomes dispersed and more dependent on self-maintenance activity, while still associating with the flock in general. As they integrate with the flock, the chicks become established within its peck order. A stable flock of about 40 chickens maintains a stable peck order. Depending on the strain of bird, egg-laying commences by about six months of age.

Turkey poults

The poult, like the chick, is active within the shell before hatching. After hatching the poult is very mobile. Great social cohesion within poult groups is notable from the first day after hatching but attachment to the hen turkey is also evident. Vocal and visual signals are used in the maintenance of close contact. As with the chick, this affinity facilitates the learning of certain critical activities, particularly feeding. Some artificially incubated poults are unable to initiate feeding or drinking and may die as a consequence of the lack of maternal association and the learning facility which this provides. Forced feeding can be practised with some success. Recent investigation of this problem has found that experimental poults, if exposed to lights flashing for about 20 min per hour for the first six days after hatching, fed more promptly and consumed more feed, particularly on the first day. A preference for green coloured lights was shown. It is interesting to speculate that the resemblance of this stimulus to the flash of metallic green from the colour of wild turkey plumage may be more than coincidental. After three months of age social hierarchies become formed in turkey groups and an established peck order is operational by five months of age, at which time groups show subdivision by sex.

Vocalisations

Vocal activity is a prominent characteristic of pigs, particularly during their suckling phase of development (Grauvogl, 1958). The division of piglet vocalisation into five different classes has been defined as follows by Jensen and Algers (1983):

> Class 1 ('croaking'). Tonal, short sounds, poor in formants. Frequently uttered at the beginning of a nursing. The most typical feature was that the starting and finishing frequencies were approximately equal, while the maximum lay higher, and was reached at the middle of the short duration.
>
> Class 2 ('deep grunt'). Non-tonal, short grunts, rich in formants. Uttered throughout nursing. No measurable pitch change. Its most typical feature was the low frequency, making it the only class of piglet calls with a basic frequency below 1 kHz.
>
> Class 3 ('high grunt'). Grunts resembling 'deep grunts' except for the basic frequency, which lay approximately 1 kHz higher.
>
> Class 4 ('scream'). Long, tonal calls with a considerable positive pitch change. Often uttered in within-litter aggressive interactions. Negative pitch change occurred only in a few instances.
>
> Class 5 ('squeak'). Calls resembling the 'screams' except for the moderate positive pitch change. Like the 'scream', it was often uttered in aggressive interactions between littermates.

The within-class variability was very low and few intermediate patterns occurred giving this vocal pattern stability. Piglet calls during nursing do not form a continuum of sounds but consist of five discrete classes with a certain within-class variation. Part of this variation is due to differences between individuals but a few differences also occur within individuals. Some of the variation within the piglet call-classes relates to frequency and duration. The specific part of a piglet's vocal signal is rather constant, however, and variations only alter the communication specificity to a small extent. Piglets which are hurt show screams of higher and more variable pitch (Wemelsfelder and van Putten, 1985).

Class 1, "croaking", shows clear pattern-constancy; Classes 4 and 5 showed two considerable variations in duration and frequency. Classes 2 and 3 seem to be uttered with some consistency with slight individual variations.

Grunts seem to play a role in individual recognition and in localisation.

Lambs can find their dams when they are out of sight, by identifying their voices (Shillito, 1975; Shillito-Walser *et al.*, 1981a). This ability improves with age, up to three weeks, and seems to vary between breeds. A lamb answers bleats more quickly when they are made by its own dam. When a ewe hears her lamb bleat she may help her lamb to find her by bleating promptly in reply. Ewes are inclined to bleat when they hear a lamb bleating, but become more specific in replying as their own lambs get older. As a result, lambs of six weeks can use vocalisations to find their ewes very easily.

Mares can recognise their foals' voices but foals respond mainly to the loudest vocalisations, irrespective of whether they come from their own mare or another. Olfaction is the final clue in recognition by the foal but the behaviour and posture of the mare assists the foal in recognising her visually.

Behavioural aspects of weaning and puberty

Weaning and puberty are the two principal events in the course of development of the young animal. Successful weaning marks the survival of the animal beyond the immature period of dependence on its mother; the passage of puberty puts the subject into the ranks of reproducing adults. Both events are often associated with temporary but acute turmoil and changes in behavioural orientations (Fraser, 1968).

Weaning

Conditions of domestication almost invariably ensure that weaning is not naturally determined. Most systems of livestock husbandry enforce relatively early separation between calf and cow, piglet and sow, lamb and ewe. In dairy cattle management the young animal is taken away from the mother soon after birth. In other farm species the young are left with their mothers until the dam's peak of lactation has passed and until the young animal has developed feeding activities alternative to nursing.

These systems of artificial weaning are usually carried out abruptly. The separated dam and young vocalise continuously, calling for one another. The normal forms of behaviour become disturbed and grazing and resting may virtually cease. After a few days the separated parties re-adopt normal behavioural activities and the divisive process is concluded. This sudden withdrawal of nursing facilities usually hinders, temporarily, the growth of the young animal, but there appear to be no other untoward sequelae to sudden weaning after a long suckling phase. Piglets, however, do not sleep deeply for the first night after weaning. In dairy calves the term weaning is applied to the cessation of milk feeding. In a group-feeding situation, abrupt weaning may cause fewer problems than gradual weaning (Barton, 1983a,b).

Although it is not often that sheep and goat mothers are left with their young long enough for natural weaning to occur, this occasionally happens in both species. Such weaning occurs when the young are between three months and six months old and the natural weaning process is a progressive one. Mothers tend to lose interest in their young quickly after natural weaning and the young are then liable to become separated from the flock. Lambs of four to six weeks of age suckle about six times per day. Evidently by four weeks of age the gradual weaning process of the young sheep has begun.

Two points regarding natural weaning are worth noting:

1. Before weaning, whether this takes place suddenly or gradually, the young animal must adopt the feeding behaviour which it will retain into adult life. Much of this adult feeding behaviour is acquired by imitation of the parent in the selection of feed and manner of eating. It is likely that the roughage of adult feedstuff, in contrast to

milk, will better satisfy hunger and so condition the young animal to its ultimate feeding behaviour.

2. The aggressive behaviour sometimes shown by the mother to her own young at the time of the latter's weaning seems in sharp contrast to the general character of maternal behaviour, although an aggressive facet is often apparent in the mother's responses to alien young. The ewe normally allows only her young to suckle and she vigorously drives away and avoids others. This acceptance of her own young and active rejection of strange young depends on the bonding process of the early sensitive period during the first few hours after parturition. In dramatic forms of weaning what appears to be happening is a reversal of the cognitive processes of the critical sensitive period as a result of which the mother's own young become regarded more like aliens. Whatever the nature of the developments of any counter-critical period might be in the mother, it would appear that the fairly sudden undoing of these developments is involved in weaning aggression.

Puberty

Puberty has been variously defined as follows:

1. the period when the sexes become fully differentiated;
2. the period when secondary sexual characteristics become conspicuous;
3. the stage when there is an ability to elaborate gametes;
4. the ability and desire to effect sexual congress;
5. the time when reproduction first becomes possible;
6. the period of activation of the neural tissues which mediate mating behaviour;
7. the termination of infant sterility.

Puberty is taken here to mean the period when effective mating can occur such as the age when oestrus is first noted in the female. The age of puberty in the cattle, sheep, horse and pig is affected by genetic and experiential factors.

The contribution of experiential influences to the development of hormone-induced behaviour is a complex process and not one of simple learning. Mounting behaviour by young male animals is not indicative of the emergence of puberty in view of the common occurrence of pre-pubertal mounting. Mounting can be seen in very young lambs, pigs, calves and kids. Young male domestic chicks show copulation behaviour as early as two days of age (Andrew, 1966). In lambs and kids mounting occurs in the first few weeks of life and in kids, for example, it is quite evident that active mounting has been a frequent activity by six weeks of age. This is greatly in advance of puberty, which in the goat has been estimated to occur at about 155 days of age. Observations on sexual behaviour in goats have established that both sexes show the complete pattern of sexual behaviour before they are full grown. Although kids readily mount each other at an early age, the earliest ages at which male goats can copulate successfully is five to six months.

A similar picture is presented by the pig, young boars being capable of mounting long before they are capable of copulation. About 50% of young male pigs exhibit mounting behaviour before two months of age although puberty in the boar is commonly estimated at seven months of age.

In cattle also it is clear that active mounting behaviour occurs so far in advance of puberty as to bear little or no relationship to it. Prior to puberty the majority of bull calves can show good mounting orientation. Improvement occurs in the mounting orientation of calves as they acquire further sexual experience. Most bull calves at the rear of the stimulus animal orientate themselves appropriately on the first breeding occasion but 30% mount inappropriately. The very young and those in early puberty have a proportion of individuals with poor mounting orientation and will frequently attempt mounting the stimulus animal from the side. Such lateral mounting in an adult animal is indicative of immaturity in its reproductive responses.

Observations have been made on the comparative aspects of behaviour in young bulls and castrates in free association in feeding yards. Young bulls and castrates begin to show differences in behaviour as early as six months of age. Young bulls show more general activity, in mounting and riding predominantly, while castrates do not exhibit these features but show instead more nosing and licking. Evidently there is a pre-pubertal differentiation in behaviour between both groups. Masturbatory activities in young bulls are usually not noted until about eleven months of age—a period which corresponds very precisely with the generally accepted age of puberty in the bull.

The age of puberty may vary little from one individual to another but can be affected by various environmental factors, particularly nutrition. The pig is exceptional, however, since young females receiving a low level of energy intake reach puberty at approximately the same age as those receiving a high level of energy intake. Male pigs which have been undernourished also appear to reach sexual maturation in the usual time. Although boars with slow rates of growth take longer to acquire an ejaculatory capacity than fast-growing boars, no effect of restricted feed intake on sexual behaviour is apparent after seven months of age.

With cattle the picture is different. High planes of nutrition tend to accelerate puberty and poor nutrition delays it somewhat. Inbred bulls take longer than others to reach puberty. Even when reared on different planes of nutrition, identical twin bulls develop their sexual responses in very similar fashion.

Experimentally, other factors of environ- mental origin can exert some influence on the time when puberty is attained in some animals. Ninety per cent of young gilts, subjected to transportation, exhibited early oestrus while among control gilts of the same age, but not subjected to the same experience, only 28% showed such evidence of puberty (du Mesnil du Buisson and Signoret, 1962). It is concluded that external stimuli can lead to the early manifesta- tion of first oestrus in swine and this tends to occur four to six days after the stimulating experience; the most effective experience of this nature is exposure to the boar. In sheep, puberty is determined more by seasonal factors than by age alone and this is most evident at latitudes furthest from the tropics.

The reproductive responses of both sexes are not usually fully developed with the first manifestation of puberty. In males libido continues to develop for some time after puberty has been reached and in the female, oestrus is often of less duration and intensity at puberty than in the sexually mature age groups.

When young and old ewes are run together with the same ram, the older ewes show longer and more intense oestrus than the younger ones and older ewes do not show short, weak oestruses in the way that young ewes frequently do. Heifers show variable characteristics of oestrus.

Post-natal progress into sexual maturity is clearly rather more than the attainment of puberty and it is this degree of survival into the prime state in the individual which determines the ultimate breeding capacity. Fewer males than female animals, under natural, competitive conditions, reach this level of survival, but larger male numbers are needed at subordinate levels to apply the competitive pressures and offer reserve forces, thereby ensuring that reproduction is effected qualitatively and quantitatively.

27 Play, practice and exercise

All young animals must learn a variety of skills in order to survive in the wild. Such learning has been emphasised in chapters and sections on feeding, predator avoidance, body care, and so on. Animals which live socially have a much more complex array of skills to learn. Each individual must learn about how to communicate, how to act during social interactions and how to assess its social role, as well as about each other individual in its social group and about all their relationships. Many of the activities which may help in such learning are referred to as play. The term is difficult to define as it has been used for activities which may immediately, or ultimately, be involved in any one of the functional systems in animals. The vigorous activities of young animals include movement or manipulation of objects, chasing, fighting without causing injury, advancing towards then retreating from another individual without contact, acrobatics of various kinds, and many variations. The idea that these activities might have a function in the improvement of physical fitness and social skills was proposed by Brownlee (1954) as a result of his work with cattle, and was reiterated by Dolphinow and Bishop (1970) and Fagen (1976). Such functions seem likely and are supported by work on children (Bruner *et al.*, 1974), but they are difficult to demonstrate experimentally (Chalmers, 1979).

The term play will be used in this chapter for convenience but the usage of the word does not imply that the examples quoted are similar in motivational state or in function. A wide range of actions, which are carried out principally by young animals and which may provide useful practice or exercise, are included under this general heading. Actions with an obvious and immediate function are not normally referred to as play.

Activities which are referred to as play occur most often in healthy young animals and its absence may be an indicator of reduced health. Social play, such as chasing and mock fighting, is common (Fig. 27.1). Solitary play can take the form of manipulatory or locomotor movements. Elements of sexual behaviour appear in the infantile play, of lambs for example, as early as two weeks of age. On these occasions lambs will mount each other, clasp and perform pelvic thrusts. Mounting and biting at play feature commonly in foals. This may become aberrant biting if the infantile behaviour is encouraged to persist into adulthood. Many play movements are truly patterned, for example, by the regularity of gaits employed, and these patterns are similar for every individual member of the species concerned.

In their accompanying emotions and in the duration of action, the various play activities differ from the "serious" counterpart activities. In the "serious" situation, when an animal has fled beyond the reach of its opponent, flight

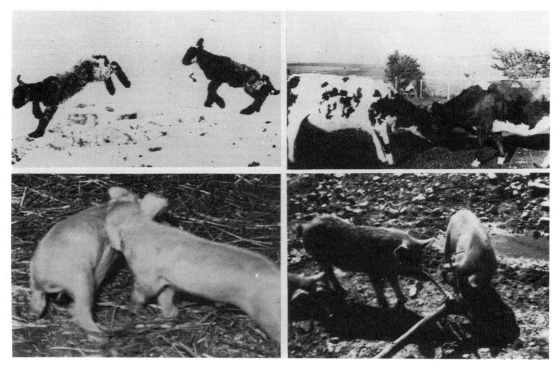

Fig. 27.1   Forms of play in sheep, cattle and pigs. Top left: leaping and chasing in lambs. Top right: mock fighting in cattle. Bottom left: fighting in piglets. Bottom right: pigs playing with an uprooted tree.

ceases. When an animal has repelled its opponent, fight ceases. Such cessations are not observed in play, which may continue for extended periods. Again, in "serious" situations there are the emotions of anger, fear, etc. which are absent in play.

The progress of kinetic development is rapid in the first few hours following birth in all the farm mammals. Neonatal behaviour contains several major kinetic features. The day-old calf, lamb, foal and kid all show bursts of sudden capricious behaviour as spontaneous acts of locomotor play in the form of leaping and infant play appears to be important in the development of kinetic competence and early social organisation. Solitary play is a form of exercise. Equine play is a good demonstration of play as a purely kinetic activity. For example, 75% of the kinetic activity of foals is in the form of play.

Systems and motives concerned in play

The various forms of movement which obviously aid survival are not simulated in play. The play movements in the young often simulate those seen in the adult activities of fighting, avoidance, predation and sex-mounting. Many activities in play occur as flight and hiding. Typically, these adult activities are not functional in the young animal. Since it is fed and protected by its dam, it normally does not require to fight nor does it require to initiate flight. As the sex organs are still immature, true sex-mounting is not seen in the young. Yet, although these activities are not required to be carried out by the young, the neuromuscular mounting requirements are in existence and are included in the agenda of practice.

The simulating nature of play movements is well illustrated in the play forms peculiar to each of the different species of domesticated mammals. Young horses use their teeth but do not head-butt in play; adult horses use their teeth but do not head-butt their opponents in fighting. In contrast, cattle do not use the teeth but use head-butting, both in play and in real fighting. Pigs show up-thrusts of the head both in play and in true fighting. Thus, in all these species, similarly patterned muscular activities are to be seen both in "serious" adult activities and in the corresponding simulated play activity. Real injury is seldom inflicted in a play-fight and no escape is truly achieved in a play-flight.

Many major behavioural systems have specific sensory goals such as repletion in ingestion or comfort in tactility. So, also, it would appear that the system of neuromuscular play is satisfied when the system is activated in exercise. It would appear that animals are reinforced in playing, as they play repeatedly and spontaneously. When play is denied, as in chronic confinement, even in the adult, an outburst of play activity is usually seen in these animals on being released.

Although the kinetic manifestations of play simulate those seen in the "serious" activities of fight, avoidance and sex-mounting, the evident emotions in these various activities differ between the "serious" situation and play. In fight there is anger, in flight there is fear and in sex-mounting there is excitement of a certain kind. In play there is only one evident emotion common to all the kinetic manifestations which is none of the above but seems to be coupled to reactivity. Thus there are vocal manifestations in play. Foals may squeal in play and calves in groups often 'baa-ock' in play. Vocalisations are used to communicate and to summon others. Communal activity is a notable feature of social play, particularly in lambs (Arnold *et al.*, 1981).

Play requirements

Exploratory play behaviour in lambs is often expressed as a social exercise (Morgan and Arnold, 1974). Groups of lambs will collectively inspect a new object. They run and chase each other over and around novel features such as mounds, bales of hay and rocks. On the other hand, lambs reared in isolation tend to withdraw from novel environments and are slow to initiate investigative movements towards new objects. Significantly they also vocalise less without companions. Lambs reared in peer groups, but without their mothers, behave similarly to lambs reared with their mothers, indicating that the main effect on playful investigation in the isolated lambs is not the result of maternal deprivation but of social deprivation.

In play-flight, as in true flight, an extent of firm surface is required for the extensive nature of such play and the kinetics of neuromuscular systems involved. In play-butting, as in true butting, objects are needed at which the play acts can be directed. Such objects can be animate conspecifics or inanimate items. Isolated calves use food buckets, straw bales and any other movable object which is accessible. For play sex-mounting, congeners are the usual objects used, but inanimate objects may also be mounted in play.

Enriched environments are inducive to play. Enriching factors for play include environmental objects, dietary enrichment, social stimulation, weather improvement, cessation of stress and release from confinement. The tendency to play in young cattle is increased by good feeding and decreased by poor feeding. Calves gallop-play more vigorously on bedded cement flooring than on bare cement flooring. Enrichment and deprivation are thus both relevant to the playing animal and to its play environment.

Play movements are not perfectly performed on the first occasion of their expression but are modified through learning (Fagen, 1981). Proficiency in play behaviour is attained remarkably quickly after animals learn the attributes of their associates and the environment. For example, playing lambs learn in galloping play to distinguish between soil and cement flooring. Calves, in butting play, quickly learn to distinguish between hard butting objects and soft butting objects. Goring play is better learned with movable than immovable objects.

Play goals and roles

The opinion has been expressed by Brownlee (1984) that although the main goal of play is to obtain physiological benefits that arise from the activity of the organs concerned, physiological benefit is not the immediate goal of play. In ingestion, an immediate goal is to taste food. So in play, an immediate goal is consummatory contact with items in the environment. Physiological benefits ensue as a consequence. Specific contact is only the initiation of the play process, for play continues beyond initiating contact. During the extended play periods, the secondary physiological benefits continue to accrue. Increased knowledge of the attributes of the animate and inanimate environment are secondary benefits which also accrue. These secondary benefits show that play has mixed goals and roles. That play leads to no primary adaptive goal is shown, for example, by the play-flight of the calf or lamb being followed by a return to near the starting set-point. On the other hand, various physiological consequences of high levels of activity result from play.

When, during prolonged confinement, muscles are deprived of optimal blood flow by the absence of such exercise as would result from play activity, there is usually an outburst of such activity on release of the affected animal. This may indicate needs for periodically increased vascularisation. The supplemental nutrition of the play muscles, through active hyperaemia resulting from play, is a physiological process in keeping with the overall roles of play in creating, temporarily, a generalised hyperaemia and contributing to normal body functioning.

Species-typical play

Calves

The characteristic aspects of behaviour displayed in play activities by cattle are prancing, kicking, pawing, snorting, vocalising and head-shaking. These are seen particularly in young calves, although adults do occasionally indulge in playful activities. Further manifestations of play include trotting, cantering and galloping with the tail at various angles of elevation; bucking, kicking one hind foot, head-butting, pawing loose soil or bedding, and mounting. Male calves do more mounting and pushing than female calves, and overall spend more time in play (Reinhardt *et al.*, 1978).

Playful kicking, which is not aggressive, may be made to one side with both legs aimlessly, but at other times kicking at a given object, usually with one hind leg, may occur. Calf play also includes butting each other or inanimate objects; they paw the ground, goring bedding, threatening attendants and making snorting noises in the course of playful actions. Playful mounting behaviour is also commonly seen in calves. Bursts of play often occur when calves are released from confinement, when freshly bedded, when introduced to other calves and with other changes in their routine or environment. Play occurs most frequently in younger calves and in those in good health.

In playful fighting, the participants appear less concerned with which will win, than with participation in the activity itself. Playful fighting is distinct from aggressive interactions in that, while playfully engaged, either animal's attention is easily distracted. Sequences of events in play are notable. For example, play pushing is typically initiated between two calves; the pushing pair may attract a third calf. As all three push one another, other couples in the common group may also be induced to start pushing. Although pushing and mounting are very often in random sequences, they are characteristically integrated into running, jumping, kicking games in which many calves in a herd participate.

Foals

Foal play begins by nibbling at the legs and mane of the mother. Among foal groups social play usually increases with age while solitary play declines. The latter is reduced to a very low order of activity by two months of age. Solitary play persists, however, in lone foals and their social play may relate to other animals and humans. Foals may also play with inanimate objects (Schoen *et al.*, 1976; Tyler, 1972).

In addition to grooming with their dams, foals in groups also groom one another. Grooming bouts often initiate play and oral snapping actions are often seen in foals when they are initiating play. The most common form of play between foals involves nipping of the head and mane, gripping of the crest, rearing up towards one another, chasing, mounting and side-by-side fighting. There are sex differences in foal play, with colts mounting more frequently and engaging in general play more vigorously than fillies. Play in foals tends to be more frequent in males than females. The response of fillies to colt play is often withdrawal or aggression. Most play involves nipping or biting various parts of the body, but running about alone or in groups, or chasing with much head tossing, sudden stops and starts, and kicking of the hind legs in the air is also typical.

Play is frequently mixed with exploratory and investigatory behaviour so that one blends into another. Play activities around the mother and alone diminish with age. Play occurs in bouts and foals initiate play bouts with each other more frequently as they mature and leave the mare. Play around the mother is reduced markedly between the first week and the fourth week of life. Foals three and four weeks of age often have play bouts lasting 10–15 min. Such bouts are usually initiated by one foal, developing the bout from a mutual grooming episode by changes to acts of nipping. A bout may be ended mutually by the two foals separating or, more often, by one foal simply turning away from the other. Most foals play with foals which are of similar age, but occasionally they play with foals differing in age by two to three months.

Lambs

For the first few weeks of life lambs stay quite close to their own ewes. By one month of age young lambs spend two-thirds of their time in the company of other lambs. By this age play is well developed. The gambolling form of play in this species is very typical. The play involves upward leaps, little dances and group chasing. Play is reduced as lambs grow and is becoming rare by four months. In general it appears that lambs are born in an advanced stage of development, both physical and behavioural. For example, they can stand, walk and suckle within the first hour. Their senses of sight and hearing are evidently better developed than those of some other neonates, such as the foal. The course of their development in play is therefore fairly rapid throughout the nursing phase.

Play in lambs is characterised by the use of a wide variety of motor patterns (Sachs and Harris, 1978; Shillito-Walser *et al.*, 1981b). It has been observed that sequences of play begin when three or more lambs engage in forms of locomotor-rotational or contact activity. The more lambs in a common group the greater is the number of events that occur during play. The amount of time spent in play has rarely been measured. It appears that lamb play reaches its highest frequency when the lambs are ten days old and then declines as an activity as lambs spend more time grazing.

Piglets

Piglet play develops notably in the second week of life. Play in young pigs is a very prominent feature of their total behaviour. It is mainly in the form of play fights. Cheek-to-cheek fighting, in which each piglet bites and roots at the other's face, neck and shoulders, is standard practice. By several weeks of age chasing and gambolling are the common forms of piglet play. The chases are usually brief. Playful individual behaviour involves rooting and mouthing of novel items. Oral manipulation and exploration of the environment is a major feature of pig behaviour, extending into adult life. Play in piglets is arrested during illness, as it is in other sick, young animals. In this respect indices of play can provide parameters of health which could be put to greater use in the practice of preventive paediatric veterinary medicine. Social play in piglets is an activity similar to other behaviours, such as cooperation, communication or altruism, in which encounters between pairs of individuals have a positive effect on their fitness (Dobao *et al.*, 1985).

Kids

Play is often described as part of the behaviour of young goats and all Caprinae. This feature may be the origin of the expression capering. Kids exhibit group play, in which many young or even an entire herd run and caper together. It has been noted that the Caprinae, believed to be the most "advanced" group of bovids, also exhibit the most elaborate and antic play. Locomotor-rotational movements are characteristic of kids which they exhibit in play around their mothers, running or galloping in circles, making high, arching jumps, running and jumping games. Little dances are also featured in kid play.

Social play in the Caprinae is as elaborate as solo play. In such play kid groups may chase, butt and ride each other, or gallop back and forth, jumping and sliding. They may jump on and off their mothers' backs, and race or bound. They make sudden stops, toss and shake their heads and whirl on their own axis, sometimes falling. They may spring vertically or chase dead items of herbage. Both males and females play-fight.

Species-general play

Common features of play occur in Artiodactyls, the order of ungulates having an even number of toes (or cloven hooves). Artiodactyl play includes solo locomotor-rotational running (often in arcs, circles or figures-of-eight or with rapid turns at high speed), leaping, kicking and jumping with head-shakes, head-tosses or body-twists. These and other characteristic and well-known artiodactyl patterns of movement are commonly termed gambols and capers. Solo gambols and capers are not the only form of artiodactyl play, however. Interactive play may take the form of chasing and reverse chasing and may include body contact in the form of pushing, butting, neck-wrestling, mutual rearing, or riding. This form of play is especially frequent in group-living species and may merge into low-intensity agonistic fighting. Social interactions involving physical contact between young male artiodactyls sometimes combine structural and functional characteristics of play with low-intensity agonistic fighting. This may determine position or rank in animals just entering subadult society (Fagen, 1981).

Contact with items other than conspecifics is another feature of artiodactyl play. Inanimate objects such as plants, or parts of plants may be tossed, shaken, pawed, pushed, jumped over, or butted repeatedly. As in other mammals, this item-orientated play behaviour may be a substitute for a conspecific or may be designed for physical training, and may relate to auto-grooming, scent-marking or investigating.

All the domesticated hoof-stock share similar characteristics of play. The lamb, foal, or calf may run round, leap vertically in the air again and again, gambolling and capering, twisting its body and kicking out with its hind feet. Such play is distinguished from avoidance of a predator, a conspecific, or a parasite and from captivity artifacts by its non-threatening context, by the playing animal's loose body tone, by its sensory inattentiveness, and by the repetition and ease of interruption of its activity.

Infant animals often repeat the same developing locomotor or manipulative behaviour with slight variation at a given stage of mastery. Such behaviour is widespread in animals and includes jumping vertically, running away from the mother and back to her, and various repetitive manipulations of objects. Such behaviour of "mastery" merges into another category of play behaviour called diversive play or diversive exploration. These varied and vigorous effector interactions with an inanimate object follow initial sensory inspection.

No matter what function of play is at issue, the interests of any two individuals in play will rarely coincide. Conflicts over social play may arise when potential partners disagree about the time or place at which play occurs. Two animals of the same age, size and sex may both benefit from moderate-intensity fighting, but if one animal has just fed or has not played for a long time, and the other is about to feed or has just played, then the second may resist the play solicitations of the first. Again, mothers may intervene in the play of their offspring and each individual will prefer to play at a closer distance to its own mother than to its playmate's mother. Any social play interaction necessarily involves a compromise between partners. This need to compromise makes play a challenge to social cooperation.

Individuals will play with partners that are close relatives (Wald, 1958). Preferences for play forms and play partners may not always coincide between playing partners and a certain amount of conflict over play results occasionally.

Social play at its cooperative best is a remarkable phenomenon. Evenly matched and closely related partners cooperate in apparent mutual physical and skill development. This play is non-injurious and does not harm social relationships. It may strengthen long-term prospects for cooperation of individuals remaining as one group. Even when an older animal plays cooperatively with a young one, special communicative signals and stabilising techniques ensure that play is fair to both participants.

Social play is neither essentially cooperative nor necessarily competitive. Sexual dimorphism in play activity as well as the sex and litter-mate preferences are in agreement with the hypothesis which assigns adaptive values to these social plays (Dobao *et al.*, 1985).

General considerations

Fagen's recent and definitive publication, on play as a general biological phenomenon, indicates the great scope for a fuller recognition of this category of behaviour as a vital force in maintaining development and self-determination. A great variety of meaningful features of play are pointed out by Fagen (1981).

Play is costly behaviour; it seems aimless, capricious, and inconsequential and its sequences include behavioural acts or sequences of behaviour also occurring in high-risk adult activities, but the products of these high-risk activities are absent from play. The risk of death by predation is not avoided as a consequence of play, conflict over a contested resource external to play is not settled and a zygote is not produced. Because play is so risky and requires so much time and energy, the question arises about beneficial effects which may result from play that might compensate for its apparent cost to the play animal.

There are, of course, great benefits to the animal both immediately and ultimately. Fagen outlines six benefits:

1. Play develops physical strength, endurance and skill, particularly in those acts or combinations of acts used in social interactions having potentially lethal consequences.
2. Play promotes and regulates developmental rates.
3. Play experience yields specific information.
4. Play develops cognitive skills necessary for behavioural adaptability, flexibility, inventiveness, or versatility.
5. Play is a set of behavioural tactics used in intra-specific competition.

6. Play establishes or strengthens social bonds in a pair or social cohesion in a group.

The main general benefit of play is its assistance to the animal in behavioural development, and Fagen alludes to this also. The evolutionary significance of the development of behaviour is that for a number of different and highly idiosyncratic reasons, young animals exhibiting complex behavioural development survived and reproduced better than other young whose behaviour changed less fundamentally with development. Developmental complexities in behaviour can therefore be viewed as reflecting adaptation. Such adaptation includes one or more components. A number of component skills include attentional, tactile and social ones, the development of each of which can begin in play and be followed through the whole life of the animal in many situations. Each component is characterised by its own rate of development and by its particular susceptibility to environmental influence during the lifetime of an individual.

The evolution of age-specific patterns of resource acquisition is a feature of behavioural maturation. This principle is most evident for overt social behaviours, such as fighting, sex, play or other interactions which are equally important. For example, age-dependent schedules of thermoregulation, of energy and nutrient requirements, and of motor development have much social impact in the tactics of grazing animals. They also affect both the parent-offspring relationship and relationships among siblings.

The evolutionary views on behaviour development amount to two principles of natural selection of genetically based variation. First, ontogenies result from biological adaptations keyed to the demands of particular environments. Second, genotypic and phenotypic composition of a given population determine the rate and direction of social behavioural evolution, including evolution of the ontogeny of social behaviour which is portrayed in play.

Laws of play

Numerous characteristic features of play have been reported and many of these have been abstracted and listed by Fagen. Those items which exemplify the laws of play behaviour in farm animals are listed below:

1. There is a play appetence. The animal that is ready to play is actively looking for an opportunity to play.
2. Social inhibitions exist, particularly avoidance of injuring the partner.
3. Use of inanimate objects or individuals of other species as substitute playmates indicates lack of stimulus specificity.
4. Interruption in every stage by stronger stimuli (loud noise, intruder, etc.) may occur and indicates that play is not imperative once started.
5. Transmission of playing mood to other individuals, particularly to playmates, shows relationship to "group effect" or social facilitation.
6. Inventing new individual or experimental play, sometimes leading to new nervous and muscular coordinations, shows the endogenous variability in play.
7. Play patterns may be exaggerated or uneconomical motility.
8. Play patterns may be relatively unordered in sequence from one time to another.
9. Short sequences and repetitious motor patterns are characteristic of play units.
10. Animals repeatedly returning to the stimulus source indicate that play has an orientation factor.
11. Rapid alternation of behaviour is a common feature.
12. The same behaviour directed at different stimuli shows the variable adoption of convenient stimuli.
13. It occurs in a relaxed situation in which there is no imperative maintenance.
14. It lacks a consummatory act as an endpoint.
15. The "play bout" is typically preceded by a

signal which indicates "what follows is play". These signals may recur during the bout to keep it continuing.

16. Actions repeated and performed in an exaggerated manner are very characteristic.
17. The activity appears "pleasurable" to the participants by subjective deduction.
18. Social play is characterised by the exaggerated and uneconomical quality of the motor patterns involved. This is most pronounced under the effects of social facilitation.
19. The individual movements making up the sequence may become more exaggerated showing a build-up in motivation within the play bout.
20. Certain movements within the sequence may be repeated more often than they would usually be in "serious" situations.
21. Movements may be both exaggerated and repeated as the most common characteristic.
22. Individual movements within the sequence may never be completed and this incomplete element may be repeated many times, indicating that behavioural units in play are not essentially linked as a chain.
23. The normal temporal groupings of functionally related actions can break down. Elements of a number of different types intermingle in the same behavioural sequences showing permutation of units.
24. Play lacks the immediate, biologically adaptive consequences that normally are associated with serious behaviour.
25. Play partners can change their roles frequently, for instance during playfights.
26. Play behaviour is practically repeatable ad libitum and lacks the reaction-specific fatigue that is characteristic of much behaviour.

This very substantial body of ethological laws relating to play behaviour indicates that this category of activity is of such vital importance to animal life that its structuring is detailed to ensure its epigenetic effects. It is clear that play is central to behavioural epigenesis, both as a set of epigenetic rules and as a mechanism for modifying these rules in response to individual play experience. The phenomenon of play, which may have its roots in various fetal activities already described at the beginning of this section, could become a basic factor in the determination of good welfare, particularly as it relates to normal development.

28 Welfare terminology and concepts

Welfare

In order that proper decisions can be taken about issues concerning animal welfare it is necessary to be very clear in the terminology used when considering the subject and precise in the measurement of welfare. There is confusion concerning the different concepts of wildlife conservation, animal rights or human obligations towards animals, and animal welfare. It is therefore necessary to explain how the word welfare is used and how it is related to moral questions (Broom, 1989a).

The welfare of an individual is its state as regards its attempts to cope with its environment (Broom, 1986c). When conditions are difficult, individuals use various methods to try to counteract any adverse effects of those conditions on themselves. One set of methods involves the use of the adrenal gland whose products mobilise energy resources and minimise the use of energy for certain everyday bodily processes. Another way of trying to deal with difficult conditions is to modify behaviour so that the state of the animal is returned to the tolerable range (Chapter 4). Behaviour can also be used to alter the motivational state and hence ameliorate the most extreme psychological disturbances. A coping system which has recently been discovered incorporates the use of naturally occurring opioid peptides in the brain which have an analgesic effect during pain or in other unpleasant conditions. The animal can reduce aversiveness by self-narcotisation. Whatever the method used, the individual may try to cope and succeed, or it may try and fail (see next section). The extent of what is done to try to cope can be measured, as can the effects of lack of success (Chapter 29). These measurements will show how poor the welfare is and other sorts of measures give some information about how good welfare is. Hence it can be seen that the welfare of an individual can be assessed precisely at any particular time. Welfare can be very good or very poor, or anywhere on a continuum between these extremes.

The assessment of welfare can be carried out in a scientific way without the involvement of moral considerations. The term welfare refers to the state of the animal and not to any human care for the animal. The question which is asked after the measurement is made is how poor must the welfare be before people consider it to be intolerable. A moral decision must be taken here and different people will draw the line, marking what is unacceptable, at different levels in the welfare continuum. The moral decision depends upon the availability of evidence about welfare but the process of deciding about morality and the process of assessing welfare are quite separate.

It is also essential to appreciate that questions about whether or not man should kill animals or exploit animals need not be related to questions about welfare. If an animal is suddenly shot, with no previous warning that this might happen, and it dies instantaneously, then there is a moral question about whether such killing should occur but there is no welfare problem. If an animal dies slowly with much pain, or is wounded by a shot which results in pain and difficulties in normal living, then its welfare is poor. Observation of the animal can provide some information about how poor its welfare is. An estimation of its welfare may also be obtained by extrapolation from studies of similarly wounded animals. It is much easier, of course, to assess welfare in domesticated animals, but the same distinction between moral decisions and such assessment needs to be made here. If animals are kept in order that they will eventually be eaten, their welfare could be good throughout their lives even up to the point of slaughter. Some people, however, do have moral objections to eating animals in such a situation where there is no welfare problem. Many other people object to the keeping of animals because of their welfare in the conditions in which they are kept. Most people would not tolerate the keeping of animals such that their welfare is extremely poor, especially if they are demonstrably in pain, but the level of poor welfare which people find morally unacceptable varies greatly. There are national differences here as well as individual differences, but both within and among countries, people's attitudes to welfare can be changed by informing them about the complexity and sophistication of the animal's life.

The importance of the distinctions made in the above two paragraphs is clearer if an attempt is made to assess situations from the animal's viewpoint. Consider a rabbit in a cage. Factors affecting the welfare of the rabbit include the size of its cage, the temperature, the complexity of the environment, the presence or absence of other rabbits, the amount and quality of food, the provision of water, the presence or absence of disease-causing organisms, the occurrence of physical injury, the presence or absence of toxic or irritating substances, the occurrence of frightening stimuli, etc. All of these factors will be important irrespective of whether the rabbit is kept on a rabbit farm for food, in a home as a pet, or in a laboratory for experimental purposes. The same factors also affect the welfare of wild rabbits and welfare can be very poor in the wild or in captivity. An animal which is confined in a cage is more likely to have some welfare problems but less likely to have others.

The effects on the individual must be considered when assessing welfare. It may be that for some species of animals, the welfare of most individuals in captivity will be poor, however much people try to improve them. For other species, however, the welfare of most individuals in captivity may be good. For every species, detailed study of the behaviour and physiology of individuals can reveal whether or not their welfare is poor. We have to get as close as we can to the rabbit's world as the rabbit perceives it and responds to it. Various forms of deprivation, discomfort or pain are important to the rabbit and lead to indicators which tell us that the welfare of the animal is poor. There is much evidence showing that animals have sophisticated systems for regulating their lives and that they are much disturbed if they cannot control certain aspects of what happens to them. There is also good evidence for elaborate systems for detecting and responding to painful stimuli. There is little or no evidence, however, concerning the ability of animals to predict and dread death. Hence the argument stated earlier that an animal's welfare can be good right up to the last second before death. For many farm animals, however, the welfare during the last few hours before slaughter can be poor and that in the last few minutes before death can be very poor indeed. For the individual animal it is not death itself or the purpose which that animal serves for man which are important, but the effects upon it of the conditions of housing and the treatment during various operations, handling, transport and slaughter.

The concept of welfare presented and defined here is clear enough to be of use to scientist and non-scientist alike. The word welfare has been used in a vague way by many people, especially in connection with payments by a state to people with insufficient means to support themselves. Many words are used scientifically in a precise way but have a colloquial usage as well and, with a precise definition, welfare should become one of these. The word well-being requires some comment for there is a close link between the concepts of welfare and well-being. Well-being refers to the way in which the individual feels about its state and is similar in usage to the French word *bienêtre* or the German word *Wohl befinden*.

Stress

When considering situations in which animals are affected by their environment it is useful to distinguish situations which are adverse from those which are not. If an animal is affected by environmental conditions but its regulatory systems, with their behavioural and physiological components, allow it to cope, then *adaptation* is said to occur. This situation is fundamentally different from one in which the environmental effect has detrimental consequences. A problem when deciding such an issue is how to assess what is detrimental. As pointed out by Broom (1983c, 1988f), the best measure of what is detrimental is reduced fitness of the individual. Some explanation of the concept of biological fitness is required here. The fitness of a genotype (a particular combination of genes) can be measured as being the per capita rate of increase of the corresponding phenotype (the expression of those genes in an individual) (Sibly and Calow, 1983). As Sibly and Calow have pointed out, following Charlesworth (1980), the fitness of a phenotype in a particular environment depends on several basic life-cycle variables: age at first breeding,

interval between successive breedings, survivorship from birth to first breeding, survivorship of adults between successive breedings, and number of female offspring per female breeding attempt. The fitness of individuals subjected to particular environmental conditions can be calculated by measuring the variables listed above. If the environmental effect is to delay first or subsequent breeding, to increase the chance of mortality occurring before first or subsequent breeding, or to reduce the number of offspring produced, then fitness is reduced.

The term *stress*, as applied to man and other animals, is normally used by the general public and by scientists to describe a situation in which environmental conditions are having adverse effects on an individual (Sassenrath, 1970; Weiss, 1972; Fraser *et al.*, 1975; Freeman, 1975a; Perry, 1975; Wood-Gush *et al.*, 1975; Hails, 1978; Warburton, 1979b; Stephens, 1980; Gross and Siegel, 1980; Maclennon *et al.*, 1982; Dantzer and Mormède, 1983; Price 1985b). Its use to refer to "any displacement from the optimum state" (Block, 1985) is of no value as it would include any environmental influence on an animal. There is often some reference to a prolonged inability to cope with the conditions (Archer, 1979). As Stott (1981) points out, stress and distress were originally the same word but physicists and some physiologists have used stress to refer to forces external to a system which displace it from its resting state. Such a usage causes no problems when referring to the properties of materials but it is confusing when applied to living organisms. The colloquial usage of stress is as a dynamic term implying that something is actually happening to the individual. The extensive work of Selye (1950) on the General Adaptation Syndrome provided the foundations for much of the research in this area but he used "stress" in several ways and tended to equate it with adrenal cortex activity, as have others since then (Banks, 1982). This is a confusing usage of the word, as explained below.

If the internal state of an animal is displaced from the tolerable range so that, for example, the animal becomes too hot, or too dry, or has too little air or too much irritant or poison, a regulatory response occurs. Such a response might control state by a feedback mechanism, where the displacement is detectable before the response, or by a feedforward mechanism, where the displacement is predicted and the corrective response is initiated before that displacement occurs. In either of these cases, or in the situation where a hazard is encountered, it may be necessary to mobilise reserves so as to make available extra energy. When a rapid, short-term response is required, such mobilisation of reserves is brought about by the sympathetic nervous system, the adrenal medulla and the secretion of adrenaline (epinephrine) and noradrenaline (norepinephrine). For more prolonged increases in activity the function is fulfilled by the adenophypophysis, the adrenal cortex and the secretion of glucocorticoids. Other responses also occur but secretory activity in the adrenal cortex has often been identified as the indicator of adverse conditions. This is unfortunate for several reasons. Firstly, adrenal cortex activity can vary considerably during each day, often in a way which provides little information about whether conditions are adverse (El Halawani *et al.*, 1973). Secondly, blood glucocorticoid levels can increase during courtship, mating and active food acquisition. Thirdly, the experience of situations during early life which involve adrenal cortex activity may benefit the individual later in life. As a consequence of these facts, those who defined stress in terms of the occurrence of an adrenal cortex response have been led to say that stress can be beneficial. Such statements contradict the general use of the term so it would be better to use "adaptive" responses (Dantzer *et al.*, 1983b) in such cases and to use "stress" responses only when there are adverse effects on the animal. Fraser *et al.* (1975) also emphasise that the implication that stress refers to some single physiological phenomenon, e.g. adrenal cortex activity, is undesirable. High blood glucocorticoid level can be a useful indicator of stress, however, for it may be associated with

exhaustion of food reserves and high susceptibility to disease. Eventually, however, the consequences for individual fitness of the physiological response must be assessed.

Selye divided his General Adaption Syndrome into a state of resistance and a stage of exhaustion, but he then used stress to describe the state of the animal during both of these stages. This is confusing. Ewbank (1973) and others (Broom, 1983c) have suggested that stress should refer to a mechanism, an active process, rather than a state. When regulatory systems are operating but are not coping with environmental conditions then the word stress should be used. The ultimate measure of whether or not an individual is coping is whether there is a reduction in fitness. Stress is therefore defined as follows (modified after Broom, 1983c, 1985). *Stress is an environmental effect on an individual which over-taxes its control systems and reduces its fitness.* The restriction of the word to times when control systems within the body are activated implies that regulatory responses are initiated and hence effects of the environmental factors are prolonged rather than instantaneous. This definition also emphasises that the word stress should be used only when the effects on the individual are detrimental and the ultimate measure of this is a reduction in fitness. The environmental factors which lead to stress are *stressors* (Freeman, 1975a, b) and the individuals under stress show *stress responses*. Using the definition of stress proposed here, no environmental conditions are said to stress individuals if the ultimate effects are beneficial. Hence the definition avoids the necessity for contradictory concepts like good stress and bad stress or over-stress and under-stress (Ewbank, 1973a; Thompson *et al.*, 1980).

The fitness related variables considered in turn below are mortality, delays in breeding, and number of offspring per breeding attempt but first some general comments are necessary. When examples of the effects of environmental conditions on fitness in man, zoo animals, farm animals or pet animals are considered, it is apparent that effects on the potential reproductive success must sometimes be assessed. Human beings seldom breed at their maximum rate, even when the constraints of providing for offspring are taken into account so fitness assessment is not straightforward. If a condition affects mortality before reproduction occurs, for example by increasing the risk of a heart attack, then actual fitness is reduced. The condition should also be considered as stressful, however, if its effects are to reduce fertility, or to change development so that reproduction would be impaired, even if the individual does not intend to reproduce. Similarly, for animals which are kept by man and slaughtered before reproduction, or not allowed to breed, reproductive potential can be assessed. This would involve experimentation with such animals or extrapolation from studies of other animals of that species, age and sex.

Mortality

In man, mortality rates differ according to lifestyle. Individuals in certain forms of employment are more likely than are others to die at an early age, and hence to reduce their likelihood of breeding. At the time that the conditions lead to an increase in the probability of mortality the individual is under stress. The chances that mortality will occur will also increase after certain events during human life such as bereavement, losing a job, divorce, etc. (Hawkins *et al.*, 1957; Holmes and Rahe, 1967). These events are stressful both in common parlance and in terms of the above definition. Many wild animals die when brought into captivity and pigs may die during or following transport. As many as 7% of pigs died during transport to some slaughterhouses in the Netherlands in 1970 (van Logestijn *et al.*, 1982). In each of these examples stress occurs when individuals are trying to cope with adverse conditions. If mortality occurs following some sudden event it is unnecessary to use the concept of stress. A similar argument applies if mortality is due to a pathogen and there is no other

environmental effect. When conditions increase the likelihood of disease or parasitism, however, they would often be considered to be stressful.

The link between stress and disease has been explored extensively in man (Wolff and Goodell, 1968), in laboratory animals (Weiss, 1972), and in some farm animals (Gross and Siegel, 1980; Siegel, 1987). Conditions which cause prolonged or frequent high levels of glucocorticoids in the blood lead to a reduction in circulating lymphocytes, thymus involution, loss of mass of spleen and peripheral lymph nodes and a general reduction in immune competence in mice (Riley, 1981). Other conditions which activate the sympathetic nervous system adrenal medullary response may, if frequent enough, increase arteriosclerosis, nephritis and heart disease (Henry and Stephens, 1977). A series of studies by Gross and Siegel (Gross and Siegel, 1979, 1980, 1981; Gross *et al.*, 1980; Thompson *et al.*, 1980), showed that the mixing of chickens from one stable group with those in another, which leads to adrenal cortex activity, could change the functioning of the immune system, sometimes increasing susceptibility to disease. In a variety of situations in which the life of the chicken was disrupted in some way, the probability of mortality due to disease was increased.

Where an environmental condition does increase susceptibility to disease, the individuals subject to that condition will not contract the disease unless they come into contact with the pathogen. It would be illogical, however, to say of two chickens whose conditions rendered them vulnerable to death by Marek's disease that one which contacted the pathogen had been under stress whilst another which did not contact the pathogen had not been under stress. It is the susceptibility to disease of animals of that genotype when placed in those conditions which should be considered and hence disease challenge experiments, such as those used by Gross and Siegel, provide information which can be used to assess whether a condition of rearing or treatment of the animals is stressful. The link between conditions or treatment of animals and disease can also be explored by epidemiological studies or studies of effects on immune system function (Ekesbo, 1981; Kelley, 1985; Siegel, 1987; Broom, 1988c). Animals in certain conditions could be said to be under stress if there is a higher incidence of a disease which reduces fitness or if the immune system functions sufficiently badly for fitness reduction to be likely in the event of disease challenge.

Delays in breeding

The delay before breeding may be increased by slow growth rate or by specific effects on behavioural or physiological aspects of the reproductive procedure. Slow growth could be due entirely to lack of food in an individual whose metabolic functioning was efficient. It adds little explanation to say that such a starved animal is under stress. Where lack of food leads to the activation of responses which reduce the efficiency of utilisation of food, however, stress may be involved. Other conditions may also reduce food intake or impair metabolic functioning in young animals, so that if food is limiting then first reproduction will be delayed. For example, McDowell (1968) showed that growing heifers were under stress when kept at high temperature since their feed conversion efficiency was reduced. Social factors which reduce growth rates include being forced to mix with strangers, which slowed the growth rate of heifers without affecting food intake (Haggett *et al.*, 1982), and individual housing, which slowed growth rates in chickens (Gross and Siegel, 1981). The rearing of young animals in isolation may have effects on individuals which are not apparent until they mix with others. Calves reared in isolation for 8 months grew normally until they were mixed with group-reared animals. Their inability to compete was apparent and their growth rates declined when in competitive feeding situations (Broom and Leaver, 1978; Broom, 1982). Similarly, mice grew normally in isolation but showed impaired growth and increased mortality, both when put

with other mice and when isolated again (Henry and Stephens, 1977). Isolation-rearing left these animals unable to cope with social interaction so the condition of isolation-rearing and exposure to a normal social situation was stressful for them. The interval between successive breedings can be extended, and hence fitness reduced, by a similar, wide range of factors to those which delay initial breeding.

Reduction in number of offspring

Animals provided with breeding opportunities may fail to breed, or may produce fewer young, because of any of the following: inadequate reproductive behaviour, failure to come into oestrus, failure to conceive, abortion, or early death of offspring. The conditions provided by zoos are not adequate for the breeding of many species. This might occasionally be due to some dietary deficiency but most of the inadequacy is in some aspect of the physical or social conditions. Even when the materials which seem to be needed for breeding to occur are present, many animals, such as the giant panda and some birds of prey, seldom breed. Hence it can be said that the animals are under stress in these conditions. It is often not clear which aspect of the conditions is the stressor but research undertaken with the aim of identifying such problems has resulted, in recent years, in improved zoo management and more species now breed in zoos. Some pet animals also fail to breed, the tortoise being a notable example. Most farm animals breed well in captivity but some for which there is not normally any attempt at breeding might fail to do so, for example turkeys which are too heavy to mate or veal calves whose prolonged confinement and poor diet would probably impair reproductive output as well as survival to breeding age.

The effects of sow housing conditions on reproductive success have been studied in some detail because of their economic importance. England and Spurr (1969) found that only 6% of gilts kept in pens in which they could move around failed to show oestrus but 17% of those confined in narrow individual stalls failed to do so. Bäckström (1973), in a study of 9600 sows, compared sows confined during pregnancy with those free to move in a pen. He found that confined sows showed greater udder disease incidence (11.2%) than free sows (6.7%), more prolonged farrowings (5.4% : 2.3%), more stillborn piglets (6.3% : 5.1%) and more piglet mortality due to mummification, splay legs or sow illness (8.0% : 5.6%). Similar results have been obtained by Svendsen and Bengtsson (1983) and by Sommer *et al.* (1982), hence many sows in confinement could be said to be under stress. Unfavourable temperatures can also affect the number of offspring produced. When environmental conditions result in high body temperatures in cows (Fallon, 1962; McDowell, 1972) and ewes (Dutt *et al.*, 1959), conception rates are low.

Practicality of stress assessment

The use of fitness reduction as the criterion of adversity when assessing whether an environmental condition is stressful is rigorous and biologically meaningful, but not always easy. It is important to appreciate that energy and other resources are often used without there being any reduction in fitness. The idea of "cost", as it is used in optimal foraging studies, often does not mean any real reduction in fitness so such "costs" would not be criteria for stress. When assessing the effects of an environmental condition on fitness it is necessary to consider each life-history variable in turn and also interactions between them (Sibly and Calow, 1983). A good performance as measured by one variable need not mean high fitness if it is involved in a trade-off with others. As mentioned above when considering the effects of isolation-rearing in mice (Henry and Stephens, 1977), isolated animals may have low mortality rates and good growth rates but they are not able to translate this into reproductive performance. Hence measurement of mortality

rate would not give a useful indication of fitness. Similarly, a good growth rate and early first breeding might be counteracted by a smaller number of offspring produced at that breeding, reduced survivorship to subsequent breedings and reduced future offspring production. In general, a small reduction in performance according to one variable might be counteracted by a good performance according to another. A delay in first reproduction might mean an increase in litter size. An increase in mortality likelihood in a spawning salmon or rutting red deer stag which puts all its energy into offspring production need not be an indicator of stress because fitness may be increased. Studies like that of Bäckström (1973), in which each variable was measured, are especially valuable and research should be concentrated on obtaining such data.

In most studies of the effects of environmental conditions a detectable increase in mortality, or delay in reproduction, or reduction in number of offspring produced will indicate fitness reduction. Measures of physiological functioning, growth rate, level of injury or susceptibility to disease can often be interpreted in terms of effects on fitness and hence can be indicators of stress. One observation of a high blood glucocorticoid level or of a brief check in growth rate provides little reliable information about whether conditions are stressful, however.

A problem in the identification of stress which arises in some circumstances, is the situation where environmental factors which do over-tax control systems and reduce fitness are present at the same time as other factors which increase fitness. When animals are brought into captivity, fitness may increase because predators are removed and both regular food and potential mates are provided. Against this background, however, certain environmental factors may be stressors. When considering whether some factor in a condition or treatment is a stressor it is necessary to compare two or more conditions without that factor and to decide which is more stressful. The crucial question is whether conditions can be altered in a way which increases fitness and reduces stress. It is obvious that stress could be reduced if animals in a certain condition die after one-quarter of a normal life-span or seldom reproduce. It is clear that individual rearing is stressful for rhesus monkeys since individually reared monkeys fail to show normal sexual behaviour and fitness is obviously reduced (Harlow, 1965). If a stud bull is kept in isolation it might fail to show normal sexual behaviour, but it may sire many offspring. In order to answer the question as to whether the isolated bull is under stress, the fitness of bulls kept in small pens and bulls kept in fields should be compared. Comparisons of fitness are possible when looking at different conditions of animal housing. The assessment of fitness is generally easier for females than for males but it is very difficult when some procedures, such as artificial insemination, are used.

Needs

The basic set of functional systems, such as temperature regulation, acquiring and processing food, etc. which allows animals to survive and reproduce is described in Chapters 1 and 4. These systems within the animal include behavioural, physiological and anatomical components but they depend for their functioning on aspects of the animal's environment, such as the presence of food. As a consequence of our studies of the functional systems of animals we can identify the resources or stimuli in the environment which are required by animals and the bodily qualities which are regulated. The general term *need* is used to refer to a deficiency in an animal which can be remedied by obtaining a particular resource or responding to a particular environmental or bodily stimulus. The need is a consequence of the functional systems and, in the case of behavioural components of such systems, depends upon the motivational state of the animal. As explained in Chapter 4, at any moment an individual will have a variety of needs, some of greater urgency than others. Each is a consequence of the general biology of the animal and, in particular, of its motivational mechanisms (Baxter, 1988; Hughes and Duncan, 1988; Broom 1988b). Hence it may be very important for an individual to be able to interact socially with other animals, or to move away from potential danger as well as to be able to eat certain food or to groom itself.

If an animal is not able to satisfy a need, the consequence, either shortly or eventually, will be poor welfare. There may be a reduction in the fitness of the individual. In fact our ideas of what are the needs of any particular kind of animal are often deduced from situations where there is some inadequacy in its environment. Another way of investigating the needs of animals is to examine what animals do when they have some free choice. These methods of finding out about needs are discussed in Chapter 29 on indicators of welfare.

Various qualifying words are often put before the word "need" in discussions about welfare and in legislation relevant to welfare. The term "biological needs" has been used and it emphasises that the animal has a very wide range of needs. It is a logically correct term but since all needs pertain to the biology of the animal the prefix could be regarded as redundant. Since the responses to most needs are physiological or behavioural, both "physiological needs" and "behavioural needs" have been described. All needs necessitate some physiological state, even if it is only in the brain, so the term "physiological needs" is scarcely necessary, except perhaps to emphasise that the animal has some deficit which is easily measured physiologically. Needs which can be satisfied by carrying out some behaviour, e.g. grooming or interacting socially, have been referred to as "behavioural needs". In some cases 'behavioural needs" have been distinguished from "physiological needs", even though satisfaction of the "physiological needs" would involve behaviour such as drinking or eating. As the behaviour is a means to satisfying the need the term "behavioural need" is not really logical. It is better to say that the animal has a need and to explain the inadequacy in the animal's environment which is leading to poor welfare. A final term which has been used is "welfare need" which could be of use in emphasising those needs which are of particular importance if poor welfare is to be prevented. This term could often be replaced by the word "need", however.

Freedoms

Whereas the term "need" refers to a characteristic of an animal, the idea of "freedoms" for animals carries an implication of moral obligation towards that animal (Broom, 1988). The proposal that farm animals should be given certain "freedoms" was put forward in the Brambell Report in 1966. In a more recent wording of the five "freedoms", necessary to avoid welfare problems, Webster and co-workers (1986) list: freedom from hunger and malnutrition, freedom from thermal or physical distress, freedom from disease or injury, freedom to express most normal behaviour, and freedom from fear. These concepts are also incorporated in the welfare codes for various farm animals in the United Kingdom (Ministry of Agriculture, Fisheries and Food, U.K., 1983). The categories differ in breadth but they are based on knowledge about the needs of animals. They provide a useful general guide to the farmer or to others involved in farm animal husbandry as to their obligations towards the animals. It is often necessary, however, to discover whether some degree of freedom is essential for the animal. In that circumstance the effects of inadequacies of freedom must be studied before advice can be given on whether that condition for the animal will result in poor welfare. In the assessment of systems for managing and housing animals, decisions about adequacy must ultimately be taken using scientific information about the extent of poor welfare.

One consequence of the idea that animals should be given freedoms such as "freedom to express most normal behaviour" is that the total behavioural repertoires of animals have been considered in discussions about animal welfare. Fraser (1988) explains that if animals are prevented from showing any of a wide range of activities within their repertoire, there may be adverse effects on them. Taken to an extreme, this approach could lead to requests that the most trivial activity should be possible for an animal but the advantage of requiring a careful investigation of the behavioural repertoire of an animal is that there is then less likelihood that some important need will be prevented. Again the ultimate criterion should be evidence of poor welfare if the animal cannot perform the activity.

Obligations and rights

The idea that people who keep or interact with farm animals have obligations towards them as regards ensuring that their welfare is not poor has been mentioned in the section on "freedoms". Most people believe that animals should not be subjected to pain or severe discomfort and that their normal biological processes should be taken into account when conditions for housing or managing them are designed. These attitudes are based on self-interest to some extent but self-interest does not account for all of the feeling of obligation. There is variation amongst individuals and amongst people from different countries in their ideas as to the extent of their obligations towards animals (Teutsch, 1978, 1987). Attitudes range from those who believe that animals can be used or treated in any way to those who would sooner cause injury or hardship to another person than to an animal.

As mentioned above in the section on the concept of welfare the question of whether or not animals should be killed, which need not be one concerning welfare, is a matter where some people hold strong views. Whilst the killing of animals for food or because they are pests is accepted by the majority of people, far fewer would condone the killing of animals for no purpose which benefits man. The number of people who do not like the idea that animals should be killed for human food has increased in recent years. The vegetarian will not eat meat whilst the vegan will not eat any animal product. Amongst those who are vegetarian or vegan there are many who have great concern for the welfare of animals but many others who will eat meat have just as much concern.

The idea of obligation to animals is widely accepted but some argue that human actions should be modified according to "animal rights". The term "right" is sometimes used in the same way as "freedom" and implies an obligation. It is, however, regarded as a characteristic of the animal rather than a description of a moral relationship with man. The term "animal rights" poses a problem because of the legal usage of the term "right". Laws are passed with human considerations as the objective so in a legal sense animals do not have rights. Since the consideration, when animal rights are discussed, is usually how humans treat other animals, rather than how two non-human species interact, it is generally simpler for people to understand the idea of human obligations than that of animal rights.

29 Welfare measurement

As explained in the previous chapter, welfare varies on a continuum from very good to very poor. The two general approaches to the measurement of welfare involve trying to assess poor welfare by using various indicators or trying to recognise good welfare (Smidt, 1983; Broom, 1986c, 1988d). As explained below, we can now use many indicators of poor welfare but there is much still to be discussed in this area of scientific research. It is likely that we cannot recognise poor welfare in some animals because we have not yet learned what measurable changes occur when the animal is utilising a particular system for trying to cope with adversity. An example of how we can be unaware of a coping system is that, until recently, we did not know that animals might cope with difficult conditions by self-narcotisation using naturally occurring opioid peptides. The recognition of good welfare is not carried out directly but depends, principally, on the absence of indicators of poor welfare and on the assessment of the preferences of animals. Preference assessment is discussed in detail below. It is essential that the importance to the animal of any preference is evaluated.

Assessing poor welfare

When animals are in conditions which they find difficult they may fail to cope with those conditions or they may succeed in coping. When they fail to cope, individual fitness is reduced and they are under stress (see previous chapter). If fitness is reduced by a condition, then the welfare of the individuals subjected to that condition is poor. The extent of the decrease in reproductive potential due to reduced life expectancy or reduced reproductive efficiency can be measured. If adaptation occurs, the animal succeeding in coping, then the amount that the individual has to do in order to cope can also be measured. If coping is easy then there is little effect on welfare. If it is difficult, then welfare is poor, and the extent to which it is poor can be assessed from the measurement. Once the welfare is evaluated, moral decisions about what is acceptable can be taken. Most people would consider it unacceptable if there was a clear increase in mortality or a condition which an animal could cope with only by grossly abnormal physiology or behaviour for, say half of its life. Many people would find a much smaller extent of poor welfare to be unacceptable. In the remainder of this section the various indicators of poor welfare are considered in turn. Short-term welfare problems of farm animals are considered first and the long-term problems such as housing conditions are discussed. This distinction is made because there are some differences in which measures are most useful in each case.

Assessing short-term welfare problems: handling and transport

When animals are handled, transported, exposed briefly to a predator or subjected to some operation they show a range of behavioural and physiological changes which have the general effect of helping them to survive the treatment. Although the changes may be biologically adaptive in some situations, they do not always have beneficial effects. The behavioural responses are diverse and most are altered according to the stimuli received. The initial responses involve orientation to one of the stimuli, suppression of normal activities and preparation for flight, defence or hiding. If the situation continues and the physical conditions are outside the tolerable range then regulatory behaviour, for example huddling in cold conditions, occurs. Both suppression of activities such as feeding or grooming and increases in modifications of posture or signalling may continue throughout the period of difficult conditions. Alternatively all active behavioural responses may cease and the individual may relapse into quiescence.

Physiological responses to difficult conditions include orientation, regulatory responses, suppression of function such as that of the gut and preparations for flight or defence. Changes which can be measured include those in heart rate, ventilation rate, adrenal functioning and brain chemistry. Heart rate responses often involve an initial bradycardia (slowing of heart rate) and some animals such as the ptarmigan (Gabrielsen *et al.*, 1977) use bradycardia when a predator is close. The major response, however, is tachycardia (increase in heart rate).

For example, Stephens and Toner (1975) reported the heart rate of a calf was 90 beats per minute when standing quietly, 135 bpm when a person entered its pen and 145 bpm when it was restrained by a person. Similarly, van Putten and Elshof (1978) found that the basal heart rate of an undisturbed slaughter weight pig was 138 bpm, but this increase by a factor of 1.5 when an electric prodder was used on it, by 1.65 when it was made to climb a loading ramp, and

by more if the ramp was very steep (van Putten, 1982). A problem with such studies is that whilst some of the increase in heart rate is a response to the treatment, some of it is a consequence of greater activity.

In a recent study by Baldock *et al.* (1988) those aspects of sheep heart rate increase which were a direct consequence of increased activity were allowed for statistically so that the non-motor heart rate response to various situations could be calculated. Sheep showed a large heart rate response to the approach of a dog, to introduction to a new flock and to being visually isolated from their companions. A smaller response was shown to spatial isolation, being loaded onto a vehicle and being transported in a vehicle (Baldock and Sibly, in press) (Table 29.1).

Work by Duncan and Filshie (1979) on hens demonstrated that different strains of hens showed different responses to a traumatic event—the close approach of a person. A strain of hens which had been described as flighty because of its behavioural response to man was compared with a strain considered to be placid. The flighty strain did show a much greater behavioural response but its heart rate response rapidly declined after the person had moved away. The supposedly placid strain showed a greater heart rate response which took very

Table 29.1
Sheep heart rate responses

Treatment	Heart rate (taking account of activity)
Spatial isolation	0
Standing in stationary trailer	0
Visual isolation	+20
Introduction to new flock (0–30 min)	+30
Introduction to new flock (30–120 min)	+14
Transport	+14
Approach of man	+50
Approach of man with dog	+84

Data from Baldock and Sibly (in press).

much longer to decline to normal levels. Work by Freeman and Flack (1980) showed that the magnitude of the adrenal cortex response to handling varied considerably from one breed of chicken to another. Such studies emphasise the need for combining behavioural and physiological indicators of welfare for all strains are clearly very much affected by the approach of the person or by handling. Duncan (1986) has also been able to use heart rate changes in assessing the responses of broiler chickens to an automatic broiler harvester. This was found to cause much briefer tachycardia than the catching of the birds by people.

There have been many studies which included the measurements of levels of adrenal products in the blood as an indicator of the responses of animals to short-term periods of difficulty. An example of a study in which this measure was combined with other physiological measures involved the assessment of the effects of different handling procedures and of transport on hens which were being removed from battery cages and taken to slaughter (Broom *et al.*, 1986, in prep.). Handling and transport of hens led to higher ventilation rates, increased blood cortisol levels, and increased utilisation of noradrenaline in the brain as measured after death. In this study the rough handling which is normal when hens are being removed from battery cages to vehicles had much greater effects than did gentle handling or a short period of transport. The duration of a journey and conditions during the journey affect adrenal and other responses. Freeman *et al.* (1984) monitored the effects of transport on blood corticosterone levels in broiler chickens and compared transported birds with non-transported controls. With control corticosterone levels at a mean of about 1.3 ng/ml, levels for transported birds were 4.5 ng/ml after 2 h and 5.5 ng/ml after 4 h in summer (20°C) and 3.9 ng/ml after 2 h and 6.2 ng/ml after 4 h in winter (2°C). Other effects after 4 h of transport were substantial increases in levels of free fatty acids and cholesterol in the blood and a reduction in blood glucose. When calves are transported there is, similarly, an

increase in blood glucorticoid, in this species cortisol, and a decrease in glucose. Mormède *et al.* (1982) showed that after a journey of more than 300 km and a night spent in transit young calves showed acute dehydration and reduced blood glucose levels which were still apparent one week later and also high levels of respiratory disease. As Kent and Ewbank (1983, 1986a, b) have demonstrated, using control calves starved for the same duration as that of a journey, some of the changes during transport are a consequence of lack of food. Plasma cortisol rose to a maximum 10 min after the start of a journey (Fig. 29.1) and plasma glucose rose in the first few hours and then dropped until the calves were fed. Other changes, seen in white blood cells, were an increase in neutrophils and a decrease in lymphocytes during transport.

Another kind of physiological indicator of welfare problems during transport and handling is the quality of the meat after slaughter. The biochemical changes in muscle, especially in glycogen metabolism, are affected by the responses of the animal to conditions during the hours before slaughter (see reviews by Hails, 1978; Tarrant, 1981 and von Mickwitz, 1982). If such conditions are very difficult for pigs there is a high likelihood that their meat will be pale, soft and exudative (PSE). This condition arises when there is very rapid glycolysis, with consequent high production of lactic acid and fall in pH,

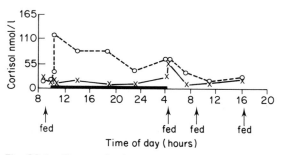

Fig. 29.1   Changes in plasma cortisol during road transportation of three-month-old calves. Values for transported calves significantly different from values for calves starved for the same period (after Kent and Ewbank, 1986b).

immediately after death. The result of this is that the water binding capacity of muscle proteins declines, water leaks out of the meat and the colour becomes paler and greyer. Another condition which can arise in cattle, pigs, etc. is dark firm dry meat (DFD). This occurs if muscle glycogen reserves are depleted before death so that little lactic acid can be produced in muscles after death and pH remains high. Both PSE and DFD meat cause substantial economic losses, especially "dark cutting" of beef. Similar problems which are a consequence of poor welfare during handling and transport can arise in poultry (Ehinger and Gschwindt, 1981). The occurrence of PSE meat in pigs occurs more after long journeys or adverse temperature conditions during the journey (Lendfors, 1970; Augustini *et al.*, 1977) and is much more likely in some breeds than in others (see later in this chapter). The likelihood of occurrence of DFD meat is also greater in pigs after long journeys and is greatly increased in beef if bulls are mixed with strange individuals during a journey or at lairage (Tarrant, 1981). Other welfare indicators which are apparent from looking at carcasses after slaughter are bruises and wounds caused by being thrown about on a journey, being maltreated by people, or by fighting consequent upon social mixing.

All of the physiological and meat quality indicators mentioned above can be complemented by measures of behaviour. The work of Kenny and Tarrant on bulls has clearly demonstrated that both fighting and withdrawal from other animals at lairage have parallels in carcass characteristics. The mixing of bulls has serious consequences for welfare and economic losses. Similar results have been obtained for fattening pigs by Guise and Penny (in press), who has found that the mixing of pigs on the farm prior to transport, on the vehicle, or at lairage leads to fighting, emotional disturbance and reduced meat quality. Behaviour observations can show which animals are likely to be most affected by transport and associated procedures. Animals which are very disturbed by these conditions show less normal behaviour such as

grooming and either over-react or do not respond to events around them. Much remains to be found out about behaviour during procedures such as handling and transport but work by van Putten, Grandin and others has provided information about how farm animals react to different characteristics of races and loading systems (see next chapter). Animals can be transported in such a way that their welfare remains good throughout—see for example Jackson (1974)—but many factors must be taken into account when designing vehicles and accommodation for transporting farm animals (Hails, 1978; Pearson and Kilgour, 1980; van Putten, 1982; CEC, 1984).

Assessing pain

It is easy to appreciate why some pain detection system should have evolved in animals. If the body of an individual has been damaged in some way it is useful for the brain to receive information about this so that appropriate action can be taken. The normal sensory system can give some indication of sensory overload but an extra system, including the section of the brain which deals with the input, is also needed. When considering how a pain system might have evolved in a particular species of animal, however, it is important to consider all aspects of that animal's life. A perceived pain stimulus is only of value if the individual needs to take some action and the action must depend on the circumstances. A limb which is pricked or cut should be removed from the source of damage and a cut should be kept from further contact which might make the injury worse. Whether or not it is of evolutionary advantage for the wound to feel painful or for the animal to respond to the extent of vocalisation as part of the pain response would depend on the circumstances. A young animal might call out loudly and solicit the help of a parent, whereas an animal which is very close to a dangerous predator might do best to keep quiet. For man, being a very social species with a long juvenile period, actions which communicate to others that pain is being experienced might often be advantageous. For species which are very vulnerable to predation or which are less social, dramatic displays associated with feeling pain might be wholly disadvantageous. These differences in how natural selection might have acted so as to affect responses, help to explain some of the curious differences amongst species in the behavioural responses produced when in pain. There can also be some differences in the responses of an individual to the same painful stimulus in different conditions. Hence it is clear that when trying to decide whether or not an animal is in pain, the various selection pressures acting on such animals and the context at the time of observation must be taken into account. As Morton and Griffiths (1985) point out, pain in an animal may not be obvious and in some situations where extrapolation from other species suggests that pain is likely to be experienced, we should assume that the animal is in pain and act accordingly.

Each person has an idea of what constitutes pain, but it is difficult to define pain. Zimmermann (1984, 1985) defines it by saying: "Pain in animals is an aversive sensory experience caused by actual or potential injury that elicits protective motor and vegetative reactions, results in learned avoidance behaviour and may modify species specific behaviour, including social behaviour". However, as Zimmermann himself points out, seeing a predator or detecting sudden auditory or olfactory stimuli may have these effects without being painful. A more useful definition is: *pain is a sensory stimulus which is itself aversive*.

We know from studies of man and other mammals that a pain detection or nociceptive system exists. Electrical recording studies show that there are neurons which fire when the skin is pricked, burned, chemically damaged or given electric shocks. There is a set of neurons in the spinocervical tract which respond in this way. It is possible to identify peptides which are involved in the transmission of such information using monoclonal antibodies and peptides can

be added, using iontophoresis, which will have effects on records from these neurones. The tract can be traced from receptors in skin, for example A-delta fibres associated with acute prickling pain and C fibres associated with burning sensation, into regions of the brain. Such studies are of especial interest because they show that a nociceptive system, with its tracts and transmitter chemicals, is present in a wide range of animals. All vertebrates have such a system, which varies little from one mammalian species to another, and invertebrates have some components of it. This physiological and biochemical evidence suggests strongly that pain can be experienced by all animals but it is very difficult to use such methods to identify pain in situations to which farm animals are exposed.

The other major sources of information about how pain is experienced are reports from human subjects and behavioural studies of man and other species. A type of observation which long caused confusion, but which is now largely explained, is that of situations which would be expected to cause extreme pain but which were not reported as being painful or which did not lead to obvious behavioural responses. For example the man in battle whose leg is shot off but who reports not knowing that this had happened until he looked at it, or the chimpanzee which picks in an apparently unconcerned way at a severe injury. It is now known that extreme pain may not be detected because of the secretion of naturally occurring analgesic opioid peptides such as β endorphin and the enkephalins (Hughes *et al.*, 1975). The major analgesic effects are mediated via the μ receptors in the brain. Such a system makes it possible for animals which are severely injured not to show responses which would make them very vulnerable to predation. It also reduces the likelihood of extreme adrenal responses which may in themselves be damaging to the animal. Any injury which is severe enough for this natural analgesia to occur must result in poor welfare, but we would not say that the individual was in pain. The nociceptive pathways may be active but pain is not experienced because of the analgesia.

Experimental studies of nociception are of some value in indicating what operations and procedures might be painful in farm animals. A widespread laboratory technique is to assess pain felt by a rat by measuring how long it allows its tail to be heated before it flicks it away and this test can also be used for pigs (Dantzer *et al.*, 1986). Such tests can be used to assess the effects of artificial analgesics. Many more extreme tests such as the induction of arthritic pain or of burning sensation by injection of formalin subdermally have been carried out. There is little doubt from such tests that the species of animals tested have a nociceptive system, experience pain and are affected by a similar range of artificial analgesics but most people would consider that such studies are immoral unless a major benefit for such animals might ensue.

Studies of normal farm procedures have been carried out, for example Gentle (1986) has studied chickens after beak trimming. He has established that nociceptors exist in the beak where it is trimmed and their response characteristics are similar to those of mammals. After beak trimming, neuromas appear. These are thought to be a major source of post-amputation pain in human patients and are often found to be associated with self-mutilation in mammalian studies. It is clear that beak trimming (or de-beaking as it is sometimes called) shows all signs of being a painful operation with prolonged painful effects as well as effects on feeding and exploratory behaviour. Any advantage in reducing damage to other birds must be balanced against such effects.

The most valuable indicators of pain, especially for a farmer or veterinary surgeon, are particular behavioural characteristics (Morton and Griffiths, 1985; Sanford *et al.*, 1986). The investigation of an animal should commence by obtaining information about food intake, water intake, defaecation, vomiting or any other signs which the stockman can report. The first assessment of behaviour should be made before the animal is disturbed. It should be possible to obtain information on respiration rate, posture, ease of movement, or movement which favours some part of the body, before close approach to the animal. When nearer to the animal its appearance and its responsiveness to various stimuli can be assessed. Finally, close examination to ascertain clinical condition and source of pain if any can be carried out. If the animal is thought to be in pain the effects of administering analgesics can be monitored. Morton and Griffiths (1985) propose that the various bodily and behavioural signs can usefully be given scores so that an accumulated score of pain level can be obtained (Table 29.2). Examples of behaviour indicating pain in farm animals include a rigid posture, grunting and grinding of teeth in cattle and goats, kicking at a painful abdomen in horses, a penguin-like stance in hens with abdominal pain, and reluctance to move in pigs and other species. Also apparent from longer periods of observation are lack of normal social behaviour in all species. A knowledge of normal behaviour is clearly necessary if responses to pain are to be detected. Extreme pain is associated with being comatose, unresponsive or moribund and must often mean that previous signs of pain have been missed and natural analgesics are now acting. Such extreme effects are unlikely to be affected by giving analgesics but the effects of many other conditions or procedures can be greatly reduced in this way.

Farm operations which may have painful effects on animals are seldom studied in this way. A recent attempt to investigate a very widespread operation is the work of Wemelsfelder and van Putten (1985) on castration of piglets. The piglets are castrated in order to avoid the boar taint which is present in the meat of some boars. It is carried out without anaesthetic during the fourth week of age in the Netherlands so the authors compared castrated males with females from the same litters. Piglets which are handled scream so Wemelsfelder and van Putten investigated whether the screams of castrated piglets were different. They found that the mean frequency of the normal handling scream was

Table 29.2
Relationship between signs and degree of pain, distress and discomfort

	Normal (0)	Mild (1)	Moderate (2)	Severe (3/4)
Appearance		Coat loses sheen, hair loss, starey — harsh _____		
		Failure to groom, soiled perineum _____		
		Discharge from eyes and nose _____		
		Eyelids partly closed _____		
			Eyes sunken and glazed _____	
		Hunched up look _____		
		Respiration laboured, abnormal panting _____		
				Grunting before expiration; grating _____ teeth
Food/water intake		Reduced _____		Zero (prolonged) _____
		Faecal/urine output reduced _____		Zero _____
Behaviour		Away from cage mates, isolated; _____	Unaware of extraneous activities _____ or bullying from mates	
		Self mutilation _____		
		Restlessness, reluctant to move, recumbent _____		
		Change in temperament _____		
		Squealing, howling, etc., especially when provoked _____		
Clinical signs	Strong pulse _____		Weak pulse _____	
Cardiovascular		Cardiac rate increased or decreased _____		
		Abnormal peripheral circulation _____		
		Pneumonia, pleurisy _____		
Digestive		Altered faecal volume, colour, consistency _____		
		Abnormal salivation _____		
		Vomiting (high frequency) _____		
			Boarded abdomen as _____ in peritonitis	
Nervous (musculoskeletal)			Lameness and arthritis _____	
		Twitching _____	Convulsions _____	

This table refers principally to laboratory animals but is relevant to farm animals also. From Morton and Griffiths (1985).

3500 Hz but the scream when the first cut was made during castration was 4500 Hz and that at the second cut was 4857 Hz. In addition there was a broadening of the number of frequencies occurring in the sound and more frequent changes in sound distribution over the frequency range. The behaviour of recently castrated piglets differed from that of females in that they were less active and showed more trembling, leg shaking, sliding and tail jerking. These differences were especially pronounced on the first day, when some animals also vomited, but were still elevated for one week after the operation. Healing is complete by two weeks. For 2–3 days after castration, the male piglets took longer to lie down and showed qualitative changes in lying which involved sparing the hindquarters. It is clear that this operation has substantial effects on the piglets and a growth check is associated with the operation and accompanying disturbance. Whilst we cannot know exactly what the piglet feels, it seems reasonable to assume that considerable pain is experienced for several days.

Other species show less pronounced behavioural responses than pigs do. Sheep in Australia are subjected to two operations which would be expected, from the knowledge of pain receptors and the responses of other animals, to be extremely painful. One of these is mulesing, which involves removal using scissors of the skin surrounding the base of the tail and anus. This produces a circle of raw flesh 10–15 cm in diameter and much bleeding. In Merinos, this area of skin is especially susceptible to fly strike, in which blowflies lay their eggs in folds of skin and their larvae eat into the animal. This is a very serious welfare and economic problem as it kills many sheep. After mulesing and healing, there is less damp folded skin for the flies to attack as there is scar tissue formed around the anus and tail. Another operation, the aim of which is to minimise tooth problems in old age, is tooth grinding. The teeth of the young sheep are ground down to a length of a few millimetres using a grindstone. No anaesthetic is used in either of these operations and healing takes some time to occur. Yet the sheep do not show a large behavioural response to the treatment. Whilst more detailed studies might reveal behavioural responses so far undescribed, when the farmer sees that some sheep resume grazing within minutes of the operation, he concludes that the sheep do not feel much pain. It is fundamentally unlikely, given the nociceptive system of sheep, that they do not feel pain in the same way that other mammals would, but they certainly make little noise and change their behaviour less than many species would in this situation. It may be that a sheep wounded by a predator, and man is certainly treated as a predator by most sheep, survives better if it does not show an extreme behavioural response. In this case the sensation may be the same but the response different. It is also likely that opioid peptides are acting rapidly in these situations (Shutt *et al.*, 1987). In this situation, as in many others on farms, where we lack knowledge about whether or not an animal is experiencing pain we should assume that it is in pain and change procedures or use analgesics accordingly.

Assessing long-term welfare problems

When difficult conditions are encountered for long periods the same responses as those described for short-term problems occur at first. Some of these continue, but others cease to occur after a period of time and may be replaced by different responses. Such changes necessitate the use of different measures and some early attempts to assess the effects of long-term problems have given spurious results as a consequence of a failure to recognise this factor. We are still learning about the mechanisms used by animals to try to cope with adversity but our current knowledge is sufficient for some useful assessment of the conditions in which animals are kept.

As discussed in the previous chapter, one possible consequence of attempting to cope is failure. Increased mortality, delays in breeding and reduction in number of offspring are important indicators of poor welfare. These may be measured directly or they may be strongly suggested by poor growth, inadequate reproductive functioning, poor lactation or maternal behaviour, high levels of injury or high incidence of disease. Such measures will not be detailed again here but poor welfare is just as readily demonstrated by such measures as by the physiological and behavioural measures described below.

The adrenal system functions when more available energy is required and, as mentioned above, not all adrenal cortex activity occurs when the conditions are adverse. The adrenal medulla responses are very brief and adrenal cortex responses, although considerably more prolonged, decline after a few hours. This leads to problems in the use of measures of adrenal function as indicators of long-term welfare problems. If adverse conditions continue for many hours, however, bursts of glucocorticoid production can be detected. Ladewig (1984) found that after bulls were tethered, there was a peak of cortisol in the blood every few hours. Free-moving bulls also showed peaks of cortisol production at intervals but these were less pronounced and less frequent. Frequent sampling is needed to discover that more cortisol peaks are occurring in a given condition and single or occasional samples are of little use because of these substantial peaks and troughs and because of substantial diurnal variation in cortisol levels. As frequent blood sampling is often impractical, some method of discovering the activity of the adrenal cortex enzymes is desirable. A method which can be carried out on live animals is the ACTH challenge technique. If an animal has used its adrenal cortex frequently then its cortical enzymes are likely to be more active than are those of an animal which uses its adrenal cortex less often. Hence an injection of a large dose of ACTH will reveal the maximum amount of glucocorticoid which can be produced. The method has been used on farm animals by Friend *et al.* (1977) and Dantzer and Mormède (1983) and has shown that cattle social mixing and calf confinement do result in higher levels of adrenocortical enzyme activity. Table 29.3 shows that pigs housed at higher stocking densities show a larger cortisol response to ACTH. Negative results of this test need not mean absence of welfare problems, however, because although some animals in adverse conditions do cease to use the adrenal response after a while, this does not mean that they do not find the conditions difficult.

Frequent adrenal activity has another effect on animals and that is to suppress the functioning of certain aspects of the immune system. Siegel (1987) explains this as follows for poultry. When glucocorticoids bind to protein in lymphoid cells they alter enzyme activity and

nucleic acid production. Glucose uptake and protein synthesis are reduced so that the production of interleukin II is reduced. The primary immunological effect of corticosterone in chickens appears to be on T-cell populations. Other examples of effects of adverse conditions on the immune system of farm animals are the reduction in recently tethered sows of antibody production to sheep red blood cells (Metz and Oosterlee, 1981) and reduced delayed type hypersensitivity to foreign protein and reduced contact sensitivity to dinitrofluorobenzene in calves kept at $-5°C$ or $35°C$ (Kelley *et al.*, 1982). Hence it might be possible to use a measure of immune system functioning as an indicator of welfare. Any system of housing or management which resulted in the individual being less good at combatting disease could be said to be worse for the welfare of the animals (Broom, 1988b). A system which can be criticised because it results in impaired immune systems functioning is not made better by using vaccination, or other methods of combatting any disease which does arise. An alternative to looking directly at the immune system is to monitor the incidence of disease. The welfare of most diseased animals is poor and a system which leads to higher levels of disease than does another system is less good for the welfare of the animals. In any comparison of systems, however, it is essential to be sure that other factors which might affect the incidence of disease are balanced effectively.

There are many behavioural measures which allow some assessment of the abnormality of behaviour (Wiepkema *et al.*, 1983). Some of these use individual measures whilst others are actions on the part of one animal which injures another, e.g. tail biting in pigs. An example of a housing system which leads to abnormal behaviour is the confinement of dry sows in stalls or tethers. A general measure of behaviour is level of activity and confined sows have often been described as being inactive. It is difficult to be sure that a low level of activity is an indicator of poor welfare, but van Putten (1980) has also suggested that confined sows are

Table 29.3
Plasma cortisol level after ACTH challenge in pigs housed at three stocking densities

| | Floor area (m²) per pig | | | |
	0.51	1.01	1.52	SE
Males	158.9	85.9	87.7	29.9
Females	107.1	58.1	90.0	12.4

Modified after Meunier-Salaun *et al.* (1987).

"apathetic"—unresponsive to events in the world around them. In a series of experimental studies on the responsiveness of sows in stalls (Broom, 1986d, e, 1987a) their behaviour was assessed from video recordings of the animals during the presentation of stimuli. The sows were very responsive to stimuli associated with food presentation but were unresponsive to an unknown person who stood in front of them, unless that person's face was within 50 cm. Stall-housed sows were also less responsive than were group-housed sows to another novel stimulus: the pouring of a fixed quantity of water at room temperature on to the sow's back whilst she was lying with her eyes open (Table 29.4). These studies provide quantitative evidence to show that confined sows are less responsive to events in the world around them than are group-housed sows.

The other major behavioural response of confined sows is to show one or more forms of stereotypy. A stereotypy is a repeated, relatively invariate sequence of movements which has no obvious purpose (Chapter 32). It could not form part of one of the normal functional systems of the animal (Broom, 1983b). Common stereo-typies of confined sows are bar-biting, drinker-pressing, head-weaving, chain-playing and sham-chewing (Cronin and Wiepkema, 1984; Rushen, 1984b; Broom and Potter, 1984) (Table 29.5). These activities increase in frequency with the time that the animal is confined and individual sows may alter over from one stereotypy to another during their period of

Table 29.4
Responsiveness of stall-housed and group-housed sows. Behaviour in the 20 min after stimulus presentation

	Stall-housed	Group-housed	
Median time to sit or stand (s)	27.5	349	P = 0.096
Median number of other activities	2.5	6.5	P = 0.004
n	24	12	(2-tailed)

After Broom (1988d).

Table 29.5
Duration (min) of stereotypies shown by stall-housed dry sows during 8 h after morning feeding has finished

	Median total	Range
Drinker-pressing	10.3	2.3–74.3
Bar-biting	2.5	0.1–10.4
Rub nose on bar	4.2	0–25.5
Sham-chewing	26.4	0–89.5
Others	0.8	0.1–5.0
Total stereotypies	51.0	33.3–114.4

After Broom and Potter (1984).

Table 29.6
The incidence of stereotypies shown by tethered sows during pregnancy

	Period of pregnancy (days)				
	1–20	31–50	51–70	71–80	81–100
Mean proportion of observation time showing stereotypies	7	41	57	57	42
Number of different stereotypies per sow	1.4	2.3	2.7	3.2	3.6

Data from Cronin and Wiepkema (1984).

confinement (Cronin and Wiepkema, 1984) (Table 29.6). The type of stereotypy which is shown by the sow may alter if her diet is changed by increasing its bulk (Broom and Potter, 1984) and a large increase in the amount of food provided can reduce the amount of time showing stereotypies (Appleby and Lawrence, 1987). The duration of stereotypies is often 10% of waking time and can be as much as 80% of waking time. Stereotypies may be pathological signs or a method of coping with difficult conditions. Calves which did not show stereotypies had more abomasal ulceration (Wiepkema *et al.*, 1984) and tethered sows which did not show stereotyped chain-playing had higher cortisol levels in the blood than those that did show it (Dantzer and Mormède, 1981).

Other behavioural indicators of poor welfare include inability to carry out normal behaviour, misdirected behaviour and attacks on conspecifics. Behaviours such as standing and lying can be difficult if the floor is slippery or uneven. Andreae and Smidt (1982) studied cattle on slatted floors and found that lying down was often preceded by many unsuccessful attempts to lie down and the whole attempt to lie might last as long as 20 min. Sometimes the normal front legs first method of lying was so hazardous because of floor characteristics that the cattle lay down rump first. Rearing conditions can lead to many abnormalities of behaviour; for example calves reared in isolation seemed not to know what social response should be shown to strange calves and were unsuccessful when competing for food (Broom and Leaver, 1978; Broom, 1982). Misdirected behaviour includes sucking at various objects after early separation from the mother. Dairy calves separated from their mother after 24 h may lick and suck at their own coat, at parts of their pen or at the ears, navel, penis or scrotum of other calves. Each of these actions, like behaviour which damages other individuals, can be quantified and used as a welfare indicator.

A possible solution to the problem of how to deal with being confined or kept for long periods in difficult conditions is to utilise naturally occurring analgesics in the brain and self-narcotise. Opioid peptides such as β endorphin and metenkephalin have analgesic effects in situations which are either painful or otherwise particularly difficult for the animal. It is possible that both inactivity, associated with unresponsiveness, and stereotyped behaviour are associated with brain chemistry changes which make the problem seem less bad. A link between certain sorts of stereotyped behaviour and the dopamine systems in the brain has been known for some time from studies such as those of Sharman and Stephens (1974) and Fry *et al.* (1976). It is not clear what in the dopamine system can usefully be measured as an indi-

cator of poor welfare, however. The link between stereotypies and analgesic peptides came initially from studies on rats. Since naloxone blocks the receptors in the brain to which β endorphin attaches when it has an analgesic effect, this raises the possibility that stereotypies are used because they promote the action of analgesic peptides. In his study on tethered sows which showed much stereotyped behaviour, Cronin found that such activity was abolished temporarily by naloxone, but other behaviour was not much affected. Such experiments are difficult to interpret, however, because naloxone may have other effects and analgesia in pigs may not be opiate mediated (Dantzer *et al.*, 1986). The assessment of self-narcotisation as a coping method is clearly of great importance in welfare research.

Recognising good welfare

The majority of this chapter is about the use of measures which demonstrate that the individual is having difficulty coping with its environment. It is also desirable to be able to recognise that welfare is good by positive evidence rather than by the absence of negative evidence. Our ability to make direct measurements which identify pleasure is, however, extremely limited. There are centres in the brain which can be stimulated electrically by the animal itself in the appropriate operant situation. Animals, including farm animals (Baldwin and Parrott, 1979), may work hard in order to be able to self-stimulate in this way so these have been called pleasure centres. It is very difficult, however, to relate such centres to everyday life. Some behaviours, such as tail wagging by dogs, are assumed to indicate pleasure because of the situations in which they occur and also because the animal may work in order to be in that situation. Tail wagging may sometimes be used to appease a dominant dog or owner rather than to indicate pleasure, however. If, indeed, an individual does feel pleasure, communication of that pleasure to others may be of no advantage, so natural selection will not have favoured such communication and individuals may avoid communicating it. Hence pleasure detection and assessment will often be difficult. Research on behaviour like tail wagging and on the practicality of direct behavioural or physiological indicators of pleasure is much needed.

The major technique which is available to discover what is good for animals is to observe their preferences and to measure how hard they will work for the preferred event or object. One technique which has long been used is to watch the animals in an environment which is rich in the complexity of stimuli and opportunities for activities which it offers. The stimuli which are chosen and the ways in which the animals spend their time provide information about the preferences of the animals. Studies like this with farm animals, e.g. Wood-Gush (1983), Jensen (1986), Jensen *et al.* (1987), McBride *et al.* (1969), Duncan *et al.* (1978), can be used when designing farm accommodation for these animals, for example the family pen for pigs (Stolba, 1982). Different types of farm housing conditions can also be compared. The simplest experiment of this kind merely involves giving the animal the choice of two conditions where the choice is expressed by moving from one place to another. Hughes and Black (1973) found that, contrary to the previous expectations of some people, hens preferred to stand on a hexagonal mesh floor rather than a coarse rectangular mesh or a perforated steel sheet. Hughes (1975) and Dawkins (1976, 1977) found that, after a brief period of becoming accustomed to new conditions, hens preferred a large cage to a battery cage. In similarly designed preference tests piglets were found to prefer to lie on perforated plastic or concrete rather than wire mesh, to spend more time in a pen with a straw container, and to avoid lying in pens with 0.23 m² per piglet if an adjacent accessible pen offered more space (Marx and Schuster, 1980, 1982, 1984).

The simple preference test experiment has been criticised in two ways. Firstly, as Duncan (1978) pointed out, the animal may not choose

what is best for it. In most situations the repeatedly expressed choices of animals are those which increase their biological fitness but some animals do choose to do things which harm them, for example over-eating. Hence choice tests alone are sometimes inadequate. A much more general criticism is that the action required in order to make the choice in an experiment is often very easy. As a result there is little indication of the importance of the choice to the individual. An individual may make a clear choice between two foods which are both very palatable and very beneficial to it. If the preferred food of these two could be obtained only by expending energy for a long time or by taking a risk, the preference might well be reversed. Hence, in order to be able to apply data from preference tests to practical situations where an improvement in welfare is sought, the strength of a preference must be assessed by discovering what costs the individual is willing to incur in order to be able to express the preference.

One situation in which the strength of a preference could be assessed was that studied by van Rooijen (1980, 1981). Gilts given the choice of two pens with different floors on which to lie had another gilt beside one pen but not beside the other. Since pigs like to occupy the pen next to another pig, the preference for flooring was balanced against the social preference. The preference for earth over concrete was sufficient to overcome the social preference (Table 29.7) but that for straw over wood shavings, although

Table 29.7
Relative times gilts spent in two adjacent pens with different floors

gilt A		Barrier	gilt B	
Earth	Concrete		Concrete	Earth
78	3		9	72

gilt C		Barrier	gilt D	
Concrete	Earth		Earth	Concrete
4	81		79	4

Modified after van Rooijen (1980).

Table 29.8
Relative times gilts spent in two adjacent pens with different floors

gilt A			gilt B	
Wood shavings	Straw	Barrier	Straw	Wood shavings
21	94		79	33

gilt C			gilt D	
Straw	Wood shavings	Barrier	Wood shavings	Straw
50	63		54	64

Modified after van Rooijen (1980).

apparent from Table 29.8, did not overcome the preference for being near another gilt. A more precise comparison of one preference with another was the assessment by Dawkins (1983) of the importance of litter to hens by balancing it against the extent to which the hens had to work for food. The extent to which individuals will work for a resource has also been used in several other welfare studies. Wood-Gush and Beilharz (1983) found that piglets in small cages utilised earth if it was provided and Hutson (1989) has found that they would press a key in order to gain access to earth in which they could root. The importance of the earth to the pigs was such that they would press keys many times in succession in order to reach it. Recent work by Duncan and collaborators (Duncan and Kite, 1987) with hens has involved the use of a weighted door to assess how much the bird would do to reach an objective on the other side. Where animals do show that they are willing to work hard in such ways it is reasonable to conclude that their welfare is improved by their achieving that objective. The experimental studies must be carried out at different times of day and over long periods since some objectives, although they are utilised only occasionally, have a very great effect upon welfare. A problem where such studies are carried out on animals which have been living in difficult conditions for long periods is that they may have adopted coping strategies which make it unlikely that they will learn the task or show sufficient activity to carry out the task. Here again it is necessary to incorporate studies of poor welfare with investigations using preference tests.

Conclusions

Since welfare is defined in terms of the state of the individual it can be measured. Much remains to be discovered about the methods which animals use to cope with difficult conditions but we already have an array of measures which we can use to assess welfare. Where measurements are aimed at discovering whether or not welfare is poor and how poor it is, it is better to make several different kinds of measurement. Each individual animal has several alternative methods of trying to cope with adversity and individuals differ in the methods which they favour. Hence the use of only one physiological measure of response to apparently difficult conditions might give the impression that most animals are unaffected by the conditions. If other physiological, behavioural and fitness measures had been taken, however, it might have been apparent that all animals had been affected but that they had used different coping procedures. A consequence of this situation for investigatory studies of animal welfare in different housing or management systems is that a team of people with different expertise is needed for an adequate evaluation of the system. It may still be useful to use one measure, however, for a single measure can indicate that welfare is poor and can give some idea of how poor it is. A problem arises when a welfare indicator does not show that welfare is poor, for this need not mean that there is no welfare problem. For example, the fitness measures such as survival, growth and reproduction have often been quoted, in this way, as showing that welfare is good. Whilst an inability to grow or reproduce, given a suitable partner, indicates that welfare is poor, the reverse does not apply since an animal which is growing and reproducing may be able to do so only by extensive use of behavioural and physiological coping procedures and may be very susceptible to disease if disease challenge occurs.

The assessment of welfare by endeavouring to discover by direct measurement when the welfare of an animal is good is clearly desirable and attempts to do this should be encouraged. The easier procedure of assessing what the animal regards as being better for its welfare by measuring its preferences and their importance to that animal is valuable as it leads to possibilities for designing better housing and management conditions. These conditions can then be compared with those in existing conditions by looking for indicators of poor welfare in animals in both conditions. Any recognition of good welfare should be carried out at various times during the animals' daily routine and should be combined with the use of indicators of poor welfare because an individual's welfare might be good at one time during its life in given conditions but poor at other times. A brief period of enjoyment could be recognisable even when most of the individual's life is difficult. A general conclusion about such welfare assessment is that in the search for conditions which lead to improved welfare, the use of indicators of poor welfare is always necessary at some stage in the study.

Some of those who are concerned about welfare express the opinion that the only adequate conditions are those which exist in the wild. This argument often leads people to assume that extensive conditions are good and intensive conditions are bad for welfare. Extensive conditions, and indeed the conditions in the wild, can lead to major welfare problems, for example those resulting from predation, extreme physical conditions or disease. The welfare of housed animals can be good and it is important to try to devise conditions for animals which are based on precise measurements of their welfare rather than on preconceived ideas about the surroundings in which they will look right. Having said this, however, our current knowledge indicates that the welfare of very many animals on farms is so poor that there is a need for urgent action to change this situation.

30 Humane control of livestock

A great variety of ways exist in which the behaviour of livestock can be controlled. Many of these are time-proven and well known to experienced stockmen. Anticipating an animal's movement is undoubtedly the best means of exercising some control over its behaviour. This is particularly true when the handling of loose animals is being attempted. The handling of such animals presents problems to those who deal with livestock. Loose animals are best controlled when they are gathered into tight groups of their own kind. Pigs, sheep and cattle can be more easily managed collectively.

The breed of animal, its temperament and the type of environment in which it was raised can affect behaviour during handling. Animals which have been raised on open range or away from people will have a large flight distance and may panic and become agitated when a handler approaches within 15 m. The problems posed by this involve serious disturbance for the animals and sometimes danger for the stockman. For example, Zebu cattle in Queensland are not only difficult to round up after spending a long period in extensive paddocks or range areas but may attack the stockman. Similar animals which have been handled regularly are much more docile. Animals which have been raised in close confinement on either solid concrete or slatted floors can also be difficult to control when they are being moved onto other surfaces or manipulated either individually or collectively in unfamiliar premises. The animal may be disturbed either by changes in physical conditions or by human presence. Hemsworth *et al.* (1981a) reported that pigs which were regularly handled when young were much easier to handle when older. The effects of previous experience needs to be considered carefully when designing animal husbandry systems. It is also of great importance to be aware of the animal's flight distance and individual space requirements in order to reduce problems with baulking and alarm behaviour when subjected to handling for shipment, sale or slaughter.

Directing

In order to be designed appropriately, handling facilities on the farm and at lairage should be based on the known behavioural characteristics of farm animals. Given adequate opportunity, cattle, sheep and pigs readily learn about their immediate environment. For example, cattle learn quickly about electric fences and can be contained by them in a field, in a collecting area or in a passageway (McDonald *et al.*, 1981). If, however, they were confronted with an electric fence for the first time when being moved in a strange area, the presence of the electric fence might hinder the process of moving the animals. The animals need time to learn about the fence and they also need the opportunity to avoid the fence. Moving electric fences, like the "electric dog" are sometimes used in dairy parlour collecting yards. The "electric dog" is a row of electrically live wires hanging downwards and moved towards the cows in the rear of the yard. It has a large adverse effect on some cows so that their milk let-down may be prevented and they may become extremely unwilling to move towards the parlour.

Every dairy farmer has to be able to move dairy cows in milk to and from the milking parlour. If the races and collecting yards which are used or the methods of moving the animals are inadequate and disturbing to some or all of the cows there will be welfare problems. Such welfare problems will often be associated with reduced milk yield. Cows may be reluctant to enter a milking parlour because of the behaviour of the cowman or because of design faults in the parlour which result in uncomfortable milking stalls or stray voltages. Such problems can lead to the use of excessive force by stockmen in the collecting yard.

The problems associated with the design of races for moving cows to the milking parlour are very similar to those of designing races used for other purposes such as movement towards vehicles prior to transport. The most extensive study of how to design good races is that of Grandin (1978, 1980a, b, 1982, 1983). She reported that cattle often balk if they encounter dark areas or areas of extreme lighting contrast. Races with sharp angular turns in them may also pose problems for cattle which are being driven and long straight races may also result in animals being either reluctant to move or moving too fast. As a consequence of these observations, Grandin recommends that races should be evenly lit, have solid walls if animals unfamiliar with them have to use them, and should be gently curved rather than having sharp corners or long straights (Fig. 30.1).

Negative stimuli such as intense sound should not be able to reach collected animals. In no event should disturbing sounds be located at a source which is in the direction that collected animals will be required to go. Shouting represents disturbing sound and induces negative reactions ranging from avoidance to flight. When such reactions are impeded, panic, which is an extreme fear reaction, is liable to ensue (McFarlane, 1976a, b).

The same principles apply when animals are being moved in slaughterhouses. Grandin's behaviour observations have allowed her to make useful recommendations in this area and she has outlined a number of design features for lairages. She points out that cattle can be most efficiently handled in yards and races which have long narrow diagonal pens on a 60 degree angle. Cattle which are waiting to be sorted can be held in a wide curved race with a radius of 5 m. From the curved race, the animals can either be sorted into diagonal pens or they can be directed to the squeeze chute, dipping vat, or restraining chute at the abattoir. The handler should work from a catwalk located along the inner radius of the race. This facilitates the movement of the animals which tend to circle around the handler in order to maintain visual contact. The curved holding race terminates in a round crowding pen which leads to a curved single race. Again, sharp contrasts of light and dark should be avoided. Single file races, forcing pens, and other areas where cattle are crowded should have high solid fences. This prevents the animals from observing people, vehicles and other distracting objects outside the facility.

Where space is limited the desired effects of positive movement can be obtained using a compact serpentine race system 80 cm wide with an inside radius of only 3.5 m or even 1.5 m and two 180 degree curves. Holding lanes should be at least 3 m wide. Evidently cattle will move quite easily by single file through narrow, curving races with a small radius and with straight, solid sides. To induce cattle to enter such a race from the collecting pen the first several metres should be straight before the first curve occurs. In such situations cattle move more easily when the handlers are positioned on the inner curvature walkways and move steadily. Such facilities at a slaughter plant can allow a line to move through slaughter at the rate of 150

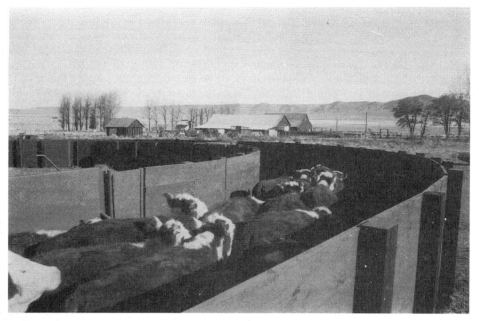

Fig. 30.1 Cattle moving easily through a wide curved race with solid sides (photograph by T. Grandin).

cattle per hour using only two people in the moving operation.

Similar arrangements are recommended for pig slaughtering operations. Pigs move most readily in single-file races with solid side fences and open barred tops. Crowd pens for pigs should have level floors and ramps should be avoided. Pigs have 310 degree panoramic vision, and puddles and shadows should be eliminated in order to avoid negative visual stimuli. Pigs tend to move from a darker area to a brightly illuminated area under artificial lighting and lighting should be so arranged as to give an increasing gradient of illumination in the direction of movement. Pigs which have been raised in dimly illuminated confinement buildings refuse to move towards direct sunlight if this enters the premises.

Cattle kept in pens spend more time against the perimeter than towards the centre. Perimeter space largely determines the long-term holding capacity. Since rectangular pens have less perimeter than polygonal pens the latter have welfare benefits and should be given first consideration in the design of a modern livestock pen. Crowded beef steers tend to position their heads around the enclosure perimeters. Thus, in some pen designs, the ratio of perimeter to area should be maximised to increase the efficiency of area usage. Attention to this phenomenon has been drawn by Stricklin, and colleagues (Stricklin, 1978; Stricklin *et al.*, 1979; Stricklin and Kautz-Scanavy, 1984) but applications of recommendations for circular or polygonal pens are still awaited in the cattle industry.

Loading, transport and slaughterhouse problems

When animals are to be transported, the first step towards this is often to put the animals in pens ready for the arrival of a transporter vehicle. If pigs or bulls are to be moved the mixing of animals from different social groups should be avoided if possible. Such mixing should also be avoided on the vehicle and in lairage if the animals are to be left there for more than a few minutes. Studies of bulls by Kenny and Tarrant (1982) and Tennessen (1983) show that mixing at lairage causes much fighting, high levels of bruising and other injury and a great increase in the incidence of dark firm dry (DFD) meat. Both bruising and DFD meat are of economic importance as well as indicating severe welfare problems prior to slaughter. Pigs going to slaughter will also fight, and may be much disturbed even if they do not fight, if mixed with strangers on farm, in vehicle or at lairage. The effects of this mixing are poor welfare and carcass down-grading due to wounds on the skin or pale soft exudative (PSE) meat (see Chapter 29). The physical conditions and the provisions of food and water on the farm before transport are also important.

When animals are loaded on to a vehicle the ease of getting into the vehicle and the characteristics of the vehicle are of critical importance in determining how easy it will be to load the animals and how great will be the effects of the procedure on those animals. Pigs, cattle or sheep

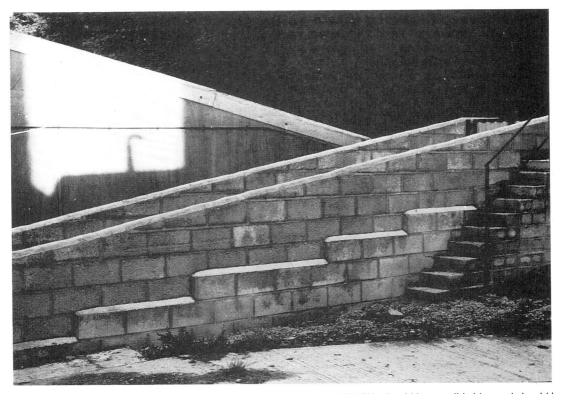

Fig. 30.2 Loading ramps for pigs should have a slope of about 1 in 7 (14%), should have solid sides and should be wide enough for at least two pigs to walk comfortably side by side.

can readily be driven up a ramp of gradient 1 in 7 (13°) with solid sides to it. It is very difficult, however, to get the animals to ascend the tail board of a lorry which is at a gradient of 30–45° to the ground. As van Putten (1982) points out, pigs may see this as an impassable barrier. Purpose-built ramps are the best answer to this problem (Figs. 30.2 and 30.3). Any ramp should be non-slippery and should be kept clean so that it remains so. It should be at an angle of not more than 15° to the ground and, at least for pigs, should allow two or three to mount at the same time (van Putten, 1982). An alternative to a ramp is to use an hydraulic loading platform. When animals look into a vehicle, if it is dark and obviously a dead end they will be reluctant to enter. A well-lit vehicle is entered more willingly, especially if the place which the animals should be leaving can be darkened first.

Vehicles are often not well designed as regards flooring, ventilation and ease of subdivision. Just as important as vehicle design, as regards the welfare of animals during transport, is the behaviour of the transport staff. Problems arise because of rough treatment during loading, over or under stocking of compartments on the vehicle, inconsiderate driving or leaving the animals in conditions which are too hot or too cold and windy for them. The other major transport problem is the effect of very long journeys, especially where there are no stops for food and water. This area has been reviewed in a Commission of the European Communities Report (1984).

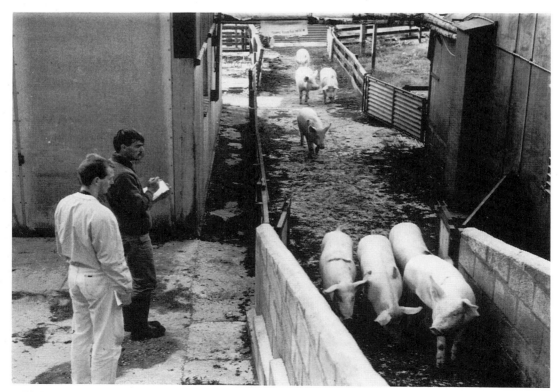

Fig. 30.3   Pigs moving up loading ramp while observers record their behaviour.

An example of a study of animals during a journey is that of Kent and Ewbank (1983). They found during an experimental transport period of 18 h that cattle lay, ruminated and ate significantly less than normal. Transported cattle lay more towards the end of the journey, particularly when the vehicle was stationary or travelling on smooth road. During the journey, 79% of ruminating occurred while the animals were standing, compared with only 3% while standing on a normal day. After transportation, the animals grazed and lay down alternately throughout the first 17 h. The lying periods increased in length as the day progressed. The first drinking behaviour in the transported cattle occurred 8 h after the journey and the amount of time spent idling was halved on the day following transportation. During the second 24-h recovery, the transported cattle lay 2.7 h longer than normal (see review by Trunkfield and Broom, in press).

Recent work on the handling and transport of poultry shows that such procedures are especially traumatic for these animals. Chickens show a substantial increase in heart rate when a person walks towards them (Duncan and Filshie, 1979) and an even greater increase when they are picked up by a person (Duncan, 1986). The rough handling involved when hens are taken from battery cages and several are carried together by their legs to a crate prior to transport leads to a large increase in plasma corticosterone (Broom *et al.*, 1986). Handling plus a journey results in elevated corticosterone and reduced noradrenaline levels as these are used up in the brain and frequent broken bones (Freeman *et al.*, 1984; Broom *et al.*, 1986). Longer journeys and longer waits before slaughter lead to poorer meat quality, lower blood sugar, lower haemoglobin levels and lower blood counts. (Ehinger and Gschwindt, 1979, 1981; Gschwindt and Ehinger, 1979). It seems that rough handling and long journeys have the greatest adverse effects on welfare. A gentler handling procedure is clearly required and birds should be taken to a nearer slaughterhouse rather than a very distant one. The handling of broilers seems to have less adverse effect if an automatic broiler "harvester" is used rather than a catching gang (Duncan, 1986).

Cattle soon become cooperative with handlers and with each other when travelling long distances by rail. When travelling together in an enclosed area, they rarely move about to alter their position or seek another part of the wagon and do so only when the train has stopped or is stopping or starting. They travel facing the side of the wagon and with their bodies at right angles to the direction of travel. This appears to be the most convenient position when seeking optimum comfort and space for balance and for minimising injury should they lose their balance. It has been found that cattle with horns usually adopt a position where their heads are resting upon the backs of the adjacent animal; this permits easier breathing and avoids goring.

On long journeys it is often over 24 h before any of the animals seek rest by lying down, but others avoid doing so for the entire journey. They usually lie down in groups of three or four after one animal has made the initial move and tend to do so at one end of the wagon. The remainder of the group will avoid trampling these animals as much as possible, quickly moving any hoof which is brought down on the body of a recumbent animal. When given the opportunity to rest while disembarked at yards in sidings, they move to the water trough or walk about for a very short period, even when food is clearly visible, and feed only after their thirsts have been quenched. At the beginning of the journey, urinations and defaecations in the wagon are frequent, but decline as the animals adjust. Cattle which have had neither food nor drink during a long journey sometimes expel small dry pellets of dung and may still urinate.

The hazards to which animals being transported by sea are vulnerable are numerous. When entering equatorial regions cattle are subject to heat stress. There is a constant danger of injury in rough weather. Horses need plenty of head room at sea. Contrary to a common belief, horses should not be continuously secured by short head ropes at sea, but should be given sufficient halter-length to lie down. Horses and cattle are highly susceptible to injury and illness during sea voyages.

Transportation by air is only permitted by very specific international regulations governing space, ventilation, stalls, flooring, etc. Horses should not be tranquilised since some react atypically and become manic. Provision should be made for appropriate humane slaughter should an animal become ill, injured or unmanageable with risk to other animals or aircraft safety. The International Air Transportation Association (IATA) provides detailed specifications and requirements for shipping procedures, crating, etc. for livestock.

When cattle arrive at an abattoir they are often injured or bruised during unloading because of too much haste on the part of animal handlers or inadequate ramps. Grandin (1979, 1980b) reported that 66% of bruises of the loin area occurred during loading or unloading of trucks.

In an efficient slaughterhouse the period during which animals are moved from pens to the point of slaughter can be very brief and the stunning and slaughter procedure itself can result in no pain for the animal. If the animals are kept in a confined race for a period of more than one or two minutes before stunning, or if stunning is carried out inadequately, or if there is inversion before slaughter, the welfare is poor. Inadequate equipment or lack of care by slaughtermen resulting in failure to stun properly can result in extreme pain and discomfort for the animals. Animals are not stunned during the Jewish schechita or the Muslim halal ritual slaughter procedures. There is a period of consciousness after the throat is cut which may last for from 30 s to several minutes during which the animal must be in great pain and distress (Daly *et al.*, 1988). As the heart still beats after stunning and blood drains from the animal just as effectively whether or not the animal is stunned there is no logical reason why stunning should not be carried out before the

throat is cut. Stunning of animals has been reviewed by Eikelenboom (1983).

Herding

Moving a number of sheep from one place to another is best done with one group as a flock. The larger the flock the more cohesion there is to hold individuals together. Small numbers present a problem. Too much driving pressure on the flock will result in some individuals reacting in panic and seeking an escape route by themselves (Syme and Elphick, 1982). If any succeed others will follow. Small numbers of sheep can be moved best by presenting them with an escape route to the desired point of collection (Hutson and Hitchcock, 1978).

Undue pressure on sheep with a sheep dog should be avoided, although well-trained dogs are essential for effective movement of sheep. If only for the retrieval of break-away individuals, a second shepherd and dog should be involved in the movement of sheep in a semi-urban environment. When being herded, sheep will trot much of the time and should be allowed to proceed at their own pace and only receive lateral spatial pressure occasionally, for directional purposes.

Cattle should not be driven at a running pace since they will split up at speed and resist being turned by a dog or driver. Halting a runaway bovine animal is difficult but can often be done by someone obstructing its route with outstretched arms waving. Animals in great alarm cannot be so stopped and may run till exhausted. Dogs, for example the Queensland cattle dog, can be used to herd cattle but some cattle will not respond to a dog, particularly if they are unaccustomed to control by dogs. Cattle are best moved in open country by horse riders.

A runaway horse cannot be stopped by a person obstructing its path. At best it can be diverted into an enclosure but some horses will run with abandon and at general risk. These are best directed towards open space. Horses in groups should only be moved by horse riders in sufficient numbers. If they are to be taken a significant distance, or along a route with gates or exits, prior planning is required to organise the operation. Under difficult circumstances horses should be moved by lead-rein, or handled individually.

Inspecting

Use of crushes

The use of direct force in controlling the behaviour of animals is best exemplified by the variety of "crushes", "races" or "stocks" that are in use on many farm premises for the tight restriction of movement in the larger farm animals. Crushes of various types are in operation for controlling cattle, for example, but the best forms of crushes allow an animal to be funnelled down a narrowing serpentine passage into the crush section. At the exit of the crush there should be a small collecting yard where animals which have already passed through the crush may be seen by the animal entering or within the crush. Crushing arrangements which make use of this broad principle allow large numbers of cattle to be examined individually and closely in a short space of time with the least amount of danger to themselves and to those handling them. Such crushing techniques allow mass treatment of herd or flock for operations such as vaccination, drenching, ear-tagging, blood sampling, tuberculin testing, pregnancy diagnosing, branding, spraying and de-horning. Many of these operations can cause animals to become so alarmed that they respond behaviourally in ways which frequently cause injury to themselves. Whilst restrained within stocks, cattle frequently attempt to escape by pushing forwards. They also frequently attempt to push their hind limbs against one side or other of the stocks. The stocks should therefore be constructed with solid sides so that it is impossible for an animal to put its hind leg between spars since, when this happens, serious

injury to the limb is likely. After stocks have been in use by a number of animals they tend to become slippery underfoot with the dung of these animals and it may be necessary to improve the footing within the stocks by the addition of ash or sand from time to time. When crushes possess some yoke arrangement which grips a restrained animal by the neck, it is important for there to be an efficient quick-release mechanism which allows the animal's neck to be released quickly should its limb slip from under it and cause it to fall within the stocks. This is particularly important when large animals such as bulls are being put into stocks. Their weight prevents them from being raised manually should they fall to the ground. Fixed crushes in which a string of animals can be restrained tightly behind one another, perhaps with intervening bars separating two or three of them, are best known as races. This form of restraint is very suitable for a close inspection of a large number of animals in a short time.

Stocks for horses are sometimes employed when an animal is to be examined per rectum, for example. Such stocks are also suitable means of restraint when some operation to the feet is being carried out on a fractious horse. Stock sizes vary with the type of horse to be examined. It is also essential that they should be extremely solid. A horse in close restraining stocks, which finds the stocks moving or hears the parts moving, is very likely to become over-excited and to lash out in a frenzy of kicking in a manner which is difficult to control.

Close approach

It is principally with regard to cattle that the problem of handling or directing loose animals is greatest. In many forms of cattle husbandry, calves are already well grown before they need to be handled for the first time. Such calves are difficult to catch and eventually to control. A full-grown calf, unaccustomed to being handled, may show different forms of behaviour when approached. An initial state of alertness is usually observed. The animal directs its attention exclusively towards the source of the approaching danger and its behaviour reveals that it is conscious of the principal stimulant in its immediate environment. Its head is directed towards this source and its eyes, ears and tail are moved in ways which indicate its total concern with the person approaching. Closer approach towards the calf usually induces a state of alarm or fear. A group of animals will quickly share this state of alarm by generating signals which are understood by all the others of the group. Close herding results: the animals pack more tightly together; they move more rapidly, their heads are held up; there is likely to be some bellowing. Further stimulation of these animals will result in the development of a state of panic during which calculated behaviour is abandoned and a resort to flight takes place. This change sometimes occurs very gradually among calves, but on other occasions it can occur in an instant. Rapid changes in such a state of alarm are more common among calves which have some prior experience of aversive husbandry.

In this condition they offer more resistance to handling. To control the behaviour of calves in this state, the approach by the handler towards the calf should be quiet, even in pace, but cautious. During this type of approach the calf will start to move away, either forwards or backwards. The handler should then modify his approach, either to the left or to the right, so as to cut off the intended route of escape. After one or two intention movements the animal will then direct its flight towards a corner. The expert handler makes use of this knowledge of animal behaviour to time his attempt at catching the animal to coincide with the time when the animal's head is directed towards a corner. When the calf is being caught it is important to grip its lower jaw and to raise it and pull it sharply to one side. Gripping the lower jaw is more effective in controlling cattle than catching the nose. Small calves in particular resent their noses being held. This part of the body is apparently very sensitive and the restriction of breathing also induces further panic.

In directing the movements of animals individually or in groups, the expert handler makes use of the fact that animals apparently regard as part of the approaching person anything which is held in the hand and extended outwards on either side. In this way one person can extend human presence considerably to either side and thereby cut off a very large escape area for an animal which is loose.

The general rule is not applicable to pigs which do not appear to be susceptible to this form of control. Pigs are best blocked from their escape route by placing some solid object, such as a board, at ground level directly in the line of escape. Once a pig has selected a line of escape it is not so likely to deviate from this line as are other animals and when this route is blocked by such visual obstruction the pig is usually stopped in flight.

Holding

A knowledge of the natural mechanics of movement in each species is extremely helpful in exercising control over their behaviour. There are many ways, some of them traditional, in which an animal's behaviour can be controlled effectively by applying some modest amount of force to a part of its body in such a way as to put the animal to a mechanical disadvantage. The most anterior part of the animal can be secured to effect overall control. Raising the head frequently restrains the general forward movement, for example, although this is not so effective with the horse. Taking some form of tight control over the muzzle controls behaviour very effectively. In the horse the application of a twitch, a loop of cord put around the muzzle and twisted tight, is the way this is done. This procedure may induce analgesic opioid peptide action in the brain. While the majority of horses respond to increasing twitching by immobilising themselves, a few will become even more fractious when such a form of restraint is imposed upon them. Snaring the snout of the pig is a similar way of controlling the behaviour of this animal, and it is probably the most effective of all in this species. Unfortunately, snaring the snout—even quite lightly—causes some pigs to vocalise with shrill screams.

The limb movements of an animal have to be controlled in many circumstances when kicking or stamping would endanger other animals in close proximity or persons handling the animal. Raising one fore leg by flexing at the knee with a rope will rapidly restrain stamping. Kicking with the hind limbs can be controlled in a variety of ways. Restraint in the region of the hocks which, to a large extent, immobilises the Achilles tendon, can be used as a method of controlling kicking. Full-grown cattle can have their hind limbs fairly effectively immobilised by the application of restricting ropes which apply pressure around the abdomen of the animal while drawing the head backwards with a rope round the horns. Raising the tail-head vertically in cattle can also immobilise the hind limbs for short periods.

Animals which are being given medical treatment of various kinds may have to be lifted from the ground to reduce opposition. This, of course, is applicable only in the case of small livestock. The way in which a calf or foal can be restrained is by lifting it bodily with the arms encircling the fore and hindquarters.

The purpose of all these forms of restraint is to immobilise the animal for short periods of time, so that some procedure considered necessary for its welfare can be carried out. Minimum discomfort to the patient and maximum safety to the operator are the criteria. These procedures should not be based on the infliction of pain upon the animal. It is emphasised, therefore, that such procedures are intended not to cause harm to the animal but to place it briefly in a state of mechanical disadvantage in the interests of its own welfare.

Training

Farm animal behaviour can be controlled quite readily following fairly simple training proce-dures. Animals quickly learn the routines of feeding, for example, and it is usually possible to lure animals into required situations by methods which they come to recognise by repetition. Animals also learn to associate certain sounds with certain husbandry routines. A great reper-toire of conditioned reflexes quickly becomes established in most farm animals in this way and by the use of the human voice (Kiley-Worthington and Savage, 1978; Murphey and Duarte, 1983).

Skilful exploitation of domesticated condi-tioning, which is known to have occurred from experience, can allow the experienced stock handler to exercise a good deal of control over the behaviour of his animals. The use of calls, sounds of buckets, whistles, etc., can provide quick labour-saving methods of assembling animals. For example, Wisniewski and Albright (1978) found that dairy cows could easily be trained to enter a milking parlour when a light was switched on or a buzzer sounded. All farm animals show a tendency to herd together and one can easily impose upon an untrained animal the training which a group of others have acquired by including it for a short time within the group, and then permitting it to share in the experiences of the group as a whole. An untrained animal can be initiated to a task by pairing it with another animal already fully trained, for example in training cattle to lead (Kilgour and Dalton, 1984, p. 49).

In training, behaviour is typically "shaped" by initially rewarding the generic action and subsequently presenting the reward only on the production of more specific actions. Repetition is important, as is consistency, and in this respect animal training resembles drilling. The standard training procedures are analogous to "shaping" in experimental animal psychology. A start is made by rewarding each successive activity which approximates the behaviour which is desired. Reward is given only to the behaviour which is close to the objective of the training. The skill of the trainer lies in recognising small progressive responses and rewarding each of these. Even the smallest progress in training may be the key to the desired performance. As training becomes completed the desired responses alone will be reinforced by reward.

In training which involves an elimination of undesired behaviour, such as biting, the conditioned painful response must be paired very closely in time with the misbehaviour. For instance, horses can usually be trained to stop biting by being pricked with a sharp nail or pin in the upper lip at the instant of an attempted bite. If punishment is to be used for misbehaviour it must come as soon as possible, preferably within seconds, after the animal's offence. The punishment conditions and the avoidance of pain reinforces the modified behaviour. It cannot be overemphasised that punishment must be very closely paired in time with the misbehaviour if the animal is to learn appropriately. Punishment in training should be in such limited form that cruelty is not practised.

Pharmacological control

The use of drugs to influence or to modify the behaviour of an animal is sometimes necessary to avoid excessive force. The range of modern chemical agents of varied pharmacological activities makes it possible to alter an animal's behaviour by tranquilisation, sedation or immobilisation (Cooper *et al.*, 1982). Today, tranquilisers are commonly used when individual animals have to be subjected, for a period, to forms of total restraint or handling to which they are unaccustomed, and which would likely induce in them a state of panic which would be detrimental to their health were it attempted by other means. Tranquilisation during transportation, or mixing, for example, has much to commend it in circumstances when animals would react adversely under these circumstances.

Tranquilisers produce psychological calming of anxiety without physiological depression or clouding of consciousness. However, if tranquilisers are used to produce manageability, high doses are usually necessary which may result in ataxia, depressed response to stimulation and to respiratory depression.

Tranquilisers do not exert hypnotic or analgesic effects. Increasing the dose does not produce greater sedation, even though the psychological depressant effects are magnified. The psychological state of the animal prior to administration of tranquilisers may markedly affect the degree of sedation achieved. Animals that are vicious, intractable and in a state of excitation may not become manageable, except with very high doses which would be totally incapacitating. Neuroleptanalgesia is a state of sedation and analgesia produced by the combined use of a tranquiliser (neuroleptic) and a narcotic, in which, although the patient remains arousable and responds to certain stimuli, various manipulations, including minor surgical interventions, can ordinarily be performed. The most commonly used preparation is Innovar-Vet (droperidol and fentanyl). Total immobilisation is a very radical form of restraint and is one which is extremely useful and warranted in many emergencies for the welfare of the subject (De Vos, 1978; Herbert and McFetridge, 1978).

Succinylcholine, curare and gallamine are neuromuscular blocking agents, which act peripherally at the neuromuscular junctions. The agents are used as adjuncts to light general anaesthetics where profound muscle relaxation is desired. Because these agents produce motor paralysis only, and do not produce either sedation or analgesia, their use on conscious animals is not justifiable on welfare grounds.

Veterinary anaesthesia was presented as a discipline over 40 years ago. For procedures not requiring full general anaesthesia chlorohydrate was available in those days. It is still available for use in large animal sedation. Since then a great revolution has taken place which has created the discipline of psychopharmacology. An early development launching this contemporary specialty was the availability of neuroleptic and anxiolytic agents. Subsequently opioid and psychoactive agents and anaesthetics expanded the field. These developments brought drugs into veterinary use for various types of control of the animal ranging from mild sedation, tranquilisation, temporary taming, short-term immobilisation to general anaesthesia. In most cases the agents can be given by small intramuscular doses which makes administration comparatively simple. Even oral or intravenous administration of drugs is technically simplified by the known dose–response relationship. Only in a few cases do unfortunate side-effects develop and in such cases these are limited to certain species. For example opioid drugs may have manic effects on a small number of horses—particularly when given in light doses.

The administration of these drugs, although simple, requires a sound knowledge of the animal's behaviour and physiology. It is particularly important to appreciate the normal inclinations of certain types of animals to react strenuously in fear or rage when control is attempted on them. Such circumstances in which restraint is initiated represent fearful stimuli to many animals. Although each species responds characteristically to such stimuli, many individuals vary in the nature and degree of response. Violent responses are stressful to the animal and chemical restraint of stressed animals cannot be approved, on welfare grounds, unless a true emergency exists which requires control of the animal. Even then the physiology of exertional stress must be borne in mind so that it will be appreciated that the animal will be significantly at risk from the procedure even though the controlling agent has minimal lethal potential.

During exertion there is increased production of carbon dioxide from glycolysis in the vigorously contracting musculature. This carbon dioxide is taken up by the red blood cells and transported to the lungs. If the increased carbon dioxide content is not removed by the lungs the hydrogen ion concentration increases in the blood and the pH decreases, resulting in acidosis. Profound hypoxia also occurs in all tissues.

Exertional stress is in fact a generalised state of acidosis which is a broad condition that cannot be characterised by any single physiological parameter. Instead, clinical–behavioural signs must be relied upon to determine the condition. With exertional stress the affected animal hyperventilates severely. This hyperventilation may result in small pulmonary haemorrhages and frothy, blood-tinged fluid appears around the nostrils. The head is held down, the mouth is held open and the tongue typically hangs inactively out of the mouth. In addition, there is profound muscular incoordination. Finally the animal falls and is unable to rise. In association with these signs other clinical features exist relating to caridac function and loss of swallowing capacity. Few animals survive exertional stress in advanced degree. Some which appear to survive are likely to die subsequently from acute heart failure or other pathophysiological developments. Among those which survive this secondary crisis a number develop localised necrosis of skeletal muscles. This latter condition is commonly termed "capture" or "exertional" myopathy.

In spite of these hazards it is occasionally necessary to treat or handle fractious animals. Using modern drugs it is feasible to do this through chemical control (Iversen and Iversen, 1981). The potential in this method to complicate physical exhaustion and stress must be considered. The following drugs are used internationally for the chemical tranquilisation and restraint of large animals. They should be used only by qualified veterinary surgeons or with veterinary advice.

Acepromazine maleate (Acepromazine)
Chlorpromazine (Largactal)
Diazepam (Valium)
Etorphine (M99: Immobilon)
Fentanyl and Droperidol (Innovar-Vet)
Carfentanil (Janssen)
Ketamine (Vetalar)
Xylazine (Rompun)
Methohexitone (Brietal)

Relevant features of these above agents are as follows:

Acepromazine

This neuroleptic is a potent phenothiazine derivative which is frequently used for tranquilization and restraint. It should not be trusted on its own as an agent to calm fractious animals since they can still respond to any threatening stimulus while under the influence of the drug. Since the drug causes hypotension animals may suffer hypoxia in situations where they are frightened and metabolise large quantities of oxygen. In such an event shock and hyperthermia may result.

Chlorpromazine

This agent has been used in animals for 30 years and is valuable in controlling animals which are intractable. To some extent it makes the animal more tame and therefore more amenable to handling in a conscious state for a short period of time. It is an anti-psychotic phenothiazine which creates a dramatic increase in dopamine activity. Phenothiazines without anti-psychotic potency do not have this characteristic.

Diazepam

This agent markedly eliminates or diminishes states of anxiety. It can be given to the animal over a prolonged period of time in order to obtain enduring results. Although it reduces anxiety it does not provide analgesia. Diazepam allows the handling of animals which are only lightly restrained. Given in high doses it can cause respiratory problems.

Etorphine

Etorphine hydrochloride is often presented as a product combined with a tranquilising agent. It is an opioid agent which is approximately a thousand times the pharmacological strength of morphine. For this reason effective doses can be given in small quantities by the intramuscular route to cause immobilisation of the animal. Within a few minutes of administration the animal falls to the ground; this condition can be reversed by the intravenous administration of its antagonist (diprenorphine). Recovery takes place within seconds and the animal is able to rise and walk (King and Klingel, 1965).

Carfentanil

Carfentanil has recently been used with a great effect in the immobilisation of wild animals and recalcitrant animals. It is a new ultra-potent morphine-like agent belonging to the fentanyl family of narcotics. Carfentanil, like the other immobilising agents, can be administered intramuscularly by projected hypodermic syringes darted at the animal by pressure gun, jab stick or cross-bow. Carfentanil can be given alone or jointly with R51703 (Janssen Pharmaceuticals). The antagonist for carfentanil is diprenophine (M50–50). Immobilisation with carfentanil, which is eight times more potent than etorphine, requires doses of very small volume and immobilisation lasts one to three hours. Diprenorphine, like naloxone which is an antagonist to etorphine acts as a competitive inhibitor at the opioid receptor sites in the central nervous system.

Effective "antagonists" such as nalorphine hydrochloride, levallorphan tartrate and naloxone hydrochloride are available to reverse the effects of narcotics. These agents do not reverse the sedative or depressant effects of other drugs. Naloxone hydrochloride must be available when using etorphine, in case of accidental human administration.

R51703

For many years now various drugs have been used in order to make wild animals tame for brief periods (Ooms *et al.*, 1981). The most recent of these is R51703 (Janssen). The administration of this drug to an intractable animals results in a calm, tranquil, alert and apparently tame animal which can be approached, handled and moved in specific directions without difficulty. R51703 is a central serotonin receptor blocker which exhibits remarkable taming properties in aggressive male cattle. Its most prominent characteristics are anxiolysis, sedation, some analgesia and anti-aggressive quality. It is found to be safe and free of serious side-effects. It can also be used as an immobilising agent. For short-term management of problem animals, drugs of this nature can be very useful.

Ketamine

This drug is principally used as a short-term anaesthetic but may not provide adequate analgesia in some species such as pigs, goats and poultry. The usual effects of ketamine and other phencyclidines is restraint characterised by catatonic immobility. Convulsions may occur. To compensate for its deficiencies this drug is usually administered in combination with another such as diazepam, phenothiazine, or a narcotic.

Xylazine

The main desired effects of xylazine in fractious animals are sedation and muscular relaxation. It is best given in combination with other sedatives since high doses have undesirable side-effects such as long recovery periods associated with struggling. It is nevertheless a very useful drug for the prompt control and immobilisation of large animals. Its anxiolytic properties are valuable.

Methohexitone

This rarely used drug is an ultra-short-acting barbiturate. It has considerable potential as an agent for rapid immobilisation without the drawback of prolonged recovery. Duration of effect is less than five minutes.

Numerous animals have been killed as a result of unwarranted chemical restraint. Malignant hyperthermia has been observed in response to anaesthetics, muscle relaxants and to stress in swine. A predisposition to such hyperthermia is probably inherited, and is commonest in the Landrace, Pietrain and Poland China breeds.

The behaviour of the species in question, the condition of the individual animal, the physiology of exertion and the circumstances of capture and control should all be thoroughly evaluated before chemical restraint is used. The mortality rate in such a procedure is much reduced when these factors are all taken into account and the procedure is carried out with the availability of equipment and materials for intensive care (Sedgwick, 1979).

31 Welfare and behaviour in relation to disease

Disease and welfare

Animals which are diseased very often have difficulty in coping with their environment, or fail to do so, hence their welfare is poorer than that of a healthy animal in otherwise comparable conditions. The effects on an animal of laminitis, mastitis, pneumonia or severe diarrhoea are easy to appreciate. Whether the disease causes pain or other kinds of discomfort or distress, veterinary treatment which reduces the effects of the disease is clearly improving the welfare of the animal. It is important to emphasise, as have Jackson (1988) and Webster (1988), that it is not the diagnosis of the disease which improves welfare but the consequent treatment. As Webster points out, "the fevered pneumonic calf, shivering in the corner of a damp draughty barn, feels rotten, and is in no way comforted by the fact that its condition has been diagnosed by a trained veterinarian''. If the consequence of disease diagnosis in a pig is preventative measures in the whole pig unit, the welfare of the animals already diseased is not improved. An important moral question for all veterinarians to ask themselves is whether or not they put the welfare of the individual farm animal first when confronted with an animal which is diseased or injured. The patient should be considered before the client who may or may not wish to pay for treatment. Similarly, the moral question for a farmer is whether or not they should allow an animal to suffer when the suffering could be reduced or prevented by seeking veterinary advice and treatment.

One of the consequences of the poor welfare associated with disease is that resistance to other disease is reduced. This has been known for a long time in the medical and veterinary professions and is part of the more general process whereby poor welfare, whatever its cause, can lead to increased susceptibility to disease. The relationship can account for the downward spiral towards death which has often been described in animals which are initially affected mildly by disease or difficult conditions. This positive feedback effect, which may or may not go as far as death, is shown in Table 31.1.

Welfare and disease susceptibility

The evidence linking welfare with susceptibility to disease is of three kinds (Broom, 1988c); first, clinical data concerning which individuals show signs of disease; second, experimental studies and surveys which compare levels of disease incidence in different husbandry systems or

Table 31.1
The interaction between poor welfare and disease over time

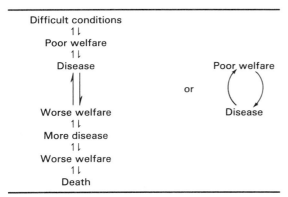

Difficult conditions
↓
Poor welfare
↓
Disease

Worse welfare
↓
More disease
↓
Worse welfare
↓
Death

or

Poor welfare

Disease

After Broom (1988c).

after different treatments; and third, studies of immune system function after different treatments.

Every veterinary surgeon can give examples of situations in which a number of animals live in apparently similar conditions but only one or two show signs of disease, or most show signs of disease but only one or two die. The individuals which are affected more by disease are those which, using physical or behavioural signs, had looked weaker and less well able to cope with the environment, for example in calves (Morisse, 1982). In group-housing situations, the more susceptible animals are often those which are obviously at the bottom of a social hierarchy with the consequence that they are chased a lot, injured by others, excluded from favoured places and sometimes prevented from obtaining an adequate diet. There is little, well-documented scientific evidence concerning this effect in farm animals, but much clinical evidence suggests that research is desirable in this area. For example, what is the reason why runt piglets are more likely to develop chronic enteritis than their larger siblings? Studies of man and of laboratory animals have concentrated much more on the question of why it is that certain individuals succumb to disease whilst others do not.

Some housing systems for farm animals or treatments such as handling, transport or farm operations lead to more welfare problems than do others. Hence there is the possibility of relating variation in welfare to variation in disease incidence. In some studies an experimental treatment can be related directly to disease effects, for example Pasteur (Nichol, 1974) found that chickens whose legs were immersed in cold water became more susceptible to anthrax. In other studies it is noticed that changes in husbandry methods are associated with changes in disease incidence, for example Sainsbury (1974) reported a gradual increase in chronic infections of poultry over a period when the frequency of intensive production practices was increasing. Direct comparisons of disease incidence levels in different housing systems are also possible but any apparent relationship between poor welfare and disease incidence must be interpreted with care as other factors which vary with conditions may affect disease incidence. Ekesbo (1981) has emphasised that environmentally evoked diseases are caused by a combination of factors. Examples of studies investigating the effects of housing conditions on disease incidence are those of Bäckström (1973) and Tillon and Madec (1984) on pigs and Gross, Colmano and Siegel who carried out disease challenge studies on chickens treated in ways which increase plasma corticosterone levels. When chickens were introduced to strange birds they displayed, fought and showed increased adrenal cortex activity. Frequent social mixing of this kind resulted in reduced resistance to *Mycoplasma gallisepticum*, Newcastle disease, haemorrhagic enteritis or Marek's disease (Gross, 1962; Gross and Colmano, 1965; Gross and Siegel, 1981). In contrast, such social mixing led to increased resistance to *Escherichia coli* and *Staphylococcus aureus* (Gross and Colmano, 1965; Gross and Siegel, 1981). When antibody activity was measured it was clear that chickens subjected to social mixing showed less activity against both viral antigens such as Marek's disease and particulate antigens such as *E. coli* (Gross and Siegel, 1975; Thompson *et al.*,

1980). The social mixing leads to increased adrenal cortex activity and this can help in counteracting inflammatory responses. Hence the pathological effects are reduced following high adrenal activity when there is invasion by organisms like *E. coli* or *S. aureus* which induce local or general inflammation and endotoxin formation. Where the principal means of defence against the pathogen is immunological, treatment such as social mixing, which leads to high adrenal activity and impaired immune system function, results in greater susceptibility to pathogen attack (Siegel, 1985).

A wide variety of studies have demonstrated that the efficiency of both antibody responses and cell-mediated immunity can be affected by exposing animals to difficult conditions (Kelley, 1980). In young calves and piglets, immunoglobulin absorption may be affected by various factors (Kruse, 1983) including impaired absorption in the absence of the mother (Selman *et al.*, 1971; Fallon, 1978) and if exposed to cold (Olsen *et al.*, 1980; Blecha and Kelley, 1981). Metz and Oosterlee (1981), who investigated the differences between sows tethered in a farrowing crate and sows in a straw-bedded pen, found that the antibody response to sheep red blood cells was greater, in tests on both sows and their piglets, when the sows had been kept in a straw pen than when they were tethered in a farrowing crate. Kelley (1985) reviewing the effects of adverse temperatures on the immune system, concludes that thermal exposure can affect the function of T-cells and have little effect on antigen-specific B-cells. Restraint of animals also had adverse effects on T-cell-mediated immune events. The mode of action of glucocorticoids on the immune system is via the reduction in production of interleukin II (see Siegel, 1985), and β endorphin is a modulator of cell-mediated immunity.

Importance of behavioural signs

Features of behaviour can be manifestations of ill-health. In fact, altered behaviour is usually the first indication of illness. Animal behaviour and veterinary diagnosis have long been closely associated; there are numerous references to the behaviour of sick animals in the classical literature of Ancient Greece. Practising veterinarians will always rely heavily on behavioural observations in arrival at a diagnosis of illness. In many common animal diseases the diagnosis is based primarily on behavioural evidence. Examples include: deficiency diseases such as aphosphorosis, metabolic diseases such as hypomagnesaemia and hypocalcaemia, and the infectious conditions such as encephalitis.

The working veterinarian is regularly presented with clinical cases having histories which are characterised by their behavioural base. It is common for animal illness to be first manifested behaviourally such as in loss of appetite, altered activity, diminished body care or behavioural atony (Fraser, 1984). Clinical veterinary work has a very real and special relationship with pathognostic behaviour in animals. Those who practise professionally the art and science of clinical veterinary medicine and surgery acquire competence at the interfaces between illnesses and their behavioural signs through years of training, experience and witness.

When the internal milieu of the animal has become abnormal, the bodily feedbacks to the central nervous system are also abnormal and in consequence the homeostatic integrity of the animal is impaired and dynamic irregularities become evident (Fraser and Herchen, 1978). The veterinarian considers these for purposes of diagnosis and prognosis. For example, the veterinary clinician may find that: the hyperexcited state in a cow is from hypomagnesaemia; the stiffened bull's gait is the result of traumatic reticulitis; the dirty coat and nose of a steer, from arrested body care, is the effect of a septicaemia; the aggressively prancing mare has an ovarian tumour; the depressed steer is toxic; the asymmetric fore limb posture of the horse is due to navicular disease; the subdued sheep has toxaemia; the pig which has ceased eating has an infection; the calf with abnormal reactions has a neural impairment; the horse walking stiffly has tetanus; and so on.

Clinical veterinary ethology

The link between altered behaviour and the diseased state is so close that there is a tendency for obviously abnormal behaviour (which presumably occurs in response to an abnormal physical state) to be used as the identification for particular diseases. For this reason a number of diseases are known by behavioural descriptions. Examples of these include staggers, sway-back, nymphomania, louping-ill (leaping), star-gazing, gid (giddiness), wobbler, wanderer, circling disease, daft lambs, doddler calves, and other more vague clinical syndromes such as "the wanderer foal", "the fading piglet" and "the downer cow" (Innes and Saunders, 1962).

A scientific interest in the altered behaviour arising from changes in health, i.e. the objective study of behaviour in diseased animals, can be termed clinical veterinary ethology. At present, the study of this subject is developing rapidly. Considerable knowledge of a practical nature now exists and the more academic aspects of this branch of ethology are progressing.

A principal objective of clinical veterinary ethologists is the accurate assessment and description of the frequency, form and spatial organisation of abnormal behaviour. By this means, clinical veterinary ethology develops a more penetrating clinical acumen, and leads to a deeper understanding of animals in a diseased or distressed state. Efficient information transfer in teaching situations also becomes possible using rational methods.

Posture

The postural characteristics of animals are among the most common behavioural features to undergo change in diseased conditions. It is therefore essential to appreciate normal posture as a basis for recognising postural abnormalities for clinical purposes. The following are the main circumstances under which animals adopt abnormal postures:

1. Mechanical conditions involving loss of support or stability by the animal.
2. Nervous conditions in which there is a reduction in adequate neural function to maintain muscular tone.
3. Permanent adaptive changes which the animal may have acquired as a result of prior experience of any disabling circumstances.
4. Painful conditions which make it impossible for the animal to maintain its natural posture.

Mechanical conditions influencing postural behaviour are many and the following few examples are given as illustrations. For example, fracture of the metacarpus in the horse makes it impossible for the animal to take any weight at all on the affected leg. Fracture of the humerus also leads to lack of mechanical support and a grossly altered posture. Severance of the flexor tendons in the horse leads to a sinking of the fetlock and a turning up of the toe. Spastic paresis of the leg in cattle results in a contraction of the gastrocnemius muscle as a result of which the affected limb becomes shorter. Congenitally contracted tendons in foals also make normal posture impossible.

Nervous conditions which can create abnormal posture include radial paralysis in the horse following prolonged recumbency during anaesthesia, for example. A lesion in the cervical vertebrae causes the condition of wobbler in the horse the main characteristic of which is a stiff neck. Abscessation of the lumbar vertebrae can cause an animal to adopt the "dog-sitting" position for lengthy periods. Abnormal carriage of the head is often a sign of cerebellar or vestibular disease and involvement of the vestibular nerve or the cerebellum can be suspected when a head tilt is present in swine. Unilateral head tilt is usually present in otoencephalitis. Facial nerve paralysis in swine occurs sometimes, with this condition to give a dropping ear on the affected side. Leaning or falling to the affected side may also occur. A wide based stance is characteristic of cerebellar dysfunction in animals.

Permanent adaptive changes may arise in a condition such as laminitis which can occur in all the hooved animals; those which have experienced laminitis for some period of time sometimes learn to walk, almost on "tip-toe" with the fore legs. This position appears to minimise pain. The adoption of this posture also means that the hind legs of the animal are brought further forward beneath it. Spinal abscessation in the pig may be the result of tail-biting and this may cause the posture of a hind leg to be altered. The common condition of foot-rot in sheep can lead, in some cases, to a state of osteomyelitis. In this condition, the affected animal frequently adopts a kneeling posture. Cattle which are kept in stalls and have experienced a form of chronic laminitis sometimes learn to stand back in the stall so that their heels overhang the standing. This posture allows the animal's weight to be transferred to its toes thereby reducing pain. Cattle which have suffered acute pain in both medial digits may stand with fore legs crossed to take all the weight on the lateral digits.

Painful conditions which cause abnormal posture in horses include also suppurative arthritis and osteomyelitis of fetlocks. The latter condition causes a tucking-under of the hind legs. Gonitis (inflammation of the stifle joint) occurs principally in horses, causing them to point the ground with the toe of the affected hind limb. Arthritis also leads to abnormal posture in other animals, for example pigs with arthritis will arch their back, presumably to minimise skeletal and abdominal pain.

The behaviour of an animal in pain has certain specific features which are recognisable. The facial expression of an animal in pain is often quite characteristic; usually there is a fixed stare with the eye. The eye is not as mobile within its orbit as in the healthy animal. The eyelids tend to be slightly puckered. The ears of animals in pain, notably horses, are usually held slightly back and fixed in that position for long periods. Animals suffering pain usually have dilated nostrils. These facial signs collectively give an animal a facial appearance of concern. In pain the animal is often seen to turn its head to one side or another, looking at one or other flank.

In colic or abdominal pain, the animal (and the horse in particular) shows various abnormalities of posture. Animals with persistent pain may show unusual recumbent behaviour; at other times they may adopt an unusual stance. Horses may back into a corner of a loose box, and both horses and cattle can sometimes be observed standing pushing their heads against a wall when a painful condition is present in the abdomen. Abdominal pain may cause the animal to lie down frequently, rising repeatedly after short intervals. In between these periods of recumbency, a horse with colic may scrape at its bedding with a fore foot, whilst slowly pivoting around on its hind legs.

In conditions of severe pain, animals often show a full distension of the nostrils, rolling the eyes in the head, extending the head and neck vigorously and groaning. Some horses lie on their backs in a position of dorsal recumbency with all four legs held in the air. This abnormal posture may be maintained for up to 15 min. More violent manifestations of pain are shown by horses on some occasions: the animal may throw itself down, may roll from side to side, may rise and walk into objects in its premises. In this state the horse seems oblivious to its surroundings and all of its behaviour is indicative of severe pain. Painful conditions of the skeleton frequently result in changes of posture and locomotion.

Diagnosis from locomotion

When the locomotor behaviour of the animal is to be examined animals should be singled out and observed in good light moving about on a clean, dry and level surface. Horses, of course, are led by hand at different gaits when special examination of locomotor behaviour is being carried out to detect any evidence of lameness.

Lameness can be defined as impaired movement or deviation from normal gait. More frequently in the veterinary context lameness refers to abnormal gait caused by painful lesions of the limbs or back or to mechanical defects of the limb. Neurological deficits which produce lameness are usually defined separately after their differential diagnosis.

Pigs are not amenable to handling and so detailed physical examination should be deferred until the animal can be removed and inspected alone. Assessment of behaviour can then be completed with minimal interference after the pig has settled down. A specific diagnostic challenge is commonly posed by pigs with disorders which present lameness or other locomotor signs. The manner in which this problem can be approached has been defined by Wells (1984) who employs a behav-ioural–neurological system within a clinical appraisal of locomotor problems in pigs.

It is recommended by Wells that when considering locomotor aspects of central nervous and neuromuscular diseases, it is a useful concept to divide clinical neurological signs into intracranial and extracranial catego-ries. Signs indicative of intracranial or brain disease include changes in mental state, seizures or convulsions, abnormal head posture, incoor-dination of head movement and cranial nerve deficits. The absence of cranial signs in neurolo-gical disease suggests that the lesion is in the spinal cord, peripheral nerves or skeletal muscles. Frequently some cranial signs will accompany abnormalities of both posture and gait. This should immediately arouse suspicion of multifocal, diffuse or systematic distribution of lesions in the nervous system (Oliver and Lorenz, 1983).

Alterations of mental state such as depres-sion, disorientation, coma or hyperexciteability may accompany locomotor signs. Depression and disorientation are features of Aujeszky's disease and encephalomyelitis. A "euphoric" state is reported to occur in pigs poisoned with arsanilic acid. Hyperexciteability is the initial feature of toxicity from an organoarsenical feed additive.

In most animals a progression through disorientation to seizures or fits is seen in many inflammatory conditions of the brain and its meningeal sheath such as in bacterial meningitis. Seizures are characterised by marked diffuse increase in muscle tone, falling into lateral recumbency and rhythmic clonic convulsions simulating running or pedalling movements of the limbs. Depression or even coma may follow a seizure. Opisthotonus (dorsiflexion of the neck) with extension of the limbs is also seen with meningitis.

Several metabolic and other systemic dis-orders have secondary effects upon the central nervous system including locomotor deficits, although their primary pathophysiology is not within the locomotor apparatus. Nervous signs of generalised metabolic derangement are often mediated through the central nervous system and are often intermittent, always generalised, and produce a wide spectrum of inconsistant neurological signs. These include confusion, coma, syncope, collapse, seizures, tremors, vision disturbances, quadriparesis, paraparesis and episodic weakness (Palmer, 1976).

Hypoglycaemia, though not a specific disease, is frequently the main metabolic manifestation of starvation in piglets during the first week of life. Confusion and ataxia progress to quadri-paresis, sometimes seizures and to death in coma. In the ataxic stages piglets stand base-wide and may rest their noses upon the floor apparently to gain further support.

Ataxia means incoordination of muscular action or gait. Signs include wide-based stance, swaying movements, falling, rolling, dysmetria (imprecise gait), crossing of the limbs and exaggerated abduction of the limbs on turning. Ataxia is one of the most common clinical signs in nervous diseases in sheep, pigs and cattle.

Paralysis is defined as loss of motor or sensory nerve function; paresis is partial paralysis. A general muscular weakness may appear as appar-ent quadriparesis and in practice may be indis-tinguishable from true neurogenic paresis. In such cases when a neurogenic component of the "paralysis" can be ruled out the term muscular weakness is thought to be more appropriate than paralysis.

Assessment of gait should take account of length of stride. Dysmetria may take the form of movements that are too long (hypermetria) or too short (hypometria). Hypermetria, called "goose-stepping", is a relatively common sign of locomotor dysfunction in the pig. Goose-stepping is sometimes due to hock-joint abnormalities preventing its movement. A dysmetric gait often includes a long stride with a prolonged supporting phase. Painful skeletal lesions give a short stride with a reduced support phase.

Recumbent animals may also indicate paralysis or muscular weakness. Paraplegia causes a dog-sitting posture. If spasticity is present the hind limbs are extended forward in the sitting position. Pain in a limb will produce abnormal limb positioning; often flexion or abduction to avoid weight bearing. Shifting of weight from one leg to another in the standing position is seen in polyarthritis. When there is pain involving all four feet, as in laminitis of an acute form, a posture is adopted with the back arched and the feet bunched together under the abdomen. Such animals are reluctant to move. A similar stance is typical of laminitis in all stock.

Diagnosis from other behaviour

A list of specific features can be given as indications of the scope for clinical applications of ethology. Lameness in cattle can be caused by a great variety of circumstances, e.g. one particular type of condition, namely abcessation of the solar matrix, results in the affected limb being cast inwards or outwards, depending on which digit is affected. The lameness pattern in this condition is quite different from that seen in laminitis.

Myelin disorders produce generalised tremors in piglets at or near birth. While the piglet is active the trembling is constant but it subsides when the piglet is at rest. Severely affected piglets can tremble so violently that they are unable to suck. An intermittent tremor is seen in some adolescent Landrace pigs, but the condition sometimes resolves itself spontaneously after a few months. Generalised tremor is present in neuromuscular weakness such as occurs in the hereditary myopathy of the Pietrain breed, the so-called "Pietrain creeper syndrome". Tremor is a regular abnormal movement caused by involuntary changes in muscle tone. It is seen sometimes in diffuse brain diseases, in particular viral encephalitis.

Tetanus produces a distinctive behaviour with rigid stance and stilted gait as its principal initial features. In tetanus there are spasms of generalised muscle contraction brought about by the effects of tetanus toxin absorbed into the nervous systems. If muscle spasms are prolonged they are termed "tonic" and if rapid they are termed "clonic". In tetanus the spasms are largely tonic with intermittent clonus. There is hyperesthesia and external stimuli provoke signs. Signs progress over one to two days from a still gait to lateral recumbency with opisthotonos and extensor rigidity of all limbs. The ears are erect, there is elevation of the tail and there is loss of voice. Muscle spasm also occurs in generalised seizures but the tonic phase is usually brief. The clonic limb movements of running or pedalling are characteristic.

Cerebral cortical necrosis affects behaviour significantly, causing lack of coordination and patterns of recumbency, which are quite characteristic.

In muscular dystrophy, affected calves walk in a characteristic style with the scapulae rising as much as 10 cm above the vertebral column giving a "broken front spring" appearance.

Cattle with hypocalcaemia adopt a very characteristic recumbent posture and many of them show an equally characteristic "S" bend of the neck whilst recumbent.

In hypomagnesaemia, it is common to observe greatly increased excitability in the behaviour of the affected animal. This excitability is evident in such behavioural features as unusual and excessive flicking of the eyes and ears and in an unusual style of walking.

Urolithiasis occurs quite commonly in rams which are housed and heavily fed. The condition is associated with characteristic behaviour including grating of the teeth, straining and arching of the back.

In gangreneous mastitis, affected ewes characteristically draw one hind leg behind the other while walking. A animal's general posture indicates a toxic state and the head is often held low.

In other animals, conditions such as ear infections and mouth ulcerations create characteristic behavioural signs.

Since this section is concerned with illustrating the connection between farm animal behaviour and illness, two examples have been chosen which detail this relationship. These examples are among the most common bovine clinical conditions which are dealt with in the routine of veterinary fieldwork, namely cystic ovarian disease and milk fever.

Cystic ovarian disease in cattle

This is characterised by the presence of enlarged and cystic follicles on the ovary. The behavioural correlates in this condition are well known. Natural oestrogen levels in the blood are raised and oestrous behaviour is affected. Oestrous periodicity seems normal in approximately 33% of cases, but alongside this there may be a continuously low degree of clinical oestrus as a background to the pattern of overt oestrous periodicity. In about 80% of clinical cases restless behaviour is very conspicuous. There is a typical feminising behaviour with increased production of vaginal mucus and frequent acceptance of mounting by other cattle. This appears to be related to the fact that the rate of thyroxine secretion in cattle with cystic ovarian disease is about double that in normal animals. The remaining 20% of clinical cases show different behavioural abnormalities.

One facet of this disease is the "virile cow syndrome" (adrenal virilism). The first change to this is usually a deepening of the voice and an increase in vocal activity so that the animals are heard roaring in masculine tones. Sometimes stockmen call such animals (which are almost as hyper-reactive as bulls) "growler-cows". Increased pawing activity may be seen in some of these animals. Among the various forms of masculine behaviour, digging with the fore feet is almost consistently observed.

Milk fever in cattle

Milk fever is a complex disturbance of the mineral concentrations and ratios in the blood of cows. The typical case occurs post-partum and within 96 h of parturition. The behaviour observed during this condition is caused by a biochemical disturbance in the plasma minerals and the physiological processes ensuing from this upset. This alteration of mineral levels in blood can explain the overall picture in a cow with milk fever. Calcium is essential for normal neuromuscular excitability, normal muscle contraction and normal transmission of nerve impulses. When the plasma-calcium level is decreased all three of these activities are increased to an abnormally high level. Thus the behaviour of the animal takes the form of increased nervous excitability, incoordination of movements, paresis and eventually coma. To a certain extent general behaviour can thus be explained; but the clinician can distinguish three main behavioural stages in milk fever. These are detailed below.

In the early stages of the disturbance the general behaviour is that of *discomfort and anxiety*. The cow is disinclined to move, has a depressed facial expression with staring eyes; she grinds her teeth and often makes intermittent paddling movements with her hind legs. There is complete bowel stasis, normally with a full rectum. Often the cow produces exaggerated abdominal efforts to defaecate to little or no avail; quite often there is a full bladder due to the animal's inability to evacuate.

As the condition progresses, the pattern of behaviour can vary further and the *excitable stage and paresis* develops.

1. The cow, in her natural surroundings at pasture, may start to show some increased excitement, by sweating and becoming more alert, under the effect of the decreasing plasma-calcium level. She may even show some degree of incoordination in her movements. In general as her powers of balance recede she is inclined to wander stiff-legged, swaying a little, to a corner of the field; she then subsides to a position of sternal recumbency.

2. The cow indoors often shows a more excitable behaviour pattern during the progress of the condition. She appears to be hypersensitive to noise, her ears are alert and continually on the move (like "radar vanes"). Unless the conditions indoors are very quiet she is disinclined to lie down as her sense of balance recedes. She adopts a variety of postures in attempting to retain her balance. If approached while standing she often tends to be aggressive. She may attempt to kick out, even though she may almost collapse in the effort, or may lower her head to butt the intruder. If her feet should slip she will show exaggerated posturing of the legs and body to retain balance. She tends to remain standing as long as possible and can be seen trembling and stiff-legged until she collapses in the stall.

Once the cow is recumbent, she becomes more placid, although sometimes showing hyperexcitability and sweating if approached. If she is disturbed at this stage, she shows excessive irritability and may eventually roll into lateral recumbency with legs extended in spasms. As *coma* supervenes, she either remains in sternal recumbency and lowers her head and neck to the ground, or rolls over onto lateral recumbency.

The variety of behavioural features, as seen by the clinician, appears to revolve round the degree of excitability in the cow. This degree of excitability appears to be influenced by the surroundings and management of the animal. Once the disturbance is set in motion the behaviour appears to be governed partly by the surroundings, partly by the management of the animal and partly by apparent fear, engendered by these factors and by presence of man.

Depression

Throughout veterinary literature, among the identifying signs of many clinical conditions in animals, mention is made of depression. For example, depression is described as a major diagnostic clinical finding in such conditions as Shipping Fever in cattle, the Mastitis–Metritis–Agalactia (MMA) Syndrome in sows, Newcastle Disease in poultry. By the clinical use of the term is meant a marked reduction in general activity, diminished responsiveness to exteroceptive stimuli and an appearance of reduced awareness in a generalised behavioural atony (see also Chapter 29). Head-pressing is a notable example (Fig. 31.1).

The typical behavioural picture of the depressed animal is a passive one. Positive, reinforcing stimuli lack influence. The bulk of the depressed animal's activity is likely to be passively derived from prompts, commands and aversive stimuli rather than through spontaneous relationship with the environment. In depression the suffering animal shows a depletion of the behavioural repertoire characteristic of the normal behaviour. The principal features of maintainance behaviour such as trophic activities and restorative functions, together with collateral social behaviour, show dissolution of hierarchical organisation, adding to the picture of suffering. Loss of maintenance priorities, through changes in "motivational time-sharing", and the intrusion of anomalous behaviour, appear to be the essential criteria of

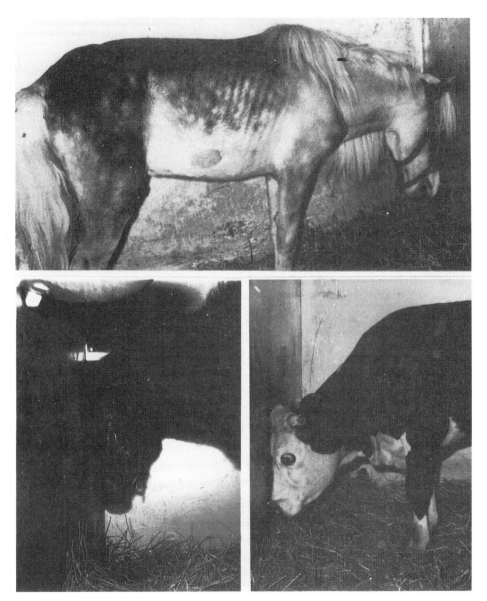

Fig. 31.1   The head-pressing syndrome in equine and bovine cases of toxic conditions.

that general state of animal illness widely referred to clinically as depressed.

Because the established concept of depression in animal illness recognises the behaviour of the animal as globally changed rather than regionally modified the main significant measure is behavioural infrequency. It shows in the reduced frequency of maintenance activities—at the level of first or second orders of behavioural homeostasis. But frequency can also measure high incidences of irregular acts such as agitations or stereotypies and apparently these also can indicate a form of suffering. The stereotyped continuation of an activity disorder could be likened to an agitated state since the two essential criteria are met, namely:

1. loss of priority organisation in maintenance behaviour: and

2. the substitution of anomalous, active behaviour at a high level of precedence and of frequency.

The depressed behaviour of an animal can therefore be recognised by a decrease in the frequency of certain classes of maintenance behaviour and an increase in the frequency of certain anomalous forms of behaviour. Consistent with this postulate is the observation that significantly elevated cortisol levels are found in young pigs showing the lowest level of playing and the highest level of abnormal activity (Schmidt, 1982). Further examples of suffering which are made explicit by behavioural changes are discussed in the next chapters.

32 Abnormal behaviour 1: Stereotypies

What is abnormality?

In order to recognise that behaviour is abnormal, the person observing must be familiar with the range of normal behaviour of that species. For some abnormalities, indeed, recognition depends upon a knowledge of the behaviour of that particular individual. One of the qualities of a good stockman is an ability to identify abnormal behaviour using knowledge acquired as a result of looking carefully at the animals. A difficulty for the stockman arises if many of the animals kept show the same kind of abnormal behaviour since such a situation can lead the stockman to believe that behaviours like bar-biting in sows are normal. A wider knowledge of the behavioural repertoire of such animals is necessary in order to establish what is normality. In order to obtain this for farm animals it is necessary to study the animals in a relatively complex environment where they have the opportunity to show the full range of their behaviour. This need not be the wild environment but it should include the components of it which are important for the animal. An extensive knowledge of the biology of such animals and a detailed ethological investigation are therefore needed in order to be able to decide what behaviour is abnormal.

The most obvious kind of abnormality is a distinct pattern of movements but even this will usually have components which are shown as components of some normal behaviour. The most common abnormalities are those where the frequency of the movements, the intensity of the actions, or the context in which the behaviour occurs is different from the normal. The animal may show the behaviour in an attempt to cope with some aspect of its environment. In some cases that abnormal behaviour may help the individual to cope but in other cases it may confer no beneficial effect. Some abnormal behaviour has an obvious detrimental effect on either the animal which is showing it, for example horses eating wood, or on other animals, for example pigs tail-biting. The word "vice" is sometimes used to refer to very many kinds of abnormal behaviour. However, when used in a human context, this word implies that blame should be attributed to the individual showing the behaviour. Since almost all of the so-called vices shown by farm animals have been shown to be a consequence of the ways in which the animals are housed or managed, it is an illogical term and will not be used in this book. The use of such a term can have the effect on the person who manages, owns, or advises about the animals that the abnormal behaviour concerned is not their responsibility but rather is a fault of the animal. Such attitudes have been an important factor in the perpetuation of many systems which result in poor welfare.

In this chapter, stereotyped behaviour is described. There follow chapters on other abnormal behaviour classified according to what it is directed at: the individual's own body, the inanimate surroundings, or other individuals. Chapter 35 concerns behaviour in which there are inadequacies of normal function and Chapter 36 deals with abnormal reactivity. The content of each of these chapters is a description of the abnormal behaviour and comments on the causative mechanisms where this is possible. It should be emphasised, however, that whilst some kinds of abnormal behaviour are a direct result of some specific problem for the animal, the actual abnormality shown is often very individual in its characteristics. The level and quality of the abnormality can vary greatly from one individual to another (Fraser and Herchen, 1962; Broom, 1987a).

Stereotypies

It has long been known that some caged animals in zoos and some human prisoners in isolation cells will pace out the same route over and over again. Similarly, birds in small cages will fly or hop from perch to perch, again following a route, and both monkeys in cages and autistic children will rock backwards and forwards for long periods. Hediger (1934, 1950) and Meyer-Holzapfel (1968) gave many examples of such behaviour in zoo animals and Levy (1944) described examples of head-shaking in battery hens and various movement patterns in children. Brion (1964) described crib-biting and sucking by horses and Fraser (1975) described bar-biting by pigs. Such repeated actions which have no obvious purpose are called stereotypies. Their occurrence and causation is described in detail by Ödberg (1978), Broom (1981, p. 98; 1983b) and Dantzer (1986).

A stereotypy is usually recognised because a sequence of movements is repeated several times with little or no variation. However, the behav-

Table 32.1

Examples of sham-chewing (no food present) by sow in stall

	Sow lying
2 s	Mouth stretch
35 s	Chewing with tongue extrusion or nose wrinkling at intervals of 4,9,4,5,4 s
4 s	Pause
48 s	Chewing, etc.
13 s	Pause
19 s	Chewing, etc. — sequence continues
	Mean duration 17.5 min

Table 32.2

Example of drinker-pressing by sow in stall

	Sow standing
5–8 s	Press drinker with snout
1–2 s	Pause
5–8 s	Press drinker (water pouring onto floor)
1–2 s	Pause; pattern repeated 7–15 times
5–8 s	Press drinker
	Swing head to left, nose in neighbour's pen

ioural repertoires of animals include many examples of repeated action patterns, for example walking, flapping flight and various displays, which would not be called stereotypies (Broom, 1983b). Hence it is necessary to include in the definition of a stereotypy some reference to its apparent lack of function. Does it form part of one of the normal functional systems of the animal (see Chapter 1)? Detailed studies using video-recording show how much variation there is in stereotyped behaviour. Table 32.1 is an example of a description of sham-chewing and Table 32.2 describes drinker-pressing, both shown by sows in stalls.

Just as action patterns, which are part of normal behaviour, are seen to be somewhat variable when analysed in great detail (Chapter 2; Broom, 1981, p. 62), so the repeated movements in stereotypies show some variation. When the descriptions of behaviour are subjected to analysis using information theory, however, the stereotypies are found to include much more redundant information, i.e. the same sequences occur, than do non-stereotyped behaviours (Stolba *et al.*, 1983). When Cronin (1985) analysed sequences of the behaviour of tethered sows he found that some sows chewed on their tether chain in a rigid sequence of actions whereas there was more variation in the sequences shown by other sows (see Fig. 32.1). These other sows, however, showed action patterns which were themselves repetitive and repeated each of these action patterns even if the order was not constant, so the behaviour would still be called a stereotypy. These examples emphasise that stereotypies are relatively invariate rather than absolutely invariate. Hence by definition, *a stereotypy is a repeated, relatively invariate sequence of movements which has no obvious purpose*. The repetition may be regular, but it need not be, and the sequence of movements may be very short, as in the head-shake of a hen, or long and complex, as in some route-tracing by bears in zoos or in the elaborate weaving sequences by some pigs in stalls or mink in cages.

As a way of trying to understand the significance and motivational basis of stereotypies, various physiological investigations have been carried out. Several different psychostimulant drugs which interfere with the metabolism of the catecholamine neurotransmitters dopamine and noradrenaline (= norepinephrine) affect the incidence of stereotypies in various animals including farm animals (Sharman and Stephens, 1974). The possible mechanisms involved are reviewed by Dantzer (1986) who concludes that ''there is good evidence that performance of stereotyped behaviour depends upon brain dopamine systems involved in the control of movement''. Opiate peptides in the brain may also be linked with stereotyped behaviour in some way, for Cronin *et al.* (1985) found that when naloxone, which blocks the μ receptor sites for β endorphin, etc., is administered to stereotyping sows they cease the behaviour. It could be that the tethered sows use stereotypies to induce the action of the analgesic opiate peptides in the brain, as Cronin *et al.* suggest, but this is not certain. It is likely that there is some interaction between the opiate peptides and the system in the brain which results in stereotyped behaviour. The electrical activity of the brain during stereotypies has not been studied in great detail but the pattern during rumination, a repeated behaviour which has a function, is rather similar to that seen in a dozing human. Houpt (1987) has pointed out that ruminants show fewer stereotypies than do other farm animals,

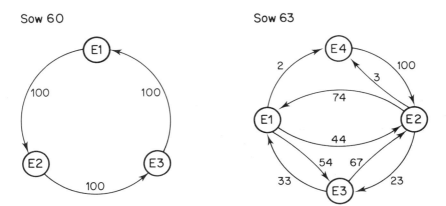

Fig. 32.1 Quantitative description of stereotyped sequences in two pregnant tethered sows. Each element corresponds to a specific motor act (e.g. E3 is sham-chewing in both sows). Numbers along arrows indicate the percentage of occasions that individual elements succeeded other elements (from Cronin, 1985).

including young calves, so it could be that rumination can fulfil a function similar to that of stereotypies.

Stereotypies occur in situations where the individual lacks control of its environment. In some cases the animal is obviously frustrated and in other cases the future events are rather unpredictable. Many examples of such situations are included in the rest of this chapter. Ideas about the causation of stereotypies and their possible function for the animal have been complicated by the fact that some situations where stereotypies are shown are barren environments but others include disturbing or threatening factors. Hence the stereotyped behaviour might increase the total sensory input in the barren environment but produce a more predictable and familiar input in the disturbing situation. These two, apparently different effects are discussed in more detail by Broom (1981, p. 99; 1983) and by Dantzer (1986).

The behaviour sequence which becomes stereotyped is sometimes an incomplete form of a functional behaviour pattern (van Putten, 1982). It might arise from direct attempts to remedy some problem, such as to remove a bar which is preventing escape or to obtain the last available particle of food. By the time that the stereotypy is established, no simple function is served. The combination of motor command and resulting sensory feedback may have some beneficial effect on the animal showing the behaviour or it may be just a sign of a behavioural pathology. Repeated sensory inputs could possibly have a direct narcotising effect on the perpetrator, or they could have an effect via an analgesic peptide as Cronin *et al.* (1985) suggest. The observation that animals showing stereotypies are often difficult to disturb is of interest here for they may have their brain state modified in a way which reduces responsiveness. They could reduce the need to use adrenal cortex responses, as seemed to be the case in the chain-playing pigs studied by Dantzer and Mormède (1981), and could have some effect which reduces the incidences of other adverse changes such as abomasal ulceration in calves

(Wiepkema, 1987). Stereotypies may be a means of alleviating the effects of adverse conditions but this is by no means fully proven and Dantzer (1986) considers that in many cases the stereotypy has become a useless and energetically costly sign of brain function pathology. Whether or not they are of any help to the animal they are clearly an indicator of poor welfare. For some stereotypies, any occurrence is an indication of poor welfare, but for others, a higher frequency of occurrence is necessary before it is quite clear that there is a problem. Details of frequency of occurrence of stereotypies are included in Chapters 29 and 37–39 on welfare of particular species of farm animals.

The remainder of this chapter includes descriptions of a wide range of stereotypies occurring in farm animals and is organised according to the nature of the movement. The first few stereotypies involve the whole body. There follow stereotypies involving much of the body or part of the body. Finally those in which the oral region is used are detailed.

Pacing or route-tracing

The repeated action patterns are those used in walking or other locomotion but the animal follows a path which returns to its point of origin and which is often repeated with only minor modifications. The route-tracing of zoo animals in cages, of some confined domestic animals and of confined or disturbed people has often been described. Some obvious frustration is normally evident, most frequently that the animal cannot escape from confinement in a cage or pen, but occasionally that access to a social partner, a sexual partner, food or some other resource is impossible.

In the horse stereotyped pacing is recognised as "stall-walking". In this anomalous behaviour the horse constantly paces or circles around the horse box. The behaviour is shown under conditions of minimal exercise in chronic confinement in a horse box. The condition closely resembles weaving with the precision and repetition in which the animal performs its rhythmic movements. As distinct from weaving in a tie-stall, the stall-walker makes use of the larger areas afforded by a loose box. This greater latitude allows the animal to perform slightly more elaborated ambulatory actions than weaving. The quantity of work performed in stereotyped pacing is often very considerable and in many cases it leads to loss of weight in the animal through energy depletion. Since the amount of the area available to the animal is essentially limited, considerable spinal flexion is required in circling and turning and this can lead to painful back conditions which can adversely affect the performance of the animal when ridden.

Stereotyped pacing also occurs in poultry. The condition can be induced by thwarting birds that are very hungry and which have a high expectation of food provision. Duncan and Wood-Gush (1971, 1972) trained hens to feed from a dish in a particular position and then thwarted feeding by putting a transparent perspex cover on the dish (Table 32.3). In poultry the stereotyped pacing resembles escape movements. Affected birds typically show repetitive pacing movements occupying the full range of one side of the pen or cage. When the condition has become established in the bird's behavioural repertoire it shows a strong tendency to persist although it may reduce in frequency if thwarting circumstances are eliminated.

Hens also pace before oviposition if no nest material is available. If hens have nest material

Table 32.3
Conditions leading to stereotyped pacing by hens

	Mean number of stereotyped pacing routines in 30 min
Deprived, fed	13.3
Not deprived, not fed	18.7
Deprived, frustrated (food under perspex cover)	161.0

Data from Duncan and Wood-Gush (1972).

they will build a nest before egg-laying and their frustration if this is not possible is probably the major factor leading to stereotyped pacing at this time (Wood-Gush, 1969, 1972; Brantas, 1980).

Rocking, swaying and weaving

The individual remains in one place when carrying out this stereotypy but the body is moved backwards and forwards or from side to side, with or without head-swinging. Monkeys in captivity, especially those deprived of their mother or of companions for some long time, show rocking behaviour. So too do autistic children and other children in very disturbing circumstances. Horses, calves and adult cattle which are tethered or in small pens will sometimes rock and sway.

Weaving is recognised as a behavioural disorder of certain horses. The main feature is swinging the head and neck and anterior parts of the body from side to side so that the weight rests alternately on each fore limb. In most cases the fore feet remain on the stable floor during the behaviour but in extreme cases each foot is raised as the weight passes on to the other foot. For further details see Sambraus (1985).

Although it is difficult to ascertain the cause of the condition in any given case, lack of variety in the environment is a likely cause (Houpt, 1981) as it occurs most commonly in riding horses which have been stabled for long periods in idleness. Many animals which exhibit weaving become physically exhausted and lose weight progressively. Once the condition is acquired it is extremely difficult to control and it is believed that the anomaly can be induced in other horses in a stable through mimicry. To some extent weaving can be controlled by tying the horse with cross reins so as to limit the lateral movement of its head but this probably is of no benefit to the horse. Ideally, affected animals should be turned out to pasture but when this is not possible through lack of space, enforced exercise can be provided by lunging or the use of a mechanical exerciser. The animals should be maintained in a loose box permitting ambulatory movement.

Rubbing

Some part of the body is moved back and forwards against a solid object and the movement is repeated so many times that it could not function merely to alleviate a local irritation.

Cattle which are confined to stalls for extended periods, such as the winter, may rub their heads repeatedly against some part of the stall. This behaviour is more noticeable in horned breeds and more in bulls than in other stock.

Head-rubbing in pigs is sometimes observed in animals subject to chronic restriction within narrow single stalls. In this behaviour the upper snout region of the sow is rubbed repetitively and vigorously along the underside of a bar across the front of the stall. The behaviour can become so vigorous that the animal may bump its head against the side of the stall at the end of each sideways rub. A few cases of such "head-banging" have been reported in which the animals have seriously injured themselves. The resultant trauma has warranted the humane destruction of some of these animals. It would appear that the control of this behaviour, as with similar somatic, stereotyped actions, calls for relief of the chronic restraint imposed upon the affected animal.

The behaviour of tail-rubbing in the horse is non-specific. It may occur as a sign of parasitism, including *Oxyuris* in the rectum, fungal infection of the perineum, or louse infestation in the region of the tail head. Persistent tail-rubbing may occur in horses without any causative infection or infestation and in these cases the condition is one of anomalous behaviour in which one feature of normal grooming is carried to excess.

The behaviour shows in horses backing into a post, tree, fence, or a portion of a building and moving the hindquarters rhythmically from side to side while the tail is pushed into the perineal region. Persistent rubbing may continue for periods of a minute or more and may be repeated. As a result of this activity the long hairs growing from the root of the tail become worn down and broken off to appear as short bristles. To eliminate the possibility of parasitism in the condition, appropriate clinical examination should be given and appropriate anthelminthic or other anti-parasitic treatment provided as necessary.

Pawing and stall-kicking

The foot is repeatedly moved along the ground or applied vigorously to the wall of the enclosure around the animal. Both are actions reported for horses. Although pawing is a normal behaviour of horses shown in such activities as clearing snow from herbage and pawing at a recumbent foal the behaviour can be shown in abnormal form when it is performed with vigour in a persistent, stereotyped fashion. Minor episodes of pawing may occur when horses are frustrated in obtaining food. The anomalous condition is shown in pawing which is so frequent and vigorous that holes may be dug in the stall floor and the hoof worn down severely. The continual pawing on a hard floor can result in various forms of leg strain and injury. Attempts to control this problem through negative conditioning have not been successful. It occurs most frequently in confined and isolated horses so may be alleviated by turning the affected animal out to pasture in the company of other horses.

Some stalled horses repeatedly lower the head, pull back the ears, arch the back and kick with a hind leg against the wall or door behind them so that a loud bang is produced. The noise may initially attract attention which the horse may be seeking but the action can lead to injury and damage. The splintering of woodwork can result in exacerbation of injuries and the production of material which the horse may later ingest. Attempts to prevent stall-kicking usually involve the use of hanging mats or barriers which might reduce injury and nuisance but do not address the cause of the problem. As with other stereotypies shown by stalled horses, putting the animal out at pasture, or providing frequent exercise and more companionship, are the real answers.

Head-shaking or -nodding

The head is moved vertically, laterally or with a rotary movement of the neck. Head-shaking occurs in the domestic fowl and takes the form of a rotary movement of the head with a series of rapid side to side turns which end with a slight downward movement (Levy, 1944). These spasms of movement last only for a second or so but may be repeated in succession for several minutes. They are shown without regard to the posture or position of the bird. There are close parallels in the movements of jungle fowl (Kruijt, 1964).

Observers have assumed that this condition is caused by frustration of movement. Increased head-shaking sometimes results from the close presence of an observer from which the bird cannot escape. For example, it has been found that in certain strains of birds the incidence of head-shaking increases five-fold in the presence of an observer in an obvious position (Hughes, 1980). There appears to be more head-shaking in caged birds than in floor-housed hens and more in Rhode Island Reds than in White Leghorns (Bareham, 1972). Variations in head-shaking incidence with space allocation and group size have not been consistent from one study to another (Bessei, 1982). Hughes (1981) found that head-shaking was affected by the presentation of novel stimuli, transfer to novel conditions and social rank. His results and those of Kruijt (1964) and Forrester (1980) suggest that head-shaking is linked to attentional mechanisms and the preparation for making a response. Hence the behaviour may have a function when shown occasionally but should be

regarded as abnormal and a stereotypy when shown often.

The behavioural anomaly of head-nodding in the horse occurs as stereotyped behaviour in various forms. The most common is repeated "bobbing" up and down of the head. As with some other stereotypies, such as weaving, it has been suggested that there may be a self-hypnotic component in this behaviour. When animals show this anomaly they certainly appear to be in a light somnolent state, showing little attention to their environment.

Control of this condition is difficult when it has become established in the horse's behaviour. A heavy fringe on the brow band of a head stall can distract a horse in this practice. This may also help to disperse flies about the head which might also be involved in the aetiology of this condition.

Wind-sucking

Air is sucked into the alimentary canal and swallowed or expelled. This behaviour, sometimes called aerophagia, is often combined with head-nodding and may also be a component of crib-biting in horses and tongue-rolling in cattle.

In pure wind-sucking, the horse hods its head and neck several times before making the intake effort. In the initial act of wind-sucking the head is jerked upwards, the horse opens its mouth, takes in air, raises the floor of the mouth and contracts the musculature of the pharynx so that air is then forcibly swallowed as the neck is flexed. The characteristic wind-sucking sound is made as some horses expel some of the air; in others the sound occurs as they swallow it. The action is repeated.

As a consequence of persistent wind-sucking the musculature of the throat increases in size due to hypertrophy from excessive use. Stomach dilation with bloating may also occur and this, in turn, can lead to gastrointestinal catarrh and episodes of colic. Horses which practise aerophagia intensively reduce their intake of feed and may scatter it, with a resultant nutritional deficiency causing reduced physical condition. It is known that horses are more likely to show wind-sucking if those stalled nearby do so and experience shows that foals may acquire the aerophagic habit from affected mothers. This latter finding has led to the belief that aerophagia may have a recessive–hereditary basis with certain animals being predisposed to the condition when subjected to the common precipitating factors of chronic inactivity and confinement (Hosoda, 1950). This may be so but the behaviour is not normally seen amongst horses at pasture.

A common method for preventing aerophagia is use of the wind-sucker strap. This is a strap which is fastened tightly around the throat which has a heart shaped piece of thick leather which sits between the angles of the jaws with the pointed end protruding towards a pharyngeal area. With this device in place difficulty and apparent discomfort are caused to the horse when the neck is flexed in the attempt to suck wind. Some horses will continue to practise the abnormal behaviour in spite of this device so that they eventually acquire pressure sores on that part of the neck where the strap presses.

Various surgical methods have been attempted to prevent wind-sucking. One of these involves the creation of fistulae, on each side of the mouth, between the buccal cavity and the outer cheek. Such fistulae prevent the formation of a vacuum in the mouth which is required in the act of swallowing air. In addition, a wind-suck operation has been devised in which the small muscles surrounding the pharynx are partially removed. Even this radical operation, however, fails to give totally satisfactory results. In general it is found that animals which respond most satisfactorily to methods of prevention are those which have not practised the anomaly for long periods (Sambraus, 1985). None of these actions is likely to be of any help to the horse and it would clearly be much better to change the environment of the animal.

Eye-rolling

The eyes are moved around in the orbit at a time when no visible object is present and moving in such a way as to lead to such movement. Veal calves confined in crates sometimes stand immobile for extended periods and do not show the normal variations between lying and upright positions. During some of these episodes the head is held motionless and the animal rolls its eyes within the orbits so that only the white sclera is shown; such eye rolling being frequently repeated.

Sham-chewing

Jaw movements like those shown when chewing food are shown at a time when the animal has no food in its mouth. This condition is typically seen in sows kept singly in stalls in which no litter is provided. The animal chews vigorously at a time when all food available has been eaten and, since pigs are not ruminants, there can be no oral content except saliva. Affected animals have chewing characteristics of their own but constant features involve periodic chewing, mouth gaping and frothing. The chewing motion causes frothing and foaming of saliva. This foam collects on the outer edges of the lips (see Fig. 32.2) and the corners of the mouth and drops to the ground where such material can remain in portions, for some time, as evidence of this activity. Sham-chewing occurs most often while the sow is lying in a prone position or on its haunches in a dog-sitting position. It can be maintained as a prominent activity enduring throughout consecutive days. Broom and Potter (1984) reported that sows spent from 0–90 min sham-chewing (median 26 min) during the eight hours of daylight and Sambraus (1985) describes sows which were sham-chewing for many hours, day after day.

While clinical sequelae to sham-chewing have not been clearly identified it has been widely noticed that affected animals are often classed

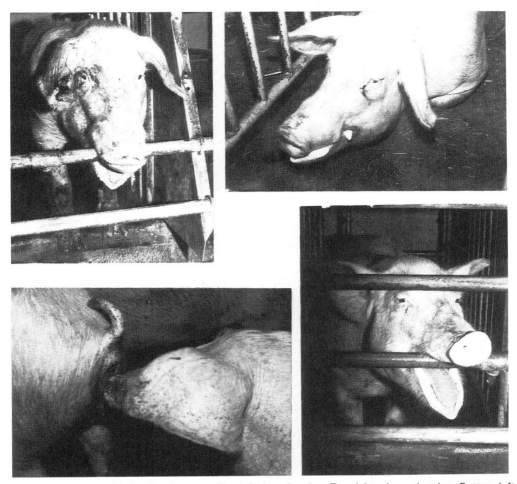

Fig. 32.2 Anomalous oral behaviour in swine. Top left: bar-chewing. Top right: sham-chewing. Bottom left: anal nosing and coprophagia. Bottom right: bar-whetting (photographs by H.H. Sambraus).

within the "thin sow syndrome". Even when such animals are provided with additional feed, significant weight gain does not occur. Such animals also are in a condition of sub-fertility due to delayed occurrence of oestrus or anoestrus following weaning (Sambraus, 1985).

Sham-chewing may be reduced if the sows were given straw or sawdust to chew and root.

When sow diet was supplemented by the same weight of oat hulls, the total frequency of stereotyped behaviour was not altered but sows lay down for longer and, as a consequence, showed more sham-chewing but less of the stereotypies shown whilst standing (Broom and Potter, 1984). A change to a group-housing system is the best way to alleviate the adverse effects on sows which result in sham-chewing.

Tongue-rolling

The tongue is extruded from the mouth and moved by curling and uncurling outside or inside the mouth with no solid material present. This stereotypy has been described in detail for cattle and it includes components of the movements involved in the prehension of forage plants during grazing. The tongue is typically extruded and rolled back into the open mouth, after which partial swallowing of the tongue and gulping of the air takes place (Fig. 32.3). Tongue-rolling may be associated with aerophagia of a particularly rapid type in which as many as two ingestions of air per minute may occur, together with frothing at the mouth. Durations of tongue-rolling episodes range from a few minutes to several hours. It occurs most commonly immediately before and after feeding. Tongue-rolling might have an origin in forms of calf feeding in which suckling is deficient. A form of tongue-rolling has been observed in early-weaned piglets and veal calves. In the latter the condition is in the form of rolling the tongue back into the mouth, sucking on it and then extending it sharply out of the mouth. This has been termed "tongue-beating".

The condition occurs in all ages and breeds but younger adult cattle and certain breeds such as Brown Swiss are thought to exhibit it most frequently. It is believed that there may be a hereditable factor in this condition but it is also believed that nutritional deficiencies can precipitate it. It occurs more often in cows within herds

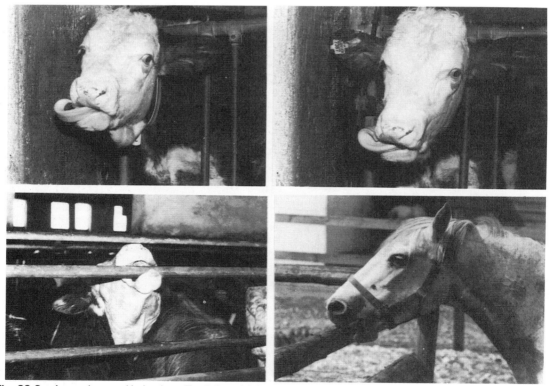

Fig. 32.3 Anomalous oral behaviour. Top left and right: tongue-rolling. Bottom left: bar-biting. Bottom right: wood-eating (photographs by H.H. Sambraus).

which are continuously confined indoors. When a feed is provided in a form low in roughage and not requiring significant oral activity in prehension and mastication, the condition may be encouraged. Since cattle actively use their tongues in grazing by encircling tufts of grass to be consumed, the mechanism of this behaviour exists in this species but not in other grazers, such as sheep and horses, in which grazing does not involve grasping with the tongue.

Attempts to control the condition have been only partially successful. Due to the aerophagic component of this anomaly, wind-sucking straps have sometimes been fixed to affected animals. Other control methods include the insertion of a metal ring through the frenulum of the tongue. Therapeutic success has been reported through the provision of diets improved by salt mixtures. The provision of freedom of movement is also believed to be helpful in the control of this condition. To prevent the spread of the anomaly, by associative induction, some specialists recommend the isolation of affected animals. Due to the suspicion of a hereditary predisposition some advisors recommend that tongue-rolling cattle should not be used for breeding. None of these measures is likely to be of any help to the animals.

Licking or crib-whetting

In stereotyped licking the tongue is applied repeatedly to an area of the animal's own body or to an object in the surroundings with the same pattern of movement. This action may result in injury to the tongue, a wearing away of the area licked or ingestion of substantial quantities of hair or other materials (see Chapter 33). Stereotyped licking occurs in situations where animals have inadequate quantities of food, no teat from which to suck, or insufficient total sensory input.

Some horses subject to chronic confinement show a form of anomalous oral behaviour in which the body of the tongue is slowly, but repeatedly, drawn across the edge of some part of the stall such as the crib or manger. The animal keeps the tongue still and firm during this action so that the behaviour does not represent true licking. It is difficult to extinguish this behaviour from the animal's repertoire of activities in the stable and prophylactic control calls for appreciation of the animal's potential needs. In some cases the provision of a salt block for licking seems to alleviate the habit. This gives rise to a suspicion that this anomalous tonguing may represent a salt desire.

Bar-biting, tether-biting or crib-biting

The animal opens and closes its mouth around a bar, tether or stable door engaging the tongue and teeth with the surface and performing chewing movements. Bar-biting has been described for pregnant sows housed in stalls or tethers which are very restrictive and do not allow the animal to turn around. The crate front and sides are made of metal piping. Tethers are commonly metal chains which the sow can bite and move up and down. Floors may be solid concrete or slats.

When engaged in bar-biting (Fig. 32.2) the sow takes into its mouth one of the cross bars at the front of the crate and bites it, rubs it with the body of the tongue or slides the mouth across the bar in rhythmic side to side motions (whetting). While biting the bar the sow may take a firm grip on it with its jaws or may press the body of the tongue against the bar. In some instances the sow disengages from the bar-biting and rubs its nose—above the snout—underneath the bar in side to side motions. Tether-biting occurs in much the same way but movements after the tether chain is taken into the mouth are more variable as the tether can be moved more than a bar can. The sequences of movements include series of elements which are repeated exactly and others which are more variable. Breaks in these activities occur so that they are produced in episodes of activity. Although trauma to the sow is not usually observed as a result of this condition, there are times when the related condition of snout-rubbing is injurious.

The anomalous behaviour of bar-biting and tether-biting can be partially controlled by improving the husbandry condition so as to provide the animal with oral occupation. This can be done by providing straw or sawdust as litter which the animal can chew or in which it can root. Bar-biting, crib-biting and other stereotypies are more frequent if straw or other manipulable material is not present (Fraser, 1975). Bar-biting and other stereotypies were not reduced by eating straw or oat hulls (Fraser, 1975; Broom and Potter, 1984) so it appears that the possibility to manipulate is important rather than the bulk of the diet. Substantially increased food rations do reduce its incidence however (Appleby and Lawrence, in press). Further details of such studies are reported in Chapter 38. Bar-biting may also be shown by cattle which are kept in close confinement (Fig. 32.3).

Horses crib-bite by grasping the edge of the manger or some other convenient fixture with the incisor teeth. The upper incisors are most often used alone. The subject presses down, raises the floor of the mouth, the soft palate is forced open and a swallowing movement occurs as a gulp of air is passed down the oesophagus into the stomach. (A "wind-sucker" achieves the same result but does not require a resting-place for the teeth.) Accompanying each effort of crib-biting there is usually a distinct grunt. In some cases horses may rest their teeth against the bottom of the manger, the lower edge of the rack or the end of a shaft or pole. In rare cases the mouth may be placed against the knees or cannons. Some horses which have been crib-biters may change to wind-suckers when remedial measures are attempted. Again, some wind-suckers in due course come to crib-bite. Some horses engage in these activities when alone in the stable but others will show it when in the company of other horses. Some affected animals will never show any signs of the disorder when under close supervision but most disregard the presence of humans and continue to practise the anomaly. Occasionally a horse will engage in this behaviour when at work, but the majority of cases only show the condition when in the stable. Young idle animals, standing in the company of confirmed crib-biters, may have the condition induced by association.

In crib-biters the incisor teeth, particularly of the upper jaw, show signs of excessive wear. This tooth wear may progress to such an extent that the incisors no longer meet when the mouth is shut and grazing then becomes impossible. The muscles of the throat increase in size. In the advanced condition, the animal becomes physically unfit.

Control of this condition is difficult and a change to less confined housing conditions is probably necessary. The most common measure is to fasten a strap round the throat, sufficiently tight to make arching of the neck uncomfortable, but not tight enough to interfere with respiration. Such straps usually require to be removed during feeding. In some types there is a metal "gullet-piece" which has a recess into which the wind pipe fits, and which allows the device to be worn without danger. Another preventative device consists of a hollow cylindrical perforated bit, which prevents the animal from making its mouth air-tight so long as it is worn. A thick rubber or wooden bit which prevents the jaws from closing is sometimes successful, but entails a certain amount of acute discomfort, and is not recommended on humane grounds. Very often crib-biters will cease the habit if housed in a bare-walled loose box, being fed from a trough which is removed as soon as the feed is finished. Preventive measures which have the desired effect at first often lose their efficiency after a time.

Surgery is sometimes performed. This is a highly specialised procedure which involves section of the throat muscles essential to the behaviour. It is a very drastic method of preventing an action which is induced by inadequate management and housing conditions.

Drinker-pressing

Pressing an automatic drinker repeatedly without ingesting the water. This stereotypy is shown by pregnant sows kept in stalls or tethers and provided with a nipple drinker. The drinker is one of the most interesting items in the animal's surroundings and some individuals spend long periods manipulating it (Table 32.2). In a study by Broom and Potter (1984) sows spent from 2 to 74 min pressing their drinkers during eight hours of daylight. The median time spent was 10 min which is considerably longer than is necessary for drinking.

33 Abnormal behaviour 2: Self-directed and environment-directed

The general principles of what constitutes behavioural abnormality are discussed in the previous chapter. Farm animals show some behaviour which is, for the most part, normal in its pattern but which is abnormal in respect of the object to which it is directed or the extent to which it occurs. In this chapter, those behaviours, other than stereotyped behaviour (Chapter 32), which are directed towards some part of the animal's own anatomy or some inanimate feature of the animal's surroundings, are discussed. Chapter 34 concerns abnormal behaviour directed towards other animals.

Self-mutilation

Self-injury through vigorous body friction or flank-biting is a serious behavioural anomaly in horses. Animals affected with this disorder may bite at their sides or rub their neck crests damaging the coat, the mane, the skin and occasionally causing flesh wounds. It is a form of behaviour which is characterised by its intensity and is sometimes accompanied by vocalisation. The disorder appears to occur more commonly in stallions than in mares or geldings.

As a means of control, affected animals can be given freedom of grazing since the condition typically occurs in circumstances of confinement and isolation. Tranquilisation may be necessary to terminate an episode. The provision of a stable companion can also be helpful in controlling the disorder (Houpt, 1981). While affected animals are not usually found to have any pathological skin condition, parasitism or gastrointestinal clinical condition, these matters should be taken into account in the assessment of the case.

Occasional individuals of all farm animal species show rubbing behaviour which results in the development of a wound and in certain circumstances animals will peck, bite or kick at themselves to an extent which results in injury. This behaviour is often associated with some localised infection, parasitism or pain (see Chapter 36), but extreme self-mutilation, like that shown by monkeys which are confined and deprived, may sometimes occur. The removal of hair, wool or feathers is considered in the next section.

Licking and eating own hair, wool or feathers

Many young calves housed in individual crates spend long periods of each day licking those parts of their bodies which they can reach. This behaviour, which may be stereotyped in form, results in the ingestion of large quantities of hair which aggregates into hair balls or bezoars in the rumen. Balls as large as 15 cm in diameter have been found in the rumens of calves (Groth, 1978) and these clog the rumen and openings to it. Digestive problems and even death can result from this. The excessive licking occurs most in early weaned calves—all dairy calves would come into this category—and more in individually housed than in group-housed calves. Ingestion of such material is occasionally shown by young lambs and by poultry but this is more frequently a different kind of behaviour which is addressed to other individuals. Some caged birds, e.g. parrots, do pull out their own feathers, with or without eating them.

Sucking and eating solid objects

Recently weaned mammals will often suck and lick the walls and bars of their pens in a non-stereotyped way. Such behaviour is particularly frequent in young calves and piglets which are weaned at a much earlier age than would occur naturally. Calves separated from their mothers in the first few days after birth will nibble, chew and suck at any object in their environment but they suck more on teat-shaped objects, especially artificial teats and the appendages of other calves (Waterhouse, 1978; Broom, 1982; van Putten and Elshof, 1982). Such behaviour will be discussed further in the next chapter.

Amongst older animals of all species, chewing at or eating solid objects is occasionally recorded. The seeking out and eating of wood, cloth and old bones and other objects by cattle and sheep is sometimes referred to as pica. In some circumstances such behaviour is a result of phosphorus deficiency which can be remedied by ingesting some of the materials for it is frequent amongst free-range animals on phosphorus-deficient land. Control of this abnormal behaviour should obviously take the form of supplying phosphorus to affected animals. It has been found that merely offering a phosphorus-rich supplement, such as bone meal, may not be sufficient to rectify a serious deficiency. Some deficient animals fail to ingest a sufficient quantity of the supplementary feed to attain satisfactory body levels of phosphorus. In such instances phosphorus would be required to be given by injectable solution.

Abnormal chewing and eating of wood, or lignophagia is not uncommon in horses in confined quarters or paddocks. It is not restricted to stalled horses since it can, as often, be observed in horses in outdoor enclosures Fig 32.3. Even in pastures, wood-chewing may take the form of debarking tree trunks. It is believed, however, that close confinement aggravates the condition (Sambraus, 1985).

Wood-chewing can lead to serious intestinal obstruction (Green and Tong, 1988). Although wood-chewing horses do not usually ingest most of the wood they chew, some splinters may be consumed and some can cause damage within the mouth. Excessive tooth wear also occurs. Affected animals may transmit the habit to associating horses. This can lead to the destruction of wooden fences, partitions and doors.

The condition appears to be associated with a desire for roughage or cellulose. Lack of roughage in the diet undoubtedly predisposes a horse to wood-chewing. Horses fed on concentrate diets with a low supply of roughage show the condition much more frequently than horses fed hay in abundance. A wood-chewer may chew 0.5 kg of wood a day from stall edgings. It has been found that ponies confined to stalls and fed a high concentrate diet spend 10% of their time wood-chewing. When a high roughage diet was given wood-chewing dropped to 2% of eating time.

Control of wood-chewing can be attempted by regular creosote painting of the wooden surfaces available to the horse but this would not prevent debarking of trees. Access to extensive pasture should be helpful in treating this condition in theory, but in practice the habit can persist and trees can be ringed by debarking. The wood chewing habit can be inhibited by the inclusion of sawdust in a high concentrate diet and this can be considered as a control measure when access to pasture is not possible.

Eating litter, earth or dung

Many animals are kept on bedding which is a potential food source for them so it is not surprising that pigs, cattle and horses will eat some of their straw bedding. This is not abnormal behaviour unless carried to an extreme. However, some litter which is used for animals is almost or completely non-nutritive and yet animals which are confined in a small space will eat their bedding, even after it has become soiled. Almost every horse in the confines of a stable can be observed to eat soiled litter on occasion, but with some horses this activity occurs habitually. The habit develops, notably in horses and in poultry, even in circumstances of husbandry which provide them with an abundance of proper feed. It is generally noted that litter-eating is practised on wood particles and chaff so that it may represent, to some degree, a depraved appetite for cellulose (Anon., 1981).

Litter-eating as seen in chicks and turkeys occurs most commonly when they are reared on chaff or wood litter. The incidence of this behaviour is highest within flocks which are not provided with sufficient feed trough space. The incidence is also higher in some breeds and strains of birds than others and this indicates a genetic predisposition to the condition. Some specialists believe that the condition can be alleviated by supplying an abundance of grit to birds and it may be that the depraved appetite component of litter-eating represents a search for mineral material.

Birds which practise litter-eating are liable to develop impaction of the gizzard or other alimentary region and this in turn causes death in many cases. When horses practise litter-eating they become increasingly indiscriminate with regard to the nature of the litter eaten and may eat mouldy, contaminated bedding. Colic is liable to occur in such cases with severe illness and death as possible consequences.

In the horse several causes of litter-eating are recognised. Imbalanced rations, feeding at the wrong time of day and heavy worm burdens

have all been found to contribute to this condition. Horses kept outdoors graze most of the day and eating is clearly their major occupation. Within stables this occupation is curtailed and grain or compounded food is often consumed quickly. If such food is not followed up with the provision of clean hay, for ingestive occupation as much as balanced nutrition, horses are likely to seek other available materials to consume.

In the control of litter-eating in poultry it is important to ensure that there is abundant feed trough space so that birds in low positions within the peck order have an opportunity to find secure space somewhere at the feed trough. Without adequate trough space they are likely to be driven away despotically and start to eat litter in compensation. In the horse, control of this abnormal behaviour requires close attention to all aspects of the diet. Appraisal of feed is necessary to ensure adequate quantity and variety. Supplementary feed should be provided in the form of salt licks and mixtures rich in minerals and vitamins. Fresh feed, such as grass or greens or carrots, should be offered regularly. Feeding times should be observed on a precise timetable with late-night or early-morning feeding being included in the schedule. Horses found to have a worm burden should obviously receive effective, appropriate anti-helminthic treatment.

Horses and cattle sometimes practise the habit of eating soil, sand or dirt. Animals with this practice are susceptible to alimentary dysfunctions. The condition has been termed geophagia and has been thought to be the result of mineral-deficient diets. Phosphorus and iron deficiencies are known, in some cases, to be responsible for soil-eating, but other affected animals do not appear to have a nutritional deficiency. Close confinement and lack of exercise appear to be the most common causal circumstances.

Excessive eating of sand or dirt can result in sand impaction of the caecum and colon in the horse. Sand impactions have also been enountered in cattle in the abomasal region as a consequence of this habit. Sand impaction appears to be more common in some geographical regions than others; it is, for example, more frequently encountered in Florida than in other parts of the USA.

Control of this condition should take into account the possibility of a mineral deficiency and a supplementary ration of bone meal should be provided to eliminate the possibility of phosphorus deficiency. In addition affected animals can be examined for anaemia and worm burdens and appropriate treatment provided when indicated. Confined animals should be provided with enforced exercise.

Coprophagia, the eating of faeces, occurs most notably in horses. The habit is so common in foals under conventional management that it is generally considered as normal behaviour in these animals, although apart from the possibility of helping to establish an adequate gut flora it would seem to be maladaptive. Coprophagia in the adult horse is anomalous and is induced by particular circumstances, as revealed in the case histories of affected animals. Coprophagia also occurs in pigs in association with the anomaly of anal massaging (Sambraus, 1979).

Adult horses practising coprophagia are typically under chronic enclosure in loose boxes. They have often undergone a change in use or management, say for example from regular exercise to no exercise or from regular routine to neglected routine. Affected animals consume their own faeces in substantial quantity. Faecal material is not left in its normal form but becomes broken up and consumed to varying extent. In some cases most of the faeces are regularly consumed.

Control of this condition in the horse can be done by muzzling the subject. Horses in loose boxes showing coprophagia can be removed to tie stalls or cross-tied but it is best to remedy the underlying husbandry defect.

Overeating

Overeating, or hyperphagia, and rapid eating are habits observed in some horses and occasion-ally in cattle. Many horses are extremely greedy and rapid eaters. In the course of bolting their food some of these animals may choke. Since the food consumed is not fully masticated digestive disorders can occur. Sometimes when cattle gain access to a feed bin containing concentrate rations they will consume excessive quantities and this can lead to serious digestive illness. When grain is consumed in excessive quantity in cattle it leads to a condition known as "grain overload". This condition is usually fatal.

The control of hyperphagia involves tactical feeding of horses. Spreading the grain in a thin layer in the trough or placing large smooth stones in the bottom of the trough are methods used to make grain difficult to consume rapidly. Supplying the grain in feed at several different times in the day may be helpful. Feeding hay before grain is also helpful. Controlling grain overload in cattle involves securing feed bins and ensuring that cattle quarters do not permit easy access to such bins. Cases of grain overload require radical therapy and may call for rumenotomy. Occasionally hyperphagia is a consequence of malfunction of the hypothalamus and may not be treatable.

Polydipsia

As mentioned in the previous chapter, some confined sows spend long periods showing stereotyped drinker-pressing but this is not polydipsia, or excessive drinking, because little of the water is ingested. Polydipsia nervosa is seen in some horses which are isolated and confined in stalls with water supplied ad libitum. Some horses will consume about 140 litres daily, or about three to four times the normal quantity. This excessive consumption can be spread over a period or may be concentrated within a relatively short time of two or three hours. An associated polyuria may be the first indication of the anomaly. Excessive drinking is also encountered in other species which are subject to close confinement and in these cases also the water consumption by the individual usually represents a two- to four-fold increase in the normal water intake. It has been observed in sheep subject to chronic close confinement in stalls and in metabolism crates. It has also been recorded in pigs kept in single stalls. In the latter case the quantity of water consumed was approximately double the normal volume. It occurs also in caged poultry.

While it is difficult to be precise about the adverse effects of this anomaly on the animal, the constant flushing of ingesta probably reduces the nutritional value of the ration. In some instances polydipsia has been noted among subjects in the "thin sow" syndrome. Autopsies performed on horses which have died from gastric or intestinal volvulus sometimes show a significantly large volume of water in the part of the alimentary canal which has undergone the twist. In some quarters of veterinary expertise there is a strong suspicion that the sudden intake of an abnormally large quantity of water may allow a segment of the alimentary canal to become heavily loaded and liable to twist. This seems as probable an explanation as any other of the precipitant factors in màny cases of gut-twist in the horse.

Polydipsia does not appear to be an anomaly which becomes fixed securely in the animal's behaviour. The condition therefore lends itself to control by appropriate management which would include the provision of rationed water. Polydipsia is most common in close confined animals given little exercise and the habit can be controlled and broken by providing better housing and regular exercise.

34 Abnormal behaviour 3: Addressed to another animal

Animals which are kept with other members of their own species, or which have an opportunity to interact with members of other species, can direct abnormal behaviour to those other animals. Much of this behaviour involves behaviour patterns which are in the normal repertoire but which are inappropriately directed. The behaviours described in this chapter are grouped according to the apparent motivational state of the animal. Animals sometimes treat other animals, or parts of their anatomy, as if they were objects to be investigated, obtained, or eaten, just as were the objects described in the last chapter. Other types of abnormal behaviour are directed inappropriately towards other animals as if they were a sexual partner, a mother, or a rival.

Animals treated as objects

The behaviour which precedes activities described in this section is often indistinguishable from that which precedes activities reported in Chapter 27. The animal approaches another individual, or more often a particular part of that individual, as if it were exploring its environment or looking for food. In circumstances where the animal approached is unable to move away because of lack of space or the close proximity of other animals, an action may be completed which is damaging to that animal.

Egg-eating

In such behaviour it is an egg, rather than a freely moving animal, to which the actions are directed. Egg-eating is a habit found in chickens kept in pens and cages. It appears to occur equally readily among flocks on deep litter and on wire mesh floors. The behaviour begins with a bird pecking at an egg until it is broken. The contents of the egg are then partially ingested. When a bird acquires this habit it is likely to increase the practice and other birds may also acquire the habit through mimicry. In some cases significant amounts of eggshell are eaten and this leads to the suspicion that the diet of affected birds may be deficient in grit. To some extent problems of this nature popularised the introduction of battery caging some decades ago but Sambraus (1985) considers that it is more of a problem in cages.

Control of this condition involves the elimination of affected birds but this may be difficult in a large flock as the perpetrators are difficult to identify. It is sometimes found possible to inject strong food dye into the substance of an egg and have this egg left lying on the ground. An egg-eating bird choosing this egg will be marked by coloration about the head. It is advisable to provide a supply of grit or oyster shell chips in dealing with problems of this nature. It is important to lay out the grit in long troughs so that birds at any level in the peck order can have occasional access to it. In cages the problem is reduced if eggs can roll away out of reach of the birds. The provision of nest boxes in larger cages reduces egg-eating as floor eggs are eaten most frequently. Where birds have access to free range or smaller outside runs, egg-eating is reduced if they can be turned out regularly by mid-day, for laying should be over by this time.

Wool-pulling and wool-eating

Wool-pulling is a form of abnormal behaviour which occurs in sheep within restrictive enclosure and indoor management systems. It is clear that crowding within pens is a contributing factor but it is also believed that a deficiency of roughage in the diet may contribute to it. In addition to pulling wool from associating members of a group the individual sheep also ingests some of the wool. It is therefore a compound anomaly and it should be distinguished from wool ingestion in young lambs which is the result of anomalous sucking.

Wool-pulling in adult sheep is usually practised by one individual within the group. In time the anomaly is induced in others by association. The sheep which receive most wool-pulling are usually those which are lowest in the social hierarchy within a group. The condition is therefore related to social dominance. In a pen in which there is intensive wool-pulling activity the amount of fleece lost is greatest in the animals low in the dominance order. The wool-pulling animal is usually identifiable through having an intact fleece. When wool-pulling first begins, affected animals are observed to pull with their mouths on the strands of wool on the backs of others. As afflicted sheep receive more attention from the wool-puller the long wool becomes denuded from the back area. Over this

region the fleece may be reduced to wool fibres of approximately three centimetres while fleece of normal length is still borne elsewhere on the body. As the anomaly intensifies, afflicted animals can lose wool so extensively over the entire body that they begin to appear semi-naked as a result of pink skin showing through the sparse remaining wool fibres.

Since this condition is clearly associated with overcrowding within indoor pens, control of the condition is possible through reduction in pen densities. Pens of about 20 m² can contain about 10 mature sheep but wool pulling is likely at this stocking level. A reduction to 50% of this density is effective in controlling wool-pulling. At this lower level of population concentration the anomaly can be eliminated, especially if there is also the provision of a regular supply of quality roughage. Hay is ideal but straw can also be useful for this purpose. While nutritional deficiencies have been suspected these have not been proved and it would appear that any nutritional need associated with this anomaly relates to an inadequacy of structured feed rather than any specific nutrient factor. Control can also be effected by releasing animals into outdoor, extensive husbandry conditions for long periods.

Young animals sometimes remove parts of the coats of their mothers whilst in close contact with them, by licking and sucking on parts of the maternal body other than the mammary gland. Young lambs may begin wool-eating as early as one or two weeks of age. The lamb sucks, chews and ingests the wool from parts of its mother's fleece on such regions as stomach, udder and tail. The accumulation of ingested wool in the lamb's stomach (abomasum) leads to the formation of compact fibrous balls (bezoars). Lambs with such wool balls may suffer severe colic attacks resembling fits. Affected lambs harbouring bezoars become anaemic, unthrifty and progressively lose bodily condition. Affected lambs stand for long periods in a stationary posture displaying distended stomachs with their backs arched. Complete alimentary obstruction, for example, in the region of the pyloris or small intestine, can cause death. Flock mortality rates can be as high as 10% (Hutyra *et al.*, 1959).

There appear to be seasonal fluctuations in the incidence of this condition in flocks of breeding sheep. Such fluctuation in incidence may also relate to deleterious features of husbandry such as the failure to clip excess wool from the ventral regions of ewes before lambing. Causal features may relate to a system of enclosure imposed on the ewe and lamb. It has also been suggested that since many of these lambs show preference for soiled wool there is an implication of depraved appetite with a specific suspicion of phosphorus deficiency, but this latter factor has not been proved to be significant in the etiology of this anomaly.

Since suspicion concerning nutritional factors exists in the ewe's condition, control of this condition justifies supply of good nutrition to breeding ewes including mineral and vitamin supplementation. Spatial arrangements suited to the resolution of the behavioural problem are a more rational method of control.

Feather-pecking, body-pecking and eating pecked matter

Feather-pecking is a form of anomalous behaviour which is common in poultry. Under conditions of intensive management it can occur in all ages and many species including chicks, adult hens, turkeys, ducks, quail, partridge and pheasants. The normal exploration and food investigation behaviour of such birds involves pecking, so it is not surprising that in a barren environment they investigate the feathers of other birds in this way. Hens crowded together on wire floors have few objects at which to peck. In these conditions birds peck on the backs, tail, ventral region and cloaca of associate birds. Mutual pecking, in which chicks in close parallel and opposite positions peck at each other, is common. In other cases several birds may be involved so that chains of peckers may form. Young birds have been observed to show no resistance or other response when their feathers are pecked but adult birds try to avoid being pecked and often assume a stooped submissive position (Wennrich, 1975a). In these cases it appears that social dominance dictates the right of one bird to peck at another. When feather-pecking within a pen escalates, the activity within the flock can lead to unrest which may depress egg yield (Kiel, 1963). Feather-pecking is especially prevalent in intensive husbandry systems and is seen most often in those breeds, such as light hybrids, which are "flighty" and hypersensitive to environmental stimuli. Environmental factors which are considered to initiate this behaviour including poor ventilation, high temperatures, low humidity, excessive population density, and excess illumination. Possibly one of the chief precipitating factors is inadequate trough space per bird. Feathers which are pecked from other birds may sometimes be eaten. Feathers may be picked out from preferred sites of other birds such as the tail and pinions which are the largest feathers in the body. In smaller chicks feathers are pecked mainly from the back and ventral region of the body. Pecked feathers are eaten and the manner in which feather-pecking behaviour proceeds for ingestive purposes is the same as that involved in food seeking and intake. Attempts to prevent the behaviour include increasing the searching aspect of feeding, for example by putting grains in the diet. Feather-eating is rare except in the intensive husbandry systems of battery cages or deep-litter pens.

Birds which feather-peck may subsequently start to peck and remove blood, skin and flesh from other birds (Brantas, 1975; Blokhuis and Arkes, 1984). Body-pecking and consequent cannibalism can begin when wounds arise due to feathers being pulled out when blood-filled new quills from the wings or tail are pecked and start to bleed (Sambraus, 1985). As many authors have noted, the outlet of the uropygial gland which protrudes slightly and the protruded cloaca after egg-laying elicit body-pecking. Feather-pecking does not lead inevitably to body-pecking and many more birds show feather-pecking. Body-pecking may also arise quite independently for it is shown in groups of young birds which are laying for the first time and which may not show feather-pecking. Neither feather-pecking nor body-pecking is preceded by threatening behaviour and both are preceded by body orientation and movements which are typical of investigatory behaviour. The bird pecked usually has little opportunity to escape but the failure of the pecker to respond differentially to an inanimate object and to another bird which responds, even by submission, is clearly abnormal. Pecked birds too are abnormal in their behaviour, for they cease to show much escape behaviour when pecked often, presumably because they have learned that previous escape attempts have proved fruitless.

Body-pecking is shown by domestic fowl, turkeys, pheasants, quail and ducks. One bird usually initiates the body-pecking but other birds are likely to join in so that pecked birds may be subjected to a barrage of pecks. The most severe effects often ensue after the cloaca has been pecked. Wounds in the cloacal region can rapidly become severe and the intestines can extrude through a cloacal wound. These are likely to be the subject of more pecking and in due course be pulled out and ingested. Mortality is therefore frequent once a wound has been produced.

Other parts of the body are also subjected to pecking. Head-pecking occurs in older birds confined together in cages whilst pecking at toes and back are sometimes widespread amongst younger birds. In toe-pecking the active bird pecks at the toes of associate birds and, on rare occasions, their own. While toe-pecking may not lead to significant wounds in the case of young chicks, wounds on the toes result from this behaviour in adult hens. Following injury there is bleeding and portions are then picked off the wound. The resultant open wound is liable to infection and further haemorrhage. Birds so afflicted show depression behaviour, retreating to a corner of the pen, refusing to eat and losing weight. In the absence of appropriate husbandry

intervention casualties occur. Head- and tail-pecking are often observed in young in over-crowded conditions. Injury and haemorrhage of head caruncle regions is not uncommon among male turkeys after fighting. Toe-pecking occurs more frequently in deep-litter pens than in caging. This may be due to the feet of associating birds being less accessible within crowded cages. It is believed that hybrid strains of birds show this behaviour more often than others.

The causation of feather-pecking and body-pecking with consequent cannibalism is described in Chapter 39 and in detail by Hughes (1984, 1985) and Blockhuis and van den Haar (1989).

The control of feather- and body-pecking is most commonly effected by beak-trimming, also called debeaking. Beak-trimming involves the removal of the anterior part of the upper mandible. By removal of this portion of the beak, pecking becomes inefficient but, as noted in Chapter 39, this is a painful procedure for birds. Beak-trimming does not eliminate aggressive picking entirely, or prevent the development of the peck order, but treated birds are less able to pull feathers. Another method used to control the condition is to limit the vision of birds. This can be done by darkening poultry pens and changing the light to a red hue through the use of infra-red lamps or painting window panes red. The vision of each individual bird can be restricted by fixing aluminium rings to the upper beak or applying ''poly-peepers'', although the use of such devices is banned in some countries. Where poly-peepers are in general use feather-pecking is minimal. None of these procedures can be carried out without some adverse effects on bird welfare and changes in the bird's environment which minimise the likelihood of the behaviour are preferable in the long run.

Anal massage

Young pigs rub their noses on other pigs, and whilst some of this behaviour is similar to teat-searching and udder-massage (see later section on belly-nosing), other behaviour appears to be of a more general investigatory nature. The anomalous behaviour of anal massage by snout-rubbing and ingestion of faeces seen in pigs occurs typically among growing pigs kept in crowded conditions. It is more noticeable where tail-docking at an early age is used for the control of tail-biting. Within their dense groups affected animals move from one animal to another, nosing the anal regions with upward massaging motions of the snout. Although some animals approached in this fashion avoid the contact, others do not. Anal massage is carried out with considerable pressure so that the snout of the active animal is pushed deeply into the perineum of the associated animal. Such an animal frequently responds to such pressure by reflex defaecation. When faeces are expelled as a result of this activity faecal ingestion occurs. This coprophagia may be carried out by the snout-rubbing animal alone or it may be joined in the activity by other pigs in the group (Sambraus, 1979).

Individual pigs implicated in this anomalous behaviour are active in going from one animal to another in a group, attempting this behaviour. Any animal which is seen to strain to defaecate may become the subject of intense snout-rubbing. Some pigs do not avoid snout-rubbing by showing any resistance and animals which tolerate such attention often acquire swelling wounds of the anus or adjacent perineal area. Such afflicted pigs become weak, have difficulty in standing, lose appetite and physical condition. Badly afflicted animals may die.

The control of anal massage and associated coprophagia can be attempted by easing crowded conditions. Since there is a suggestion that the anomaly can be induced in pigs in adjoining pens by visual association, solid walls between pens are preferred. This reduces association between pigs in different pens and appears to reduce the transfer of excitability and imitation. Anomalous snout-rubbing may be reduced by supplying pigs in pens with objects to occupy them by chewing and rooting.

Tail-biting

Of all the abnormal behaviours of farm animals tail-biting in pigs has attracted most attention due to the problem it has created in the pig industries. The behaviour is seen among growing pigs grouped in pens but it is sporadic in its occurrence. Tail-biting was recognised as a problem in pig rearing for many years but was not considered as a serious matter until the modern pig industry became established following World War II (Dougherty, 1976). The behaviour first appears with a pig taking the tail of another crossways into its mouth and chewing on it lightly. The animal receiving this attention usually tolerates it. In due course the tail-biting attention becomes more severe with resultant wounds on the tail and haemorrhage. It is believed that haemorrhage encourages more active tail-biting and other pigs in the group begin to chew on the damaged tail. The injured tail becomes progressively eaten away to its root. At this point associating tail-biting pigs may begin to bite the afflicted animal on other parts of the body such as the ears, the vulva and parts of the limbs. All of this behaviour is associated with much unrest in the pen-mates.

A pig injured as the result of excessive biting becomes submissive and then depressed in behaviour, reacting only slightly to being bitten. Wounds may become contaminated with infection resulting in abscessation of the hindquarters and the posterior segment of the spinal column. Secondary infection may occur in the lungs, kidneys, joints and other parts as a result of pyaemia.

It is difficult to induce tail-biting and hence difficult to study it experimentally (Ewbank, 1973). A variety of conditions are thought to predispose to tail-biting including breed type (e.g. Landrace), dense grouping of rapidly growing pigs of about 50 kg in weight, insufficient trough space, insufficient drinking facility, adverse environmental features (high levels of noise, noxious gas, humidity, temperature) (Gadd, 1967). Combinations of these and other factors lead to unrest within the group. The unrest evidently creates irritability, over-excitability and increased activity. It is believed that this is the development of motivational factors leading to tail-biting in an impoverished environment with little opportunity for diversive activities.

Oral activity is greater in the pig than in other farm species and pigs try to explore items in the environment with the snout or mouth by rooting and chewing. It is noticed that under extensive husbandry systems pigs engage in considerable mouthing activities including such acts as picking up and carrying sticks in the mouth and chewing up material for bedding. Phases of greater activity have been noted within pens of fattening pigs three to five months of age and about 50 kg in weight. Much activity within pig groups occurs during the morning and when temperatures are high. The cannibalistic behaviour of tail-biting is independent of a social hierarchy and it is found that it is frequently the smaller animals in a group which develop the habit (van Putten, 1978).

In the control of tail-biting, amputation of the distal half of the tail has become a widespread practice. It has been found that it is not necessary to remove the entire tail to prevent the anomaly developing. It appears that the distal half of the tail in the pig is comparatively insensitive. By removal of this part, the entire remaining section of the tail is sufficiently sensitive that pigs react effectively when a tail-biting attempt is made on them.

Other methods of controlling this behaviour involve husbandry (Bryant, 1972). Affected animals can be removed from the group to make a group of individuals all showing this behaviour. This can be done since mutual tail-biting does not usually occur when such animals are penned together. Atmospheric factors within the building should receive attention so that uncomfortable environmental factors are eliminated. Pens of growing pigs should be under-populated at the start when the group is first formed. This will ensure that the pen will still be adequate in size for the group when its

members have subsequently grown to twice or more their original sizes. General improvement and the quality of husbandry and the use of straw bedding are also frequently found to be beneficial in controlling this condition. Animals which have the opportunity to root in earth seldom show tail-biting so the proviion of earth may help to reduce the incidence of this and other abnormal behaviours in pigs.

Animals treated as sexual partners

Many farm animals are kept in single sex groups and seldom or never encounter a member of the opposite sex. Hence it is inevitable that sexual behaviour will often be directed to individuals of the same sex. Such behaviour may be considered abnormal in that it cannot result in offspring production but the normal development of sexual behaviour often involves parts of adult sexual behaviour being directed towards various individuals of either sex. Hence some homosexual acts or sexual behaviour towards other species is to be expected among young animals and may also have a function when shown by older animals. Homosexual interactions are very frequent among groups of cows. Cows and heifers in oestrus are mounted by other cows and this behaviour is used as a sign of oestrus by stockmen (Chapter 19). Occasionally such mounting can lead to injury but, partly because of its use to the stockman, it is not usually considered to be a problem. It has been suggested by Parker and Pearson (1976) that mounting by females is an effective way of attracting dominant males. Any benefit is derived by the mounted cow, which is in oestrus, but Parker and Pearson point out that the mounting is often reciprocated when the mounting cow is herself in oestrus. It is, however, questionable as to whether such mounting should be regarded as normal behaviour for it rarely occurs in wild or semi-wild cattle. Hall (in press) found that female–female mounting was not shown by Chillingham wild cattle in England except by animals found to be partially masculinised. Hence this behaviour must be considered to be abnormal, especially the high frequencies of mounting seen in the absence of a bull.

Sexual mounting of males by other males occurs frequently when young or mature male animals are held together in monosexual groups (Stephens, 1974). When this is a continuing arrangement as, for example, in the husbandry of large numbers of young bulls or rams being raised for breeding, it is found that the sexual orientation of these animals is inevitably directed to their own kind. The resultant behaviour evidently becomes established, by habit, in these animals. When exposed subsequently to female stock in conventional breeding arrangements some of these animals are incapable—for varying periods of time—to alter their sexual orientation. Homosexual rearing may lead to impotence in stud animals which will persist for a variable period in rams, bulls, boars and male goats, although it is not usually permanent (Price and Smith, 1984).

Control of this condition is difficult in forms of husbandry which are characterised by dense grouping of male animals. Such grouping is, in a sense, sometimes desirable in husbandry since these circumstances can induce the effect of "bachelor grouping" in which suppression of libido is a notable feature. Given exposure to female stock, libido can be stimulated and aggressive interaction between males may result in husbandry problems. Mixed grouping is not therefore feasible. Outbreaks of mounting and riding in entire bull calves, which can result in injuries, are prevented when the calves are kept with their dams, who inhibit such outbreaks of socially maladaptive behaviour. Since social facilitation is also a likely component of this problem (Stricklin, 1976), reduction in group size whenever possible helps to control the condition. A very notable form of homosexual behaviour exists as "the buller steer syndrome".

In beef cattle production it has been known for many years that some bullocks, or steers, will stand to be mounted by other steers under conventional pasturage conditions. In extensive grazing the condition does not represent a serious problem and these animals, or "bullers", do not suffer from excessive mounting. Under commercial feedlot conditions the incidence of bulling has increased and serious economic losses continue to occur from this syndrome of anomalous behaviour. It is recognised that these bullers characteristically stand to be mounted but will also engage in mounting other bullers. In addition, some steers, despite the fact that they are castrated, are active "riders" on bullers. In cattle feedlots some riders repeatedly mount a few specific bullers. This may continue until the riders lose weight and the bullers become exhausted, injured or collapse. Death may also occur following injury to bullers and it has been estimated that the economic loss in feedlot systems in North America due to bulling is second only to respiratory disease. Its incidence has been generally estimated at about 4% (Klemm *et al.*, 1983, 1984).

Although the buller syndrome can occur in feedlots where synthetic hormones are not used, the incidence of the condition rises in such feedlots following hormonal administration, such as injection with progesterone and oestradiol, or oral administration of DES (stilboestrol) (Schake *et al.*, 1979). A common denominator in the buller steer syndrome is that both bullers and riders are castrated with a growth-promoting female sex hormone compound. Physiologically, buller steers have been found to have more creatinine, 17-hydroxy-corticosterone and oestrogen in their urine and blood globulin than normal steers. In spite of these features, there is general acknowledgement that other factors contribute to the aetiology of the syndrome and increasingly it has been recognised that a further common denominator in affected groups is a high population of animals within a group. While crowding may be a contributing factor it is now thought that total population size within a feedlot is more important. It would appear that crowding stress, together with a mixture of other husbandry factors, such as hormone administration, vaccination and dipping, constitute the causal circumstances. To compound the group stress, repeated introduction of new steers into feedlots is now found to increase the buller incidence.

While it has been commonly believed that bullers are steers which are excessively feminised and give off sexually stimulating pheromones, this is now questioned. It has become recognised that both bullers and riders are much more aggressive animals than sexually neutral steers in the same feedlot. It is commonly observed that bullers are the largest and most aggressive steers in a feedlot. Although bullers may be submissive to riders, this is a relative state since they are found to be more non-sexually aggressive in most instances.

It would appear that bullers and riders are those animals which involve themselves in intense social interactions. The vast majority of steers in cattle pens, by contrast, avoid social interactions in a manner typical of normal social bovine behaviour. As a result it now appears that competitive activity results in the behaviours of bulling and riding and that, among both groups, riders are those in a marginally higher social position than bullers. Amongst competing animals, riding may be used to impose social dominance. At high stocking densities social contests may occur more intensively, resulting in a greater amount of riding.

The quality of contact must be quickly recognised as the real nature of this social–sexual problem, which may prove to have a hyposerotonergic basis. Aversive social encounters are a prominent feature of chronic, restrictive enclosures of high-density groups. The agonistic content in dominance hierarchies is roughly in proportion to social concentration. In addition, social rank disparities are greater, and occur more frequently, when the number of animals in a given space increases. More aggression occurs when the amount of space for a given quantity of animals, in number or bulk, decreases. In other words, as animal volume per unit of group space increases, so the quality of social exchange declines.

There is no doubt that the buller steer syndrome is a welfare problem as well as an economic problem. The behaviour is part aggressive and part sexual. Control of this condition really requires reduction of population pressure and withdrawal of hormonal stimulus. Partial control can be exercised through supervision. It is the practice in most large feedlots to observe steers closely at least once each day. This allows steers in the process of becoming bullers to be identified quickly and removed from the system before injuries occur. Removed steers can be placed in a separate lot with fewer animals and this allows the condition to subside. It has been found that recovery from the syndrome is possible following a short period of isolation. Animals housed indoors are sometimes deterred from mounting by bars placed over the pen, which physically prevent mounting, or by electric wires over the pen. Both of these measures fail to deal with the root of the problem and the electric wires may lead to severe effects on some individuals.

Animals treated as mother

Young mammals which are separated from their mother at an earlier time than the normal weaning age often show teat-seeking and sucking behaviour which is directed towards inanimate objects (Chapter 33) or pen-mates. Sometimes this behaviour, which is called belly-nosing and intersucking in piglets and calves, persists into adulthood.

Belly-nosing

Belly-nosing is a behaviour shown by piglets which is an up and down movement of the snout and the top of the nose on the belly of other pigs and on the soft tissue between their hind legs and between their fore legs. This behaviour was described by van Putten and Dammers (1976) and Schmidt (1984) and it is similar in form to the massaging movements directed by piglets towards the udder of the sow. Belly-nosing is not shown before weaning but is shown by piglets which have been weaned much earlier than the normal weaning age (Fraser, 1978b).

Since many piglets are weaned at 3–5 weeks of age, which is 2–3 months before weaning would occur in the absence of human influence, the behaviour is very widespread. Some piglets kept in flat-deck cages are pursued and belly-nosed for long periods and their nipples, umbilicus, penis or scrotum may become inflamed. In some cases, male piglets urinate when belly-nosed and the belly-noser ingests the urine (M. A. Barton, personal communication). High levels of belly-nosing were negatively correlated with weight gain in the study by Fraser (1978b). Various authors have suggested that animals which are often belly-nosed may be weaker than the average but it is not clear that belly-nosing is the cause of the weakness.

The control of belly-nosing can be simple for the behaviour is seen much less in animals weaned later than 6 weeks of age. The incidence of the behaviour is also reduced by the provision of straw which the piglets can manipulate (van Putten and Dammers, 1976; Schouten, 1986). In the study by Schouten belly-nosing was seen most frequently during the transition from an active to a resting phase. Piglets in a bare crate spent several minutes in this transition and often showed belly-nosing at this time. Those provided with straw usually lay down simultaneously and started chewing straw. As a consequence the duration of belly-nosing was significantly greater in the piglets without straw.

Intersucking by calves

Calves separated from their mothers suck and lick at their own bodies, at objects in their pens (Chapter 33) and at parts of the bodies of other calves. They commonly suck on the navel, prepuce, scrotum, udder and ears of other animals. Sucking the scrotum is very common among male calves. The testes are pushed up by the nose of the sucking calf which then sucks on the empty scrotal sac. The posture and position of the sucking animals is that of the naturally suckling calf and includes the pushing movements the calf normally directs at the cow's udder. The calves which are sucked usually show a passive response. Such calves suck others in their turn and this leads to "chains" of sucking and sucked calves in which several animals may be involved. If the coat of the other calf is sucked significant quantities of hair may be ingested leading to formation of balls (see Chapter 33). If the penis is sucked, urine is often produced and then drunk by the sucking calf. This can lead to liver disorders and to reduced nutrient intake. Another adverse consequence of intersucking is that the part of the calf sucked may become inflamed, damaged and infected (Kiley-Worthington, 1977).

Experimental studies have shown that injurious intersucking is more common in bucket-fed calves than in those fed from the mother or an artificial teat (Czako, 1967; Kittner, 1967; Scheurmann, 1974). The presence of the teat is important but the time taken to feed is also a factor. Calves suckling their mothers spend 60 min per day doing so but bucket-feeding calves spend only 6 min per day (Sambraus, 1985). Hence in the control of this anomaly the best results are obtained by providing feeding conditions which resemble those of normal ingestive behaviour in young animals. It is found that feeding calves with milk through automatic nursers with teats whose aperture is such that the sucking time of each feed period is sufficiently prolonged will reduce the likelihood that other objects or calves will be sucked. Sucking periods lasting approximately 30 min appear to eliminate intersucking. Another remedy is tying up calves for an hour following bucket-feeding, for this evidently allows time for the desire to suck to diminish so that intersucking is not shown so often after that time period. The supply of supplemental roughage, such as 150 g of a supply of straw, can also result in a reduction in intersucking. Urine drinking can be reduced by the plentiful supply of water from a normal drinker for the calves. Mees and Metz (personal communication) provided calves with water trickling down a wall or pipe and the animals licked that water rather than showing urine drinking.

Intersucking or milk-sucking by adult animals

This behaviour involves a cow or bull sucking milk from the udder of a cow. The forms of this anomalous behaviour can vary (Grommers, 1977). Among adult milking cattle, sucking the udders of other members of the dairy herd is seen periodically. Such intersucking by adult cattle involves the withdrawal of milk from a lactating animal and is a behavioural abnormality of occasional occurrence under a variety of circumstances of husbandry. Among "suckler" herds of cows with nursing calves, "sneak sucking" may occur by alien calves or by an adult animal such as a bull. On rare occasions milking cows are discovered with the habit of sucking milk from their own udders.

Cattle which suck milk from herd mates characteristically choose the same lactating animal and this leads to a paired arrangement. Within such pairs it is sometimes found that animals will mutually suck each other, either simultaneously or alternately. Intersucking instances usually take place during periods of idling by the herd. They are therefore more easily seen among cattle awaiting the evening milking or resting in the early afternoon when grazing animals often loaf.

The loss of milk from intersucking can become significant and frequent sucking by an adult can lead to teat damage, pathological changes and deformation of the udder. Within some very large dairy herds this behavioural anomaly can represent a serious problem with as many as 10% of lactating cattle becoming involved in affected dairy herds. The anomaly is worsened by the influence of social facilitation and by the large numbers in modern herds.

Factors leading to milk-sucking are various. It is believed that the anomaly may relate to hereditary predisposition in some cases; the condition is seen more frequent in the Jersey breed than in the Holstein, for example. Little doubt exists, however, that the anomaly is husbandry-related in many cases and that the condition can increase in frequency as a result of imitation. In contrast with the condition in the young calf, intersucking behaviour in the adult animal is more common in open husbandry systems. Wood *et al.* (1967) report that those calves which show intersucking may go on to intersuck milk as adults and other authors have suggested that various forms of experience with or without teats in calfhood may increase or decrease intersucking as an adult. The behaviour is sufficiently unpredictable, however, that is a difficult subject for experimentation. Waterhouse (1978, 1979) reared calves individually with a non-nutritive teat on the wall of the pen for three months but neither those calves nor any without such a teat showed intersucking as adults.

In the interests of control it is advisable to have close supervision of the herd when an adult intersucking case has been suspected. By this means, confirmation of the subject can be obtained and spread of the condition by mimicry can be arrested. As a preventive measure, an increased provision of roughage can be made in the diet. Such roughage should be offered during periods when idling occurs. Since there is strong suspicion of a heritable nature it may be unwise to breed from animals showing the adult disorder.

Attempts to control anomalous milk-sucking in the past have taken the form of applying devices, which carry pointed prongs, to the face and nose region of the sucking animal. The attempt is to ensure that the animal seeking to suck will cause an avoidance reaction in any animal approached. Unfortunately, some of these devices can hinder the affected animal's natural feeding. Furthermore, if the affected animal is persistent, it can inflict wounds on other animals. A modern electrical device secured to the forehead and giving an electrical shock to the wearer when the circuit is closed by head pressure is reported to give good results. Since the shock is received by the sucking animal the method is more appropriate than older methods in which the aversive stimulation was directed at the receiving animal. In the latter case the affected animal was not subject to treatment. Even with modern devices, intersucking is a problem which may persist in some cases so that the culling of affected animals becomes necessary.

Animal treated as rival

Some aggressive behaviour shown towards members of the same or other species is normal. It serves a function in defence of the individual, defence of the young, or establishment of ownership or social position. Problems arise in farm animal husbandry where a situation which is conducive to aggressive behaviour is created and that aggression is particularly severe in its effects or too frequent. Aggressive behaviour which leads to welfare problems is discussed in Chapters 37–39. Some of this behaviour would be considered to be abnormal because of its intensity or frequency. Threats or attacks directed towards man are a cause for concern but many of these are not abnormal behaviour. A cow with a calf or a bull which attacks a stockman is not behaving abnormally. The process of domestication has not led to the elimination of all defensive or competitive behaviour directed towards man although it has reduced it considerably. Certain forms of husbandry make such behaviour much more likely to occur than do others.

The threat display of a bull is a sequence of actions which all of those who might encounter a bull should know.

1. The animal turns towards the source of stimulus with the long axis of the body acutely angled. The animal's head and neck are slightly deviated, more obliquely from this line. In this position the animal presents the lateral aspects of the head, neck and shoulder closer to the stimulus than the hind parts, which are turned away slightly.
2. The line of the back, from the withers to the tail head drops as a result of the hind legs being drawn slightly forward below the abdomen.
3. There is fixation and protrusion of the orbit.
4. Hair on the dorsal aspect of the neck is erected.
5. Muscular rigidity is demonstrated by the tenseness of the posture.
6. Deep monotonal vocalisations or snorts may accompany the display.

In the case of the horse there is muscular tension, extending the head, laying back the ears and exophthalmos, which causes the sclera of the eyeball to become visible. This latter feature has been termed by horsemen as "showing the white of the eye". In other animals such as boars, tenseness of posture through muscular rigidity is a prominent feature of threatening.

The horned ungulates defend or attack by striking aggressively with the head. In polled animals the blow delivered is in the form of a knock while in the horned animals the effect may be one of goring, i.e. horning. Some individuals may show heading behaviour. These animals use their heads in threat displays where the head is worked into the ground and the earth is loosened. Butting by bulls and male goats is a very well known behaviour problem. It would appear that the habit occurs most often in animals confined by themselves and which have previously experienced some degree of socialisation through close human contact. In some instances the behaviour is directed at physical structures such as doors or gates.

Biting is exhibited occasionally by horses. Stallions are particularly prone to this but young horses and chronically enclosed horses may also exhibit the behaviour (Houpt, 1981). The biting is usually in the form of snapping and nipping with the incisor teeth on the body of any person coming within reach or approaching the animal. This biting behaviour is aggressively directed in some instances to other horses. The typical biter exhibits the behaviour with the warning signals of ears laid flat, lips retracted, teeth bared and tail often switching. Biting attempts are usually very sudden.

Rearing and striking with the fore feet is a dangerous habit of some horses, more commonly seen in stallions and in light horses than in others. Striking out with one fore limb may be done, of course, without rearing. Animals which have this tendency, or disposition, in their behaviour may exhibit it when first approached or may show it after they have been held by the head in restraint for a period.

In kicking with the hind feet together the feet can be used to strike out explosively to reach another animal or person within four to six feet. Sometimes the kicking is directed at stall partitions (Chapter 33). This of course is a natural method of self-defence among horses and becomes anomalous when it is practised habitually and aggressively. The head is lowered, the body is lifted behind the withers and both hind limbs are vigorously extended backwards. Kicking with one hind foot is again a natural defensive action in ungulates when the individual space of the animal, in the region of its posterior pole, is invaded. It is usually delivered sharply in one downwards or backwards direction without full extension of the limb.

One particular version of a single hind limb kick is the "cow kick", so named because it is the common natural method of kicking in cattle. In the cow kick one hind limb is briefly projected forward, outward and backward. Another hind limb kick involves the extended projection of the limb forward, sideways and backward at full stretch. Such kicks often are delivered with precise aim. This contrasts to kicking backwards both hind feet at 180 degrees to the spine. Such extended hind limb kicking is a feature of mule behaviour and this type of kick is sometimes termed a "mule kick". Some horses are able to reach as far forward as the shoulder during such kicks.

The control of all of these aggressive actions is complex. In some cases, avoidance of the specific eliciting circumstances is the answer. In others training procedures are necessary and many books have been written on this. For most animals, early experience is of importance and housing conditions can have a considerable effect. Bulls and stallions which have been confined for a long period are often particularly dangerous to man. Long-term isolation of dairy bulls during rearing and during adulthood often results in animals being dangerous to man and to other cattle, whereas bulls kept in groups are much less aggressive (Hunter and Couttie, 1969).

35 Abnormal behaviour 4: Failure of function

The conditions which are imposed on farm animals lead to some abnormalities of sexual behaviour, parental behaviour and basic body movements which are inadequacies of function rather than stereotypies or active misdirection of behaviour. Individual variation within a farm animal species also accounts for some anomalous behaviour. In this chapter such abnormalities are described, factors affecting their occurrence are discussed, and possible control measures are considered.

Inadequacies of sexual functioning

Failure to reproduce or delay in reproduction is an important economic problem and such failure often involves behavioural inadequacy (Lindsay, 1985). Such abnormalities in behaviour can be most conveniently dealt with according to the phase of the reproductive cycle that is affected. Oestrus and libido are, of course, the important prerequisites for reproduction and it is in these areas that some of the principal anomalies of reproductive behaviour occur.

Silent heat

In some animals the physiological changes of oestrus occur without the behavioural features usually associated with them being evident. This condition is termed "silent heat" and its occurrence emphasises the dichotomy which can occur with respect to physiological oestrus and behavioural oestrus (Fraser, 1968). Silent heat, which is something of a misnomer, emphasises the fact that normal oestrus is principally a behavioural phenomenon.

The terms "silent heat", "quiet ovulation" and "suboestrus" are extensively used synonymously for this condition, which is of common occurrence (Rottensten and Touchberry, 1957). Among dairy cattle an overall incidence of 20–30% has been recorded by various observers in a variety of countries and it has been reported to occur more among high-producing cows (Morrow, 1966). The incidence in cattle is highest among heifers low in position in the social hierarchy of the herd. Silent heat is not uncommon in mares, ewes and sows.

The anomaly relates to absent or weak manifestation of overt behavioural oestrus in animals which have all the other, physical, characteristics of the phenomenon including uterine turgidity and congestion, with follicular ripening leading to ovulation. The physical characteristics in this condition are so complete that these animals are capable of being fertilised if bred artificially. Mares with this condition, for example, are found to have a normal level of fertility if forcefully bred. Similarly in cattle, if the condition can be satisfactorily identified, artificial insemination at an appropriate time can be associated with normal levels of fertility.

Silent heat is a normal physiological condition in sheep at the commencement of the breeding season. It is also considered to be a normal function of ovarian activity in the early post-partum period of cattle. This may be true also of pigs. The condition is anomalous in its occurrence at other times and has long been recognised as a breeding problem which was historically termed "breeding shyness".

The incidence of the condition is sometimes found to be very high in contemporary systems of dairy cow management which involve large numbers of animals being managed in a single group. In these groups the population density is such that there is ongoing social confusion which leads to instability in the social hierarchy. As indicated above, this form of social stress is known to be a cause of oestrus suppression. Excessive noise, temperatures above 30°C and other extreme weather conditions can all lead to suppression of oestrus behaviour (Hurnick, 1987).

Control of this condition must relate to improved management of breeding animals so as to minimise the amount of social stress.

Male impotence

During the breeding of farm animals under conditions where male and female are together for a short period only it is sometimes found that the male animal does not respond to the breeding female. Among cattle there sometimes occurs a condition of "somnolent impotence" in bulls which have an abnormally protracted reaction time at breeding. In this condition the bull lays its chin on the hindquarters of the cow and directs little attention to the latter. The animal maintains an inactive stance with which there is an appearance of somnolence, created by the eyes being partially or periodically closed

much of the time. This condition has been recognised as a breeding problem of considerable significance. It appears to occur more in beef breeds than in others and, to date, has been most often recognised in the Hereford and Aberdeen Angus breeds. In these breeds the condition is refractory to treatment and, in such circumstances, becomes a state of behavioural sterility which usually leads to the animal being culled (Fig. 35.1).

Coital disorientation

During the controlled breeding of the larger farm animals it is standard practice to have the

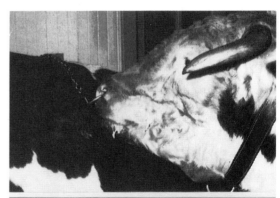

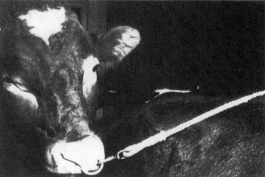

Fig. 35.1 Somnolent impotence in bulls characterised by inactivity and inattention to the "teaser" or oestrous cow.

female secured and the male led to her on a lead rope. This action initiates reaction time, which is the time lapsing between initial contact and mounting. Immediately following contact it is normal for the male animal to align himself in the same long axis as the female. The active alignment is normally carried out positively and briskly. Once assumed, alignment is generally fully maintained up to the time of mounting. In a number of cases male animals show positional disorientation such that the animal's long axis is markedly deviated from the female axis. Such deviation is maintained throughout the reaction time which, under these circumstances, is normally so protracted that mating fails to occur.

Coital disorientation can be seen occasionally in young and inexperienced male animals but this is not normally an inactive condition or one that is maintained for long. In the truly anomalous condition the animal is inactive and is found to be behaviourally impotent in most cases. The condition can be encountered in all farm species of livestock, notably bulls and goats, and has been studied most specifically in the male goat which has a seasonal phase of comparative impotence in many individuals.

Features of the studied condition are as follows:

1. The two factors of disalignment and impotence are very closely related in that they usually appear concurrently.
2. Those subjects which show most impotence throughout the year manifest most occurrences of deviated posture.
3. A fairly obvious prodromal relationship exists in which the appearance of disalignment occurs in the subject's behaviour some time (usually a matter of weeks) before the appearance of impotence behaviour.
4. Each subject when deviating does so constantly to a given side, some always to the left and others always to the right.
5. The stance of disalignment is adopted positively, as is characteristic of proper alignment, shown by these subjects at other periods of sexual potency.

6. This form of deviated posture is maintained for lengthy spells within the reaction time, or throughout it, in contrast to any accidentally created disalignment which, in other circumstances, is quite quickly corrected.
7. The angle of deviation is not always the same; in some subjects it is 45° from the true position, in others it is up to 90°; at 135°, all sexual activities cease in the affected animal.
8. When pronounced deviation disappears, it does so by degrees over a variable period of time. In these circumstances intermediate degrees of deviation are observed, until proper positioning is re-established.

Intromission impotence

Another form of male impotence involves intromission failure. In this condition, which has been observed in bulls and rams, the subject can mount but fails to achieve intromission in spite of active pelvic thrusting movements. The condition has previously been termed "psychic impotence" due to the fact that no physical impairment is attributable to these animals as a cause of the condition (Kendrick, 1954). The behaviour of animals with this condition, as given in a variety of reports, shows remarkable consistency. The bull shows a high degree of libido, prompt alignment behind the cow and a short reaction time. The bull mounts readily but only partially covers the cow. The bull's hind feet are not brought forward close to the hind feet of the cow (Fig. 35.2). As a result, close genital apposition does not occur and the bull thrusts in vain for a time before dismounting. Such episodes can be repeated many times without effect. The condition exists as a behavioural entity which is encountered in several dairy breeds of cattle and in the Suffolk breed of sheep.

In the case of bulls the condition can be found in animals which have previously had a satisfactory history of normal copulatory function.

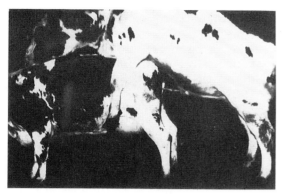

Fig. 35.2 Anomalous reproductive behaviour: intromission impotence in a bull.

In the case of rams the condition has been encountered in young animals within certain breedlines. The anomaly may not be of permanent duration. It frequently persists for six months to a year but often becomes resolved spontaneously.

Some aspect of previous experience is often the cause of inadequate sexual behaviour in male farm animals. A lack of interest in receptive female animals may occur because sexual behaviour is directed towards males (Chapter 34) or towards other species. The lack of libido, or inadequacy of mating movements described above may be reduced in the breeding group by selection, but control normally necessitates a change in management practice. Some animals are seasonal breeders, such as red deer (Lincoln, 1971) and some breeds of sheep (Ortavant and Thibault, 1956), so there is testis growth and regression during the year. Domestication has minimised such seasonality in farm animals but physical conditions, nutrition and fluctuating social contact are still factors which would have affected sexual activity in the wild and still do so now. Some rams are slow to attain puberty and are reproductively inactive when others of the same age are active, but no hormonal deficiency is detectable (Mattner *et al.*, 1973; Knight, 1973). General social deprivation, or specific deprivation of contact with and odours of females, could reduce the ability of rams to respond to the smell of oestrous ewes (Zenchak and Anderson, 1980) or their behaviour. The sexual behaviour shown by young farm animals could make later sexual behaviour less efficient. Silver and Price (1986) showed that orientation for mounting by beef bulls is more frequently correct after juvenile mounting experience. However, Orgeur and Signoret (1984) showed that rams isolated in early life still showed normal copulatory behaviour provided that they had had contact with females during adolescence. Boars which had been reared in isolation with solid-walled pens reacted inadequately in mating tests but contact with other boars through wire mesh during rearing improved later mating behaviour markedly (Hemsworth *et al.*, 1978; Hemsworth and Beilharz, 1979). Such research, which is discussed in more detail by Beilharz (1985) and Price (1985), emphasises that remedies for male sexual inadequacy involve avoiding prolonged isolation-rearing and giving animals complete or partial contact with both sexes during development.

Inadequacies of parental behaviour

Parental behaviour in farm animal species is largely maternal, in practical terms, for the only behaviour of males which benefits the young is defending the group against attack and such behaviour is relevant in only a very limited range of farming situations. Inadequacies or abnormalities of maternal behaviour are often of very great importance to the welfare of the young and the economics of the farming enterprise. Selection of farm animals for breeding has been based on the production characteristics of the progeny, on milk output, on reproductive output and on absence of handling problems. A characteristic which has been largely neglected is quality of maternal behaviour. As a consequence there are breeds of farm animals, like Merino sheep, in which the mothers often neglect or desert their young. High mortality in young calves and piglets is partly a consequence of inadequate maternal behaviour. Some of this inadequacy is a consequence of the housing system but there are genetic differences between good and bad mothers. Genes which result in poor maternal behaviour would have a very low incidence in wild populations.

Neonatal rejection

Various forms of neonatal rejection can occur on the first day post-partum in farm animals. Notable among these cases are active desertion or persistence of aggressive reactions by the mother towards the newborn. Together with maternal failure, neonatal rejection is the principal form of abnormal maternal behaviour among farm species. In the sow this condition can take the form of cannibalism, to be discussed later. While most cases of neonatal rejection occur spontaneously, some are due to short-term separation from the newborn animal early in the post-partum period. Immediate separation of kids or lambs from their mothers at parturition for periods as short as one hour can lead to a rejection of the young by the mothers (Hercher *et al.*, 1958). This fact is substantially true for other farm species.

Desertion of lambs by ewes, involving the ewe walking away from the lambs, has been recorded to be as high as 22% in Corriedales (Winfield, 1970) and 21% in primiparous Merinos (Shelley, 1970). Lower frequencies are recorded in other studies (Arnold and Morgan, 1975) with Merinos but desertion is more frequent in many of the fine-woolled breeds than in other breeds. When fine-woolled Merinos have twins they very often move off after giving birth to the second lamb and are followed by only the first-born, so that the second lamb dies unless found by a shepherd (Stevens *et al.*, 1982). Ewes of British breeds do not move off unless both lambs follow them. Nutritional factors are also likely to be important and it might be considered adaptive, rather than abnormal, for a ewe on a low protein diet to desert her offspring if she would not be able to feed it (Arnold, 1985).

In a number of cases the reaction of the mother to the newborn is very aggressive and includes attacks on the latter in the form of butting, striking, driving away or biting. Since the newborn animal will persist in orientating itself towards the maternal figure, the repeated approach of the young animal to the aggressive mother worsens the condition and makes the affected maternal subject hyper-reactive. The losses which result from this are considerable.

Among sheep it is found that neonatal rejection occurs more frequently in ewes with their first lambs than with experienced ewes (Shelley, 1970). This again is a general fact among the other farm species, indicating that maternal inexperience may be a predisposing factor to this anomalous behaviour. Aggressive responses towards offspring are shown by some mothers. Donaldson (1970) describes such attacks by primiparous dairy cows. She also reports that mothers which had themselves been individually housed when young and handled often (J.L. Albright, personal communication) were less likely to ignore their young than were group-reared, non-handled calves. Broom and Leaver (1977) and Broom (1982), however, found that isolation-reared heifers turned away from their calves more than did group-reared heifers after the initial licking period and drew parallels with the inadequacies in social responsiveness to peers shown by the isolation-reared heifers. The finding that reduced early social experience can lead to rejection of young has been reported for monkeys (Harlow and Harlow, 1965; Chamove *et al.*, 1973), but more investigation is needed on the importance of this factor in farm animals. Surveys of foal rejection by mares emphasise the importance of previous experience with young, in that most problems occurred with primiparous mares (Houpt, 1984; Houpt and Olm, 1984). Disturbance at the time of foaling, either by stallions or by people, seemed to be a contributory factor and the prevalence of this problem with Arabian mares suggests that there is a genetic predisposition to show such abnormal behaviour in these animals.

Control of neonatal rejection may in the

future by helped by changes in breeding and in rearing procedures, but at present it can be effected only through intensive care to the parturient animal. Such care can ensure that the newborn animal and the mother do not become separated and that the mother's attention is directed to the young animal. An abnormal maternal aggressive attitude to the neonate calls for an immediate intervention to protect the young. Tranquilisation of mothers affected with this condition, which may be analogous with puerperal psychosis, is sometimes necessary.

Maternal failure

Some animals which do not actively desert or aggressively reject their young fail to show adequate maternal responses to them. The failure to supply maternal attention towards the newborn is frequently first shown in a delay or a failure to groom and clean it immediately following its birth. When such failure occurs the neonate is left in a wet condition and the mother fails to acquire the olfactory and gustatory stimulation from the neonate which should initiate bonding and assist in identification of her progeny. The next feature which is deficient in the behaviour in this syndrome is the reluctance by the maternal animal to accommodate the suckling attempts by the neonate. As the newborn commences teat-seeking behaviour, the mother shows persistent negative reactions, moving the udder away from the neonate. Such turning has the effect of keeping the young animal in front of the mother's head and prevents it from suckling. Another inadequacy involves movement whenever the young tries to grasp the teat. Such behaviour, like desertion and aggression to young, is most frequently shown by primiparous mothers and is often only temporary. Such young mothers are often very attentive to their young but older mothers may sometimes not restrict the movements of the young adequately or not return to them often enough so that the young are more likely to become associated with mothers which are not

their own (see next section). Careful stockmanship is necessary in order that problems of maternal failure can be detected and remedied.

Stealing young

Pre-parturient ewes, cows and mares often approach, sniff and remain close to the newly born young of other members of their group. This is not abnormal behaviour but it can lead to problems if the mother of the young animal approached does not retain close contact with it because of weakness, maternal failure or social subordination. An alien female can dispossess the mother in these circumstances and this is sometimes facilitated by movement of the young animal away from the mother to other adults nearby. Young ungulates commonly attempt to suckle from alien adults but these attempts are usually rejected (Sambraus, 1971; Lent, 1974). The intense interest shown by many ewes in alien lambs (Welch and Kilgour, 1970) and cows in alien calves (Edwards, 1983) can be followed by acceptance of suckling attempts and the young being stolen from its mother. Edwards (1983) found that 33% of calves born in group-housing suckled from an alien female during the first 6 h of life and older cows were more likely to steal calves. The resulting problems are common to cattle, horses and sheep wherever large numbers of pregnant females are enclosed together. For example, lamb-stealing leads to confusion over lamb ownership. Sometimes newborn lambs with disputed ownership find themselves with foster mothers not yet in lactation. At other times the disputed or stolen lamb fails to acquire its due share of colostrum. Even when a newborn lamb is adopted through lamb-stealing, the foster mother may later reject her own lamb when it is born or may have no colostrum left for it (Edwards, 1982, 1983). In these various circumstances lamb deaths frequently occur. Some lamb-stealing is done by ewes which have lost their own lambs in stillbirth. While the stealing may not be entirely detrimental to the stolen lamb it may affect the maternal behaviour of the deprived ewe if this is her first lambing; in the next season such a ewe will be inexperienced and more likely to show anomalous behaviour at lambing.

The control of these problems can be effected by separating the cow, mare or ewe from the group before or very soon after parturition. Animals giving birth indoors can be put in separate calving boxes, preferably in sight of other animals, shortly before giving birth. The separation can be brought about by erecting a hurdle pen around the mother.

Killing young and maternal cannibalism

Violent behaviour is sometimes shown by parturient farm animals, as it is by many wild animals. Although the original function of such behaviour is defence of the offspring, it is a practical problem when the aggression is directed at stockmen and it can be directed at the young themselves. The control of such puerperal aggression against people or offspring involves prompt restraint and the provision of anti-psychotic therapy, such as chlorpromazine. Alternatively, given appropriate therapy with a neuroleptic agent such as azaperone, most cases are found to be normal in behaviour when they recover consciousness.

Maternal chewing of their own newborn is seen in pigs and sheep. The most dramatic form of maternal cannibalism occurs in the sow and involves the biting, killing and eating of newborn piglets by sows (Fig. 35.3). Within the general anomaly, three subtypes of behaviour, varying in degree of expression, can be recognised in affected sows (Sambraus, 1976, 1985).

1. In the simplest form of the condition, the sow is hyper-reactive following the birth of the piglets and responds with agitation to their activities, including their vocalisations. Piglets become crushed by the sows' agitated movements. The accidentally killed piglets may be eaten or partially eaten.
2. The second syndrome of cannibalism

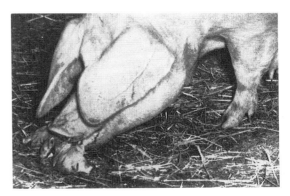

Fig. 35.3 Anomalous reproductive behaviour: cannibalism in a sow.

resembles the anomaly of neonatal rejection occurring in other species. In this the sow shows persistent active avoidance of her piglets. Avoidance leads to aggression directed towards piglets approaching the sow closely. Such piglets are then likely to be bitten and killed. Dead piglets may be eaten or partially eaten.

3. The third cannibalistic syndrome in the sow resembles the general condition of puerperal aggression occurring in other species. The sow is hyperactive following parturition and shows aggression towards people or piglets coming within her range. The affected sow snaps aggressively at any intruding piglet. The aggressive biting usually leads to the death of the whole litter. As with the other two allied syndromes of cannibalism, piglets killed by biting may be eaten, partially eaten, or left.

All these forms of cannibalism in the sow are associated with hyperexcitability and are limited, chiefly, to sows with their first litters, although it can first appear in experienced breeding sows. Although the anomalous behaviour is usually shown soon after the birth of the piglets the sow may accept the piglets normally at first and exhibit cannibalism a day later. More usually the condition develops immediately following the parturient process. Once the cannibalism has started, the anomalous behaviour is likely to continue until the litter is lost entirely. On rare occasions a single piglet will be killed and eaten with the remainder of the litter untouched. In a number of rare instances sows have killed and eaten individual piglets which are already well grown, as old as two weeks of age.

Although some killed piglets may be left uneaten, the consumption of piglets by sows, under any circumstances, must be considered as cannibalism since the normal behaviour of sows encountering dead piglets is to leave them uneaten. At parturition it is normal for a sow to be in a more excitable condition and to be more reactive and quick to defend herself and her litter. It may be that the degree or direction of the excitability is the source of maternal cannibalism in sows. It is unknown whether hormonal factors play a part in this condition but certain genetic factors are suspected since the condition occurs more in some breeds than in others. The more affected breeds, however, are those which show great excitability in general. The genetic predisposition may therefore be more general than specific in nature (Kiel, 1963; Behrens, 1968).

Certain husbandry conditions are found to be associated with maternal cannibalism in the sow. For example, if a sow is placed in a novel environment at the time of parturition it appears that cannibalism is more likely to occur. This implies environmental maladjustment as a factor. In this regard it has also been widely observed that the supply of straw to pre-partum sows, which allows them to engage in nest building, seems to lessen the likelihood of cannibalism (Brummer, 1972; Sambraus, 1976).

In the control of this condition in pigs, it has been widely found in clinical work that deep sedation of the affected animal removes the nervous cause (Boothroyd, 1965). Following such sedation, affected animals are usually no longer aggressive and often accept the remains of their litters with normal maternal behaviour. Pharmaceutical products which are neuroleptics have been found generally effective for this purpose, for example acepromazine or azaperone. Chlorpromazine, as an anti-psychotic pharmacological agent, is effective and would seem a rational choice of drug (Lewis and Oakley, 1970). The sow should be given sufficient medication to eliminate consciousness for a short period and this should be done as early as possible after the start of the condition. While it was once considered that maternal cannibalism in swine was a form of depraved appetite a wide range of nutrient deficiencies were suspected in its cause. Such factors as protein deficiency, calcium deficiency and avitaminosis were believed to be causal factors. Such views are not held today, nor could they be easily held in view of the progress that has been made in the commercial compounding of well-balanced rations for pigs. In view of a substantial amount of unpredictability in this condition it is doubtful if it can be entirely controlled, but attention should be given to the provision of quiet farrowing quarters for gilts having their first litters. Such quarters should be provided several days in advance of the anticipated birth, i.e. about 112 days after breeding (gestation mode = 115 days).

A form of maternal cannibalism occurs in ewes lambing in crowded indoor conditions. The anomaly is "covert" in that ewes will not normally engage in this activity while observed openly. The anomaly takes the form of persistent nibbling of the lamb's appendages. Such ewes may eat off the tails and feet of their newborn lambs. While this may not lead to the death of the lamb, those with severely damaged feet require to be destroyed. In addition to serious hoof injury, tails which have been chewed down to the stump can become seriously infected with resultant inflammation of tissues in that region. Lambs so affected are liable to strain excessively and this can cause rectal prolapse.

The condition of cannibalism only occurs where ewes are maintained in indoor husbandry systems. It is believed that an excited state is established in such ewes, similar to that described for affected sows, as a result of housing conditions which restrict movement.

Control of this condition can be effected simply by adequate provision of outdoor space. Parturient ewes indoors require quarters in which a lambing pen is incorporated. Since this condition, like all others affecting some aspects of abnormal appetite, creates grounds for suspicion about nutritional factors, it is important to provide well-balanced rations to lambing ewes for this and other reasons of perinatal health.

Abnormalities of basic movements

Some forms of farm animal housing prevent certain movements from occurring or make normal sequences of movement difficult to carry out. Movements which are prevented include wing-flapping and flying by hens in battery cages, walking by calves in crates, sows in stalls or tethered animals and running by many housed farm animals. Abnormalities in grooming by calves in crates or confined sows which cannot reach the back of the body have been described in Chapter 33. Hens in battery cages have insufficient room for normal preening with associated stretching (Chapter 39). In a study by Müller-Fickenwirth and Fölsch (1988), hens kept on wire showed the first part of the elaborate dust-bathing sequence of hens on litter, but as food was the only material which they could use, the sequence was abbreviated and abnormal. Other examples of this kind are described in Chapters 37–39.

Abnormal lying and standing

Hooved animals kept on slippery slatted floors have especial difficulty in lying down and standing up again. Such problems are described in detail for cattle (Andreae, 1979; Andreae and Smidt, 1982). Cattle normally lie after a brief period of sniffing the ground, lowering the front quarters (Fig. 11.2). The sequence of movements shown by fattening bulls on slatted floors is shown in Fig. 35.4. The period of ground

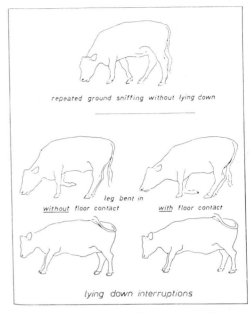

repeated ground sniffing without lying down

leg bent in

without floor contact   *with floor contact*

lying down interruptions

Fig. 35.4   Young cattle on slippery slatted floors show alterations in behaviour which inhibit, delay or prolong lying. For comparison with normal lying, see Fig. 11.2. (From Andrae and Smidt, 1982).

sniffing before lying is prolonged, presumably because the animal is apprehensive about the slipperiness of the floor. There are also many interruptions in the sequence of movements once the body starts to be lowered. The ground sniffing intention movements occurred a mean of seven or eight times before lying was completed when bulls were put onto slatted floors and 40% of the lying sequences were interrupted. On deep straw, intention movements were followed directly by lying on most occasions and less than 5% of lying sequences were interrupted. Bulls did adapt to slippery floors to some extent but many of them did so by lying down hindquarters first (Fig. 35.5). This very unusual way of lying may be less hazardous for the animals in these difficult circumstances.

The lying behaviour of sows in stalls and in farrowing crates is different from that of sows in a larger area because lateral movements are not possible. The sow normally moves her body to

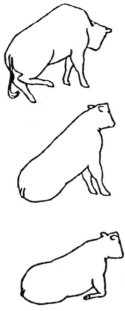

Fig. 35.5 In the same situation as that in Fig. 35.4, some young cattle lie down rump first, presumably to minimise painful events when trying to lie on the slippery floor (see also Fig. 11.2). (From Andrae and Smidt, 1982).

the side in the course of lowering her body to the ground but if bars prevent this from happening she is forced to drop down from a greater height. Such movements are more likely to result in sow injuries and much more likely to lead to piglets being squashed by the sow. Another factor which contributes to this abnormal lying behaviour is weakness of leg and other muscles consequent upon lack of exercise. Sows which have been in stalls or tethers for a long time may be unable to lie down slowly and carefully because of their inactivity during the non-farrowing period. Other abnormalities of lying behaviour are a consequence of lameness or other localised body pain.

Dog-sitting

Among breeding sows, restrained for most of their pregnancy in narrow single stalls devoid of bedding, the condition of dog-sitting is observed (Fraser, 1975). The anomalous behaviour is, however, not restricted to stalls since it can be observed in mature pigs kept in high-density groups within pens, again in the absence of bedding. In the typical posture the animal is very inactive, remains in a seated posture on the haunches, maintains the head in a lowered position and has half-closed eyes. The animal gives the overall appearance of somnolence and the term "mourning" has been applied to this behaviour.

A form of dog-sitting is sometimes observed in veal calves permanently confined in narrow crates. Here it is observed that the behaviour of such a calf has been influenced negatively by its husbandry circumstances. Again, occasional adoption of a dog-sitting posture can be seen in heavy livestock such as bulls, but this may not be abnormal.

Somnolent dog-sitting in sows kept on solid floors, which are constantly soiled, sometimes results in ascending infection of the urinary tract. This can lead to cystitis and nephritis and in due course these inflammatory conditions can result in wider systemic infection resulting in abortion in some cases and in other cases to sudden death associated with pyaemia. In some pig housing systems the incidence of serious clinical sequelae to this anomalous behaviour may be as much as 2%. Some cases of dog-sitting are associated with the "thin sow" problem.

The control of anomalous dog-sitting require changes in housing systems. Dog-sitting is one of several indicators of poor welfare which, on ethical grounds, call for husbandry alteration (Sambraus, 1981).

The control of abnormal lying and standing involves removal of the causes. Slippery slatted floors should be avoided and conditions which lead to leg weakness should not be used. Farm animals need exercise on adequate flooring and suitable lying conditions.

36 Abnormal behaviour 5: Anomalous reactivity

Very low or very high levels of activity and responsiveness are also abnormalities of behaviour. Just as in certain circumstances people can become very lethargic or hyperactive, so too can farm animals. The causes are occasionally specific neurological disorders but most frequently they are an inadequacy in rearing or housing conditions.

Prolonged inactivity

Motionless sitting, standing or lying is reported as abnormal behaviour in various farm animals by Wiepkema *et al*. (1983). There is much variation amongst species and amongst individual wild animals in the proportion of time which they spend active. Any estimate of the degree of abnormality to ascribe to animals which seem inactive must involve a comparison with animals of that genetic type in conditions which allow a wide variety of activities. Prolonged inactivity has been reported for sows in stalls and tethers, for example Jensen (1980, 1981) recorded that tethered animals were lying for 68% of the day-time period whilst the pigs in an area of woodland and field studied by Wood-Gush and Stolba spent 50% of the day-time rooting and only a short period lying (Wood-Gush, 1988). Various factors must affect the level of activity

but it is frequently found that confined animals are less active. Prolonged lying in sows can lead to urinary tract disorders (Tillon and Madec, 1984) and this is discussed further in Chapter 38.

When calves are kept in small crates such that they are unable to turn around, lying down is sometimes difficult and it reduces sensory contact with events in the building. The calves often stand for long periods, lean against the side of the crate, or adopt a semi-seated posture against the rear of the crate. During this chronic standing they may show some stereotyped behaviour (Chapter 32) or may remain completely immobile for very long periods.

Chronic standing in horses is more common in separate stalls than in groups. It is also sometimes encountered in horses which appear to have acquired orthopaedic conditions of the hindquarters and hind legs. As a rule such animals are aged. As a result of their localised clinical or subclinical conditions, difficulty is experienced by these animals in rising and lying. Since the horse, in rising, finally gets to an upright stance by a forceful extension of the hindquarters, chronic orthopaedic lesions in these parts are likely to be the seat of pain during such sudden movement. Experience of such pain would condition the horse against lying. This problem has long been recognised by horse keepers; it was once a particular problem among heavy horses.

The only way to prevent prolonged lying in pigs or chronic standing in calves is to provide conditions which allow more movement and the expression of a greater variety of normal behaviour. For horses with orthopaedic lesions it was not an uncommon practice in former times for horsemen to provide such animals with a strong chain or timber across the rear posts of a horse stall for the animal to lean its hindquarters against so as to permit rest and sleep.

Tonic immobility

The gross display of submissive inertia in animals is termed tonic immobility (Fraser, 1960a). When this condition occurs as a behavioural problem it takes the form of lying or freezing in protracted recumbency. The condition may be compounded by the presence of a concurrent illness contributing to recumbency. In cattle the principal characteristic is persistent ventral recumbency with occasional vigorous extension and depression of the head and neck; this latter characteristic is shown usually in response to stimulation such as prompts, commands and other aversive initiatives. The recognition of anomalous tonic immobility or tonic dyskinesis is essential in the rational handling of fallen, or "downer", livestock of all species to ensure that their circumstances are given appropriate consideration (Fig. 36.1; Fraser and Herchen, 1962).

The general nature of the anomalous behaviour of protracted voluntary lying or extended freezing is characterised by an abnormally low level of reactivity to such stimulation as would otherwise be effective in making the animal change position or posture. The condition may be a normal response, notably in poultry, but all cases requires a full clinical examination to ensure that no structural or pathological

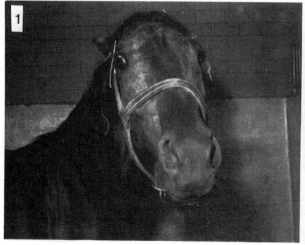
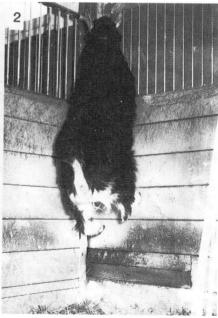

Fig. 36.1 Abnormal reactions in restrained animals. 1, startle reaction and threat (fight or flight) in a mare, 2, leaping in flight in a goat.

condition is contributing to the recumbency. The freezing response is a normal response of birds to close contact with a predator and in young domestic chicks its duration is affected by the treatment received by the birds and by their previous experience (Broom, 1969a, b; Rose *et al.*, 1985). If a domestic chicken or adult fowl is handled by a person and then laid down on the ground and its head covered for a few seconds it will show tonic immobility for a period of seconds or minutes (Ratner and Thompson, 1960). It seems that this behaviour is the normal response to capture by a dangerous predator. It is not, therefore, abnormal for the species but it is a response that a wild jungle fowl is unlikely to show often during its lifetime. Hence it is an unusual response for a bird to show and it gives some indication of how dangerous the bird judges the situation to be.

It is not clear whether the tonic immobility shown by cattle and other large farm animals is homologous with that shown by poultry but there is some similarity in the conditions in which it occurs as well as in the response itself.

Certain husbandry situations are seen to be closely associated with the appearance of this behaviour and it is reasonable to assume that they are causative, in some measure. The subject, in virtually all cases, is closely restrained or limited in movement when some stressful circumstances occur. Some specific circumstances are fairly frequently implicated during the following: (a) transportation of cattle and sheep; (b) enforced group movements, such as gathering or driving; (c) forceful manipulations on tied stock; (d) pain experiences. Other less commonly associated situations include: (e) casting; and (f) pursuit in enclosed quarters.

In farm animals, the principal identifying features are briefly as follows:

1. A history revealing a stressful event.
2. A sudden appearance of a state of locomotor inertia in the subject, shown particularly in an unwillingness to make responses which involve complex, coordinated, bodily movement.
3. An apparent absence of any physicopathological condition likely to create such kinetic deficiencies, as are evident in the subject's behaviour.
4. Associated behaviour includes general alertness denoted by localised movements of the head, eyes and ears. Adjustment limb movements also occur.
5. Sensitivity of the body surface to stimuli such as an electric goad, is present and likewise the blink, anal, pedal and other reflexes are present. On the other hand, reflexes involving changes in bodily position, e.g. some extension limb movements and righting after lateral rotation, usually show varying degrees of inhibition. A strong persistence of whichever head posture has been adopted is commonly observed.

Even transient forms of the phenomenon can allow physical injury to be superimposed, e.g. during shipping a recumbent subject closely contained in a group can be readily trampled upon by its conspecifics. Clinical consequences of the phenomenon are more usually seen in protracted cases. Workers on the experimental condition in laboratory animals have observed that the duration of the phenomenon varies considerably and there is no reason to doubt that, in farm animals also, the phenomenon can be of variable duration and may in some instances be protracted.

Clinical authorities accept that, in some cases, the "downer" cow can exist as another example of "tonic immobility" or catalepsy. When the downer cow is encountered maintaining recumbency in the face of varieties of stimulation, but apparently physically sound, many clinical workers try quickly transferring the cow to a new situation, e.g. from indoors to outdoors, or otherwise modifying the environment (e.g. presence of a dog). Frequently this makes the subject rise immediately; the condition is therefore not so much an inability to rise as a strong unwillingness to try to rise. This unwillingness not only stimulates a pathological bodily state but, as already stated, soon establishes one.

Unresponsiveness

Measures of activity level can be obtained accurately but it is difficult to know whether reduced activity means poor welfare. In descriptions of abnormal behaviour, authors such as van Putten (1980) and Wiepkema *et al.* (1983) have emphasised that confined sows may be unresponsive to events in the world around them in addition to being inactive. Such behaviour is sometimes called apathetic. In studies of sows in stalls, Broom (1986d, e, 1987a) measured their responsiveness to three different stimuli. All animals video-recorded were responsive to stimuli associated with the advent of food but they showed little response to a stranger standing in front of them or to 200 ml of water at room temperature tipped onto their backs whilst they were lying awake. Group-housed sows, in contrast, were much more likely to take notice of strangers and to sit or stand and carry out other activities when the stimulus was presented. This work shows that stall-housed sows are abnormally unresponsive to such stimuli Table 29.4. The results of such work are likely to depend upon the precise nature of the stimulus presented for a very frightening stimulus might elicit a maximal response in all sows.

Hyperactivity

Animal handling is made difficult when animals show freezing responses or startle responses but neither of these is abnormal behaviour. Shying, jibbing or baulking by horses can sometimes be extreme in the extent to which they are shown and may necessitate the use of blinkers and the avoidance of potentially startling situations (Fig. 36.1). The behaviour is within the normal range of responses to danger, however. Problems arise when individuals injure themselves because of their high reactivity or if they influence others to behave similarly. High-density housing of animals and the presence of dense flocks or herds at pasture can make such socially transmitted hyperactivity dangerous to the animals and to people. Grazing animals which are suddenly disturbed, even by an innocuous object such as blown paper, may stampede. They are more likely to be injured due to collision cr falling during a stampede. Primitive man exploited this behaviour in order to catch large herbivores, for example Indian peoples in North America caused bison to stampede over cliffs. The behaviour is present in wild populations but it can be maladaptive. Stampedes of cattle, horses or sheep can be very damaging to the animals.

Hysteria

The occurrence of the extensive alarm reaction in poultry is often termed hysteria. Flightiness in the domestic chicken appears in different types of nervous and hysterical behaviour occurring in differing environments and age groups. Hysteria in the caged laying hen is characterised by sudden flying about, squawking and trying to hide. The incidence of hysteria in penned poultry is closely related to flock density. Flocks of 40 have been found to have 90% incidence of hysteria while flocks of 20 had an incidence of 22%. Claw removal in birds has been found to reduce hysteria although some strains are resistant. Even in cages hysteria can occur but it is less of a problem in multiple-hen cages containing three to five rather than the larger numbers of birds. Undoubtedly caging controls hysteria in poultry to some extent although it can spread throughout a flock kept in battery cages. Hens in a cage adjacent to hysterical birds may or may not be affected, but individual birds apparently trigger an episode within a cage leading to hysteria among all the individuals within that cage. Following episodes of hysteria within caged birds traumatic sequelae occur in the form of torn skin over the back. In addition, there is a drop in feeding and egg production following hysteria (Craig, 1981).

In broiler chickens, and particularly in turkeys, hysteria may result in pile-ups of birds under which some die. Good stockmanship prevents hysteria responses, for example the good stockman entering a poultry house always knocks to warn the animals that human entrance is imminent. This minimises the escape response which might otherwise occur and be magnified as it moves in a wave down the house. Another method of controlling hysteria is to place baffles in the poultry house so that birds do not move too far before reaching a baffle. The consequent pile-ups are smaller and mortality is reduced.

37 Cattle welfare problems

During the last 40 years, some aspects of cattle management have been changing considerably but, at the same time, our knowledge of cattle physiology and behaviour has been improving. It is clear that cattle have complex brain mechanism regulating their behaviour processes, elaborate social structure and sophisticated learning ability (Craig, 1981; Broom, 1981; Kilgour and Dalton, 1984; Stricklin and Kautz-Scanavy, 1984). These results have made many animal scientists reconsider the effects of conditions and procedures on farms, both in terms of their efficiency as regards production and with respect to the welfare of the animals.

The general range of welfare problem areas is the same for cattle as for other farm animals (Table 37.1). Problems of farm operations, transport and disease are discussed in Chapters

30 and 31. This chapter is concerned with the effects of housing and management systems. In many aspects of farm animal management improved welfare leads to improved production. If the welfare of a dairy cow is improved there is often a greater milk yield and if the welfare of very young calves is improved, the resulting increases in growth rate and survival chances lead to economic advantages for the farmer. In other situations, however, improving welfare leads to reduced profits, for example when high stocking density is detrimental to welfare. Modern cattle husbandry systems do lead to some welfare problems, as discussed below. A general change in cattle management methods has been an increase in production pressure. Nutritional expertise has increased to the point where animals now convert feed to meat and milk very efficiently. If animals are pushed hard energetically, there need not be welfare problems and management difficulties but these are more likely and should be taken into account when deciding or advising about which system to choose.

Certain general points are relevant to the management of all cattle and so will be made before considering problems specific to calves, beef cattle and dairy cows. Feeding of housed cattle may lead to difficulties for the animals because the acquisition of food in housing conditions is very different from that when grazing. Physical difficulties may occur, as

Table 37.1
The general range of farm animal welfare problems

Ill-treatment
Neglect and poor management
Disease and lack of treatment
Inadequate housing
Poor handling and moving facilities and procedures
Transport including loading and unloading
Treatment at markets
Slaughter and pre-slaughter procedures
Farm operations
Breeding procedures and consequent difficulties
Provision for emergencies

described by Cermak (1987), but social factors are also very important. Cattle synchronise their feeding to a large extent (Benham, 1982a; Potter and Broom, 1987) so where group feeding is possible, enough feeding places for each animal are required (Metz, 1983; Wierenga, 1983). Those animals which cannot find a feeding place may not get sufficient food and it is likely that there are adverse effects on their welfare. The precise effects of the frustration which occurs when food is inaccessible because of competition remain to be determined. Competitive feeding situations where there are no individual feeding places pose extra problems for cattle. The subordinate individual has to attempt to obtain food despite the attacks or threats of other individuals. Bouissou (1970) found that the greater the extent of the barrier between feeding places for cows, the fewer the attacks which occurred (Fig. 37.1). A trough which requires subordinate cows to come close to dominant individuals results in those subordinates walking greater distances and taking longer to obtain a meal (Albright, 1969; Fig. 37.2). Calves of low social rank obtain less of the favoured food if trough space is restricted

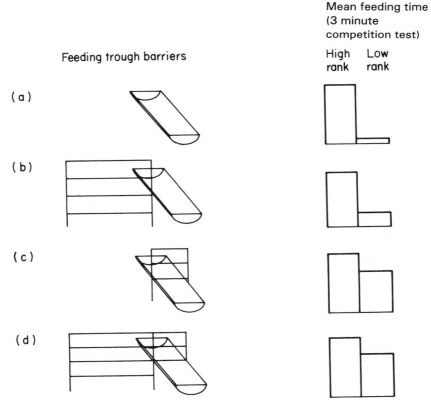

Fig. 37.1 Physical barriers affected feeding times by cows ranking high and low in a competitive order. With no barrier (a) the low ranking cows were scarcely able to feed. A body barrier (b) improved the situation slightly for the low ranking cows but a head barrier (c) and a complete barrier (d) had a much greater effect (redrawn after Craig, 1981, data from Bouissou, 1970).

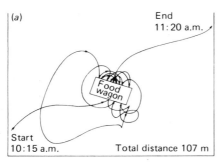 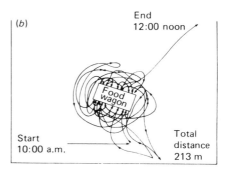

Fig. 37.2   The paths of two cows in a herd after food is provided in a food wagon are shown. Animal (a) was found to be high in a competitive order whereas animal (b), which was low in that order, walked further because of displacement at the food wagon and took longer to feed (after Broom, 1981, modified after Albright, 1969).

(Broom and Leaver, 1978; Broom, 1982). In order to minimise such welfare problems which are often associated with poor weight gain, farmers should provide feeding spaces for all individuals, preferably with barriers between the individual places. Adaptation to a single food source is possible for cattle, however, for a transponder-operated feeding stall can be successful (Albright, 1981), but certain individuals in a herd may have difficulties in such systems.

Another general problem for housed cattle is having to stand on floors which are wet, slippery, uneven, or hazardous because of sharp edges. Slippery slats can lead to difficulties in standing or lying (Andreae and Smidt, 1982; see also Figs 35.4 and 35.5). These and other inadequacies of flooring can result in limb injuries, foot lameness, tail-tip necrosis and various diseases (see papers in Schlichting and Smidt, 1987). Lameness is the greatest welfare problem of housed dairy cows and factors influencing its occurrence include floor quality and poor drainage which results in cows standing in slurry (Wierenga and Peterse, 1987).

Calf welfare

In the first few days after birth the major calf welfare problems are enteric and respiratory diseases. The calves of dairy cows may fail to obtain sufficient colostrum for a variety of reasons (Edwards, 1982; Edwards and Broom, 1982, Broom, 1983a). Management practices which maximise the chance that colostrum will be obtained and minimise contact with pathogens have important beneficial effects on calf welfare. If calves of dairy cows are normally left with their mother for the first 24 or 48 hours, the risk that the calf will not suckle early enough to obtain and absorb the immunoglobulin from colostrum can be minimised by the stockman placing one of the mother's teats in the mouth of the calf as early as possible after the calf stands. Group-calving situations where several cows calve during a short period can lead to a cow's colostrum being drunk by a calf other than her own or to calves being rejected by their own mothers. Such occurrences can be prevented by providing separate calving boxes which should ideally allow the cows some visual contact with other cows. The provision of soft bedding for the calf is also desirable and is easier where special calving accommodation is available.

Dairy calves are deprived of their mother from an early age and many are individually housed so that they are confined in a small space and deprived of all or most social contacts. In the European Community, 17 million out of a total of 22 million calves per annum are reared for veal in small crates and fed on a diet with inadequate iron and roughage (Susmel, 1987). Many animals used as replacers for dairy herds are also individually housed. The welfare problems resulting from this rearing method are substantial. Calves housed for long periods in small pens which do not allow them to turn around are deprived in various ways. Firstly the typical veal calf crate does not allow the animal to groom the hind part of its body. All calves do groom all of their body several times per day if given the opportunity to do so. The effects of being unable to groom a large part of the body are apparent in direct physical effects but the effects of the frustration which is likely to be associated with this inability is not known. The other effect on grooming when calves are housed in a small pen is that these calves show excessive amounts of grooming of those parts of the body which they can reach and this grooming often results in ingestion of much hair with consequent formation of hair balls or bezoars in the rumen. These hair balls may on occasion block the exit from the rumen. Another restriction imposed by crates or other small pens is in the postures which can be adopted when lying. de Wilt (1985) reported that a common lying posture amongst group-housed calves involves turning the head backwards whilst for 2–8% of total lying time the hind legs are stretched out. Neither of these postures is possible in a crate so some frustration and discomfort is likely as a consequence. Stereotyped behaviours (Broom, 1983a) are shown by many crate-housed calves. Some licking is stereotyped but the most common of such behaviours is tongue-rolling. Stereotyped behaviour is certainly abnormal and one of the behavioural responses to difficult conditions (Chapter 32).

Other problems associated with close confinement include thermoregulatory difficulties and inability to escape from disturbing stimuli. In hot conditions calves stretch their limbs whilst lying but this is not possible in a small pen. An animal in a small pen may be frightened by human approach or by some sound but it is not able to avoid or retreat from the disturbing stimulus. After being reared in a small crate, calves were more adversely affected by the procedures of loading and transport than were group-reared calves, in that they showed a greater increase in cortisol production (Trunkfield and Broom, 1989; Trunkfield *et al*, in preparation). Another major problem of individual housing is inability to show social behaviour. Young calves kept in groups interact with other calves frequently and associate closely. Individually reared calves cannot interact much with one another and long periods of social isolation lead to failure to develop normal social behaviour. When calves which have been reared individually for many months were put in a social situation they failed to show some ear movements and other social signals and they did not retaliate if attacked. As a consequence they were unable to compete with animals reared in groups and they failed to grow as fast in a competitive feeding situation (Broom and Leaver, 1978; Broom, 1982).

Group-housing can also lead to problems for some calves. Certain animals may show intersucking and urine-drinking. This behaviour can lead to poor growth in those animals which drink urine and to soreness in the animals which are sucked. The problem is absent from many units and it is likely that current research will allow recommendations about management practices which will largely eliminate it. It is rarer in the U.K., where dairy calves are usually left with the mother for 24 h, than in countries like the Netherlands where bucket-rearing from birth is common. In a study by de Wilt (1985) the use of teat buckets resulted in no preputial sucking whereas 48% of calves given milk in open buckets did so, but other studies in other conditions have not always given such results. Calves in groups sometimes fail to drink from teats connected to a milk reservoir but work by Barton (Barton, 1983a; Barton and Broom, 1985) showed that in these young calves, aggressive behaviour was not the cause of this. Calves showed much social facilitation of feeding and for groups of ten calves, the positioning of five milk-supplying teats close together encouraged even the weaker calves to come to the teats and drink. Another group-housing system which can work well is an electronic feeder system triggered by transponders worn by the calves. This system facilitates rationing of milk but it allows only one calf to feed at a time. Straw-based group-housing systems are used extensively by commercial veal units in the U.K. and they result in low levels of disease and good economic returns (Webster *et al.*, 1986). With further refinement of management procedures such systems are likely to replace individual crate-housing internationally as the normal method of calf housing.

Whether calves are kept in crates or in groups their diet has an effect on their welfare. The two commonest inadequacies are lack of iron and lack of roughage. The public demand for white veal results in many calves being fed an amount of iron which would inevitably result in their early death if they were not slaughtered whilst still young. The amount of iron needed to avoid anaemia and unnatural white meat is summarised in Fig. 37.3 (taken from Webster *et al.*, 1986). It is clear from this figure that some calves need more than 50 mg iron/kg dry food if they are not to be anaemic (below 9 g haemoglobin/100 ml blood). As anaemia is a pathological symptom it seems reasonable to assume that the welfare of anaemic calves is poor and hence that systems which produce white veal result in poor welfare for this reason as well as for other reasons stated above. Low roughage diets are also a consequence of white veal production. Calves are fed a diet which does not allow normal rumen development. Such conditions often result in ulceration of the abomasum. Diets which include adequate roughage have beneficial behavioural effects as well as permitting normal bodily development so all calves should be fed adequate roughage from two weeks onwards. Since white veal production is inefficient and there are inevitable welfare problems it is to be hoped that public demand for it will continue its rapid downward trend and such production systems will soon disappear.

Since young calves are so vulnerable to disease and are generally affected by adverse physical and social conditions, their welfare is often poor when they are transported and taken to market. Despite this fact, a million young calves per annum are transported from France to Italy for veal production and many young calves are taken to market in the U.K. The British calves should be more than a week old before marketing but many are not and even at one week the calves are ill-equipped to cope with the vicissitudes of vehicle and market conditions. In most European countries, calves are not marketed before weaning and the British practice is regarded as undesirable for production and welfare reasons. Calves should be sold from farm to farm, if movement at an early age is essential, or should be marketed after five weeks of age.

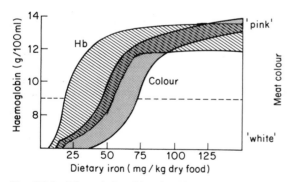

Fig. 37.3 The relationship of calf dietary iron intake with both haemoglobin concentration in the blood (if low the animal is anaemic) and meat colour. Each is shown as a band because calves vary in their utilisation of dietary iron. Some claves cease to be anaemic (more than 9 g/100 ml) at an intake of 18 mg/kg but others are still anaemic at 50 mg/kg. If most calves have white meat, many of them will be anaemic (from Webster *et al.*, 1986).

Beef cattle welfare

The housing conditions for calves destined for beef production are sometimes similar to those kept for veal production so they have similar welfare problems. Older beef animals are kept in small individual pens or are tethered in some countries and they then show much stereotyped behaviour. Riese *et al.* (1977) reported that stereotyped behaviour included tongue-rolling, weaving movements and self-licking. Wierenga (1987) reported that one-third of young, individually housed bulls spent several minutes in every hour showing tongue-rolling. Physiological responses to confinement also occur. Ladewig (1984) reported that tethered bulls showed more frequent episodes of high blood cortisol levels than did bulls able to interact socially in groups. Such abnormal behaviour and physiology is probably exacerbated by both social deprivation and inability to perform behaviours because of spatial restriction. Individual housing of beef animals is more frequent when they are bulls than when they are steers. In Germany 98% of beef animals are bulls but in the U.K. 92% are steers. The U.K. situation is likely to change following the ban on growth promoters.

Fighting and mounting can lead to welfare problems when beef animals, especially bulls, are kept in groups. The most important way of minimising such problems is to keep the animals in stable groups since social mixing leads to much fighting with consequent injuries, bruising and extreme physiological responses (Kenny and Tarrant, 1982). In stable groups, mounting may lead to more injury than does fighting (Appleby and Wood-Gush, 1986). Animals which are frequently mounted become bruised and may suffer severe leg injuries. Mounting can be greatly reduced by the use of overhead bars, which physically prevent it, or an electrified grid which deters animals which wish to mount. The brief initial experience of an electric shock has a relatively small adverse effect on welfare as compared with the serious effects on animals which are repeatedly mounted.

The stocking density of beef animals and the flooring provided also have considerable effects on welfare. High stocking densities lead to more aggression, injury and bruising. Beef animals increase rapidly in body weight but they have little exercise if they are housed in small pens and their leg growth may not be able to keep pace with that of the rest of the body. The final weights reached are much higher now than they used to be so the legs are scarcely adequate to support the body. The consequence is cartilage damage, clear indications of limb pain and obvious difficulties in standing and lying (Dämmrich, 1987). Graf (1984) found that these problems were absent if fattening bulls were reared on deep straw and that such conditions also led to fewer behavioural problems.

Dairy cow welfare

The major welfare problems for housed dairy cows are lameness, mastitis and difficulty in finding feeding and lying places. Most of these problems are associated with the design of the housing system but some are a consequence of poor stockmanship. The causes of both lameness and mastitis are multifactorial and there is an interaction between the response of the animal to its conditions and the likelihood of clinical infection. A reduction in pathogen challenge will usually help to reduce disease incidence but changes in management methods, of the kinds which have other beneficial effects on welfare, can have an effect on minimising disease which is as great or greater. Studies at the Institute for Animal Disease Research, Compton, have shown that there are positive correlations between lameness and mastitis incidence. High production increases the occurrence of both lameness and mastitis. Mastitis has declined in dairy herds where concentrate feeding has been introduced following the introduction of milk quotas; in an experimental study, Manson and Leaver (1986, 1989) found that the lameness incidence was higher in cows fed on a high protein diet. The incidence of lameness can be reduced by the use of foot baths and by hoof trimming but much remains to be discovered about the conditions which lead to individuals being likely to become lame.

Space allowances are often quoted for housed dairy cows, for example Arave *et al.* (1974) quoted 2.3 m^2 per cow, but house design and social stability must be taken into account when deciding on the best space allowance in any building. Social mixing leads to various behavioural and reproductive difficulties (Bouissou, 1976). Even when social disruption is minimal, cows need places to which to retreat so as to avoid confrontation with other individuals. Potter and Broom (1987) report that cows use cubicles and feed barrier sections for this. If there is a shortage of feeding places, due to the highly synchronised behaviour of dairy cows (Benham, 1982a; Wierenga, 1983; Potter and Broom, 1987) there are considerable effects on the cows. Metz and Mekking (1984) reported a dramatic increase in chasing and it is likely that the welfare of cows is poor when they are unable to get a feeding place because their herd-mates are feeding. Narrow passageways in a cubicle house can cause problems for cows, for example Konggaard (1983) saw more contact, yielding, turning and waiting if passageways were 1.2 m wide than if they were 2 m wide. An inadequate number of cubicles, such that not all cows can lie at once, leads to more aggressive interactions and low-ranking animals having to lie in passageways where conditions are dirty and likelihood of injury or disease is high (Kaiser and Lippitz, 1974; Friend *et al.*, 1977; Wierenga, 1987). Other welfare problems for dairy cows concern ill-treatment or neglect by the stockman and producers when it comes to milking. The use of an electric dog or of physical force in the collecting yard are not conducive to good welfare or good milk production. Good stockmen are consistent in their milking parlour procedures and deal with the cows in a quiet, predictable way.

Welfare consequences of future developments in cattle management

Conventional methods of cattle breeding have changed the animals considerably during recent years and future changes are likely to be accelerated by new possibilities for genome manipulation. For example selection for double muscling in beef cattle and the possibility of transferring genes which increase growth rate or modify final body form could both result in animals with larger, faster growing bodies. New growth promoters (e.g. bovine somatotrophin, BST), if these are allowed to be used, could have the same effect. These techniques need not have any adverse effect on welfare but any increase in production pressure could lead to more problems. In addition, body weight increase without corresponding increase in leg size and strength could result in more lameness. Any modification of animals should be checked carefully using proper scientific measures of welfare to ensure that animals do not find it more difficult to cope with their environment. Such studies should be carried out over a period as long as the maximum farm lifetime of the animal. The offspring of transgenic animals should also be studied in this way. New techniques should not be licensed for general use unless such welfare checks have been carried out and have shown that there are no adverse effects on the animals. Some modifications of animals could result in improved welfare, for example if genes were implanted which increased the efficiency with which disease could be combatted by the individual.

The crossing of breeds of animals can lead to welfare problems for cows if a large breed of bull is crossed with a smaller breed of cow, resulting in increased calving difficulty. Similar problems can arise if embryo transfer is used. Multiple implantation of embryos could lead to other problems. The actual transfer of embryos could be a major operation which is traumatic for the cow but techniques which have only a minor effect are now possible. Any embryo transfer procedure should be such that cow welfare is not worse than that of cows undergoing a normal pregnancy.

A quite different development area which can have effects on welfare is the development of microprocessors and other electronic control units. Cows can already carry transponders which allow them to be fed individually and this methodology could be improved to minimise the chances that any individuals fail to obtain food. This system of feeding cows at a single or small number of feeding stalls can lead to problems because dominant individuals may attack others or deter them from feeding. Some very timid cows might be quite unwilling to approach a feeder when an aggressive individual is near it. Recent work by Wierenga (in press) and Wierenga and van der Burg (1989) involves the use of auditory signalling devices on the cow's ear which tells each individual when to come to feed. Animals which have already fed receive no food if they enter the feeder so this system provides a means for distributing feeding times for each individual throughout the day. Such a system should work well for all animals except for those which are stimulated to feed only when another animal is feeding. Electronic systems could also allow cattle greater control over their physical environment for example by giving them the opportunity to regulate environmental temperature and air-flow rates. Lack of control is a major cause of welfare problems (Broom, 1985), so such possibilities could improve welfare. The development of robotics is likely to make possible in the near future the automatic milking of cows. Cows would be recognised individually on entry to a milking stall and a computer which had been pre-programmed with their udder coordinates would attach a milking machine to them. Provided that this could be done without any discomfort to the cow it could improve welfare since the cow could come to be milked wherever she chose to do so.

38 Pig welfare problems

The complexity of pig behaviour, and the brain mechanisms which control it, is evident from the studies described in earlier chapters. Their learning ability is considerable and their social behaviour elaborate. As a consequence, welfare problems arise for pigs if they are unable to control events in their environment, if they are frustrated or if they are subjected to unpredictable situations. For example, inability to prevent attack by another pig, to regulate body temperature, or to groom adequately can all lead to poor welfare. Such effects are additional to those which are a result of injury, disease or other pain and physical discomfort.

Pig welfare problems (Broom, 1989b) include those due to physical abuse, neglect, handling, transport, farm operations (Chapter 30), and disease (Chapter 31). This chapter is concerned principally with the effects of widely used housing systems on pigs. The largest section is that on dry sow housing and this is followed by discussion of the effects of accommodation for farrowing, piglets after weaning and fattening pigs. A final section refers to work on alternative whole systems for pig management.

Dry sows and gilts, i.e. those which may be pregnant but which are not lactating, are kept in a variety of different housing systems. These include tethers, stalls, groups with feeding stalls, groups with food, supplied on the floor or in a communal trough, groups with electronic sow feeders (Figs. 38.1 and 38.2), groups in fields or large yards, and, experimentally, in the family pen system. There is some variation within each of these categories, particularly with respect to the microclimate, the type of flooring, the use of straw or other bedding materials, the diet and the frequency of feeding. In this review, the major variables considered are the types of housing systems and the presence or absence of straw or other bedding. The studies reviewed differ in scientific quality, because of the numbers of observations, the numbers of animals studied, or the involvement of complicating variables, so an attempt is made to evaluate the results accordingly and to emphasise those studies with the most clear-cut results.

There is a range of indicators of poor welfare and some information about good welfare can be obtained from studies of what animals choose when given the opportunity. The data reviewed in this chapter are organised according to welfare indicators. At our present stage of knowledge this seems to be the most useful kind of organisation but, due to individual variation and strain variation in the kinds of coping methods used by pigs, the ideal study combines a range of different measures. Few studies have adequately combined measures so far but individual measures can give some idea of the minimum numbers of individuals whose welfare is poor in each of several systems.

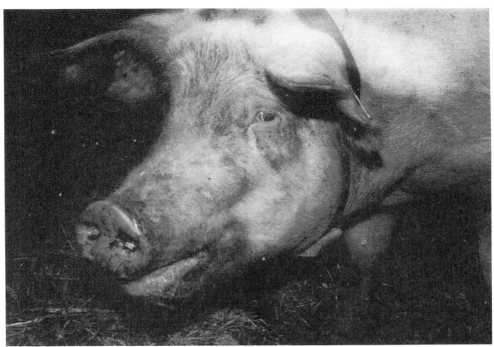

Fig. 38.1 This sow is wearing an electronic transponder which will trigger food delivery when she enters the feeding gate. The transponder may be on a collar, on an ear tag or, since it can be very small, implanted under the skin to allow electronic recognition throughout life (photograph by D.M. Broom).

Growth and piglet production

It is possible that a gilt which fails to grow or a gilt or sow which produces very small litters of piglets may have a welfare problem although other factors contribute to the wide variation in individual production. In comparative studies of production systems, however, it is often difficult to discover how many individuals do badly in this way because the data are presented as a mean of animals in a system. Hence a few pigs which produce well could mask a few bad producers. Where average production figures are used it is clear that well-managed units can do equally well whether the sows are confined or in one of the forms of group-housing. The quality of stockmanship is an important factor affecting production which will also have an effect on welfare. In general, data on growth and piglet production have not been presented in the agricultural literature in a way which facilitates the identification of individuals with welfare problems.

Reproduction problems

Some sows are culled because they do not become pregnant and others because they have small litters. These reproductive failures or inadequacies can occur because the sow encounters difficult conditions and has difficulty in trying to cope with them. Many factors lead to anoestrus in the pig (Meredith, 1982) but several authors have attributed anoestrus to housing conditions. A.H. Jensen *et al.* (1970) reported

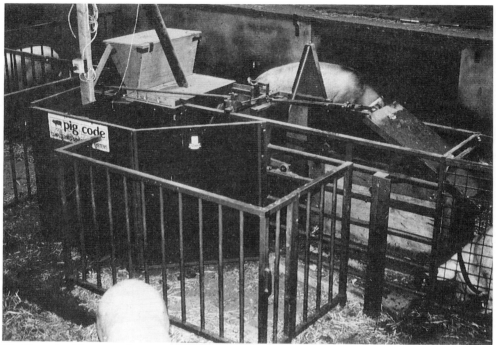

Fig. 38.2   Sows kept in groups have access to this electronic sow-feeder which delivers food to them, after their entry, only if they have not received their ration for the day (photograph by D.M. Broom).

that tethered gilts reached first oestrus 4 days later than group-housed gilts and Mavrogenis and Robinson (1976) found even larger differences in the time of first oestrus between gilts in stalls and gilts housed in groups. Individual penning of sows can lead to fewer sows becoming pregnant after service, or attempted service, than group-rearing of sows (Fahmy and Dufour, 1976). Sommer (1979), Sommer *et al.* (1982) and Hemsworth *et al.* (1982) also found that stall-housed sows returned to oestrus after their piglets had been weaned later than group-housed sows. Maclean (1969), however, reported that in groups where much "bullying" occurred the opposite result was obtained and Hansen and Vestergaard (1984) also reported that the delay before conception was greater in some group-housed sows. Many farmers with sows in stalls or tethers experience difficulty in getting some of their gilts or sows pregnant, but in these situations and some of the studies mentioned above there is doubt about the precise reason why this happens. The problem may be that reproduction is impaired by poor welfare in the housing condition but the impairment may sometimes be limited to the extent to which the pigs show signs of oestrus which can be detected by a stockman.

The effects of housing conditions on the onset and occurrence of oestrus need to be studied in a way which controls for all variables, but research does suggest that there are more problems when gilts or sows are kept in stalls or tethers than if they are kept in a well-managed group-housing system. It is important to note, however, that welfare can be poor in group-housing systems where much fighting occurs and that oestrus can be delayed in such situations.

Other measures of reproductive problems may reflect poor welfare during the gestation period and problems at farrowing. Most studies of such problems are complicated by the fact that sow accommodation during both gestation and farrowing may influence the results. Bäckström (1973) compared 1283 sows confined in a crate during pregnancy and farrowing with 654 sows free in a pen at both times. In crate-housed sows there was a higher incidence of mastitis/metritis/agalactia (11.2% : 6.7%) and greater numbers of sows whose farrowing time was longer than 8 h (5.4% : 2.3%). In a more recent study, Vestergaard and Hansen (1984) studied four groups of sows which were tethered or loose-housed during pregnancy and during farrowing. The duration of farrowing was significantly shorter (mean 234 min) in those sows which were loose-housed throughout than in those which were tethered at one stage or another (mean 335–352 min). It seems possible that lack of exercise is having some adverse effect on the sow. There was no effect of the sows' housing conditions on the numbers of live piglets born but since only 70 sows were studied such a difference would have to have been large to have been apparent. Bäckström (1973) and Sommer *et al.* (1982) did find more stillborn piglets if sows were confined. When all sows in a housing condition are considered, the mean differences between conditions are found to be small but the effects on certain sows is large. There are problems for some sows from group-housing and for rather more sows from confined conditions but we do not know enough about how this is brought about. On commercial farms which have well-managed stall units, reproductive problems are generally thought to be no more frequent than on units with group-housing. It must be emphasised, also, that in surveys such as that of Bäckström, there is a possibility that variation in unit size or in stockmanship may be contributing to the differences reported. In general, the coping systems of animals have evolved so as to minimise effects on reproductive success so if there are differences between systems, even a small effect may indicate considerable welfare problems.

Sow disease and injury

Disease itself usually means impaired welfare but disease can also be an indicator that welfare has been poor (Broom, 1986c, 1988c). Animals which utilise their adrenal cortex frequently may have impaired immune system function and greater susceptibility to disease (Kelley, 1980; Siegel, 1987). The effects of housing conditions on the health of sows and piglets was reviewed by Ekesbo (1981), who pointed out that the relative levels of disease in different systems is much affected by differences in the use of antibiotics.

If sows are exposed to very infectious diseases such as Aujeszky's or swine fever then all may become infected, irrespective of their previous welfare. Non-infectious, or less infectious, diseases such as those leading to some foot and leg problems, sores, torsion of the gut, or ulcers are more obviously related to environmental conditions and the animals' attempts to cope with them. Confined sows appear to be more susceptible than group-housed sows to certain diseases but the results of the surveys which have been done could be influenced by other variables. Whilst better studies are needed, several studies have results which should be mentioned here. In some cases, disease and injury are difficult to distinguish so these will be treated together.

The effect of housing conditions on farrowing problems has been discussed in the previous section. Bäckström (1973) found greater total sow morbidity at farrowing in crate-housed sows (24.1%) than in loose-housed sows (12.8%) as well as greater MMA incidence. The quality of management may have improved since these studies were carried out, however. Confined sows may also be more subject to urinary disease and leg problems whilst group-housed sows are more likely to receive pig inflicted injuries and sometimes have higher parasite loads. Tillon and Madec (1984) noticed that urinary tract disorders had increased in frequency in France during a period when more and more sows were confined. They reported on the relatively high incidence of such disorders in tethered sows and (Madec, 1984) suggested that sows might be more prone to urinary disorders if they have to lie on their faeces. They also found that tethered sows drink less and urinate less often than do loose-housed sows so that urine is more concentrated and bacteria have longer to act within the urinary tract (Madec, 1985). This problem is probably a consequence of low activity levels and consequent infrequent drinking, hence whilst it could be in part a consequence of the effect of the housing system on the animal, it may be reduced within that system by stockmen encouraging the animals to stand and drink. There is clearly much variation among sows here as some inactive sows drink infrequently but other active sows drink very often. Tillon and Madec (1984) also reported that in one-quarter of tether units more than 20% of sows showed serious lameness. Several other authors have reported similar findings. Bäckström (1973) found that the number of traumatic injuries caused by pen fittings and flooring was 6.1% in confined sows but 0.8% in loose-housing. Most studies of leg injuries and infections which cause lameness have related their incidence to the type of flooring. Penny *et al.* (1965) attributed high incidence of foot rot to poor concrete floors and Smith and Robertson (1971) described how poorly designed or maintained slatted floors resulted in many legs and foot injuries and high culling rates. Bäckström (1973) found that 6.3% of 588 sows on partly slatted floors had foot lesions but these were shown by only 3.3% of 3520 sows on unslatted floors. It is now clear that good slats cause fewer problems than poor slats but the incidence of sow lameness is still very high. There remains the probability that confinement and associated lack of exercise cause lameness even on good flooring. de Koning (1983) has utilised a precise method for quantifying integumental lesions and has reported that such lesions

can be of high frequency in tethered sow units.

Injuries resulting from attacks by other sows can be serious in group-housing conditions. Good management, for example a good feeding system and the maintenance of stable groups, can minimise fighting and consequent injury but injury can have a serious detrimental effect on welfare in a poorly managed system. Where sows are attacked by others the lesion can be quantified in a precise way (Gloor and Dolf, 1985). Any system for keeping sows which results in high levels of fights which cause injury, vulva biting or tail biting is clearly bad for the welfare of at least some of the pigs. This topic is considered further below in relation to behavioural and physiological measures.

Sow activity and responsiveness

Abnormally low levels of activity and lack of responsiveness to events in the surrounding world have been proposed as indicators of poor welfare in pigs (van Putten, 1980; Wiepkema *et al.*, 1983). Several authors have reported that sows confined in stalls or tethers are inactive for longer periods than are sows in groups (e.g. Ekesbo *et al.*, 1978; Jensen, 1979, 1980a, 1981; Gravas, 1982; Carter and English, 1983) but others have found no such effect or have reported the reverse (Nygaard *et al.*, 1970; Bengtsson *et al.*, 1983; see review by Cariolet and Dantzer, 1985). Some of these differences are explained by Cariolet and Dantzer's findings that sow activity is affected by parity, stage of pregnancy and extent of lameness. A more important complicating factor is that whilst some confined sows are inactive for much of the time, others show much stereotyped behaviour. If inactivity, with associated unresponsiveness, and stereotyped behaviour are alternative strategies which sows use to try to cope with adverse conditions, the gross measures of the activity of sows in a particular housing condition are not very useful. It is better to study individual animals in detail and to try to assess responsiveness in a precise way. In a series of experimental studies on the responsiveness of sows (Broom, 1986d, e, 1987a), stall-housed sows were found to be less responsive to stimuli other than food presentation than were group-housed sows (Table 29.4). There was, however, considerable variation amongst the stall-housed sows in this respect.

Stereotypies

Confined sows are not able to groom normally (van Putten, 1977), they may have difficulty thermoregulating, most are fed small volumes of food infrequently, they cannot interact normally with other sows and they cannot move away from people or other potentially hazardous stimuli. One response shown by a variety of animals to such situations where the individual has little control of its environment is stereotypic behaviour (Broom, 1983b; Dantzer, 1986), e.g. bar-biting, manipulating the tether chain or drinker, sham-chewing and various other repeated, apparently functionless movement (see Figs. 32.1, 32.2). Such behaviour is occasionally shown by group-housed sows but the mean frequency is extremely low. Examples of reported total duration of stereotypies in stall-housed sows are: 11% of the 8 h after feeding (Broom and Potter, 1984), 10–14% of 24 h (Blackshaw and McVeigh, 1984a, b), and 22% of the time active (Jensen, 1980a, 1981). For tethered sows, examples are : 1.8–28% of 2 h observation time in different units (Carter and English, 1983), 15% of 9 h of day-time (Bengtsson *et al.*, 1983) and 14.5–29% of 24 h (Blackshaw and McVeigh, 1984a, b). Some individual tethered sows watched by Cronin and Wiepkema (1984) performed stereotypies for a mean of 80% of day-time observation periods. The figures obtained in such studies depend upon the efficiency of the recording method, especially on the use of video-recording, but there is clearly much variation between sow housing units and within any particular unit, in the amount of stereotypy shown. Gilts show less stereotypy (Blackshaw and McVeigh, 1984a, b;

Cronin and Wiepkema, 1984), and such behaviour is not evenly distributed through the day (Rushen, 1984b; Broom and Potter, 1984). Many reports from farmers of low incidence of stereotypy, however, are a result of failure to notice some stereotypies such as sham-chewing and there may be some reduction in the incidence of stereotypies when human observers are present. Diet can have an effect on stereoptypies. If added roughage is in the form of a manipulable material such as unchopped straw there can be considerable reduction in stereotypy but chopped straw does not have this effect (Fraser, 1975). The addition of high bulk material to concentrates caused a redistribution of stereotypies but no net change in total duration in one study (Broom and Potter, 1984). A high level of feeding (4 kg per gilt per day) resulted in much lower levels of stereotypies than a low level (1.25 kg per gilt per day) in a study by Appleby and Lawrence (1987).

There is much debate about whether stereotypies are a method used by animals to help them to cope with adversity or a pathological consequence of trying to cope but, whatever the results of this debate, there is no doubt that an animal showing stereotypies for a long period is very abnormal in its behaviour. The stereotypies are an indicator of poor welfare and they are frequent in most sow stall and tether units. The relatively low levels at which pregnant sows are commonly fed may be a contributory factor to poor welfare but the confinement itself must be a major part of the problem for the animal.

Aggressive and other injurious behaviour

The welfare of an animal which is injured by another, or which is often pursued by another, or whose movements are severely restricted by the presence of other dominant individuals, is probably poor. Aggression does occur in tethers and stalls, but whilst its frequency may be high (Vestergaard and Hansen, 1984; Barnett *et al.*,

1987; Dolf, in press) the physical effects on the individual attacked are slight. Some farmers using group-housing systems for sows report serious fighting and extensive wounding. The extent of this fighting is greatest if there is competition for food. The system studied by Csermely and Wood-Gush (1986), which would be regarded generally as a poor one, was a group of 11 sows whose food was dropped automatically onto the floor from above. Most agonistic encounters occurred within 30 min of the food drop. The group was stable and no serious injuries resulted from the fighting but the welfare of subordinate sows was probably very poor and Csermely and Wood-Gush recommended that visual barriers should separate sows at feeding places. A group-housing system with well-designed individual feeding stalls allows all sows to feed at once with no aggression being possible during feeding, so this would seem to be a good system on welfare grounds Fig. 38.3. A modern version of this system and the electronic sow feeder system are described by Edwards

(1985). The electronic sow-feeder system (see also Lambert *et al.*, 1983a) has the advantage that sows receive their own individual ration but the disadvantage that only one sow can feed at a time so sows tend to queue for feeder access. Early versions of electronic sow-feeder systems had disadvantages which led to considerable problems of bitten vulvas and other injuries. These included poor design and positioning of the feed crate, e.g. a back gate which did not prevent contact by sows behind, a rear exit only system, a gate which allowed other sows to follow the first in, or a feeder positioned in a lying area. Work on management and studies of behaviour (Lambert *et al.*, 1983a, b, 1984, 1985, 1986; Edwards, 1985; Hunter *et al.*, 1988) in electronic sow-feeder systems has shown that efficient training, a sufficient number of feeders, once a day feeding, stable grouping, front exit feeders and a good bedded lying area or kennel can result in few welfare problems. Most sows are easy to train but up to a quarter need longer-lasting help from the stockman (Thomas and Signoret, 1989). It will probably not be possible to remove all problems—for example sows may prefer to feed in groups but only one sow at a time can feed on this system. A disadvantage of this system is that it is a little more difficult for the stockman to operate and more careful observation of sows is required in order to avoid problems.

Another group-housing system, in which boars and offspring are present with the sows, is the family pen system developed by Stolba and Wood-Gush (Stolba, 1982; Wood-Gush, 1983). The sows have a more diverse and interesting environment in this system and there are seldom any indicators of welfare problems. Even more is demanded of the stockman running this system, however, so there might be risks to welfare if an inefficient stockman was involved.

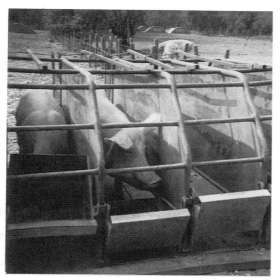

Fig. 38.3 Sows can be fed individually in feeding stalls so as to minimise aggression. Most feeding stalls are closed at the back when the food is provided. The majority of such systems are for sows kept indoors.

Adrenal and other physiological measures

Measurements of plasma glucocorticoid levels are useful indicators of the welfare of animals subjected to short-term procedures such as handling and transport. Single blood samples, however, like measurement of heart rate, are of little use when the long-term effects of housing systems are being evaluated. The evaluation of responses to a challenging situation after various previous housing conditions is of some interest, although precise interpretation is rather difficult. Barnett *et al.* (1984) compared the cortisol responses to loading and transport and to ACTH challenge in sows previously kept in tethers, pairs or groups. The tethered sows showed a greater response to the transport and some sign of a higher response to ACTH challenge, but there were also high responses from some animals in pairs. Barnett *et al.* (1981) had found that tethered sows had higher plasma cortisol levels than stall-housed sows and a further study (Barnett *et al.*, 1987) showed that this higher level could be reduced by using wire mesh between the tether stalls. These results may not, however, reflect long-term responses to the housing conditions.

The possibility that animals may cope with prolonged exposure to difficult environments by self-narcotisation using naturally occurring opioid peptides such as β endorphin has been proposed. Studies on pigs are limited to the finding that stress-induced analgesia is apparently non-opioid in pigs (Dantzer *et al.*, 1986) and to the work of Cronin *et al.* (1985) on the link between stereotypies and opioid peptides. Cronin's experiment demonstrated, by the use of the receptor blocker naloxone, that the behaviour and the inhibitor are linked in some way. It may be that sows use stereotypies as a means of self-narcotising but this is by no means proved and studies by Rushen (personal communication) suggest that stereotypies are not more narcotised. It is also possible that other behavioural indicators of poor welfare, such as lack of responsiveness, are associated with self-narcotisation, but at present we have no clear indicator of the use of such methods of coping.

Studies of preferences and the improvement of welfare

In designing their family pen system, Stolba and

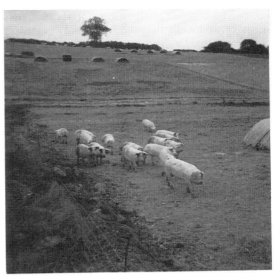

Fig. 38.4 Sows kept in a field with arks to shelter in can walk, run, root and carry out a wide range of other activities. The best fields are those with shallow soil and stones or rock near the surface for these do not get too muddy. Welfare can be poor in very cold conditions unless bedding is provided.

Wood-Gush utilised information from their studies of how sows preferred to spend their time in an extensive and varied outdoor environment (Wood-Gush, 1983). Such studies are of value when designing systems which can then be compared on welfare production grounds with existing systems (Fig. 38.4). Simpler preference studies also aid in the development of systems in which welfare may be improved. Sows in fields spend much time rooting so Wood-Gush and Beilharz (1983) assessed the usage of earth by pigs in bare environments. These pigs used the earth a lot and Hutson (1989) has found that pigs will carry out operant responses many times where the opportunity to root in earth is the reinforcer. Studies of the floor preferences of gilts have been carried out by van Rooijen (1980, 1981, 1982). In studies where floor preference was balanced against social attraction van Rooijen was able to demonstrate that earth floors were much preferred to concrete but that the preference for straw over woodchips was less clear-cut. The extensive usage of straw as a material to manipulate is clear from many studies on sows, e.g. Jensen (1979) and bengtsson *et al*. (1983). Fraser (1975) described how the provision of long straw led to a clear reduction in the duration of stereotyies in stall-housed sows and many research studies have suggested that straw is desirable as a material for bedding and for manipulation by sows and fattening pigs (Jongebreur, 1983; Gloor and leimbacher, 1984; Grauvogl, 1987). Straw may not be the only material which serves this purpose and its beneficial effects may not counteract all the effects of an otherwise adverse environment, but its use should be considered in all systems where no comparable material is present.

Farrowing sow and suckling piglet welfare

A major welfare problem in all countries is the high level of piglet mortality within the first few days of life. In the U.K. 11% of piglets born alive fail to survive to weaning. Some of these are very weak when born but almost all of them can be successfully hand-reared and will grow well (England, 1974). The most important cause of death in young piglets is overlying by the sow. Piglets may be squashed and killed or may be weakened so that they are less likely to be able to suckle and more likely to succumb to diseases. Selection by breeders has resulted in a substantial increase in the size of the modern sow, in relation to her wild ancestor, but much less change in the size at birth of the piglets. Diseases are also a major factor in piglet mortality and the likelihood of serious disease effects is dependent upon the absorption of immunoglobulins from colostrum. A summary of the factors leading to inadequate colostrum intake by piglets is shown in Fig. 29.6. Piglet weakness and mortality is clearly a major welfare problem, as well as being a great economic problem for the farmer. When sows farrow in straw-bedded pens, some piglet mortality occurs, especially if the straw is not

very deep. Mortality is higher if no bedding is present but can be reduced if the piglets can be attracted away from the sow, except when suckling, from an early age. The use of creeps, which allow piglets into an area which the sow cannot reach, facilitates this. When pig farmers tried to put more sow-farrowing pens into a building and cut labour costs by reducing the size of the pens and not using straw the piglet mortality increased dramatically. The use of a farrowing crate (Fig. 38.5) in this situation reduced mortality and various versions of the farrowing crate are now very frequently used on pig farms. Piglet survival is improved by using a warm creep area and bars on the farrowing crate which minimise the chance that the piglet will move under the sow. Overlying is still a problem, however, in part because sows cannot lie down slowly and carefully when they are in a crate but drop the hindquarters to the ground rather precipitately.

After farrowing the sow's environment is interesting because she is frequently visited by piglets. She is very restricted in her movements, however, and she cannot move much towards the piglets. Hence it would seem to be a rather frustrating situation for the sow. Before farrowing, sows will build large nests if they are given the opportunity and there are indications that the inability to build a nest is frustrating for the sow (Baxter, 1982). Overall the widely used farrowing crate is easy to manage but is far from ideal for the sow. Although it is better for the piglet than a farrowing pen of similar size with no crate in it, a large-amount of space and deep straw would seem to be better still. Research on alternative farrowing accommodation is being carried out but much more work is needed in this area.

Piglet and fattening pig welfare

A traumatic event encountered by each piglet on commercial farms is weaning. As described by Jensen (1986), piglets left with their mother are weaned long after 10 weeks of age, but the common commercial practice is to wean at three

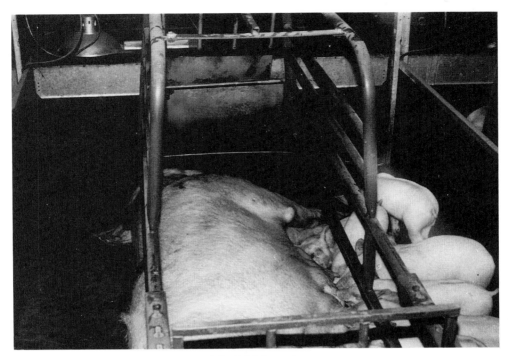

Fig. 38.5 Sow in a farrowing crate (photograph by D.M. Broom).

or four weeks of age. Such early weaning must have considerable effects on the piglets, leading to poor welfare, but only a few of these have been assessed. The absence of the mother and her teats from which milk can be obtained forces the piglet to look for food elsewhere and leads to much nosing and sucking of other piglets. Belly-nosing is an up and down massaging movement with the snout placed under the belly of other pigs which has often been described as being shown frequently by early weaned piglets (van Putten and Dammers, 1976; Schmidt, 1982). During or after belly-nosing the genitalia or navel may be sucked and urine drunk. Anal massage may also occur and can lead to lesions with bleeding (Sambraus, 1979). Piglets may be chased around in a pen by those attempting belly-nosing, etc., and it seems likely that their welfare is adversely affected by the chasing, the inability to escape and by injuries which may

result. The piglet which is attempting belly-nosing etc., or snout-rubbing and sucking on floor, wall or bars, is manifesting its desire to suck which would be directed at the sows' teats had these been still available. The persistence of such behaviour gives some indication of the extent to which the piglet feels deprived. As discussed in Chapter 32, some abnormal oral behaviours in piglets are linked to the same dopaminergic pathways in the brain as are stereotyped behaviours in older animals (Schmidt, 1982).

Another welfare problem which arises at the time of weaning is fighting. If piglets from different litters are mixed after weaning they interact in various ways including fighting, as would be expected when they have to establish new social relationships. Such fighting can result in injuries but these are seldom severe. As with belly-nosing, the major problem which arises is probably that of the individual which is continually being chased around the pen by one or more other piglets. Fighting may be reduced by the use of tranquilisers at the time of mixing piglets but it is not yet clear whether this improves the subsequent welfare of the piglets. All of the problems of belly-nosing, etc. and fighting are exacerbated if the piglets cannot escape from one another because they are in a small pen with no way of getting out of the sight of other individuals. Fighting when pigs are mixed is a greater problem with older pigs since they can inflict much more serious injuries on one another so mixing of pigs should be avoided. Since farmers cannot always do this there is a need for more investigation of how to introduce individuals in such a way that they do not injure one another.

The amount of space available to piglets or fattening pigs affects their ease of movement and ability to find an adequate resting place as well as their ability to avoid the undesirable attention of others. It is not just the area of floor which is of importance, however, but the quality of space available. When assessing the space requirements of pigs all of their movements during lying and standing need to be taken into account (Petherick, 1983). Other factors which should also be considered are the provision of adequate separate lying and dunging areas (Baxter and Schwaller, 1983), the possibility of feeding without there being a high possibility of attack by others, and the possibility of avoiding serious attack, etc. by others. A very important aspect of the family pen system designed by Stolba and Wood-Gush (Stolba, 1982; Wood-Gush, 1983) is that the animals are in an environment with many subdivisions and opportunities for individuals to get away from others. McGlone and Curtis (1985) found that the provision of "pop-holes" into which piglets could put their heads reduced the adverse effects of fighting and it seems likely that a pen design which included "pop-holes" or partitions which allowed chased piglets to hide might be very beneficial to their welfare. Such an improvement in the environment of these piglets might

also reduce the frequency of poor performers which take longer to grow to slaughter weight. The problems of the weakest pigs in a group apply just as much to older pigs which are usually kept in bare pens.

Another major welfare problem for fattening pigs is having to stand on inadequate floors. Pigs may trap their claws, suffer abrasion injuries or break or strain their legs because the floors are slippery. Old concrete floors and old slats cause especial problems but some of the newer floors for piglets or older fattening pigs are clearly very uncomfortable for the animals to stand and move on. Preference studies by Marx and Mertz (1987) give some useful information about what floor pigs choose to stand on. Such work should be followed up by comparisons of welfare, including the incidence of various forms of lameness, in pigs kept on each of the floors.

Handling and transport

The initial response of a pig to a disturbing situation, such as the close approach of a person or a sudden noise, is orientation to the stimulus, suppression of normal activities and preparation for flight, defence or hiding. Behavioural and physiological changes occur together and, in addition to the behavioural changes mentioned above, there is increased heart rate, increased ventilation rate, production of catecholamines from the adrenal medulla, production of glucocorticoids from the adrenal cortex and associated changes in brain chemistry. All of these can be measured and, by comparison with resting rates, levels during other activities and maximal possible responses, an indication of how hard the animal is having to work in order to cope with the conditions imposed upon it can be obtained. Of particular importance in this assessment is the time course of the response. An increase in heart rate by a factor of 1.3 for 30 s is obviously much less detrimental to the animal than an increase lasting for several hours. Heart rate is a useful measure of the response of animals to various short-term treatments provided that some account is taken of the ongoing activity (Baldock and Sibly, in press). When fattening pigs were studied by van Putten and Elshof (1978) their basal heart rate was found to be 138 beats per minute. This increased by a factor of 1.5 when an electric prodder was used, by 1.65 when the animals were made to climb a loading ramp and by more if the ramp was very steep (van Putten, 1981). Some of this increase is a consequence of the activity but some is part of the preparation by the animal for emergency responses. A larger increase in heart rate ($\times$ 2.6) was found when Augustini and Fischer (1982) studied the effects of driving pigs up a steep ramp and onto a lorry but animals loaded using a tail-gate lift showed a small decline in heart rate. The heart rate of pigs was elevated much less during transport than during loading in several studies and von Mickwitz (1981) found that the time of feeding prior to loading had a major effect.

Behavioural studies of pigs during handling and transport confirm that loading has the biggest effect on welfare. Animals resist attempts to move them, vocalise and adopt defensive postures frequently during loading. Behavioural indicators of poor welfare during the journey are usually associated with inappropriate temperature, high stocking density or poor driving (Jackson, 1973; Augustini et al., 1977; van Putten and Elshof, 1978). Fighting is rare during movement but can cause serious problems when the vehicle is stationary (Pearson and Kilgour, 1980).

Pigs may die during transport and the term Malignant Hyperthermia Syndrome is sometimes used in these circumstances. Sybesma et al. (1978) reported on genetic differences in the likelihood of death during transport. Pietrain are very vulnerable and Landrace are more vulnerable than Large Whites. Susceptible animals often show a positive response to the halothane test and in the Dutch study the death rate was 3.35% for halothane-positive pigs but 0.32% in those which were halothane-negative. The quality of meat after slaughter is also affected by the physiological changes associated with high adrenal activity and with the activity associated with fighting. Skin blemishes are also an indication of fighting or bruising due to poor driving. Hence these measurements made after slaughter provide information about the welfare of animals during the journey. Moss (1981) reported that after a two hour journey from farm to slaughter, 59% of gilts had PSE meat and the mean plasma cortisol level was 6.4 g per 100 ml. Corticosterone level should also be measured in pigs. If there was a long delay (24 h) before slaughter the PSE frequency dropped to 25% in gilts but 81% of boars had DFD meat. Guise and Penny (in press) have shown that high stocking density and mixing of animals before transport substantially increase the likelihood of carcass skin blemishes. The detrimental effects of mixing on farm or at loading are of particular interest and the authors recommend that pigs should be kept in their housing groups up to and during transport.

39 Poultry welfare problems

Human attitudes to poultry often differ from those to sheep, cattle, goats or pigs. The chicken is less often thought of as an individual and few people would ascribe much intellectual ability to it. These attitudes are partly a consequence of the very large numbers of these animals which are kept in one place, partly to the fact that they are birds and therefore harder for a person to identify with than are the larger mammals, and only slightly because of any real difference in behavioural ability. In fact when individual chickens are put into experimental learning situations which are not frightening to the birds they perform quite well. Their sensory ability is very good when compared with that of man and their social organisation is complex, requiring considerable ability in learning and memory in order to maintain it. The chicken is too often seen in a situation where its fear of man dominates most of its activities. Hence the average member of the public or chicken farmer is unable to assess adequately its behavioural complexity and awareness of its environment. These attitudes to chickens, and to a lesser extent to other poultry, have had a considerable influence on man's assessment of what conditions these animals need and what treatment they can tolerate. Those who have studied the behaviour of the domestic fowl in detail, especially those who have looked at feral fowl (McBride *et al.*, 1969; Wood-Gush *et al.*, 1978) inevitably acquire much respect for the members of this species. There are few differences in behaviour between the wild Burmese red jungle fowl (*Gallus gallus spadiceus*) and the domestic form (*Gallus gallus domesticus*) (Kruijt, 1964) and the diversity of calls, displays and other behaviour (Baeumer, 1962; Guyomarc'h, 1962; Collias and Joos, 1953) are very impressive. The modern concept of rank order, or pecking order, in a social group originated with work on chickens (Schjelderup-Ebbe, 1922; Guhl, 1968) and has been developed substantially by further work on this species (Rushen, 1984a).

The examples of welfare problems reported in this chapter are confined to the chicken because most work has been carried out on this species and because of its numerical importance. The domestic fowl is the most common bird in the world with numbers estimated at 9–10 billion. It is a very successful species which exploits man very effectively. If there are widespread welfare problems in this species, however, then a majority of the animals in the world which suffer because of man's activities are chickens. Hence the welfare of chickens is a very important subject. The two main sections in this chapter concern the effects on welfare of housing systems for hens kept for egg production and of housing for broilers kept for chicken meat production. There are some welfare problems in breeding hens, in the rearing of young chickens and in rearing turkeys, ducks and geese, so some of these are mentioned here.

The important problems associated with the handling and transport of poultry are also discussed.

Management systems for laying hens

Hens kept for egg-laying were largely maintained in free-range conditions in most countries until 1950. The birds were normally shut up in some sort of house at night but were able to roam around a farm yard or field throughout the day. There was then a change to indoor housing on deep litter for a period of 10–15 years followed by a further change to the use of battery cages in controlled indoor environments (Table 39.1).

Table 39.1
Percentages of laying hens in the U.K. kept in different ways

Year	Free-range	Deep litter	Battery cages
1948	88	4	8
1956	44	41	15
1961	31	50	19
1965	16	36	48
1977	3	4	93
1981	2	2	96

After Ewbank (1981).

The average population of laying hens in the U.K. increased from 50 million in 1938 to 70 million in 1964 but then, as egg population efficiency improved, it declined to 52 million by 1981. The cost of eggs, in relation to other comparable foods, dropped as efficiency increased so the consumer has benefited in financial terms from the improved production efficiency. In recent years, however, there has been a small resurgence in free-range and some development of indoor group housing systems because a section of the public did not wish to buy eggs from poultry units where the hens were kept in battery cages.

Free-range hens

Free-range systems are those where hens are kept with access to an open area at a stocking density defined by regulation in the European Economic Community as being no higher than 1000/ha. This space allowance of 10 m² per hen is similar to that which was used on larger units before 1950. There are problems about the rate at which the ground is fouled by droppings in a situation where no dropping removal is possible so the Farm Animal Welfare Council in the U.K. recommended a maximum stocking density of 375/ha (26.7 m² per hen). If hens are left at the higher density without being moved to a new area then the risk of disease is high. For example, Löliger *et al.* (1981) reported that the incidence of worm infestation and coccidiosis was at least 10 times higher in a well-run free-range system than in battery cages. Löliger *et al.* also reported a rather high incidence of predation by birds of prey in their German free-range units. Both disease and predation must be considered when welfare is assessed (Fig. 39.1). In addition, as Sainsbury (1980) points out, free-range birds are subject to extreme weather conditions and their welfare may be so poor during extreme winter weather that their egg production is substantially reduced. Hence welfare can be very poor in free-range units but these problems are soluble. If stocking density is high the risk that parasites and diseases transmitted via faeces will have significant effects should be cut down by moving the animals to fresh ground. The effects of inclement weather can be reduced by providing well-insulated and ventilated houses. Domestic fowl are by origin a tropical species so in winter conditions the hens may seldom venture outside. Hence these houses need to be almost as good as the indoor group-housing accommodation. Hens often stay indoors during periods of rain or wind as well as cold so the problems of aggression and house design referred to later in this chapter are relevant to free-range hens. The fact that conditions may effectively prohibit free-range hens from going outside is often not

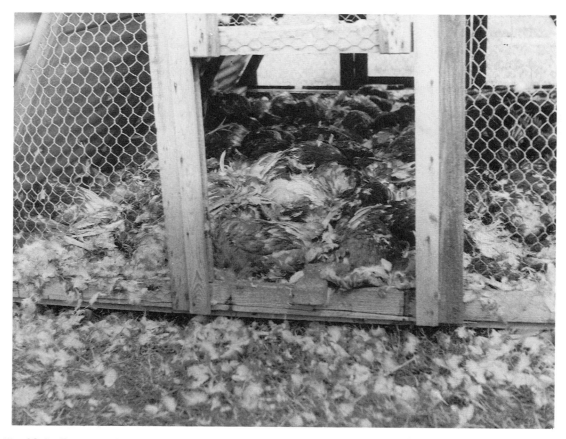

Fig. 39.1   Free-range hens are vulnerable to predation from predators like foxes.

appreciated by those who advocate such systems without qualification. Most hens, however, do utilise the opportunity to walk, flap, scratch, peck and interact socially in range conditions. No studies have evaluated in a precise way the value to the hen of being in a field rather than in a large hen house. It is clear that welfare problems can be reduced to a very low level by free-range accommodation for hens but it is quite possible that all of the advantages to the hen of free-range can obtain within a well-designed building.

Battery cages for hens

The first use of rows of cages for hens in a building where the physical conditions could be controlled occurred in the United States in the 1930s. Such rows could be called a battery of cages so the term "battery cage" gradually became widespread as the system developed. Modern battery houses (Fig. 39.2) allow the most complete separation of the birds from their faeces and this has considerable advantages for disease and parasite control. The faeces may be carried away by a belt under the cages or may fall

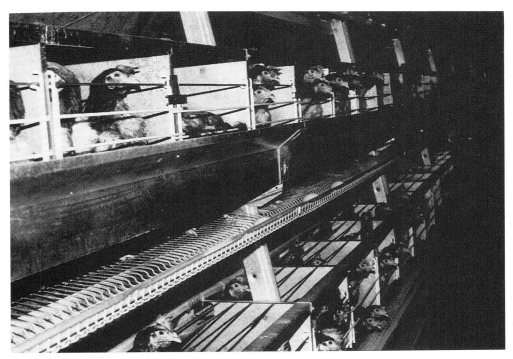

Fig. 39.2   Hens in battery cages (photograph by D.M. Broom).

directly or via deflectors into a pit. Figure 39.3 shows some designs of battery houses. Disease is further reduced by the all-in all-out management system. Hens are brought into a clean empty house shortly before they start to lay and they are all removed for slaughter at the same time when they are about 72 weeks old. The number of birds in a cage is commonly five in European countries but is often more in North America. Hence the number of birds which can be contacted directly by any individual is not large and disease transmission is further limited. The average temperature, humidity and ventilation throughout the house can be controlled with some accuracy. Water is usually available continuously from drinkers and food is supplied regularly and usually automatically by a moving chain or belt. Medication can be supplied to birds in a row of cages via food, water or fine droplet spray. The low disease, good air conditions, constant water supply and regular supply of well-balanced diet are all advantages of the battery cage system in the maintenance of good welfare. Against these advantages must be set an array of disadvantages.

An important risk for animals in any building with automatic systems is that these may fail. Drinkers may become blocked, food conveyers may fail to convey food to some cages, ventilation and heating systems may cease to work effectively. In each of these situations, and in those where birds become ill or trapped, alarm systems and careful inspection are needed. The inspection of birds in many battery cages is relatively easy. Hence the good stockman can check regularly on every bird in a battery house and identify some severe welfare problems. It is well known, however, that inspection is much

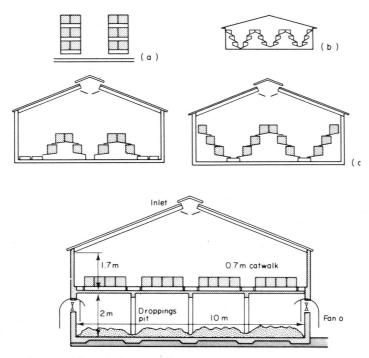

Fig. 39.3 Battery cage houses. (a) vertical cages; (b) semi-stepped cages; (c) fully stepped cages; (d) flat-deck cages over deep pit for droppings. Some modern systems have more tiers of cages (after Sainsbury and Sainsbury, 1988).

less efficient if the birds are in the bottom row of cages or in a row which the stockman cannot see. As Elson (1988) points out, the bottom row should not be too low for inspection and if there are many tiers of cages it is essential that gantries positioned so as to allow inspection of the upper tiers are present. Another risk to welfare in all houses accommodating animals is fire. All animals should be kept in such a way that they can be evacuated from their building in case of fire. It would take a long time to open all the cages in a battery house containing 100 000 birds and birds which have lived in a cage for a long period might not leave the cage readily even if the building was on fire. This is a serious inadequacy of the system as there are sometimes cases of battery houses burning down. Fire alarms and sprinkler systems could help to reduce the risk but it will always remain a serious problem.

Many of the problems for a hen in a battery cage are a consequence of things that she cannot do. She cannot move freely, flap her wings, perch, build a nest before oviposition, scratch for food, dust-bathe, or peck at objects on the ground. The consequences of such deprivation are frustration, pecking at other birds and certain abnormalities of growth and body form. The evidence concerning how poor welfare becomes as a result will now be summarised.

Free-range hens walk much more than those kept in cages or in groups on a wire floor (Fölsch, 1981). Wing-flapping is entirely prevented and there is a reduction in the total amount of comfort behaviour carried out in a cage as compared with group-housing or free-range (Black and Hughes, 1974). Battery cages provide little room for hens to stretch their legs or preen normally (Bogner, 1984; Sainsbury, 1984). We do not know much about the immediate effects on the bird of such inabilities to exercise when they want to do so. One behavioural test which can be carried out to assess how great a deprivation is involves giving the animal the opportunity to perform the activity and measuring performance after various periods of deprivation. For example, the amount of water drunk can be measured after various periods of water deprivation. Wennrich (1975b, 1977) showed that birds removed from a battery cage and put into a larger area showed much wing flapping. Nicol (1987b) studied this "rebound effect" further and compared birds kept in cages for different times. Longer periods confined in cages were associated with more prolonged wing-flapping when released. This is clearly a welfare problem but it is difficult to say how bad it is.

The long-term effects of lack of exercise are those on bones and muscles. Caged birds have lower bone weight and greater bone brittleness than birds which have more freedom of movement (Meyer and Sunde, 1974) and more caged birds are lame (Kraus, 1978). The levels of osteomalacia and osteoporosis are considerably higher in caged hens than in group-housed or free-range hens (Löliger *et al.*, 1980; Löliger, 1980, 1981) and it is suggested by Martin (1987) that there is much more muscle weakness in caged birds. The muscle characteristics of birds kept in different ways are evident from meat quality studies but do not necessarily provide information about welfare. Perhaps the most important evidence of poor welfare is the incidence of broken bones when the hens are taken to slaughter. Simonsen (1983) reported that the incidence of broken wing bones on arrival at the slaughterhouse was 0.5% in hens free to move but 6.5% in hens from cages. A further 9.5% of hens from cages had broken bones after slaughter. Nielson (1980) reported similar results. Gregory and Wilkins (in press) dissected 3115 spent hens from battery cages in

the U.K. and found that a mean of 29% had broken bones before the time that they reached the water bath stunner at slaughter. Removal of the birds from the cages and hanging on the shackling line were identified as points where damage was most likely to occur. Knowles and Broom (in prep) have found that hens from battery cages are much less active than those in a perchery or an Elson terrace system and their humerus and tibia breaking strengths are less. Exercise is correlated with bone thickness and strength in hens as in other animals. It is not known how much discomfort is associated with osteomalacia and osteoporosis but there can be no doubt that broken bones are extremely painful. Anything which regularly leads to a high incidence of broken bones is a very serious welfare problem, see reviews by Broom and Knowles (1989), Knowles and Broom (in press). The handling and transport procedures (see later) are a major problem and these are not quite the same for free moving and caged birds. However, it is clearly going to be necessary for some substantial change in housing or handling or both if this high incidence of broken limbs is to be avoided.

Hens use perches when these are available, especially at night when they often perch close together (Lill, 1968). When perches at several levels are provided, hens choose to perch high above ground (Blokhuis, 1984) but they will utilise a low perch in a battery cage (Tauson, 1984b). Lill also reports that hen arousal levels are reduced if they can perch, and provision of a perch leads to increased leg-bone strength (Hughes and Appleby, 1989). The strong preferences which most hens have, to use a perch if there is one, does suggest that the provision of perches is likely to improve welfare.

The fact that hens in free-range conditions walk considerable distances in good weather conditions is evidence for their preference for being in a larger rather than a smaller space but they use that larger space intermittently. Hughes (1975) and Dawkins (1976, 1977) examined preferences directly by giving hens from battery cages the option of remaining in the cage or using a large run. After a period of four hours during which they remained in the familiar cage for most of the time they moved outside and subsequently preferred the large run. Hens reared outside always preferred the larger area. It is necessary to know something about the importance of any preference, however, and Dawkins found that hens spent most time in the larger run even if they were fed in the cage or could be near other hens in the cage.

Domestic fowl show elaborate nest-searching, nest-building and other behaviour before egg-laying, which is essentially the same as that of wild jungle fowl (Wood-Gush, 1954, 1971; McBride *et al.*, 1969, Fölsch, 1981). Hens in a cage have no nesting material, no nest cup and no quiet, dark place in which to lay. They are often pushed aside from their planned laying place (Brantas, 1974). Although it is clear from the work of Appleby *et al.* (1984) that a dark nest site is not needed, there are various indications of the extent of the frustration felt by hens which are about to lay an egg in a battery cage (see summary by Kite, 1985). Plasma corticosterone levels increase pre-oviposition but this occurs whether or not a nest is available (Beuving, 1980) so it is probably a preparation for the egg-laying procedure. Hens give a pre-laying "Gackeln" call (Baeumer, 1962) whose intensity and duration is three times higher if the bird is in a battery cage (Hüber and Fölsch, 1978; Schenk *et al.*, 1984). This may indicate greater frustration but the clearest behavioural indicator is stereotyped pacing. At the time when a nest would normally be built the hen walks up and down in the cage in a repetitive way (Wood-Gush and Gilbert, 1968; Brantas, 1980) see p. 310.

Another abnormality of the battery cage which prevents certain normal behaviours is the wire floor. The hen cannot scratch on the ground for food or dust-bathe. The preferences of hens for different sorts of metal flooring were assessed by Hughes and Black (1973). Hughes (1976) also assessed how hens choose when offered wire mesh and litter floors. If the hen had to decide on each day which of two cages to remain in they usually choose the cage with a

litter floor but they used both wire-floored and litter-floored cages if both were available. Litter floors were strongly preferred shortly before and during oviposition and most eggs were laid on litter. Dawkins (1981) found that hens would enter a very small cage with litter on the floor rather than a larger one with a wire floor. Hens deprived of food, however, chose a wire-floored cage with food in it rather than a litter-floored cage without food; if limited time was available for feeding or being on litter they chose to feed (Dawkins, 1983). These studies provide information about the extent of the hen's preference for a litter floor but they need to be combined with work on the effects of being deprived of litter. When hens are prevented from dust-bathing they may show anomalous behaviour in the cage such as attempting to bathe in the feed (Martin, 1975; Wennrich, 1976; Vestergaard, 1980) and dust-bathing movements on cage-mates or in the air (Vestergaard, 1982; Martin, 1987). Hens kept in cages for some time and then given dust to bathe in showed an amount of dust-bathing behaviour which was proportional to the duration of the period of deprivation (Vestergaard, 1980).

Hens spend much time investigating their environment by pecking at objects and their bills are richly provided with sensory receptors. Birds in cages have little at which to peck so they direct much pecking, which may be food searching behaviour, to substitute objects (Fölsch and Huber, 1977; Fölsch, 1981). Some pecking stereotypies are also shown in cages (Martin, 1975). The fact that pecking is not just a matter of obtaining food is demonstrated by the finding that birds will work for food reward by pecking at a key even when food is present (Duncan and Hughes, 1972). Hens in cages sometimes peck persistently at cage fittings (Brantas, 1974; Fölsch, 1981) and at the feathers and vent of cage-mates. Blokhuis (1986) suggests that the major reason why feather pecking occurs in battery cages is that hens do not have enough other things at which they can peck (see summary of such ideas by Hughes, 1985). Feather pecking occurs more often after feeding and after egg-laying (Preston, 1987). It is more common if food is restricted (Bessei, 1983), if a pelleted diet is provided (Jensen *et al.*, 1962), if the light level is high (Hughes and Duncan, 1972; Bessei, 1983) and if the floor is made of wire (Hughes and Duncan, 1972; Brantas, 1974; Simonsen *et al.*, 1980). A motivational basis for feather-pecking related to dust-bathing deprivation is clear from the work of Vestergaard (1989). Feather loss leads to heat loss and to increased food intake (Wathes, 1976; Leeson and Morrison, 1978), specially before moulting (Tauson and Svensson, 1980). Pecking which has rather more severe effects on the individual pecked often starts in young hens with pecking at the vent and progresses to serious injury or death. Such pecking and real aggressive attacks on other birds are not normally a serious problem in battery cages, perhaps because the birds are on average, older and too close together for full aggressive behaviour to be shown. Al-Rawi and Craig (1975) showed that attacks by one of four hens in a cage on another were most frequent at a space allowance of 824 cm² per hen and less frequent at 412 cm² or 1442 cm² or 2888 cm² per hen.

Unchecked growth of bill and claws can be a problem in battery cages. If there is no possibility for birds to wear these down they may grow to the extent that they are seriously deformed. As Tauson (1986, 1988) has shown, the provision of an abrasive strip in the cage can solve this problem. Many other injuries or deformities which occur in cages can be rectified by improving cage design. Tauson (1977, 1978, 1985) has surveyed such problems and made recommendations about how to solve them. Birds became trapped in cages by the head or neck (29%), body or wings (28%), toes or claws (15%), hocks (13%) or other means. The most common place for trapping was a gap between the manure deflector and the egg guard and the second most common was in the front wall of the cage. Such trapping, which obviously leads to poor welfare and sometimes leads to death, can be minimised by: simplifying cage fronts, e.g. by using horizontal rather than vertical bars; using

variable manure deflectors with no distance or a large distance from the side partition; using floor mesh no larger than 25×37 mm; and avoiding dangerous gaps between partitions and cage floors (Tauson, 1988). Steep floors, e.g. with slopes of 23%, lead to high levels of foot deformities because birds' feet slip down onto cross-wires but this can be avoided by using slopes no greater than 12%. Foot deformity incidence can also be reduced by provision of a perch in the cage (Tauson, 1980, 1988). Wire mesh sides to cages cause some feather wear and Tauson (1984a) showed that the provision of solid partitions reduced feather wear by 15%.

Deep litter, perchery and strawyard

The deep litter system in which many hens are housed together on some sort of litter, or partly on slats, in a building with many nest boxes was very widespread in the early 1960s. The space allowance for hens was commonly 0.18 m² for heavy breeds and 0.14 m² for light breeds if slats were provided and 0.27–0.36 m² per bird if there were no slats (Sainsbury, 1980). This stocking density is similar to the 0.18–0.27 m² per bird in the whole of a battery house. In the deep litter system, however, the hens have most of the space available to them. The deep litter system is in widespread use for breeding birds so it is generally acceptable to the poultry industry except for the extra difficulties in collecting eggs as compared with a battery house. In the Netherlands, 15% of eggs come from deep litter houses and these cost 9–23% more in the shops than do eggs from battery cages.

The perchery is a development from the deep litter house in which birds are not just on the floor but they have rows of perches at different levels in the building which they can and do use. One problem which arises in houses with many perches is that some young birds come into the house and do not use the perches. Appleby (1985) found, however, that perch use was almost universal if perches had been available to the hens when they were young chicks. The third system of this general type is the covered strawyard developed by Sainsbury (1981; see

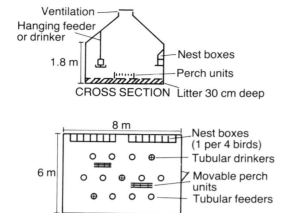

Ventilation
Hanging feeder
or drinker

1.8 m

Nest boxes
Perch units

CROSS SECTION   Litter 30 cm deep

8 m

6 m

Nest boxes
(1 per 4 birds)
Tubular drinkers
Movable perch
units
Tubular feeders

Divided sections
9 m × 8 m
to take 200 birds

Access from front
for cleaning

PLAN OF COVERED STRAW YARD

Fig. 39.4   Diagrams of the covered straw yard (after Sainsbury and Sainsbury, 1988).

Fig. 39.4). This is cheap to build and houses about 200 hens, at 0.27 m² per hen, on straw 30 cm deep. In each of these systems the hens have much freedom of movement, although there are some social restrictions on this. A variety of activities is possible and feather pecking is rare. There are, however, some welfare problems because disease and parasitism incidence can be higher, e.g. intestinal worms, and aggression may result in considerable injury to a small number of birds. Good stockmanship is necessary to identify birds with health problems or signs of injury and to separate these from the main group. The major economic problem is that some birds do not lay in nest boxes so their eggs are difficult to find and are often dirty. Some automation of egg collection from nest boxes is possible but, in general, the collection of eggs is much more labour intensive than in a battery house.

Modified cages

Some modifications of battery cages which reduce the incidence of injuries but do not give

the animal more freedom to carry out normal behaviour have been mentioned in connection with reducing the incidence of injuries. The provision of a perch in a battery cage has also been discussed. Sufficient space for birds to stretch and flap their wings could be provided in a taller cage with a floor area a little larger than the conventional cage. A moulded nest site seems to be important (Kite, 1985) but it would be difficult to provide nesting material. However there are possibilities for a modified cage which should result in better welfare. Since major problems for a hen in a battery cage seemed to be lack of space and inability to escape from a bird which is pecking it, the get-away cage was designed by Elson (1976). This was developed further in the Netherlands (Brantas *et al.*, 1978) and in the Federal Republic of Germany (Wegner, 1980). These cages (Fig. 39.5) house about 20 hens on two levels and they have nests, perches and a sand bathing area. The designs of get-away cage developed so far pose practical problems because of the large number of cracked and dirty eggs and the difficulties of egg collection. Welfare problems exist for those few individuals which fail to find the water nipples or which are attacked by other birds. Inspection of the birds is quite often difficult so these problems may not be readily discovered.

Aviaries

A range of intermediates between the get-away cage and the perchery includes the aviary, volière, volierenstall, voletage, Hans Kier unit and tiered wire floor unit. The aviary or volière (Fig. 39.6) has extra floors of wire or slats with feeders drinkers and nest boxes on each floor. The early aviaries have sometimes had severe problems of aggression, e.g. that in the United Kingdom (Hill, 1984) but later Swiss systems seem better in this respect (Fölsch *et al.*, 1983a, b). Similar problems exist in the best German Volierenstall with mortality of 1.5% (Rauch and Wegner, 1984). The Swiss voletage (Fig. 39.7),

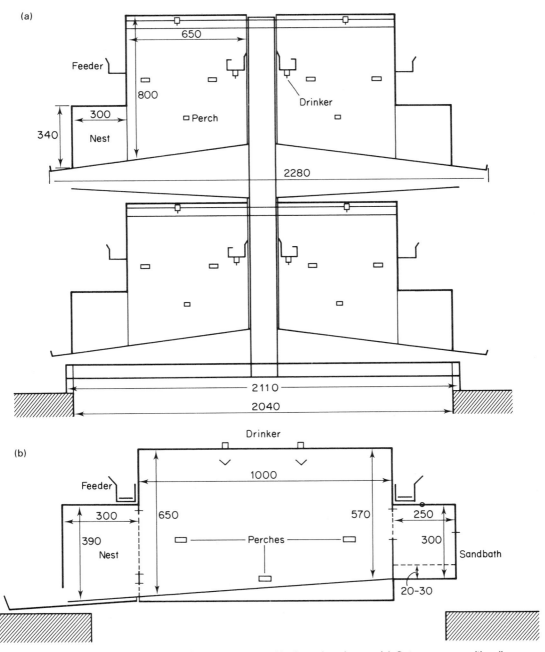

Fig. 39.5 Section diagrams of two forms of get-away cage, with dimensions in mm. (a) Get-away cage with roll-away nest ± droppings pit. (b) Get-away cage with roll-away nest and sand bath. (After Wener *et al.*, 1981.)

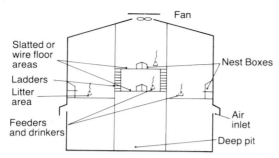

Fig. 39.6   Diagrammatic cross-section of Gleadthorpe aviary (from Sainsbury and Sainsbury, 1988).

Dutch tiered wire floor (Fig. 39.8) and Danish Hans Kier system have low aggression levels. In some Dutch tiered floor units there is no mortality but in others it is as high as 2%. In each aviary, birds are provided with at least 14 cm perching space each. The Swiss voletage is operating commercially and birds are given at least 590 cm² each of floor area, although Fölsch

et al. (1983a) recommend 1000 cm² each. The Hans Kier system has a 7 m² sloping wire floor and many perches 5 cm high. The 75 hens in the unit are allowed access to a sand-covered area which is 20% of the floor by way of electrically controllable shutters which open in the afternoon only. Norgaard-Neilson (1985) reports that feather-pecking and aggression are very low in this system. In aviaries and in other group-housing systems, aggression can be reduced by having uniform illumination with no bright patches in which hens may accumulate and fight (Gibson *et al.*, 1985). It is also important that there should be no sharp corners from which retreat is difficult when pursued. In all of these systems contact with droppings can occur so risk of coccidiosis is higher. Some systems allow for the use of belts which carry away faeces and keep the moisture level low.

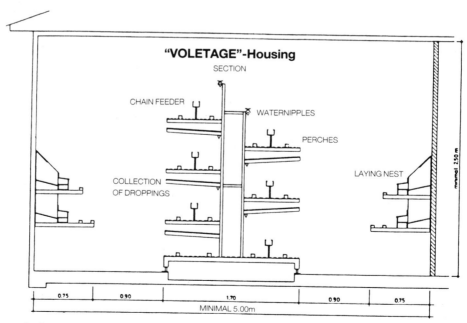

Fig. 39.7   Voletage for hens (after Fölsch *et al.*, 1983a).

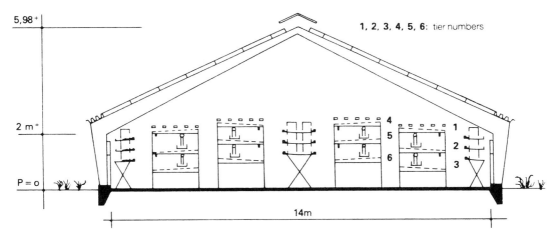

Fig. 39.8   The tiered wire floor system for housing of laying hens. Characteristics: (1) three tiers of floors; the upper floor is a resting area; (2) bordering wire floors mounted at unequal heights to create staircase effect; (3) litter covering all of the ground floor area (after Dutch Society for the Protection of Animals, 1986).

Alternative housing for laying hens—assessment on welfare and economic grounds

The welfare of the average bird in a hygienically maintained perchery, get-way cage or aviary is almost certainly better than that of the average bird in a battery cage. However the welfare of the bird which is seriously bullied by others or which is badly affected by disease is worse than those in the battery cage alternative. Recent developments in several European countries make it likely that one or several of the more spacious group-housing systems will soon be quite acceptable on practical and welfare grounds. If a system resulted in a doubling of the price of eggs then many fewer people would buy eggs so there is no chance that such a system would be accepted. If, however, there is a small increase in cost then egg consumption will not be affected, farmers can still make a living and welfare is much improved. A summary of extra costs compiled by Elson (1985) is shown in Table 39.2.

A general, gradual change throughout Europe from battery cages to a system costing up to 15%

Table 39.2
Egg production costs in different poultry systems

System	Space[a]	Cost
Laying cage	450 cm²/bird	100
Laying cage	560 cm²/bird	105
Laying cage	750 cm²/bird	115
Laying cage	450 cm²/bird + perch	100
Laying cage	450 cm²/bird + perch + nest	102
Shallow laying cage	450 cm²/bird	102
Get-away cage, 2 tier		110
Aviary	10–12 birds/m²	115
Aviary and Perchery and Multi-tier housing	20 birds/m²	105–108
Deep litter	7–10 birds/m²	118
Strawyard	3 birds/m²	130
Semi-intensive	1000 birds/ha	135 (140[b])
Free-range	400 birds/ha	150 (170[b])

[a] Space refers: in cages to cage floor area, in houses to house floor area and in extensive systems to land area.
[b] Includes land rental.
After Elson (1985).

more and resulting in the same price increase to the consumer would result in no loss in revenue to farmers. A change to an aviary, get-away cage, or perchery system would be acceptable on welfare grounds provided that problems of severe aggression could be largely eliminated. If this could not be done then an extended cage with four or five birds in it would be the next best alternative.

Housing of chickens reared for meat

There is an extensive literature about the welfare of laying hens but there have been very few studies of meat, or broiler chickens. The numbers of broilers are very large indeed so any welfare problems would involve very many individuals. The limited amount of information available is reviewed in this section and the problems associated with handling and transport in the next section.

The modern breeds of broilers grow very quickly and most are now slaughtered at seven weeks of age, by which time they have reached a weight of 1.5–2 kg. A typical broiler house is something like the deep litter house for hens. It is rectangular, being about 20 m wide and with a good ventilation and temperature control system. Before birds are put in, the clean floor is covered with litter such as wood shavings or straw to a depth of about 15 cm (Sainsbury, 1980). Day-old chicks are introduced into the house at a density which will result in a weight of birds at the end of the growing period of about 34 kg/m². Typical numbers in a house are 10 000–20 000. At the beginning of the rearing period the chickens have plenty of space but at the end of the seven weeks they are crowded close together. Little is know of the effects of this crowding.

A major problem with this rearing system is that there are many birds present and there is little or no facility for inspection so an individual which is weak, injured or sick is often not detected. Most of these individuals die and their bodies remain in the litter. In some cases, weak individuals die because they are trampled on by the other birds, for as the density approaches the final level of 34 kg of birds on each m² it is essential to be able to stand up in order to survive. A change in the numbers which can be kept in one building and in the design of the building so as to allow inspection is desirable here. Another disadvantage of having very large numbers of birds in a single building arises if the birds are suddenly frightened and hysteria develops. If this happens, many birds may move rapidly to the end of the building where there is a pile-up, under which many individuals may be crushed to death. Hysteria can be minimised by good stockmanship and the effects can be reduced by putting baffles in the house.

The rapid growth rate of a modern broiler is not uniform throughout its body. Muscle grows very quickly but bones, and in particular the leg bones, grow less fast. As a consequence, a point is reached at which the birds' legs cannot easily support its body. There is then a risk of being trampled, as mentioned above, but there will also be prolonged contact with the litter beneath the bird. Faecal matter accumulates very rapidly in a broiler house so that the litter is covered with faeces well before the end of the growing period. The faeces and their breakdown products have a corrosive effect on skin so birds which have to sit on the soiled litter for long periods get breast-blisters and hock-burns. These can be wide-spread in a broiler unit and are visible to the customer buying a chicken. One consequence of this is that legs are often cut short on carcasses so that hock-burns cannot be seen. Another consequence is that many carcasses are down-graded further so that they can only be used for chicken pieces. It seems likely that these serious skin abrasions and blisters cause considerable discomfort to the birds so the system of housing, or the breed itself, should be modified so as to avoid hock burns and breast blisters. Breeding should encourage better leg development or less muscle development. Birds should not be kept on faeces-covered litter.

Very few broilers are kept on any other system but there are a few which are free-range. In

France the "Label Rouge" is given only to free-range chickens and a study of such systems has been carried out in the U.K. by Sainsbury and Schwabe (personal communication). A different strain of bird is needed in order that it can cope with free-range conditions.

Operations, handling and transport of poultry

Beak-trimming

Since chickens which are crowded together sometimes peck one another and cause injury or death the commercial practice of de-beaking, better called beak-trimming, has developed. The procedure involves putting the young chick's bill into a cutter which cuts off about one-third of the bill by means of a heated blade which also cauterises the stump. It has been stated that the part of the bill which is removed is merely horny material with no nerve supply so the birds feel no pain at cutting or later. This is certainly wrong as Desserich *et al.* (1984) have shown in a histological study. They found that the chicken's bill has many Herbst's and Merkel's corpuscles, which are sensory receptors, and many free nerve endings in the part which is cut off during beak-trimming. The removal of the end section of the bill causes a non-regenerable loss of touch and temperature sensitivity. Work by Gentle (1986) has shown that scar tissue remains on the beak stump and that neither dermal structures nor nerves regenerate into this scar tissue. The damaged nerves develop into neuromas which continued to grow for at least 10 weeks after the operation. In general in animals, neuromas are painful so it is likely that the chickens suffer pain for a prolonged period after beak-trimming. Breward and Gentle (1985) recorded electrical impulses from primary afferent fibres originating from regenerating nerves and neuromas. They found abnormal spontaneous activity which again suggests that the birds are in pain and their welfare is poor. Studies of behavioural and white cell responses to beak trimming

also support this conclusion (Gentle and Hill, 1987; Gentle and Seawright, 1988).

Hen handling and transport

Chickens are very much disturbed by close contact with people for man is a large and dangerous animal to a chicken. Hence it is not surprising that the handling which precedes transport to slaughter has a considerable effect on the birds. The nature of that handling depends upon the conditions in which the birds are kept but it normally involves one or more birds being picked up and put into a crate which holds about 15 birds for the duration of the journey. If the hens are in battery cages the sequence of actions normally involves a person opening the cage door, grabbing one or more hens by the legs, pulling them out of the cage, passing them to another person who collects two to five birds held by one leg in each hand, carrying the birds upside down to the end of the row of battery cages or to the door of the house where a vehicle is waiting, and putting the birds into a crate. As mentioned earlier in this chapter, such handling may result in broken bones, especially if the birds have lived in a battery cage.

The effects on welfare of the rough handling which hens normally receive prior to transport can be assessed by monitoring their adrenal and other emergency responses. In a study in which normal handling and gentle handling were compared (Broom *et al.*, 1986) the plasma corticosterone levels were much higher after the rougher handling (Table 39.3), indicating that the emergency response elicited in the hens was greater. In this study, a journey of one hour in a lorry resulted in a smaller increase in corticosterone than that following normal rough handling. The significant effects of handling and transport on plasma corticosterone, plasma glucose and hypothalamic noradrenaline are shown in Fig. 39.9. Glucose production is increased following corticosterone secretion but the increase is not large because it is used up during

Table 39.3
Levels of plasma corticosterone in hens

Treatment	Corticosterone (ng/ml)
No handling, sample within 60 s	0.4
Five min. after gentle carrying to crate	1.45
Five min. after normal carrying to crate	4.30

After gentle handling as opposed to after normal handling, $p = 0.008$

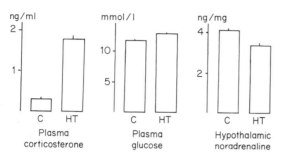

Fig 39.9 The levels of corticosterone and glucose in the blood plasma were higher in hens which were handled and transported (HT) than in hens which were not (C). The level of the transmitter substance noradrenaline was lower after handling and transport (data from Broom *et al.*, 1986).

transport. Noradrenaline is a neurotransmitter which is used up during handling and transport. These studies suggest that handling of hens has a greater adverse effect on their welfare than does a short journey. Longer journeys may pose considerable problems for hens, however, as reported in the next section on broilers. For reviews of the transportation of poultry and physical factors during the journey which affect the bird see Hails (1978) and Freeman (1984).

Handling and transport of broilers

In the U.K., each of the 400 million broiler chickens produced annually is transported twice, once as a very young chick and once to the slaughterhouse. Twenty-five million turkeys and nine million ducks are also transported. Newly hatched chicks require particular physical conditions, especially temperature but, given such conditions, there is little evidence that there are welfare problems when they are transported (Freeman, 1984). Broilers which have reached 2 kg are collected up from the floor of broiler houses, put in crates, taken by vehicle to the slaughterhouse, removed from the crates and hung by their feet on the shackling line, stunned and slaughtered. Again, physical conditions on the journey are important in relation to welfare but even if these are adequate there can be problems with limb breakages, bruises or impaired meat quality. Poor meat quality is often correlated with some emergency response and abnormal behaviour in the few hours preceding slaughter. Ehinger and Gschwindt (1979) and Gschwindt and Ehinger (1979) have demonstrated that longer journeys and long waits at the slaughterhouse have more adverse effects on meat quality.

There is a range of physiological responses to handling and transportation (e.g. Halliday *et al.*, 1977; Freeman *et al.*, 1984). The latter authors reported that untransported control birds had corticosterone levels of 1.0–1.6 ng/ml whereas levels after handling and 2 h transport were 4.5 ng/ml and after 4 h transport were 5.5 ng/ml. The normal catching procedure in which a catching gang goes into the house and birds are gathered up by their legs leads to a substantial response. An interesting recent study by Duncan (1986) involved the use of a broiler-catcher or harvester which is driven through the broiler house moving birds by rotating rubber flails onto a belt and into a crate. Birds collected up by such a broiler-catcher showed a much briefer increase in heart rate than birds collected up by people. The better welfare when the broiler-catcher is used emphasises the adverse effect on chickens of handling by people.

Glossary of terms relevant to farm animal behaviour and welfare

Abnormal behaviour, Aberrant behaviour: Behaviour which differs in pattern, frequency or context from that which is shown by most members of the species in conditions which allow a full range of behaviour (See Chapter 32).

Action pattern: A sequence of movements shown by an individual which is repeated on subsequent occasions in a largely invariate form (See Chapter 2). Other individuals may show similar action patterns.

Adaptation: (1) At the cell and organ level, the waning of a physiological response to a particular condition, including the decline over time in the rate of firing of a nerve cell. (2) At the individual level, the use of regulatory systems, with their behavioural and physiological components, so as to allow an individual to cope with its environmental conditions (see Chapter 28). (3) In evolutionary biology, any structure, physiological process, or behavioural feature that makes an organism better able to survive and to reproduce in comparison with other members of the same species. Also, the evolutionary process of leading to the formation of such a trait.

Aerophagia: Pathological and excessive swallowing of air.

Aggregation: A group of individuals of the same species, comprised of more than just a mated pair with their dependant offspring, gathered in the same place but not necessarily organised or engaged in cooperative behaviour. To be distinguished from a true social group.

Aggression: A physical act, or threat of action, by an individual which causes pain or injury or reduces freedom in another individual.

Agonistic behaviour: Any behaviour associated with threat, attack or defence. It includes features of behaviour involving escape or passivity as well as aggression (see Chapter 13).

Allogrooming: Grooming directed at another individual animal as opposed to self-grooming, which is directed at the animal's own body.

Allomimetic (allelomimetic) behaviour: Any behaviour where animals perform the same activity with some degree of mutual stimulation and consequent coordination.

Anomalous behaviour: Behaviour which is somewhat abnormal (see abnormal behaviour) particularly in respect of deviations from the normal pattern or frequency (as in general medical usage). May be a variant of a normal activity such as chewing or licking.

Anorexia: Abnormal lack of ingestive behaviour, e.g. in toxic and depressed clinical states.

Anosmia: Lack of sense of smell.

Assembly: The grouping together of the members of a society for any communal activity.

Aversion therapy: Treatment of a compulsive form of behaviour by associating the behaviour with an electric shock, or other aversive stimulation.

Aversive: Such as to cause avoidance or withdrawal.

Bond: Any close relationship formed between two individuals.

Causal factor: The inputs to a decision making centre each of which is an interpretation of an external change or an internal state of the body. (See Chapter 4).

Circadian rhythm: A rhythm in behaviour, metabolism or some other activity such that events in it recur about every 24 hours (see **Rhythm**).

Comfort-shift: A minor change of posture or position which may briefly interrupt rest.

Competition: (1) Among individuals, the striving of two or more individuals to obtain a resource which is in limited supply. Success might result from such abilities as speed of action, strength in fighting or ingenuity in searching. (2) Among genotypes, striving to carry out any life function in a way which is better than those used by other genotypes so that the fitness (reproductive success) of the genotype is increased.

Conditioning: The process by which an animal acquires the capacity to respond to a given stimulus, object or situation in a way which would previously have been a response to a different stimulus.

Conspecific: Belonging to the same species.

Consummatory act: An act which reduces greatly the levels of causal factors which promote a certain activity so that the activity is terminated, e.g. mating terminates courtship behaviour.

Contactual behaviour: Maintenance of bodily contact. The formation of simple aggregations through behaviour of this sort occurs very commonly in farm animals.

Controller: The individual in a group who determines whether or not a new group activity occurs, when it happens and which activity it is (see Chapter 15).

Cope: Have control of mental and bodily stability. This control may be short-lived or prolonged. Failure to be in control of mental and bodily stability leads to reduced fitness (see **Stress**).

Coprophagia: Eating faeces. This is normal behaviour in rabbits but occurs abnormally in other animals (see Chapter 33).

Core area: The area of heaviest regular use within the home range.

Critical period: See **Sensitive period**.

Crowding: The situation in which the movements of individuals in a group are restricted by the physical presence of others (see **Over-crowding**, Chapter 13).

Density dependence: Processes which are influenced by physiological or environmental factors so that they occur only when the density of the population increases, e.g. tail-biting behaviour in swine.

Depression: A general state of behavioural atony (sagging posture, unresponsive, apparently dispirited).

Displacement activity: An activity which is performed in a situation which appears to the observer not to be the context in which it would normally occur. Being so dependent for recognition on observer ability to determine relevance to context, the term is of very limited use (see Chapter 4).

Display: A behaviour feature which may impress or intimidate a partner, rival, or potential attacker.

Diurnal: (1) On a daily basis. (2) Occurring in daylight time.

Dominance: An individual animal is said to be dominant over another when it has priority of access to a resource such as food or a mate. A dominant individual is usually superior in fighting ability to a subordinate but this may not have been tested.

Drive: A collection of causal factors which promote related behaviours. The term often implies potential progression towards a goal. Although a definition is included here because the term drive is in widespread use, we consider it is easier to understand motivation if reference is normally made to causal factors rather than to drives.

Ecological niche: The environment in which the species performs best and which it comes to live in and occupy in nature.

Ecology: The scientific study of the interaction of organisms with their environment, including both the physical environment and the other organisms that live in it.

Ecosystem: All of the organisms of a particular habitat, such as grassland or coniferous woodland, together with the physical environment in which they live.

Eliminative behaviour: Patterns of behaviour connected with evacuation of faeces and urine.

Environment: External influences on the development of behavioural or other biological traits. External means outside the system or unit under consideration, not necessarily outside the whole organism.

Enzootic: Referring to a disorder in animals that is peculiar to a particular location or type of place and affects a small proportion of animals exposed in such a location.

Epimiletic behaviour: The provision in behavioural terms of care or attention, includes nursing in particular.

Epizootic: The spread of a disease or disorder through a population of animals (the equivalent of an epidemic in humans).

Estrous cycle: See **Oestrous cycle**.

Ethogram: A detailed description of the behavioural features of a particular species (see Chapter 2).

Ethology: The observation and detailed description of behaviour in order to find out about how biological mechanisms function. Sometimes such studies are carried out in a natural or semi-natural setting, but the study, as defined above, of animals on farms or in laboratories is ethology.

Experience: A change in the brain which results from information acquired from outside the brain. The information can originate in the environment of the individual or within the body, for example from sensory input, from low oxygen availability or from a new hormone level in the blood (see Chapter 3).

Exploration: Any activity which has the potential for the individual to acquire new information about its environment or itself (see Chapter 12).

Flight distance: That radius of space around an animal within which intrusion provokes a flight reaction (see Chapter 13).

Flight reaction: A characteristic escape reaction, specified for a particular enemy and surroundings, occurring as soon as the intruder approaches within a given distance.

Foraging: The behaviour of animals when they are moving around in such a way that they are likely to encounter and acquire food for themselves or their offspring (see Chapter 9).

Fraser Darling effect: The stimulation of reproductive activity by the presence and activity of other members of the species in addition to the mating pair.

Functional systems: The different sorts of biological activity in the living animal which together make up the life process, for example temperature regulation, feeding, predator avoidance. These functional systems have behavioural and physiological components (see Chapter 1).

Genotype: The genetic constitution of an individual organism designated with reference either to a single trait or to a set of traits (see **Phenotype**).

Geophagia: Eating soil.

Gonad: The organ that produces sex hormones and gametes, either an ovary (female gonad) or testis (male gonad).

Grooming: The cleaning of the body surface by licking, nibbling, picking, rubbing, scratching, etc. When action is directed towards the animal's own body, it is called self-grooming, when directed at another individual, it is referred to as allogrooming.

Group effect: An alteration in behaviour within a number of associating animals brought about by common participation. A simple example is social facilitation, in which there is an increase of an activity merely from the sight or sound (or other form of stimulation) coming from other individuals engaged in the same activity.

Habituation: The waning of a response, which could still be shown, to a repeated stimulus. This is distinct from fatigue.

Head-pressing: Postural disorder characterised by apparent head stabilisation through forehead contact with a vertical surface. The head is lowered and the inactive posture is maintained for long periods. Assumed to give clinical implication of cerebral disease. Noted in horses and cattle.

Hierarchy: A sequence of individuals or groups of individuals in a social group which is based upon some ability or characteristic. The term is most frequently used where the ability assessed is that of winning fights or displacing other individuals (see Chapter 15).

Home range: The area that an animal learns thoroughly and uses regularly. The home range may or may not be defended; those portions that are defended constitute the territory (see also **Core area**, Chapter 13).

Homeostasis: The maintenance of a body variable in a steady state by means of physiological or behavioural regulatory actions.

Hormone: Any substance, secreted by an endocrine gland into the blood or lymph, that affects the physiological activity of other organs in the body; hormones can also influence the nervous system, and through it, the behaviour of the organism.

Imprinting: (1) Rapid and relatively stable learning taking place in early life. (2) The infantile parameter whereby, often without any apparent immediate reinforcement, broad supra-individual characteristics of the species come to be recognised.

Individual distance: The minimum distance from an animal within which approach elicits attack or avoidance (see Chapter 13).

Ingestive behaviour: Behaviour concerned with the selection and intake of food, milk, water, etc.

Initiator: The individual in a social group which is the first to react in a way which elicits a new group activity (see Chapter 15).

Instinct: A term implying behaviour which is entirely genetically controlled. The use of this term is undesirable and confusing because neither behaviour nor any other whole animal characteristic can develop independently of all environmental influences.

Intention movements: The preparatory motions that an animal may go through prior to switching to a new behaviour.

Intersucking: Abnormal sucking activity directed to appendages of others. This occurs notably in groups of young livestock prematurely weaned and in some adult cows (see Chapter 34).

Kinesis: An undirected reaction, without orientation of the body in relation to the stimulus.

Leader: The individual which is in front during an orderly group progression (see Chapter 15).

Learning: A change in the brain which results in behaviour being modified for longer than a few seconds as a consequence of information acquired from outside the brain.

Libido: An internal state which is measured by the likelihood of showing sexual behaviour given appropriate opportunity (see Chapter 20).

Lignophagy: Wood eating.

Maladaptation: Faulty adaptation to environmental circumstances.

Mobbing: Joint assault or threat by a group of animals.

Motivation: The process within the brain controlling which behaviours and physiological changes occur and when (see Chapter 4).

Motivational state: A combination of the levels of all causal factors (see **Causal factor** and Chapter 4).

Mourning behaviour: Somnolent episodes with orbital fixation and loss of attention to environmental events. The behaviour is associated with the "dog-sitting" posture in sows confined in single stalls.

Need: A deficiency in an animal which can be remedied by obtaining a particular resource or responding to a particular environmental or bodily stimulus (see Chapter 28).

Neuroethology: The study of the overall neural control of behaviour.

Neurophysiology: The scientific study of the nervous system especially the physiological processes by which it functions.

Niche: (see **Ecological niche**).

Nursing: The behaviour of the mother mammal which allows the young to suck milk from her teats.

Observational learning: Learning that occurs when one animal watches the activities of another.

Oestrous (estrous) cycle: The repeated series of changes in reproductive physiology and behaviour that culminates in oestrus or "heat", i.e. receptivity. (The noun is oestrus (estrus) and the adjective oestrous (estrous).)

Ontogeny: The process of development of an organism from single cell to adult.

Over-crowding: Crowding such that the fitness of individuals in the group is reduced (see **Crowding**, Chapter 13).

Pain: A sensation which is itself extremely aversive. The specialised pain fibres are usually involved in pain sensation. The results of the interpretation of sensory input, such as that associated with predator detection and consequent "fear", are not included by this definition in the category of pain (see Chapter 29).

Pair bonding: A close and long-lasting association formed between a male and female.

Pandiculation: General outstretching as an action pattern.

Peck order: A stable hierarchy in which each individual is able to threaten, displace or attack individuals lower than itself with impunity. The term was coined following work with chickens but is now used for any animal (see Chapter 15).

Periodicity: A series of events separated by equal periods in a time series (see Chapter 2).

Phenotype: The observable properties of an organism as they have developed under the combined influences of the genetic constitution of the individual and the effects of environmental factors (contrast with **Genotype**).

Pheromone: A substance produced by one animal which conveys information to other individuals by olfactory means (see Chapter 7).

Pica: The seeking out and eating of foreign objects such as wood, cloth and old bones (see Chapter 33).

Polydipsia: Excessive drinking of water beyond physiological needs.

Posture: The distinctive relation of the extremities of the head, neck and limbs to the trunk of the animal's body. Posture is also manifest in the disposition of the limbs in the standing position.

Reaction time: Time between the occurrence of an environmental change and the beginning of the response of the animal.

Redirected activity: The direction of some behaviour, such as an act of aggression, away from the primary target and toward another, less appropriate object. This term must be used with care as it implies that the observer knows what the primary target is.

Reflex: A simple response involving the central nervous system and occurring very shortly after the stimulus which evokes it. It characteristically involves only a part of the organism, although the whole may be affected, and is usually a response to localised stimuli.

Reinforcer: An environmental change which increases or decreases the likelihood that an animal will make a particular response, i.e. a reward (positive reinforcer) or a punishment (negative reinforcer) (see Chapter 3).

Releaser: (see **Sign stimulus**).

Reproductive habilitation: Those events which furnish the animal with the physiological preparedness to reproduce.

Rhythm: A series of events repeated in time at intervals whose distribution is approximately regular (see Chapter 2).

Rights: There is much discussion about "animal rights" which should be clearly distinguished from the concept of animal welfare (see Chapter 28) but some definition of animal rights may be useful here. (1) A legal entitlement which can be defended using the laws of the country. In most countries animals do not have rights in this sense. (2) A privilege which is justifiable on moral, perhaps religious, grounds. In relation to animals this concept is easiest for most people to understand in terms of human obligations towards animals. In all societies the majority of people consider that they have some obligations towards animals which are separate from any self-interest.

Ritual behaviour: An originally variable sequence of behavioural actions which has become an almost unchangeable sequence. Such behaviour may lose its original meaning and acquire a use in communication.

Ritualisation: The process of producing ritual behaviour.

Scent marking: The deposition of solid or liquid pheromones, typically on a tree, bush or rock (see **Pheromone**, Chapter 7).

Self-grooming: Grooming directed at the individual's own body. This is distinguished from allogrooming, the grooming of another individual.

Sensitisation: The increasing of a response to a repeated stimulus.

Sensitive period: A time interval during development within which the behaviour, at that time or later, is especially likely to be affected by certain types of experience.

Sensory physiology: The study of sense organs and the ways in which they receive stimuli from the environment and transmit them in the nervous system.

Sign stimulus: A specific environmental feature which elicits a response from an animal.

Social behaviour: The reciprocal interactions of

two or more animals and the resulting modifications of individual activity.

Social facilitation: Behaviour that is initiated or increased in rate or frequency by the presence of another animal carrying out that behaviour (see Chapters 9 and 15).

Social organisation: The size of a social group; its composition in respect of age, sex and degrees of relatedness of group members; all of the relationships among individuals in the group; and the duration of association of the members of the group (see **Social structure,** Chapter 15).

Social structure: All of the relationships among individuals in a social group and their consequences for spatial distribution and behavioural interactions (see Chapter 15).

Socialisation: (1) The total modification of behaviour in an individual due to its interaction with other members of its society. (2) Affiliation with humans.

Society: A group of individuals belonging to the same species and organised in a cooperative manner.

Sociobiology: The study of the biological bases of social behaviour, employing evolution as the basic explanatory tool.

Souring: Regression in behaviour to poorly controlled destructive activities. Acts of uncompliance, notably in schooled horses.

Stereotypy: A repeated, relatively invariate sequence of movements which has no obvious purpose (see Chapter 32).

Stress: An environmental effect on an individual which over-taxes its control systems and reduces its fitness. Fitness reduction involves increased mortality, or failure to grow, or failure to reproduce (see Chapter 28).

Suckling: The behaviour of a young mammal whilst it is ingesting milk from the teats of its mother or another female mammal.

Symbiosis: The intimate, relatively protracted, and dependant relationship of members of one species with those of another.

Taxis: (1) Locomotion oriented systematically with respect to a source of stimulation. (2) Locomotory behaviour involving a steering reaction. (3) The spatial correction movement resulting in orientation.

Technopathies: Diseases and behavioural disorders occurring as a result of technical innovations in animal husbandry.

Territoriality: Behaviour associated with territory defence.

Territory: An area which an animal defends by fighting, or by demarcation which other individuals detect, so that the mark or other signal is a deterrent to entry (see Chapter 13).

Thigmotaxis: Movement so as to maintain close bodily contact with an inanimate surface or another animal.

Tonic immobility: A behaviour state of a few seconds or longer during which an animal makes no movement as a consequence of some temporary environmental situation or of a pathological condition (see Chapter 36).

Trail pheromone: A substance laid down in the form of a trail by one animal and followed by another member of the same species.

Trophic: Pertaining to food and feeding.

Umwelt: A German term (loosely translated as "the world around me") used to indicate the total sensory receptivity of an animal. Each species has its own distinctive *umwelt.*

Welfare: The state of an individual as regards its attempts to cope with its environment (see Chapters 1 and 28).

Whetting: (1) Rubbing horns or tusks repetitiously—as though to sharpen them. (2) Repeated stroking of a body part, e.g. tongue or poll on a stall fixture.

References

Abraham, S., Baker, R., Denton, D. A. Kraintz, F., Krantz, L. and Purser, L. (1973). Components in the regulation of salt balance: salt appetite studied by operant behaviour. *Aust. J. exp. Biol. med Sci.* **51**, 65–81.

Adamec, R. E. (1978). Normal and abnormal limbic system mechanisms of emotive biasing. In *Limbic Mechanisms*, ed. K. E. Livingston and O. Hornykiewicz, New York.

Adamec, R. E. and Stark-Adamec, C. (1983). Limbic kindling and animal behaviour—Implications for human psychopathology associated with complex partial seizures, *Biol. Psych.,* **18**, 2.

Albright, J. L. (1969). Social environment and growth. In *Animal Growth and Nutrition* ed. E. S. E. Hafez and I. A. Dyers. Philadelphia: Lea and Febiger.

Albright, J. L. (1981). Training dairy cattle. In *Dairy Sciences Handbook*. Vol. 14, 363–370. Clovis CA.: Agriservices Foundation.

Alexander, G. (1960). Maternal behaviour in the Merino ewe. *Proc. Aust. Soc. Anim. Prod.,* **3**, 105–114.

Alexander, G. and Bradley, L. R. (1985). Fostering in sheep. IV. Use of restraint. *Appl. Anim. Behav. Sci.,* **4**, 363–372.

Alexander, G. and Shillito, E. E. (1977). The importance of odour, appearance and voice in maternal recognition of the young in Merino sheep (*Ovis aries*). *Appl. Anim. Ethol.,* **3**, 127–135.

Alexander, G. and Stevens, D. (1985a). Fostering in sheep III. Facilitation by use of odourants. *Appl Anim. Behav. Sci.,* **14**, 345–354.

Alexander, G. and Stevens, D. (1985b). Fostering in sheep. II. Use of hessian coats to foster an additional lamb onto ewes with single lambs. *Appl. Anim. Behav. Sci.* **14**, 335–344.

Alexander, G. Signoret, J-P, and Hafez, E. S. E. (1974). Sexual and maternal behaviour. In *Reproduction in Farm Animals* ed. Hafez. E. S. E. 3rd Edition Philadelphia: Lea and Febiger, p. 222.

Alexander, G. Lynch, J. J. and Mottershead, B. E. (1979). Use of shelter and selection and unshorn ewes in paddocks with closely or widely spaced shelters. *Appl. Anim. Ethol.,* **5**, 51–69.

Alexander, G. Stevens, D. and Bradley, L. R. (1983a). Washing lambs and confinement as aids to fostering. *Appl. Anim. Ethol.* **10**, 251–261.

Alexander, G. Stevens, D. Kilgour, R. de Langen, H. Mottershead, B. E. and Lynch, J. J. (1983b). Separation of ewes from twin lambs: Incidence in several sheep breeds. *Appl. Anim. Ethol.* **10**, 301–317.

Alexander, G., Stevens, D. and Mottershead, B. (1983c). Problems in the accurate recording of lambing data. *Aust. J. Exp. Agric. Anim. Husb.,* **23**, 361–368.

Alexander, G. Kilgour, R. Stevens, D. and Bradley, L. R. (1984). The effect of experience on twin-care in New Zealand Romney sheep. *Appl. Anim. Behav. Sci.,* **4**, 363–372.

Alexander, G., Stevens, D. and Bradley, L. R. (1985). Fostering sheep I. Facilitation by use of textile lamb coats. *Appl. Anim. Behav. Sci.,* **14**, 49–61.

Algers, B. (1984). A note on behavioural responses of farm animals to ultrasound. *Appl. Anim. Behav. Sci.,* **12**, 387–391.

Algers, B. (1989). Vocal and tactile communication during suckling in pigs. *Sveriges Lantbruksuniversitet, Rapport,* **25**. Skara: S. L. V.

Allison, T. and Cichetti, D. V. (1976). Sleep in mammals: Ecological and constitutional correlates. *Science, N. Y.* **194**, 732–734.

Allison, T. and van Twyer, H. (1970). The evolution of sleep. *Nat. Hist.* **79**, 56–65.

Almli, C. R. and Weiss, C. R. (1974). Drinking behaviours: Effects of lateral preoptic and lateral hypothalamic destruction. *Physiol. Behav.* **13**, 527–538.

Almquist, J. O. and Hale, E. B. (1956). An approach to the measurement of sexual behaviour and semen production of dairy bulls. *Proc. 3rd Intl. Congr. Anim. Reprod.* Camb. P, Plenary papers, p. 50–59.

Al-Rawi, B. and Craig, J. V. (1975). Agonistic behaviour of caged chickens related to group size and area per bird. *Appl. Anim. Ethol.* **2**, 69–80.

Altmann, J. (1974). Observational study of behaviour: sampling methods. *Behaviour,* **49**, 227–267.

Anderson, B. (1971). Thirst and brain control of water balance. *Amer. Sci.,* **59**, 408–415.

Andreae, U. (1979). Zur Aktivitätsfrequenz von Mastbullen bei Spaltenbodenhaltung. *Landbauforschung Völkenrode,* **48**, 89–94.

Andreae, U. and Smidt. D. (1982). Behavioural alterations in young cattle on slatted floors. In *Disturbed Behaviour in Farm Animals* ed. W. Bessei, *Hohenheimer Arbeiten,* **121**, 51–60. Stuttgart : Eugen Ulmer.

Andrew, R. J. (1956). Fear responses in *Emberizia* spp. *Br. J. Anim. Behav.* **4**, 125–32.

Andrew, R. J. (1966). Precocious adult behaviour in the young chick. *Anim. Behav.,* **12**, 64–76.

Anonymous, (1981). *First European Symposium on Poultry Welfare.* World Society for the Protection of Animals, Zürich, Switzerland.

Appleby, M. C. (1985). Developmental aspects of nest-site selection. In *Second European Symposium on Poultry Welfare,* ed. R. -M. Wegner, 138–143. Celle: World Poultry Science Association.

Appleby, M. C. and Lawrence, A. B. (1987). Food restriction as a cause of stereotypic behaviour in tethered gilts. *Anim. Prod.* **45**, 103–110.

Appleby, M. C. and Lawrence, A. B. (in press). Hunger as a cause of stereotypic behaviour in pregnant sows. *Appl. Anim. Behav. Sci.*

Appleby, M. C. and Wood-Gush, D. G. M. (1986). Development of behaviour in beef bulls : sexual behaviour causes more problems than aggression. *Anim. Prod.* **42**, 464.

Appleby, M. C., McRea, H. E. and Pertz, B. E (1984). The effect of light on the choice of nests by domestic hens. *Appl. Anim. Ethol.* **11**, 249–251.

Arave, C. W. and Albright, J. L. (1976). Social rank and physiological traits of dairy cows as influenced by changing group membership. *J. dairy Sci.* **59**(5): 974–985.

Arave, C. W., Albright, J. L. and Sinclair, C. L. (1974). Behaviour, milk yield and leucocytes of dairy cows in reduced space and isolation. *J. dairy Sci.,* **59**, 974–985.

Arave, C. W. and Walters, J. L. (1980). Factors affecting lying behaviour and stall utilisation of dairy cattle. *Appl. Anim. Ethol.,* **6**, 369–376.

Archer, M. (1971). Preliminary studies on the palatibility of grasses, legumes and herbs to horses. *Vet. Rec.,* **89**, 236–240.

Archer, J. (1979). Behavioural aspects of fear in animals and man. In *Fear in Animals and Man* (W. Sluckin, ed.) Princeton, N. j.: Van Nostrand Rheinhold.

Archer, M. (1977). Grazing patterns of horses. *Br. Vet. J.,* **133**, 98.

Arnold, G. W. (1960). The effect of the quantity and quality of pasture available to sheep on their grazing behaviour. *Aust. J. agric. Res.,* **11**, 1034–1043.

Arnold, G. W. (1964). Factors within plant associations affecting the behaviour and performance of grazing animals. In *Grazing in Terrestrial and Marine Environments* (D. J. Crisp, ed.). Oxford: Blackwell.

Arnold, G. W. (1977). Analysis of spatial leadership in a small field in a small flock of sheep. *App. Anim. Ethol.,* **3**, 263–270.

Arnold, G. W. (1982). Some factors affecting the grazing behaviour of sheep in winter in New South Wales. *Appl. Anim. Ethol.,* **8**, 119–125.

Arnold, G. W. (1985). Parturient behaviour. In *Ethology of Farm Animals, World Animal Science,* A5, ed. A. F. Fraser, 335–347. Amsterdam : Elsevier.

Arnold, G. W. and Dudzinski, M. L. (1978). *Ethology of Free Ranging Domestic Animals* Amsterdam: Elsevier.

Arnold, G. W. and Grassia, A. (1982). Ethogram of agonistic behaviour for thoroughbred horses. *Appl. Anim. Ethol.,* **8**, 5–25.

Arnold, G. W. and Hill, J. L. (1972). Chemical factors affecting selection of food plants by ruminants. In *Phytochemical Ecology,* ed. J. B. Harborne, pp 71–101 London: Academic Press.

Arnold, G. W. and Maller, R. A. (1974). Some aspects

of competition between sheep for supplementary feed. *Anim. Prod.* **19**, 309–319.

Arnold, G. W. and Maller, R. A. (1977). Effects of nutritional experience in early and adult life on the performance and dietary habits of sheep. *Appl. Anim. Ethol.,* **3**, 5–26.

Arnold, G. W. and Morgan, P. D. (1975). Behaviour of the ewe and lamb at lambing and its relationship to lamb mortality. *Appl. Anim. Ethol.,* **2**, 25–46.

Arnold, G. W. and Pahl, P. J. (1974). Some aspects of social behaviour in domestic sheep. *Anim. Behav.* **22**, 592–600.

Arnold, G. W., Wallace, S. R., and Rea, W. A. (1981). Associations between individuals and home range behaviour in natural flocks of three breeds of domestic sheep. *Appl. Anim. Ethol.,* **7**, 239–257.

Arthur, G. H. (1961). Some observations on the behaviour of parturient farm animals with particular reference to cattle. *Vet. Rec.* **12**, 75–84.

Augustini, C., Fischer, K. and Schön, L. (1977). Auswirkungen unterschiedlicher Transportbelastungen auf intra vitam und post mortem erfabare parameter beim Schwein. *Die fleischwirtschaft,* **57**, 2037–2040, 2043.

Bäckström, L. (1973). Environment and animal health in piglet production. *Acta vet. Scand.* Suppl **41**, 1–240.

Baeumer, E. (1955). Lebensart des Haushuhns. *Z. Tierpsychol.* **12**, 387–401.

Baeumer, E. (1962). Lebensart des Haushuhns, dritter Teil-uber seine laute und allgemaine Ergänzungen. *Z. Tierpsychol.,* **19**, 394–416.

Baile, C. A. & Forbes, J. M. (1974). Control of feed intake and regulation of energy balance in ruminants. *Physiol. Rev.* **54**, 160–214.

Bailie, J. H. (1982). Management and economic effects of different levels of oestrus detection in the dairy herd. *Vet. Rec.,* **110**, 218–221.

Balch, C. C. (1955). Sleep in ruminants. *Nature* Lond. **175**, 940–941.

Baldock, N. M. & Sibly, R. M. (in press). Effects of management procedures on heart rate in sheep. *Appl. Anim. Behav. Sci.*

Baldock, N. M., Sibly, R. M. & Penning, P. D. (1988). Behaviour and seasonal variation in heart rate in domestic sheep (*Ovis aries*) *Anim. Behav.* **36**, 35–43.

Baldwin, B. A. (1972). Operant conditioning techniques for the study of thermo-regulatory behaviour in sheep. *J. Physiol,* **226**, 41–42p.

Baldwin, B. A. (1979). Operant studies on the behaviour of pigs and sheep in realtion to the physical environment. *J. Anim. Sci.,* **49**, 1125–1134.

Baldwin, B. A. & Parrott, R. F. (1979). Studies on intracranial electrical self-stimulation in pigs in relation to ingestive and exploratory behaviour. *Physiol. Behav.,* **22**, 723–730.

Banks, E. M. (1964). Some aspects of sexual behaviour in domestic sheep, Ovis aries. *Behaviour,* **23**, 249–279.

Baptista, L. F. & Petrinovich, L. (1986). Song development in the white-crowned sparrow: social factors and sex differences. *Anim. Behav.* **34**, 1359–1371.

Barash, D. P. (1982). *Sociobiology and Behaviour* (2nd ed.), Elsever Science Publishing Co., 426 pp.

Bareham, J. F. (1972). Effects of cages and semi-intensive deep litter pens on the behaviour and adrenal response and production in two strains of laying hens. *Br. vet. J.,* **129**, 153–163.

Barlow, G. W. (1977). Modal actions patterns. In *How Animals Communicate* ed. T. A. Sebeok, Indianopolis: University of Indiana Press.

Barnett, J. L., Cronin, G. M. and Winfield, C. G. (1981). The effects of individual and group penning of pigs on plasma total and free corticosteroid concentrations and the maximum corticosteroid binding capacity. *Gen. Comp. Endocrinol.,* **44** : 219–225.

Barnett, J. L., Cronin, G. M. Winfield C. G. and Dewar, A. M. (1984). The welfare of adult pigs : the effects of five housing treatments on behaviour, plasma corticosteroids and injuries. *Appl. Anim. Behav. Sci.,* **12**, 209–232.

Barnett, J. L., Hemsworth, P. H. and Winfield, C. G. (1987). The effects of design of individual stalls on the social behaviour and physiological responses related to the welfare of pregnant pigs. *Appl. Anim. Behav. Sci.,* **18**, 133–142.

Barnett, S. A. (1963) *A Study in Behaviour.* London:Methuen.

Barton, M. A. (1983a). Behaviour of group-reared calves on acid milk replacer. *App. Anim. Ethol.,* **11**, 77.

Barton, M. A. (1983b). The effects of management and behavioural factors on intake of acidified milk and concentrates by group-reared calves. *Anim. Prod.* **36**, 512.

Barton, M. A. and Broom, D. M. (1985). Social factors affecting the performance of teat-fed calves. *Anim. Prod.* **40**, 525.

Baryshnikov, I. A. and Kokorina, E. P. (1959). Higher nervous activity and lactation. *Int. Dairy Cong.* **15**, 46–53.

Bateson, P.P.G. (1964). Changes in chicks' responses to novel moving objects over the sensitive period for imprinting. *Anim. Behav.* **12**, 479–489.

Bateson, P.P.G. (1966). The characteristics and context of imprinting. *Biol. Rev.,* **41**, 177–220.

Bateson, P.P.G. (1978). Sexual behaviour and optimal outbreeding. *Nature, Lond.* **273**, 659–660.

Bateson, P.P.G. (1980). Optimal outbreeding and the development of sexual preferences in Japanese quail. *Z. Tierpsychol.,* **53**, 231–244.

Baxter, M.R. (1982). Environmental determinants of excretory and lying areas in domestic pigs. *Appl. Anim. Ethol.* **9**, 195.

Baxter, M.R. (1988). Needs – behavioural or psychological? *Appl. Anim. Behav. Sci.,* **19**, 345–348.

Baxter, M.R. and Schwaller, C. (1983). Space requirements for sows in confinement. In *Farm Animal Housing and Welfare* ed. S.H. Baxter. M.R. Baxter and J.A.C. MacCormack. *Curr. Top. vet. Med. Anim. Sci.,* **24**, 181–195.

Beach, F.A. (1970). Some effects of gonadal hormones on sexual behaviour. In: *The Hypothalamus,* p. 617 New York: Academic Press.

Beach, F.A. (1976). Sexual attractivity, proceptivity, and receptivity in female mammals. *Horm. Behav.* **7**, 105–38.

Beilharz, R.G. (1985). Special phenomena. In *World Animal Science* A5. *Ethology of Farm Animals,* ed. A.F. Fraser. Amsterdam: Elsevier.

Beilharz, R.G. and Zeeb, K. (1982). Social dominance in dairy cattle. *Appl. Anim. Ethol.,* **8**, 79–97.

Behrens, H. (1968). Der Kannibalismus der Schweine. *Tierzuchter* **20**, 705.

Bell, F.R. (1959). Preference thresholds for taste discrimination in goats. *J. agric. Sci., Cambridge.* **52**, 125–128.

Bell, F.R. (1960). The electroencephalogram of goats during somnolence and rumination. *Anim. Behav.* **8**, 39–42.

Bellinger, L.L. and Mendel, V.E. (1974). A note on the reproductive activity of Hampshire and Suffolk ewes outside the breeding season. *Anim. Prod.,* **19**, 123–126.

Bengtsson, A-C, Svendsen, J., and Persson, G. (1983). Jamforande undersokring an draktiga suggor i 4 olika inhysnings system: beteende-studier och renhetsstudier. (Comparison of four types of housing for sows in gestation: behaviour studies and hygiene studies). *Sveriges Lantbruksuniversitet, Institutionen for Lantbrukets Byggnadsteknik, Rapport,* **36**, 76pp Lund.

Benham, P.F.J. (1982a). Synchronisation of behaviour in grazing cattle. *Appl. Anim. Ethol.,* **8**, 403–404.

Benham, P.F.J. (1982b). Social organisation and leadership in a grazing herd of suckler cows. *Appl. Anim. Ethol.,* **9**, 95.

Benham, P.F.J. (1984) Social organisation in groups of cattle and the interrelationship between social and grazing behaviours under different grazing management systems. Ph.D. thesis, University of Reading.

Benjaminsen, E. and Karlberg, K. (1981). Post weaning oestrus and luteal function in primiparous and pluriparous sows. *Res. vet. Sci.,* **30**, 318–322.

Bennett, I.L., Finch, V.A., and Holmes, C.R. (1985). Time spent in shade and its relationship with physiological factors of thermoregulation in three breeds of cattle. *Appl. Anim. Behav. Sci.,* **13**, 227–2.

Bentley, D.R. and Hoy R.R. (1972). Genetic control of the neuronal network generating cricket (*Teleogryllus, Gryllus*) song patterns. *Anim. Behav.,* **20**, 478–92.

Berliner, V.R. (1959). The oestrus cycle of the mare. In *Reproduction in Domestic Animals,* ed. H.H. Cole and P.T. Cupps, First Edition. Academic Press, New York, p. 267.

Berlyne, D.E. (1967). Arousal and reinforcement. In *Nebraska Symposium on Motivation* (M.R. Jones. ed.). Lincoln: University of Nebraska Press.

Bessei, W. (1982). Head shaking in the domestic fowl. *Hohenheimer Arbeiten,* **121**, 147–151.

Bessei, W. (1983). Zum Problem des Federpickers und Kannibalismus. *D.G.S.,* **24**, 656–665.

Beuving, G. (1980). Corticosteroids in laying hens. In *The Laying Hen and its Environment,* ed. R. Moss, *Curr. Top. vet. Med. Anim. Sci.,* **8**, 65–82. The Hague: Martinus Nijhoff.

Black, A.J., and Hughes, B.O. (1974). Patterns of comfort behaviour and activity in hens: cages and pens. *Br. vet. J.,* **130**, 23–33.

Blackshaw, J.K. and McVeigh, J.F. (1984a). Stereotype behaviour in sows and gilts housed in stalls, tethers and groups. In *Advances in Animal Welfare Science* 1984/5 ed. M.W. Fox and L.D. Mickley, Washington: Humane Society of the United States.

Blackshaw, J.K. and McVeigh, J.F. (1984b). The

behaviour of sows and gilts, housed in stalls, tethers and groups. *Proc. Aust. Soc. Anim. Prod.,* **15**, 85–92.

Blackwell, R. E. and Guillemin, R. (1973). Hypothalamic control of adenohypophyseal secretions, *Ann. Rev. Physiol.,* **35**, 357.

Blakemore, C. and Cooper, G. F. (1970). Development of the brain depends on the visual environment. *Nature, Lond.* **228**, 477–478.

Blakemore, C. and van Sluyters, R. C. van (1974). Reversal of the physiological effects of monocular deprivation in kittens: further evidence for a sensitive period. *J. Physiol.,* Lond. **237**, 195–216.

Blecha, F. and Kelley, K. W. (1981). Cold stress reduces the acquisition of colostral immunoglobulin in piglets. *J. Anim. Sci.,* **52**, 594–600.

Block, M. L., Volpe, L. C., Hayse, M. J. (1981). Saliva as a chemical cue in the development of social behaviour. *Science, N. Y.* **211**, 1062–1064.

Blockey, M. A. deB. (1978). The influence of serving capacity of bulls on herd fertility. *J. Anim. Sci.,* **46** (3):589.

Blockey, M. A. deB. (1979). Observations on group mating of bulls at pasture. *Appl. Anim. Ethol.,* **5**, 15–34.

Blockey, M. A. deB. (1981). Further studies on the serving capacity test for beef bulls. *Appl. Anim. Ethol.,* **7**, 337–350.

Blokhuis, H. J. (1983). Sleep in poultry. *World's Poult. Sci. J.,* **39**, 33–37.

Blokhuis, H. J. (1984). Rest in poultry. *Appl. Anim. Behav. Sci.,* **12**, 289–303.

Blokhuis, H. J. (1986). Feather pecking in poultry: its relation with ground pecking. *Appl. Anim. Behav. Sci.,* **16**, 63–67.

Blokhuis, H. J. and Arkes, J. G. (1984). Some observations on the development of feather-pecking in poultry. *Appl. Anim. Behav. Sci.,* **12**, 154–157.

Blokhuis, H. J. and van den Haar, J. W. (1989). Effects of floor type during rearing and of beak trimming on ground pecking and feather pecking in laying hens. *Appl. Anim. Behav. Sci.,* **22**, 359–369.

Bloom, W., and Fawcett, D. (1968). *A Textbook on Histology* 9th edn., Philadelphia: Saunders.

Bogner, H. (1984). *Einige Verhaltensweisen von Legehennen bei unterschiedlichen Platzangebot.* München: IGN-Tagung.

Bolles, R. C. (1975). *Theory of Motivation.* New York: Harper and Row.

Booth, D. A. (1978). Prediction of feeding behaviour from energy flows in the rat. In *Hunger Models: Computable Theory of Feeding Control* ed. D. A. Booth. London: Academic Press.

Boothroyd, A. (1965). The control of gilts which savage their litters. *Vet. Rec.,* **77**, 970.

Bourne, F. J. (1969). Studies on colostral and milk whey proteins in the sow. 1. Transition of mammary secretion from colostrum to milk with natural suckling. *Anim. Prod.,* **11**, 337–343.

Bouissou, M-F. (1970). Role du contact physique dans la manifestation des relations hierarchiques chez les bovins: consequences pratiques. *Annales de Zootechnie,* **19**, 279.

Bouissou, M.-F. (1976). Effet de differentes perturbations sur le nombre d'interactions sociales éclorgées au sein de groupes de bovins. *Biol. Behav.,* **1**, 193–198.

Bouissou, M.-F. and Boissy, A. (1988). Effects of early handling on heifers' subsequent reactivity to humans and to unfamiliar situations. In *Proceedings of the International Congress on Applied Ethology in Farm Animals, Skara 1988,* ed. J. Unshelm, G. van Putten, K. Zeeb and, I. Ekesbo, 21–38. Darmstadt: K. T. B. L.

Box, H. O. (1973). *Organisation in Animal Communities.* London: Butterworth.

Boyd, J. D., and Hamilton, W. J. (1970). *The Human Placenta,* Cambridge, Heffer.

Brantas. G. C. (1974). Das Verhalten von Legehennen:quantitive Unterschiede zwischen Käfig- und Bodenhaltung. In *Ursache und Beseitigung von Verhaltensstorungen bei Haustieren,* 138–146.

Brantas, G. C. (1975). Welzijn produktie en profit. *Tijdschr Diergeneesk.,* **100**, 703–708.

Brantas, G. C. (1980). The pre-laying behaviour of laying hens in cages with and without laying nests. In *The Laying Hen and its Environment,* ed. R. Moss, *Curr. Top. vet. Med. Anim. Sci.,* **8**, 227–234. The Hague: Martinus Nijhoff.

Brantas, G. C. de Vos-Reesink, K. and Wennrich, G. (1978). Ethologische Beobachtungen an Legehennen in Get-Away-Käfigen. *Arch. Geflügelk.,* **42**, 129–132.

Breward, J. and Gentle. M. J. (1985). Neuroma formation and abnormal afferent nerve discharges after partial beak amputation (beak trimming) in poultry. *Experientia,* **41**, 1132–1134.

Brion, A. (1964). Les tics chez les animaux. In *Psychiatrie Animale,* ed. A. Brion and H. Ey, pp 299–306. Paris: Desclée de Brouwer.

Brooks, C. McC. (1981). The autonomic nervous

system, molder and integrator of function. Review of a concept. *Braz. J. Med. biol. Res.,* **14,** 151–160.

Brooks, V. B. Cooke, J. D. and Thomas, J. S. (1973). The continuity of movements. In: *Advances in Behavioural Biology: Control of posture and locomotion,* R. B. Stein, K. G. Pearson, R. S. Smith and J. B. Redford (eds). **7,** 257–272. New York: Plenum Press.

Brooks, V. B. and Stoney, S. D. Jr. (1971). Motor mechanisms: The role of the pyramidal system in motor control. *Ann. Rev. Physiol,* **33,** 337–392.

Broom, D. M. (1968a). Specific habituation by chicks. *Nature, Lond.,* **217,** 880–881.

Broom, D. M. (1968b). Behaviour of undisturbed 1 to 10 day old chicks in different rearing conditions. *Develop. Psychobiol.,* **1,** 287–295.

Broom, D. M. (1969a). Reactions of chicks to visual changes during the first ten days after hatching. *Anim. Behav.* **17,** 307–315.

Broom, D. M. (1969b). Effects of visual complexity during rearing on chicks' reactions to environmental change. *Anim. Behav.* **17,** 773–780.

Broom, D. M. (1979). Methods of detecting and analysing activity rhythms. *Biol. Behav.,* **4,** 3–18.

Broom, D. M. (1980). Activity rhythms and position preferences of domestic chicks which can see a moving object. *Anim. Behav.,* **28,** 201–211.

Broom, D. M. (1981). *Biology of Behaviour.* Cambridge: Cambridge University Press.

Broom, D. M. (1982). Husbandry methods leading to inadequate social and maternal behaviour in cattle. In *Disturbed Behaviour in Farm Animals,* ed. W. Bessei, *Hohenheimer Arbeiten,* **121,** 42–50. Stuttgart: Eugen Ulmer.

Broom, D. M. (1983a). Cow-calf and sow-piglet behaviour in relation to colostrum ingestion. *Ann. Rech. vét.,* **14,** 342–348.

Broom, D. M. (1983b). Stereotypies as animal welfare indicators. In: *Indicators Relevant to Farm Animal Welfare,* ed. D. Smidt, *Curr. Top. vet. Med. Anim. Sci.,* 81–87. The Hague: Martinus Nijhoff.

Broom, D. M. (1983c). The stress concept and ways of assessing the effects of stress in farm animals. *Appl. Anim. Ethol.,* **1,** 79.

Broom, D. M. (1985). Stress, welfare and the state of equilibrium. In *Proc. 2nd Eur. Symp. Poult. Welfare,* ed. R. M. Wegner, 72–81 Celle: World Poultry Science Association.

Broom, D. M. (1986a) (Ed.) *Farmed Animals.* New York: Torstar Books.

Broom, D. M. (1986b). The influence of the design of housing systems for cattle on lameness and on behaviour: summary of discussion on behavioural and veterinary aspects. In *Cattle Housing Systems, Lameness and Behaviour,* ed. H. K. Wierenga and D. J Peterse, *Curr. Top. vet. Med. Anim Sci.,* **40,** 179–181. Dordrecht : Martinus Nijhoff.

Broom, D. M. (1986c). Indicators of poor welfare. *Br. vet. J.,* **142,** 524–526.

Broom, D. M. (1986d). Stereotypies and responsiveness as welfare indicators in stall-housed sows. *Anim. Prod.,* **42,** 438–439.

Broom, D. M. (1986e). Responsiveness of stall-housed sows. *Appl. Anim. Behav. Sci.,* **15,** 186.

Broom, D. M. (1987a). Applications of neurobiological studies to farm animal welfare. In *"Biology of Stress in Farm Animals: an Integranted Approach"* ed. P. R. Wiepkema and P. W. M van Adrichem. *Curr. Top. vet. Med. Anim. Sci.,* **42,** 101–110. Dordrecht: Martinus Nijhoff.

Broom, D. M. (1987b). General conclusions. *Welfare Aspects of Housing Systems for Veal Calves and Fattening Bulls,* 161–166. Luxembourg: Commission of the European Communities, EUR 10777 EN.

Broom, D. M. (1988a). After the sensory analysers: problems with concepts and terminology. *Behav. Brain Sci.* **10,** 370–371.

Broom, D. M. (1988b) Needs, freedoms and the assessment of welfare. *Appl. Anim. Behav. Sci.,* **19,** 384–386.

Broom, D. M. (1988c). The Relationship between welfare and disease susceptibility in farm animals. In *Animal Disease – a Welfare Problem* ed. T. E. Gibson, 22–29. London: BVA Animal Welfare Foundation.

Broom, D. M. (1988d). The scientific assessment of animal welfare. *Appl. Anim. Behav. Sci.,* **20,** 5–19.

Broom, D. M. (1988e). Welfare considerations in cattle practice. *Proc. Brit. Cattle Vet. Ass.* for 1986–7, 153–164.

Broom, D. M. (1988f). Les concepts de stress et de bien-être. *Rec. Méd. vét.,* **164,** 715–722.

Broom, D. M. (1989a). Animal Welfare. In *The Veterinary Annual, 29,* ed. C. S. G. Grunsell, M-E. Raw and F. W. G. Hill, p. 9–14. London: Wright.

Broom, D. M. (1989b). The assessment of sow welfare. *Pig vet. J.,* **22,** 100–111.

Broom, D. M. and Arnold, G. W. 1986. Selection by grazing sheep of pasture plants at low herbage availability and responses of the plants to grazing. *Aust. J. agric. Res.*, **37**, 527–538.

Broom, D.M. and Johnson, E. (1980). Responsiveness of hand-reared roe deer to odours from skin glands. *J. nat. Hist.*, **14**, 41–47.

Broom, D.M. and Knowles, T.G. (1989). The assessment of welfare during the handling and transport of spent laying hens. *Proc. 3rd Eur. Symp. Poult. Welfare.* ed. J.M. Faure & A.D. Mills. Tours: World Poultry Science Association.

Broom, D.M. and Leaver, J.D. (1977). Mother-young interactions in dairy cattle. *Br. vet. J.*, **133**, 192.

Broom, D.M. and Leaver, J.D. (1978). The effects of group-housing or partial isolation on later social behaviour of calves. *Anim. Behav.* **26**, 1255–1263.

Broom, D.M. and Potter, M.J. (1984). Factors affecting the occurrence of stereotypies in stall-housed dry sows. *Proc. Int. Cong. Appl. Ethol. Farm. Anim.*, ed. J. Unshelm, G. van Putten and K. Zeeb, 229–231. Darmstadt: K.T.B.L.

Broom, D.M., Pain, B.F., and Leaver, J.D. (1975). The effects of slurry on the acceptability of swards to grazing cattle. *J. agric. Sci., Camb.*, **85**, 331–6.

Broom, D.M., Knight, P.G. and Stansfield, S.C. (1986). Hen behaviour and hypothalamic-pituitary-adrenal responses to handling and transport. *Appl. Anim. Behav. Sci.*, **16**, 98.

Brownlee, A. (1954). Play in domestic cattle in Britain: an analysis of its nature. *Br. vet. J.*, **110**, 48–68.

Brownlee, A. (1984). Animal Play. *Appl. Anim. Behav. Sci.*, **12**, 307–312.

Brownstein, M., Russel, J.T., Gainer, H. (1980). Synthesis, transport and release of posterior pituitary hormones. *Science, N.Y.* **207**, 373–378.

Bruce, W.N. and Decker, G.C. (1958). The relationship of *Stomoxys calcitrans* abundance to milk production in dairy cattle. *J. econ. Ent.* **51**, 269.

Brummer, H. (1972). Den Einfluss von Wasserentzug auf das Auftreten von Kronismus beim Hauskaninchen. *Tierärzlt. Umschau* **27**, 291–296.

Bruner, J.S. Jolly, A. and Sylva, K. eds. (1974). *Plays: its role in development and evolution* Harmondsworth: Penguin.

Bryant, M.J. (1972). The social environment: behaviour and stress in housed livestock. *Vet Rec.* **90**, 351–359.

Bryant, M.J. and Ewbank, R. (1974). Effects of stocking rate upon the performance of groups of growing pigs. *Br. vet. J.* **130**, 139–49.

Bryant, M.J. Rowlinson, P. and van der Steen, H.A.M. (1983). A comparison of the nursing and suckling behaviour of group- and individually-housed sows and their litters. *Anim. Prod.*, **36**, 445–451.

Burley, N., Krantzberry, G. and Radman, P. (1982). Influence of colour-bonding on the conspecific preference of zebra finches. *Anim. Behav.*, **30**, 444–455.

Calhoun, J.B. (1962a). *The Ecology and Sociology of the Norway Rat* U.S. Dep. Helth, Educ. Welf. P.H.S. Doc. 1008. Washington. D.C.: U.S. Govt Printing Office.

Camhi, J.M. 1984. *Neuroethology: Nerve Cells and the Natural Behaviour of Animals*, Sunderland Mass: Sinauer.

Campbell, D.G. and Fraser, A.F. (1961). A note of animal behaviour as a factor in parasitism. *Can. Vet. Jour.* **2**, 414–415.

Campbell, R.G. (1976). A note on the use of a feed flavour to stimulate the feed intake of weaner pigs. *Anim. Prod.* **23**, 417–419.

Campitelli, S. Carenzi, C. and Verga, M. (1982). Factors which influence parturition in the mare and development of the foal. *Appl. Anim. Ethol.* **9**, 7–14.

Cariolet, R. and Dantzer, R. (1985). Activité motrice des truises attachées durant la gestation: mise en evidence de quelques facteurs de variations. *Journées Rech. Porcine en France.* **17**, 237–248.

Carpenter, C.C. (1971). Discussion of Session 1: Territoriality and dominance. In *Behavior and Environment: the use of Space by Animals and Men* (A.H. Esser, ed.). New York: Plenum.

Carson, K. and Wood-Gush, D.G.M. (1983a). Equine Behaviour: I. A review of the literature on social and dam-foal behaviour. *Appl. Anim. Ethol.* **10**, 165–178.

Carson, K., and Wood-Gush, D.G.M. (1983b). Equine behaviour: II. A review of the literature on feeding, eliminative and resting behaviour. *Appl. Anim. Ethol.* **10**, 179–190.

Carter, A. and English, P.R. (1983). A comparison of the activity and behaviour of dry sows in different housing and penning systems. *Anim. Prod.*, **36**, 531.

ten Cate, C. (1984). The influence of social relations on the development of species recognition in zebra finches. *Behaviour*, **91**, 263–285.

Cermak, J. (1987). The design of cubicles for British Friesian dairy cows with reference to body weight and dimensions, spatial behaviour and upper leg lameness. In *Cattle Housing Systems. Lameness and Behaviour* ed. H.K. Wierenga and D.J. Peterse, *Curr. Top. vet. Med. Anim. Sci.,* **40,** 119–128. Dordrecht: Martinus Nijhoff.

Chacon, E and Stobbs, T.H. (1976). Influence of progressive defoliation of a grass sward on the eating behaviour of cattle. *Aust. J. agric. Res.,* **27,** 709–27.

Chaimers, N.R. (1979). *Social Behaviour in Primates.* London: Arnold.

Chambers, D.T. (1959). Grazing behaviour of calves reared at pasture. *J. agric. Sci., Camb.* **53,** 417–424.

Chamove, A.S., Rosenblum, L.A., and Harlow, H.F. (1973). Monkeys (*Macaca mulatta*) raised only with peers. A pilot study. *Anim. Behav.,* **21,** 316–325.

Cheng, T.H. (1958). The effect of biting fly control on weight gain of beef cattle. *J. econ. Ent.* **51,** 278.

Chenoweth, P.J., and Osborne, H.G. (1975). Breed differences in the reproductive functions of young beef bulls in Central Queensland. *Aust. vet. J.,* **51,** 405–406.

Christian, J.J. (1955). Effects of population size on the adrenal glands and reproductive organs of male mice. *Am. J. Psychol.* **182,** 292–300.

Christian, J.J. (1961). Phenomena associated with population density. *Proc. natn. Acad. Sci,* U.S.A. **47,** 428–491.

Clegg, M.T. Breamer, W, and Bermant, G. (1969). Copulatory behaviour of the ram Ovis aries. III. Effects of pre- and post-pubertal castration and androgen replacement therapy. *Anim. Behav.* **17,** 712–717.

Cole, D.J.A, Duckworth, J.E. and Holmes, W. (1976). Factors affecting voluntary feed intake in pigs: I. The effect of digestible energy content of the diet on the intake of castrated male pigs housed in holding pens and in metabolism crates. *Anim. Prod.,* **9,** 141–148.

Colgan, P. (1989). *Animal Motivation.* London: Chapman and Hall.

Collery, L. (1969). The sexual and social behaviour of the Connemara pony. *Br. vet. J.* **125,** 151–152.

Collery, L. (1974). Observations of equine animals under farm and feral conditions. *Equine vet. J.* **6.** 170–173.

Collias, N. and Joos, M. (1953). The spectographic analysis of sound signals of the domestic fowl. *Behaviour,* **5,** 175–188.

Commission of the European Communities (1984). *International transport of farm animals intended for slaughter.* EUR 9556 EN. Luxembourg: C.E.C., pp 67.

Cools, A.R. Janessen, H.J., and Broekkamp, C.L.E. (1974). The differential role of the caudate nucleus in the initiation and maintenance of morphine-induced behaviour in rats. *Arch. Int. Pharmacodyn.* **210,** 163.

Cooper, J.R, Bloom, F.E, and Roth, R.H. (1982). *The Biochemical Basis of Neuropharmacology,* 4th edn. Oxford: Oxford University Press.

Couttie, M.A. and Hunter, W.K. (1956). Sexual behaviour of Aberdeen Angus bulls. *Proc. 3rd Int. Congr. Anim. Reprod. Artif. Insem.* (Cambridge), Section III, 98–100.

Cowan, W.M. (1979). The development of the brain. *Scientif. Amer.* **241,** 112–133.

Craig, J.V. (1981). *Domestic Animal Behavior.* Englewood Cliffs, N.J.: Prentice Hall.

Craig, J.V. and Bhagwat, A.L. (1974). Agonistic and mating behaviour of adult chickens modified by social and physical environments. *Appl. Anim. Ethol.* **1,** 57–65.

Craig, J.V. and Guhl, A.M. (1969). Territorial behaviour and social interactions of pullets kept in large flocks. *Poult. Sci.,* **48,** 1622–28.

Craig, J.V., Biswas, D.K., and Guhl, A.M. (1969). Agonistic behaviour influenced by strangers, crowding and heredity in female domestic fowl (*Gallus gallus*). *Anim. Behav.,* **17,** 498–506.

Cronin, G.M. (1982). Oestrous behaviour and fertility in gilts. *Appl. Anim. Ethol.* **8,** 581.

Cronin, G.M. (1985). *The development and significance of abnormal stereotyped behaviours in tethered sows.* Ph.D. thesis, University of Wageningen.

Cronin, G.M. and Wiepkema, P.R. (1984). An analysis of stereotyped behaviour in tethered sows. *Ann. Rech. vet.,* **15,** 263–270.

Cronin, G.M. Wiepkema, P.R and van Ree, J.M. (1985). Endogenous opioids are involved in abnormal stereotyped behaviours of tethered sows. *Neuropeptides,* **6,** 527–530.

Cruze, W.W. (1935) Maturation and learning in chicks. *J. Comp. Psychol* **19,** 371–409.

Csermely, D. and Wood-Gush, D.G.M. (1986). Agonistic behaviour in grouped sows. *Biol. Behav.,* **11,** 244–252.

Curtis, S.E. (1983). Perception of thermal comfort by farm animals. In *Farm Animal Housing and Welfare* ed. S.H. Baxter, M.R. Baxter and J.A.C. MacCormack, *Curr. Top. vet. Med. Anim. Sci.,* **24,** 59–66. The Hague: Martinus Nijhoff.

Czako, J. (1967). Gegenseitiges und Selbstsaugen der Kälber. *Wiss. Fortschr.,* **5,** 218

Daly, C. C., Kallweit, E. and Ellendorf, F. (1988). Cortical function in cattle during slaughter; conventional captive ball stunning followed by exsanguination compared with shechita slaughter. *Vet. Rec.* **122,** 325–329.

Dämmrich, K. (1987). The reactions of the legs (bone; joints) to loading and its consequences for lameness. In *Cattle Housing Systems, Lameness and Behaviour.* ed. H. K. Wierenga and D. J. Peterse, *Curr. Top. vet. Med. Anim. Sci.* **40,** 50–55. Dordrecht: Martinus Nijhoff.

Dantzer, R. (1986). Behavioural, physiological and functional aspects of stereotyped behaviour: a review and a reinterpretation. *J. Anim. Sci.,* **62,** 1776–1786.

Dantzer, R. and Mormède, P. (1981). Pituitary adrenal consequences of adjunctive behaviours in pigs. *Horm. Behav.* **15,** 386–395.

Dantzer, R., Mormède, P., Bluthé, R-M and Soissons, J. (1983). The effect of different housing conditions on behavioural and adrenocortical reactions in veal calves. *Reprod. Nutr. Dévelop.,* **23,** 67–74.

Dantzer, R., Bluthé, R-M and Tazi, A. (1986). Stress-induced analgesia in pigs. *Ann. Rech. vét.* **17,** 147–151.

Dawkins, M. (1976). Towards an objective method of assessing welfare in domestic fowl. *Appl. Anim. Ethol.,* **2,** 245–254.

Dawkins, M. (1977). Do hens suffer in battery cages? Environmental preferences and welfare. *Anim. Behav.,* **25,** 1034–1046.

Dawkins, M. (1981). Priorities in the cage size and flooring preferences of domestic hens. *Br. Poult. Sci.,* **22,** 255–263.

Dawkins, M. (1983). Battery hens name their price: consumer demand theory and the measurement of animal needs. *Anim. Behav.,* **31,** 1195–1205.

Dawkins, R. (1968). The ontogeny of a pecking preference in domestic chicks. *Z. Tierpsychol.* **25,** 470–474.

Dawkins, R. (1976). *The Selfish Gene.* Oxford: Oxford University Press.

Dawkins, R. (1982). *The Extended Phenotype.* Oxford: W. H. Freeman.

Dawkins, R. (1986). *The Blind Watchmaker.* London: Longman.

Deakin, A. and Fraser, E. B. (1935). Fecundity and nursing capacity of large Yorkshire sows. *Scientif. Agric.* **15,** 458–462.

Dellmeier, G. R. Friend, T. H. and Gbur, E. E.

(1985). Comparison of four methods of calf confinement. II Behaviour. *J. Anim. Sci.,* **60,** 1102–1109.

Denton, D. A. (1967). Salt appetite. In: *Handbook of Physiology* ed. C. F. Code and W. Heidel, Sect. 6, Vol. 1. Washington, D. C. American Physiological Society.

Desserich, M., Fölsch, D. W., and Ziswiler, V. (1984). Das Schnabelkupieren bei Huhnern. Ein Eingriff in innervierten Bereich. *Tierärztl. Prax.* **12,** 191–202.

Devilat, J., Pond, W. G. and Miller, P. D. (1970). Dietary amino acid balance in growing finishing pigs: effects on diet preference and performance. *J. Anim. Sci.,* **30,** 536–543.

De Vos, V. (1978). Immobilisation of free-range wild animals using a new drug. *Vet. Rec.,* **103,** 64–68.

Diamond, I. T. (1982). Changing views of the organisation and evolution of the visual pathways. In: *Changing Concepts of the Nervous System,* New York, Academic Press.

Dickinson, A. (1985). Actions and habits: the development of behavioural autonomy. In: *Animal Intelligence,* ed. L. Weiskrantz, 67–78. Oxford: Clarendon Press.

Dickson, D. P., Barr, G. R., and Wieckert, D. A. (1967). Social relationships of dairy cows in a feed lot. *Behaviour,* **29,** 195–203.

Dietrich, J. P., Snyder, W. W., Meadows, C. E. and Albright, J. L. (1965). Rank order in dairy cows. *Anim. Zool.,* **5,** 713. (Abstract)

Dobao, M. T. Rodriganez, J. and Silio, L. (1985). Choice of companions in social play in piglets. *Appl. Anim. Behav. Sci.,*

Dolf, C. (in press) Agonistic behaviour of dry sows in single stalls and group housing under special consideration of the resulting risk of lesions. *Appl. Anim. Behav. Sci.,*

Dolphinow, P. J. and Bishop, N. (1979). The development of motor skills and social relationships through play. *Minn. Symp. Child Psychol.* **4,** 141–98.

Donaldson, S. L. (1970). The effects of early feeding and rearing experience on social maternal and milking parlour behaviour in dairy cattle. Ph.D. thesis. Purdue University.

Donaldson, S. L., Black, W. C. and Albright, J. L. (1966). The effects of early feeding and rearing experiences on dominance, aggressive and submissive behaviour in young heifer calves. *Am. Zool.* **6,** 247.

Done-Currie, J. R., Hecker, J. F., and Wodzicka-Tomaszewska, M. (1983). Behaviour of sheep transferred from pasture to an animal house. *Appl. Anim. Ethol.,* **12**, 121–130.

Dougherty, R. W. (1976). Problems associated with feeding farm livestock under intensive systems. *World Rev. Nutr. Diet.* **25**, 249–275.

Drago, F. Canonico, P. L. Bitetti, R., and Scapagnini, U. (1980). Systemic and intraventricular prolactin induces excessive grooming. *Eur. J. Pharmac.* **65**, 457–458.

Duckworth, J. E. and Shirlaw, D. W. (1958). A study of factors affecting feed intake and the eating behaviour of cattle. *Anim. Behav.,* **6**, 147–154.

Dudzinski, M. L., Schuh, H. J., Wilcox, D. Gardiner, G., and Morrissey, T. (1978). Statistical and probablistic estimations of forage conditions from grazing behaviour of Merino sheep in a semi-arid environment. *Appl. Anim. Ethol.,* **4**, 357–368.

Dudzinski, M. L., Muller, W. J., Low, W. A. and Schuh, H. (1982). Relationship between dispersion behaviour of free-ranging cattle and forage conditions. *Appl. Anim. Ethol.,* **8**, 225–241.

Duffy, E. (1962). *Activation and Behavior.* New York: Wiley.

Dufty, J. H. (1971). Determination of the onset of parturition in Hereford cattle. *Aust. vet. J.* **47**, 77–82.

Duncan, I. J. H. (1978). The interpretation of preference tests in animal behaviour. *Appl. Anim. Ethol.,* **4**, 197–200.

Duncan, I. J. H. (1986). Some thoughts on the stressfulness of harvesting broilers. *Appl. Anim. Behav. Sci.,* **16**, 97.

Duncan, I. J. H. and Filshie, J. H. (1979). The use of radiotelemetry devices to measure temperature and heart rate in domestic fowl. In: *A Handbook on Biotelemetry and Radio Tracking,* ed. C. J. Amlaner and D. W. Macdonald, pp 579–588. Oxford: Pergamon.

Duncan, I. J. H. and Hughes, B. O. (1972). Free and operant feeding in domestic fowls. *Anim. Behav.,* **20**, 775–777.

Duncan, I. J. H. and Kite, V. G. (1987). Some investigations into motivation in the domestic fowl. *Appl. Anim. Behav. Sci.,* **18**, 387–388.

Duncan, I. J. H., and Wood-Gush, D. G. M. (1971). Frustration and aggression in the domestic fowl. *Anim. Behav.,* **19**, 500–504.

Duncan, I. J. H., and Wood-Gush, D. G. M. (1972). Thwarting of feeding behaviour in the domestic fowl. *Anim. Behav.,* **20**, 444–451.

Duncan, I. J. H., Savory, C. J. and Wood-Gush, D. G. M. (1978). Observations on the reproductive behaviour of domestic fowl in the wild. *Appl. Anim. Ethol.* **4**, 29–42.

Dutch Society for the Protection of Animals (1986). *Alternatives for the battery cage system for laying hens.* p 51.

Dyck, G. W. (1971). Puberty, post-weaning oestrus and oestrus cycle length in Yorkshire and Lacombe swine. *Can. J. Anim. Sci.,* **51**, 135–140.

Edmunds, M. (1974). *Defence in Animals.* Harlow: Longman.

Edwards, F. W., Oldroyd, H. and Smart, J. (1939). *British Bloodsucking Flies,* London, British Museum.

Edwards, S. A. (1979). The timing of parturition in dairy cattle. *J. agric. Sci., Camb.* **93**, 359–363.

Edwards, S. A. (1982). Factors affecting the time to first suckling in dairy calves. *Anim. Prod.* **34**, 339–346.

Edwards, S. A. (1983). The behaviour of dairy cows and their newborn calves in individual or group housing. *Appl. Anim. Ethol.,* **10**, 191–198.

Edwards, S. A. (1985). Group housing systems for dry sows. *Farm Bldg. Progr.* **80**, 19–22.

Edwards, S. A. and Broom, D. M. (1979). The period between birth and first suckling in dairy calves. *Res. vet. Sci.,* **26**, 255–256.

Edwards, S. A. and Broom, D. M. (1982). Behavioural interactions of dairy cows with their newborn calves and the effects of parity. *Anim. Behav.* **30**, 525–535.

Edwards, S. A., Broom, D. M. and Collis, S. C. (1982). Factors affecting levels of passive immunity in dairy calves. *Br. vet. J.,* **138**, 233–240.

Ehinger, F. and Gschwindt, B. (1979). Transporteinflusse auf Schlachtgeflügel. 1. Einflussverschiedens. *Die Fleischwirtschaft,* **59**, 234–236.

Ehinger, F. and Gschwindt, B. (1981). Der einfluss unterschiedlicher Transportzeiten auf die Fleischqualität und auf physiologische Merkmale bei Broilern verschiedener Herkunft. *Arch. Geflügelk.,* **45**, 260–265.

Eikelenboom, G. (ed.) (1983). *Stunning of Animals for Slaughter. Curr. Top. vet. Med. Anim. Sci.,* **25**. The Hague: Martinus Nijhoff.

Ekesbo, I. (1981). Some aspects of sow health and housing. In *Welfare of Pigs* ed. W. Sybesma, *Curr. Top vet. Med Anim Sci.,* **11**, 250–266. The Hague: Martinus Nijhoff.

Ekesbo, I., Jensen, P. and Hogsved, O. (1978). Nygammal typ ab Sinsuggehallning nagra etologiska data. *Startryck ur Svensk Veterinartidning,* **30**, 23, 845–848.

Elson, H. A. (1976). New ideas on laying cage design:

the "get-away" cage. In *Proc. Vth. Eur. Poult. Conf.* II

Elson, H.A. (1985). The economics of poultry welfare. In *Second European Symposium on Poultry Welfare*, ed. R.-M. Wegner, 244–253. Celle: World Poultry Science Association.

Elson, H.A. (1988). Making the best cage decisions. In *Cages for the Future* Proceedings of Cambridge Poultry Conference, 70–76 London: A.D.A.S. (Ministry of Agriculture Fisheries and Food).

Engels, E.A.N., Malan, A., and Baard, M.A. (1974). The voluntary feed intake of three breeds of sheep on natural pasture. *S. Afr. J. Anim. Sci.*, **4**, 27–29.

English, P.R. Smith, W.J. and McLean, A. (1977). *The Sow-Improving her Efficiency*. Ipswich: Farming Press.

English, P.R., Baxter, S.H. and Smith. W.J. (1982). Accommodating the welfare dimensions in future systems. *Anim. Prod.*, **34**, 367.

Epstein, A.N. (1983). The Neuropsychology of Drinking Behaviour. Chapter 9 in *"Handbook on Behavioural Neurobiology"*. E. Satinoff and P. Teitelbaum (eds.), Plenum Press, New York and London.

Esslemont, R.J. and Bryant, M.J. (1976). Oestrous behaviour in a herd of dairy cows. *Vet. Rec.* **19**, 472–475.

Esslemont, R.J., Glencross, R.G., Bryant, M.J. and Pope, G.S. (1980). A quantitative study of pre-ovulatory behaviour in cattle (British Friesian heifers). *Appl. Anim. Ethol.* **6**, 1–17.

Evarts, E.V. (1973). Brain mechanisms in movement. *Scientif. Amer.* **229** (1), 96–103.

Ewbank, R. (1963). Predicting the time of parturition in the normal cow. *Vet. Rec.* **75**, 367–371.

Ewbank, R. (1973). Abnormal behaviour and pig nutrition. An unsuccessful attempt to induce tail biting by feeding on high energy, low fibre vegetable protein ration. *Br. vet. J.*, **129**, 366–369.

Ewbank, R. (1981). Alternatives: definitions and doubts. In *Alternatives to Intensive Husbandry Systems*, 5–9. Potters Bar: Universities Federation for Animal Welfare.

Ewbank, R, and Bryant, M.J. (1972). Aggressive behaviour amongst groups of domesticated pigs kept at various stocking rates. *Anim. Behav.* **20**, 21–8.

Fabricius, E. (1951). Zur Ethologie junge Anatiden. *Acta zool. Fenn.* **68**, 1–178.

Fagen, R.M. (1976). Exercise, play and physical training in animals. *Perspective Ethol.* **2**, 189–219. New York: Plenum.

Fagen, R. (1981). *Animal Play Behaviour*. New York: Oxford University Press.

Fahmy, M.H. and Dufour, J.J. (1976). Effects of post-weaning stress and feeding management on return to oestrus and reproductive traits during early pregnancy in swine. *Anim. Prod.*, **23**, 103–110.

Falk, J.L. (1969). Conditions producing psychogenic polydipsia in animals. *Ann. N. Y. Acad. Sci.*, **157**, 569–589.

Fallon, R.J. (1978). The effect of immunoglobulin levels on calf performance and methods of artificially feeding to the newborn calf. *Ann. Rech. vét.* **9**, 347–352.

Fantz, R.L. (1957). Form preferences in newly hatched chicks. *J. comp. Psychol.* **50**, 422–430.

Farneslow, M.S. (1979). Naloxone attenuates rats' preference for the signalled shock. *Physiol. Psychol.*, **7**, 70–74.

Faure, J.M. and Jones, R.B. (1982a). Effects of sex, strain and type of perch on perching behaviour in the domestic fowl. *Appl. Anim. Ethol.* **8**, 281–293.

Faure, J.M. and Jones, R.B. (1982b). Effects of age, access and time of day on perching behaviour in the domestic fowl. *Appl. Anim. Ethol.* **8**, 357–364.

Favre, J.Y. (1975). *Comportement d'Ovins Gardés*. Ministère de L'Agriculture École Nationale Supérieure Agronomique de Montpellier.

Federation Equestre Internationale (1981). *Identification of Horses*, pp. 48, F.E.I.

Fitzsimons, J.T. (1979). The physiology of thirst and sodium appetite. *Monogr. Physiol. Soc.*, No. 35, Cambridge: Cambridge University Press.

Flerko, B. (1970). Control of follicle stimulating hormone and luteinising hormone secretion. In *The Hypothalamus* p. 351. New York: Academic Press.

Fletcher, I.C. and Lindsay, D.R. (1968). Sensory involvement in the mating behaviour of domestic sheep. *Anim. Behav.* **16**, 410–414.

Fletcher, I.C. and Lindsay, D.R. (1971). Effect of rams on the duration of oestrus behaviour in ewes. *J. Reprod. Fertil.*, **25**, 253–259.

Fölsch, D.W. (1981). Das Verhalten von Legehennen in unterschiedlichen Haltungs systemen unter Berucksichtigung der Aufsuchtmethoden. In *Das Verhalten von Huhnern*, ed. D.W. Fölsch and K. Vestergaard, *Tierhaltung*, **12**, 9–114. Basel: Birkhäuser Verlag.

Fölsch, D.W. and Hüber, A. (1977). Bewegungsaktivität und Lautausserungen in Tagesrhythmus. *K.T.B.L. Schrift,* **223**, 99–114.

Fölsch, D.W. and Vestergaard, K. (1981). *The*

Behaviour of Fowl. Basel: Birkhauser Verlag.

Fölsch, D.W. Dolf, C. Ehrbar, H. Bleuler, T. and Teygeler, H. (1983a). Ethologic and economic examination of aviary housing for commercial laying flocks. *Int. J. Stud. Anim. Prob.* **4**, 330–335.

Fölsch, D.W., Rist, M., Munz. G. and Teygeler, H. (1983b). Entwicklung eines tiergerechten Legehennen – Haltungs systems: Die Volierenhaltung. *Landtechnik, 6*, 225.

Foot, J.Z. and Russell, A.J.F. (1978). Pattern of intake of three roughage diets by non-pregnant, non-lactating Scottish Blackface ewes over a long period and the effects of previous nutritional history on current intake. *Anim. Prod.,* **26**, 203–215.

Foote, R.H. Munkenbeck, N. and Greene, W.A. (1976). Testosterone and libido in Holstein bulls of various ages. *J. dairy Sci.* **59**, 2011–2013.

Foote, W.C. Sefidbakht, N. and Madsen, N.A. (1970). Puberal oestrus and ovulation and subsequent oestrus cycle patterns in the ewe. *J. Anim. Sci.* **30**, 86–90.

Forrester, R.C. (1979). Behavioural State and Responsiveness in Domestic Chicks. Ph.D. thesis, University of Reading.

Forrester, R.C. (1980). Stereotypies and the behavioural regulation of motivational state. *Appl Anim. Ethol.,* **6**, 386–7.

Fowler, D.G. (1975). Mating activity and its relationship to reproductive performance in Merino sheep. *Appl. Anim. Ethol.* **1**, 357–368.

Fowler, D.G. and Langford, C.M. (1976). The prediction of fertility and fecundity from the mating activity of ewes. *Appl. Anim. Ethol.* **2**, 277–281.

Francis-Smith, K. (1979). Studies on the feeding and social behaviour of domestic horses. Ph.D. Thesis, University of Edinburgh.

Franklin, J.R. and Hutson, G.D. (1982). Experiments on attracting sheep to move along a lane-way. III. Visual stimuli, *Appl. Anim. Ethol.* **8**, 457–458.

Fraschini, F., and Martini, L. (1970). Rhythmic phenomena and pineal principles. In *The Hypothalamus* p. 529, New York: Academic Press.

Fraser, A.F. (1957). The disposition of the bull. *Br. J. Anim. Behav.* **5**, 110–115.

Fraser, A.F. (1960a). Spontaneously occurring forms of "tonic immobility" in farm animals. *Canad. J. comp. Med.* **24**, 330–332.

Fraser, A.F. (1960b). The influence of psychological and other factors on reaction time in bulls. *Cornell Vet.,* **50**, 126–132.

Fraser, A.F. (1964). Observations on the pre-coital behaviour of the male goat. *Anim. Behav.* **12**, 31–33.

Fraser, A.F. (1968). *Reproductive Behaviour in Ungulates*. London: Academic Press.

Fraser, A.F. (1970a). Enkele studies over voortplant-ing by Schapen. (A spectrum of studies in sheep reproduction). *Vlooms diergeneesk. Tijdschr.* **39**, 17–35.

Fraser, A.F. (1970b). Some observations on equine oestrus. *Brit. Vet. J.* **126**, 656–657.

Fraser, A.F. (1973). The British veterinarian and modern sheep reproduction. *Vet. Rec.* **92**, 585–588.

Fraser, A.F. (1974). The behaviour of growing pigs during experimental social encounters. *J. Agric. Sci.* **82**, 147–163.

Fraser, A.F. (1976). Some features of an ultrasonic study of bovine foetal kinesis. *Appl. Anim. Ethol.* **2**, 379–383.

Fraser, A.F. (1977). Foetal kinesis and a condition of foetal inertia in equine and bovine subjects. *Appl. Anim. Ethol.* **3**, 89–90.

Fraser, A.F. (1978a). A general review of sexual behaviour in livestock. Eine generalle Uberprufung des Sexualverhaltens bei Nutztieren, *Proc. 1st Wld. Congr. on Ethol. Appl. to Zootechnics,* **1**, 507–512.

Fraser, A.F. (1978c). Tests in applied ethology. *Appl. Anim. Ethol,* **4**, 1–4.

Fraser, A.F. (1980b). The appraisal of vital behaviour in the neonate foal. In *Proceedings of the International Congress on Animal Production. Madrid.* pp 617–620.

Fraser, A.F. (1980c). The ontogeny of behaviour in the foal. *Appl. Anim. Ethol.* **6**, 303.

Fraser, A.F. (1981). Animal togetherness. *Appl. Anim. Ethol.* **7**, 303–305.

Fraser, A.F. (1982a). Social tolerance in livestock. *Appl. Anim. Ethol.* **8**, 501–505.

Fraser, A.F. (1982b). Kinetic behaviour and some of its ways. *Appl. Anim. Ethol.* **9**, 107–110.

Fraser, A.F. (1983). Curious idling. *Appl. Anim. Ethol.* **10**, 159–164.

Fraser, A.F. (1984). The behaviour of suffering in animals. *Appl. Anim. Behav. Sci.,* **13**, 1–6.

Fraser, A.F. (1985). Background to anomalous behaviour. *Appl. Anim. Behav. Sci.,* **13**, 199–203.

Fraser, A.F. (1988). Behavioural needs in relation to livestock maintenance. *Appl. Anim. Behav. Sci.,* **20**, 368–376.

Fraser, A. F. (1989). Pandiculation: the comparative phenomenon of systematic stretching. *Appl. Anim. Behav. Sci.* **23**, 263–268.

Fraser, A. F. and Brownlee, A. (1974). Veterinary ethology and grass sickness in horses. *Vet. Rec.,* **95**, 448.

Fraser, A. F. and Herchen, H. (1962). Tonische immobilität bei tieren und ihre bedeutung für die veterinärmedizine. *Wien Tierärztl. Monatsschr.* **49**: 271–276.

Fraser, A. F. and Herchen, H. (1978). Terminal foetal postures observed in a bovine caesarean survey. *Appl. Anim. Ethol.* **4**, 315–322.

Fraser, A. F. and Penman, J. H. (1971). A clinical study of ram infertilities in Scotland. *Vet. Rec.* **89**, 154–158.

Fraser, A. F. and Sane, C. R. (1982). Sexual behaviour in domesticated animals. Chapter 52 in: *Reproduction in Farm Animals*, ed. by Sane, et al. Bombay: Varghese Publishing.

Fraser, A. F. and Terhune, M. (1977a). Radiographic studies of postural behaviour in the sheep foetus. I. Simple foetal movements. *Appl. Anim. Ethol.* **3**, 221–234.

Fraser, A. F. and Terhune, M. (1977b). Radiographic studies of postural behaviour in the sheep foetus. II. Complex foetal movements. *Appl. Anim Ethol.* **3**, 235–246.

Fraser, A. F. and Laing, A. H. (1968). The "ram effect" and breeding results in Suffolk ewes. *Scott. Agric.* **47**, 29–31.

Fraser, A. F. Hastie, H. Callicott, and Brownlie, S. (1975). An exploratory ultrasonic study on quantitative foetal kinesis in the horse. *Appl. Anim. Ethol.* **1**, 395–404.

Fraser, D. (1974). The vocalisation and other behaviour of growing pigs in an 'open field' test. *Appl. Anim. Ethol.* **1**, 3–16.

Fraser, D. (1975a). Vocalisations of isolated piglets. I. Sources of variation and relationships among measures. *Appl. Anim. Ethol.* **1**, 387–394.

Fraser, D. (1975b). Vocalisations of isolated piglets. II. Some environmental factors. *Appl. Anim. Ethol.* **2**, 19–24.

Fraser, D. (1975c). The effect of straw on the behaviour of sows in tether stalls. *Anim. Prod.* **21**, 59–68.

Fraser, D. (1978). Observations on the behavioural development of suckling and early weaned piglets during the first six weeks after birth. *Anim. Behav.* **26**, 22–30.

Fraser, D. (1980). A review of the behavioural mechanism of milk ejection of the domestic pig. *Appl. Anim. Ethol.* **10**, 301–317.

Fraser, D. (1984). The role of behaviour in swine production: A review of research. *Appl. Anim. Ethol.* **11**, 317–339.

Fraser, D. Thompson, B. K. Ferguson, D. K. and Darroch, R. L. (1979). The 'teat order' of suckling pigs. 3. Relation to competition within litters. *J. agric. Sci. Camb.* **92**, 257–261.

Freeland, W. J. and Janzen D. H. (1974). Strategies in herbivory by mammals: the role of plant secondary compounds. *Am. Nat.* **108**, 269–89.

Freeman, B. M. (1984). Transportation of poultry. *Wld Poult. Sci. J.,* **40**, 19–30.

Freeman, B. M. (1985). Stress and the domestic fowl : physiological fact or fantasy. *Wld. Poult. Sci. J.* **41**, 45.

Freeman, B. H, and Flack, I. M. (1980). Effects of handling on plasma corticosterone concentrations in the immature domestic fowl. *Comp. Biochem. Physiol.,* **66A**, 77–81.

Freeman, B. M., Kettlewell, P. J., Manning, A. G. C., and Berry, P. S. (1984). Stress of transportation for Broilers. *Vet. Rec.* **1114**, 286–287.

Friend, D. W. Cunningham, H. M and Nicholson, J. W. G. (1962). The duration of farrowing in relation to the reproductive performance of Yorkshire sows. *Can. J. comp. Med. vet. Sci.,* **16**, 127–130.

Friend, T. H. and Dellmeier, G. R. (1988). Common practices and problems related to artificially rearing calves: an ethological analysis. *Appl. Anim. Behav. Sci.,* **20**, 47–62.

Friend, T. H., Polan, C. E., Gwazdauskas, F. C. and Heald, C. W. (1977). Adrenal glucocorticoid response to exogenous adrenocorticotropin mediated by density and social disruption in lactating cows. *J. dairy Sci.,* **60**, 1958–1963.

Fritchen, R. (1975). Toilet training pigs on partially slotted floors. *Neb. Guid. G.* 74–140, University of Nebraska-Lincoln.

Fry, J. P., Sharman, D. P. and Stephens, D. B. (1976). The effect of apomorphine on oral behaviour in piglets. *Br. J. Pharmacol.,* **56**, 388p.

Gabrielsen, G. W., Kanwisher, J. W. and Steen, J. B. (1977). Emotional bradycardia: a telemetry study on incubating willow grouse, *Lagopus lagopus. Acta physiol. Scand.,* **100**, 255–257.

Gadd, J. (1967). Tail-biting: causes analysed in 430 case studies. *Pig Farming,* **15**, 57–58.

Garcia, J., Ervin, F. R. and Koelling, R. A. (1966).

Learning with prolonged delay of reinforcement. *Psychon. Sci.,* **5**, 121-2.

Garcia, J., Ervin, F.R., York, C.H. and Koelling, R.A. (1967). Conditioning with delayed vitamin injection. *Science, N.Y.* **155**, 716-18.

Gentle, M.J. (1986). Neuroma formation following partial beak amputation (beak-trimming) in the chicken. *Res. vet. Sci.,* **41**, 383-385.

Gentle, M.J. and Hill, F.L. (1987). Oral lesions in the chicken: behavioural responses following nociceptive stimulation. *Physiol. Behav.,* **40**, 781-783.

Gentle, M.J. and Seawright, E. (1988). The effects of partial beak amputation on circulatin leucocytes in the domestic fowl. *Med. Sci. Res.,* **16**, 145-146.

George, J.M. (1969). Variation in the time of parturition of Merino and Dorset Horn Ewes. *J. agric. Sci. Camb.* **73**, 295-299.

George, J.M. and Barger, I.A. (1974). Observation on bovine parturition. *Proc. Aust. Soc. Anim. Prod.* **10**, 314-317.

Gibb, M.J. (1977). Herbage intake of grazing sheep. *Br. vet. J.* **133**, 96.

Gibson, T.E. (1988). (Ed.) *Animal Disease - a Welfare Problem?* London: British Veterinary Association Animal Welfare Foundation.

Gibson, S.W., Innes. J., and Hughes, B.O. (1985). Aggregation behaviour of laying fowls in a covered strawyard. In *Second European Symposium on Poultry Welfare*, ed. R.-M. Wegner, 296-298. Celle: World Poultry Science Association.

Glickman, S.E. and Sroges, R.W. (1966). Curosity of zoo animals. *Behaviour* **24**, 151-88.

Gliner, J.A. (1972). Predictable vs. unpredictable shock: preference behaviour and stomach ulceration. *Physiol. Behav.,* **9**, 693-698.

Gloor P. and Leimbacher A. (1984). Gruppenbucht fur Galtsauen. *Blatter für Landtechnik,* **249**, 1-6.

Gloor, P. and Dolf, G. (1985). Galtsauenhaltung einzeln oder in Gruppen? *Schrift. der Eidg. Forsch. für Betriebswirtschaft und Landtechnik FAT,* Tänikon.

Goatcher, W.D. and Church, D.C. (1970). Taste responses in ruminants: III. Reactions of pigmy goats, normal goats, sheep and cattle to sucrose and sodium chloride. *J. Anim. Sci.,* **31**, 364-372.

Goethe, F. (1940). Beobachtungen und Versuche uber angeborene Schreckreaktionen junger Auerhuhner (*Tetrao u. urogallus L.*) *Z. Tierpsychol* **4**, 165-167.

Gonyou, H.W. and Stookey, J.M. (1987). Maternal and neonatal behaviour. In *The Veterinary Clinics of North America.* 3, 2. *Farm Animal Behaviour,* 231-249. Philadelphia: Saunders.

Gonyou, H.W. and Stricklin, W.R. (1981). Eating behaviour of beef cattle groups fed from a single stall or trough. *Appl. Anim. Ethol.* **7**, 123-133.

Gonyou, H.W. Christopherson, R.G. and Young, B.A, (1979). Effects of cold temperature and winter condition on some aspects of behaviour of feedlot cattle. *Appl. Anim. Ethol.* **5**, 113-124.

Gonyou, H.W., Hemsworth, P.H. and Barnett, J.L. (1986). Effects of frequent interactions with humans on growing pigs. *Appl. Anim. Behav. Sci.,* **16**, 269-278.

Graf, B.P. (1984). *Der Einfluss unterschiedlicher Laufstall systeme auf Verhaltensmerkmale von Mastochsen.* Doktor Dissertation der Eidgenossischen Technischen Hoschschule, Zürich.

Grafen, A. (1982). How not to measure inclusive fitness. *Nature, Lond.,* **298**, 425-426.

Grafen, A. (1984). Natural selection, group selection and kin selection. In *Behavioural Ecology*, 2nd edn., eds. J.R. Krebs and N.B. Davies, pp. 62-84. Oxford: Blackwell.

Grandin, T. (1978). Design of lairage, yard and race systems for handling cattle in abattoirs, auctions, ranches, restraining chutes and dipping vats. 37-52. *1st World Congr. Ethol. Appl. Zootechnics, Madrid.*

Grandin, T. (1979). The effect of stress on livestock and meat quality prior to and during slaughter. *Int. J. Stud. Anim. Prod.* **1**, 313-337.

Grandin, T. (1980a). Observations of cattle behaviour applied to the design of cattle-handling facilities. *Appl. Anim. Ethol.* **6**, 19-31.

Grandin, T. (1980b). Livestock behaviour as related to handling facilities design. *Int. J. Stud. Anim. Prob.,* **1**, 33-52.

Grandin, T. (1982). Pig behaviour studies applied to slaughter-plant design. *Appl. Anim. Ethol.,* **9**, 141-151.

Grandin, T. (1983). In *Farm Animal Housing and Welfare* ed. S.H. Baxter, M.R. Baxter and J.A.C. MacCormack, *Curr. Top. vet. Med. Anim. Sci.,* **24**, 137-149. The Hague: Martinus Nijhoff

Grauvogel, A. (1958). Über das Verhalten des Hausschweines unter besonderer Berucksichtigung des Fortpflanzungsverhaltens. Dissertation Freien Universität Berlin.

Grauvogl, A. (1987). The significance of straw for the behaviour of piglets. In *Welfare Aspects of Pig*

Rearing ed. D. Marx, A. Grauvogl and D. Smidt. C.E.C.

Gravas, L. (1982). Production and behaviour of free moving and locked sows. *Proc. Second int. Livestock Eur. Symp.*, 411–419. St. Joseph, Mich, Am. Soc. Agric. Eng.

Green, P. and Tong, J.M.J. (1988). Small intestinal obstruction associated with wood chewing in horses. *Vet. Rec.*, **123**, 196–198.

Grommers, F.J. (1977). Sucking among cows: A contribution to prevention and treatment. *Europ. Vereinigung f. Tierzucht. 28. Jahrestagung*, Brussel.

Gross, W.B. (1962). Blood cultures, blood counts and temperature records in an experimentally produced "air sac disease" and uncomplicated *Escherichia coli* infection of chickens. *Poult. Sci.*, **41**, 691–700.

Gross, W.B. and Colmano, G. (1965) The effect of social isolation on resistance to some infectious diseases. *Poult. Sci.*, **48**, 515–520.

Gross, W.B. and Siegel P.B. (1975). Immune response to *Escherichia coli*: *Am. J. vet. Res.*, **36**, 568–571.

Gross, W.B. and Siegel, P.B. (1979). Adaptation of chickens to their handler and experimental results. *Avian Dis.*, **23**, 708–714.

Gross, W.B. and Siegel, P.B. (1981). Long-term exposure of chickens to three levels of social stress. *Avian Dis.*, **25**, 312–325.

Grossman, S.P. (1975). Role of the hypothalamus in the regulation of food and water intake. *Psychol. Rev.* **82**, 200.

Grossman, S.P. (1976). Neuroanatomy of food and water intake. In *Hunger: Basic Mechanisms and Implications*, ed. D. Novin, W. Wyrwicka, and G. Bray p. 51. New York: Raven Press.

Groth, W. (1978). Tierschutz und verhaltensbezogene Gesichtspunkte der Kälbermast. *Tierzuchter*, **10**, 419–422.

Gschwindt, B., and Ehinger, B. (1979). Einfluss von Transport und Wortezeiten vor dem Schlachten auf Fleischqualität und biochemische Merkmale bei Broilern. *Arch. Geflügelk.*, 78–82.

Gubernick. D.J. (1981). Mechanisms of maternal 'labelling' in goats. *Anim. Behav.* **29**, 205–206.

Guhl, A.M. (1968). Social inertia and social stability in chickens. *Anim. Behav.*, **16**, 219–232.

Guise, H.J. and Penny, R.H.C. (in press). Factors influencing the welfare and carcase and meat quality of pigs. I The effects of stocking in transport and the use of electric goads. *Anim. Prod.*

Guthrie, D.M. (1980). *Neuroethology: An Introduction*. New York: Wiley

Guyomarc'h, J.-C. (1962). Contribution a l'étude du comportement vocal du poussin de *Gallus domesticus*. *J. Psychol. norm. path.*, **3**, 283–306.

Hafez. E.S.E. (1962). Sexual behaviour in farm animals. In *Reproduction in Farm Animals*, Baillière, Tindall and Cox, London p. 162.

Hafez. E.S.E. (1975). The Behaviour of Domestic Animals. London: Ballière Tindal.

Hafez. E.S.E. and Dyer, I.A. (eds). (1969). *Animal Growth and Nutrition*. Philadelphia: Lea and Febiger.

Hale, E.B. and Almquist, J.O. (1960). Relation of sexual behaviour to germ cell output in farm animals. *J. Dairy Sci., Suppl.* **42**, 145–169.

Hall, S.J.G. (1983). Grazing behaviour of Chillingham cattle. *Appl. Anim. Ethol.*, **11**, 71.

Hall, S.J.G. (1989). Chillingham cattle: social and maintenance behaviour in an ungulate that breeds all year round. *Anim. Behav.***38**, 215–225.

Halliday, W.G., Ross, J.G., Christie, G. and Jones, R.M. (1977). Effect of transportation on blood metabolites in broilers. *Br. Poult. Sci.*, **18**, 657–659.

Hamilton, W.D. (1963). The evolution of altruistic behaviour. *Am. Nat.*, **97**, 354–356.

Hamilton, W.D. (1964a). The genetical evolution of social behaviour I. *J. theoret. Biol.*, **7**, 1–16.

Hamilton, W.D. (1964b). The genetical evolution of social behaviour II. *J. theoret, Biol.*, **7**, 17–32.

Handscome, S.G. (1974). While shepherds watched their clocks by night. *Farmers' Weekly* **81**, 43.

Hansen, L.L. and Vestergaard, K. (1984). Tethered versus loose sows: ethological observations and measures of productivity. *Ann. Rech. Vét.*, **15**, 245–256.

Hansen, L.L., Hagels, A.M., and Madsen, A. (1982). Behavioural results and performance of bacon pigs fed "ad libitum" from one or several self-feeders. *Appl. Anim. Ethol.*, **8**, 307–333.

Hansen R.S. (1976). Nervousness in hysteria of mature female chickens. *Poult. Sci.* **55**, 531–543.

Harborne, J.B. (1982). *Introduction to Ecological Biochemistry*. 2nd edn. London: Academic Press.

Harlow, H.F. (1969). Age-mate or peer affectional system. *Adv. Study Behav.* **2**, 333–83.

Harlow, H.F., and Harlow, M.K. (1965). The affectional systems. In *Behavior of Nonhuman Primates*, Vol. 2. (A.M. Schrier, H.F. Harlow and F. Stollnitz eds.). New York: Academic Press.

Harlow, H.F. and Zimmermann, R.R. (1959).

Affectional responses in the infant monkey. *Science, New York.* **130**, 421–432.

Harris, J.A., Hillerton, J.E. and Morant, S.V. (1987). Effect on milk production of controlling muscid flies, and reducing fly-avoidance behaviour, by the use of Fenvalerate ear tags during the dry period. *J. dairy Res.,* **54**, 165–171.

Hart, L.A. and Hart, B.L. (1988). Autogrooming and social grooming in impala. *Annls. N. Y. Acad. Sci.,* **525**, 399–402.

Hartmann, E.L. (1973). *The Functions of Sleep.* Yale University Press, London.

Hartsock, T.G. (1985). Feasibility of day-one weaning followed by fostering to reduce pig death losses. *J. Anim. Sci.,* **61**. Suppl. 1, 209.

Hartsock, T.G. and Graves, H.B. (1976). Neonatal behaviour and nutrition related mortality in domestic swine. *J. Anim. Sci.,* **42**, 235–241.

Hauptman, J. et al (1972). *Etologie Hospodavskych Zvirat.* Prague: Statni Zmedelske Nakladatelstvi.

Hediger, H. (1934). Über bewegungstereotypien bein gehaltenen Tieren, *Rev. suisse Zool.* **41**, 349–356.

Hediger, H. (1941). Biologische Gestzmässigkeiten im Verhalten von Wirbeltieren. *Mitt. Naturf. Ges. Bern.*

Hediger, H. (1950). *Wild Animals in Captivity.* London: Butterworths.

Hediger, H. (1955) *Studies of the Psychology and Behaviour of Captive Animals in Zoos and Circuses.* London: Butterworth.

Hediger, H. (1963). The evolution of territorial behaviour. In: *The Social Life of Early Man.* ed. Washburn. S.L. London: Methuen.

Heimer, L. (1978). *Limbic mechanism* In *The Continuing Evolution of the Limbic System Concept,* ed. Livingston, K.E. and Hornykiewicz, pp. 95–187. New York: Plenum Press.

Hemsworth, P.H. and Barnett, J.L. (1987). Human-animal interactions. In *The Veterinary Clinics of North America,* 3, 2, *Farm Animal Behaviour,* 339–356. Philadelphia: Saunders.

Hemsworth, P.H. and Beilharz, R.G. (1979). The influence of restricted physical contact with pigs during rearing on the sexual behaviour of the male domestic pig. *Anim. Prod.* **29**, 311–314.

Hemsworth, P.H. Winfield, C.G. and Mullaney, P.G. (1976). A study of the development of the teat order in piglets. *Appl. Anim. Ethol.* **2**, 225–233.

Hemsworth, P.H., Barnett, J.L. and Hansen, C. (1986). The influence of early contact with humans and subsequent behavioural responses of pigs to humans. *Appl. Anim. Behav. Sci.,* **15**, 55–63.

Hemsworth, P.H., Barnett, J.L. and Hansen, C. (1986). The influence of handling by humans on the behaviour, reproduction and corticosteroids of male and female pigs. *Appl. Anim. Behav. Sci.,* **15**, 303–314.

Hemsworth, P.H., Barnett, J.L. and Hansen, C. (1987). The influence of inconsistent handling by humans on the behaviour, growth and corticosteroids of young pigs. *Appl. Anim. Behav. Sci.,* **17**, 245–252.

Hemsworth, P.H. Beilharz, R.G. and Brown, W.J. (1978a). The importance of the courting behaviour of the boar in the success of natural and artificial matings. *Appl. Anim. Ethol.* **4**, 341–347.

Hemsworth, P.H., Brand, A, and Willens, P.J. (1981). The behavioural response of sows to the presence of human beings and their productivity. *Livestock Prod. Sci.,* **8**, 67–74.

Hemsworth, P.H., Findlay, J.K. and Beilharz, R.G. (1978b). The importance of physical contact with other pigs during rearing on the sexual behaviour of the male domestic pig. *Anim. Prod.,* **27**, 201–207.

Hemsworth, P.H. Barnett, J.L. and Hanson, C. (1981). The influence of handling by humans on the behaviour, growth and corticosteroids in juvenile female pigs. *Horm. Behav.* **15**, 396–403.

Hemsworth, P.H. Salden, N.T.C.J. and Hoogerbrugge, A. (1982). The influence of the post-weaning social environment on the weaning to mating interval of the sow. *Anim. Prod.,* **35**, 41–48.

Henderson, R. and Stolba, A. (1989). Incidence of oestrus and oestrus trends in lactating sows housed in different social and physical environments. *Appl Anim. Behav. Sci.,* **22**, 235–244.

Herbert, D.M. and McFetridge, R.J. (1978). In *Chemical Immobilisation of North American Game Mammals.* 44–47. Edmonton: Alberta Department of Recreation, Parks and Wildlife.

Hercher, L., More, A.U. and Richmond, J.B. (1958). Effect on post partum separation of mother and kid on maternal care in the domestic goat. *Science N. Y.,* **128**, 1342–1343.

Herrnstein, R.J. (1977). The evolution of behaviourism. *Amer. Psychol.,* **32**, 593–603.

Hess, E.H. (1956). Space perception in the chick. *Scient. Amer.* 195(1), 71–80.

Hill, J.A. (1984). Gleadthorpe aviary, first year report. *Farm. Bldg. Eng.,* **1**, 14–15.

Hillerton, J.E., Bramley, A.J. and Broom, D.M.

(1983), *Hydrotaea irritans* and summer mastitis in calves. *Vet. Rec.,* **113**, 88.

Hillerton, J.E., Bramley, A.J. and Broom, D.M. (1984). The distribution of five species of flies (Diptera: Muscidae) over the bodies of dairy heifers in England. *Bull. Ent. Res.,* **74**, 113.

Hillerton, J.E., Bramley, A.J. and Yarrow, N.H. (1985). Control of flies (Diptera: Muscidae) on dairy heifers by Flectron ear tags. *Br. vet. J.,* **141**, 160.

Hillerton, J.E., Morant, S.V., and Harris, J.A. (1986). Control of Muscidae on cattle by Stock-Guard ear-tags, the behaviour of these flies on cattle and the effect on fly-dislodging behaviour. *Entomologia exp. appl.* **41**, 213–218.

Hinch, G.N., Thwaites, C.J., Lynch, J.J. and Pearson, A.J. (1982). Spatial relationships within a herd of young sterile bulls and steers. *Appl. Anim. Ethol.,* **8**, 27–44.

Hinde, R.A. (1959). Unitary drives. *Anim. Behav.* **7**., 130–141.

Hinde, R.A. (1970). *Animal Behaviour: A Synthesis of Ethology and Comparative Psychology*, 2nd edition, New York: McGraw Hill.

Hinde, R.A. (1973). Contraints on learning—an introduction to the problems. In *Constraints on learning* ed. R.A. Hinde and J. Stevenson-Hinde, London: Academic Press.

Hinde, R.A., Thorpe, W.H. and Vince, M.A. (1956). The following responses of young coots and moorhens. *Behaviour* **9**, 214–242.

Hirsch, H.V.B. and Spinelli, D.N. (1970). Visual experience modifies distribution of horizontally and vertically oriented receptive fields in cats. *Science N.Y.* **168**, 871–879.

Hishikawa, Y. Cramer, H. and Kuhlo, W. (1969). Natural and melatonin-induced sleep in young chickens. A behavioural and electrographic study. *Exp. Brain Res.* **7**, 84–94.

Hockman, C.H. and Bieger, D. (1976). *Chemical Transmission in the Mammalian Central Nervous System*, London: University Park Press.

Hodgson, J. and Wilkinson, J.M. (1967). The relationship between live-weight and herbage intake in grazing cattle. *Anim. Prod.,* **9**, 365–376.

Hogan, J.A. and Roper, T.J. (1978). A comparison of the properties of different reinforces. *Adv. Stud. Behav.,* **8**, 155–255.

Holmes, R.J. (1980). Normal mating behaviour and its variations. In *Current Therapy in Theriogenology.* ed. D.A. Morrow pp.931–936. Philadelphia. W.B. Saunders.

Hooker, D. (1954). Early human foetal behaviour, with a preliminary note on double simultaneous foetal stimulation. *Res. Publ. Ass. Res. Nerv. Ment. Dis.* **33**, 98–113.

Hooker, D. and Humphrey, T. (1954). Some results and deductions from a study of the development of human foetal behaviour. *Gaz. Med. Port.* **7**, 189–197.

Horn, G. (1985). *Memory, Imprinting and the Brain.* Oxford: Oxford University Press.

Horne, J.A (1977). Factors relating to energy conservation during sleep in mammals. *Physiol. Psychol.* **5**, 403–408.

Horrell, R.I. (1982). Immediate behavioural consequences of fostering 1-week-old piglets. *J. agric. Sci. Camb.,* **99**, 329–336.

Horrell, R.I. and Bennett, J. (1981). Disruption of teat preferences and retardation of growth following cross-fostering of one-week-old. *Anim. Prod.,* **33**, 99–106.

Horrell, R.I. and Hodgson, J. (1985). Mutual recognition between sows and their litters. *Applied Ethology in Farm Animals* ed. J. Unshelm, G. van Putten and K. Zeeb, 108–112. Davmstadt: K.T.B.L.

Hosoda, T. (1950). On the heritability of susceptibility to wind-sucking in horses. *Jap. J. zootech. Sci.,* **21**, 25–28.

Houpt, K.A. (1981). Equine bahaviour problems in relation to humane management. *Int. J. Stud. Anim. Prod.,* **2**, 329–336.

Houpt, K.A. (1984). Treatment of aggression in horses. *Equine Pract.,* **6(6)**, 8–10.

Houpt, K.A. (1987). Abnormal behavior. In *The Veterinary Clinics of North America 3, 2 Farm Animal Behavior* ed. E.O. Price., 357–367. Philadelphia: Saunders.

Houpt, K.A. and Hintz, H.F. (1983). Some effects of maternal deprivation on maintenance behaviour, spatial relationships and responses to environmental novelty in foals. *Appl. Anim. Ethol.,* **9**, 221–230.

Houpt, K.A., and Olm, D. (1984). Foal rejection: A review of 23 cases. *Equine Pract.,* **6(7)**, 38–40.

Houpt, K.A. and Wolski, T. (1982). *Domestic Animal Behaviour for Veterinarians and Animal Scientists.* Ames: Iowa State University Press.

Houston, A.I. and McFarland, D.J. (1976). On the measurement of motivational variables. *Anim. Behav.* **24**, 459–475.

Howard, B.R. (1972). Sleep in the domestic fowl. *Proc. Soc. Med.* **65**, 177–179.

Hoyt. D. F. and Taylor, C. R. (1981). Gait and the energies of locomotion in horses. *Nature, Lond.* **292**, 239–240.

Hsia, L. C. and Wood-Gush, D. G. M. (1982). The relationship between social facilitation and feeding behaviour in pigs. *Appl. Anim. Ethol.* **8**, 410.

Hsia, L. C., and Wood-Gush, D. G. M. (1984). Social facilitation in the feeding behaviour of pigs and the effect of rank. *Appl. Anim. Ethol.*, **11**, 265–270.

Hüber, A., and Fölsch, D. W. (1978). Akustiche Ethogramme von Huhnern: die Auswirkung verschiedener Haltungs systeme. *Tierhaltung.* **5**, Basel: Birkhäuser Verlag.

Hudson, S. J. and Mullord, M. M. (1977). Investigation of maternal bonding in dairy cattle. *Appl. Anim. Ethol.* **3**, 271–276.

Hughes, B. O. (1971). Allelomimetic feeding in the domestic fowl. *Br. Poult. Sci.*, **12**, 359.

Hughes, B. O. (1975). Spatial preference in the domestic. *Br. vet. J.*, **131**, 560–564.

Hughes, B. O. (1976). Preference decisions of domestic hens for wire or litter floors. *Appl. Anim. Ethol.*, **2**, 155–165.

Hughes, B. O. (1980). Behaviour of the hen in different environments. *Anim. Regul Stud.*, **3**, 65–71.

Hughes, B. O. (1981). Headshaking in fowls. *Proc. First Eur. Symp. Poult.* Welfare, KOGE, Denmark : World Poultry Science Association.

Hughes, B. O. (1984). Feather pecking and cannibalism in domestic fowls. *Hohenheimer Arbeiten*, **121**, 138–146.

Hughes, B. O. (1985). Feather loss – how does it occur. In *Second European Symposium on Poultry Welfare*, ed. R.-M. Wegner, 178–188. Celle : World Poultry Science Association.

Hughes, B. O. and Appleby, M. C. (1989). Increase in bone strength of spent laying hens housed in modified cages with perches. *Vet. Rec.* **124**, 483–484.

Hughes, B. O. and Black, A. J. (1973). The preference of domestic hens for different types of battery cage floor. *Br. Poult. Sci.*, **14**, 615–619.

Hughes, B. O. and Duncan, I. J. H. (1972). The influence of strain and environmental factors upon feather pecking and cannibalism in fowls. *Br. Poult. Sci.*, **13**, 525–547.

Hughes, B. O. and Duncan, I. J. H. (1988). Behavioural needs: can they be explained in terms of motivational models? *Appl. Anim. Behav. Sci.*, **20**, 352–355.

Hughes, B. O. and Wood-Gush. D. G. M. (1971). A specific appetite for calcium in domestic fowls. *Anim. Behav.*, **19**, 490–499.

Hughes, J., Smith, T. W., Kosterlitz, H. W., Fothergill, L. A., Morgan, B. A. and Morris, H. R. (1975). Identification of two related pentapeptides from the brain with potent opiate agonist activity. *Nature, Lond.* **258**, 577–9.

Humphrey, T. (1970). Function of the nervous system during prenatal life. In *Physiology of the Perinatal Period*, 2, Ch. 12. New York: Appleton-Century-Crofts.

Hunter, W. K. and Couttie, M. A. (1969). The behaviour of groups of bulls at lay off. *Br. vet. J.*, **125**, 252–

Hunter, E. J., Broom, D. M., Edwards, S. A. and Sibly R. M. (1988). Social hierarchy and feeder access in a group of 20 sows using a computer controlled feeder. *Anim. Prod.*, **47**, 139–148.

Hurnick, J. F. (1987). Sexual behaviour of female domestic mammals. In *The Veterinary Clinics of North America*, 3, 2, *Farm Animal Behavior*, Ed. E. O. Price, 423–461. Philadelphia: Saunders.

Hurnick, J. F. King, G. J. and Robertson, H. A. (1975). Oestrus and related behaviour in postpartum Holstein cows. *Appl. Anim. Ethol.* **2**, 55.

Hutchison, H. G., Woof, R., Mabon, R. M., Saleke, I. and Robb, J. M. (1962). A study of the habits of Zebu cattle in Tanganyika. *J. agric. Sci. Camb.*, **59**, 301–317.

Hutson, G. D. (1980). The effect of previous experience on sheep movement through yards. *Appl. Anim. Ethol.* **6**, 233–240.

Hutson, G. D. (1984). Spacing behaviour of sheep in pens. *Appl. Anim. Behav. Sci.* **12**, 111–119.

Hutson, G. D. (1989). Operant tests of access to earth as a reinforcement for weaner piglets. *Anim. Prod.* **48**, 561–569.

Hutson, G. D. and Hitchcock, D. K. (1978). The movement of sheep around corners. *Appl. Anim. Ethol.*, **4**, 349–355.

Hutyra, K., Marek, L., Macsy, J. and Marringer, R. (1959). *Spezielle Pathologie und Therapie des Haustiere*. Jena : VEB Gustav Fischer Verlag.

van Iersel, J. J. A. and Bol, A. C. A. (1958). Preening in two tern species. A study on displacement activities. *Behaviour* 13, 1–88.

Immelmann, K. (1972). Sexual and other long-term aspects of imprinting in birds and other species. *Adv. Study Behav.* 4, 147–174.

Immelmann, K. (1977). *Einfuhrung in der Verhaltensforschung*. Berlin: Parey.

Ingram, D. L. (1965). Evaporative cooling in the pig. *Nature, Lond.,* **207**, 415–416.

Innes, J. R. M. and Saunders, L. Z. (1962). *Comparative Neuropathology.* New York: Academic Press.

Isaacson, R. L. (1982). *The Limbic System* (2nd ed.), New York: Plenum Press.

Iversen, S. D. and Iversen, L. (1981). *Behavioural Pharmacology,* Oxford: Oxford University Press.

Izard, K. (1983). Pheromones and reproduction in domestic animals. In *Pheromones and Reproduction in Mammals,* ed. J. G. Vandenbergh. New York: Academic Press.

Jackson, W. T. (1974). Air transportation of Hereford cattle to the Peoples Republic of China. *Vet. Tec.* **94**, 209–211.

Jackson, P. G. G. (1988). The assessment of welfare in diseased farm animals. In *Animal Disease—a Welfare Problem,* ed. T. E. Gibson 42–46. London: British Veterinary Association Animal Welfare Foundation.

James, H. (1959). Flicker: an unconditioned stimulus for imprinting. *Can. J. Psychol.* **13**, 59–67.

Jenkins, P. F. (1978). Cultural transmission of song patterns and dialect development in a free-living bird population. *Anim. Behav.* **36**, 50–78.

Jensen, A. H., Yen, J. T., Gehring, M. M. Baker, D. H., Becker, D. E. and Harmon, B. G. (1970). Effects of space restriction and management on pre- and post-pubertal response of female swine. *J. Anim. Sci.,* **31**, 745–750.

Jensen, L. S. Meril, L. H., Reddy, C. V., and McGinnis, J. (1962). Observations on eating patterns and rate of food passage of birds fed pelleted and unpelleted diets. *Poult. Sci.,* **41**, 1414–1419.

Jensen, P. (1979). Sinsuggors beteendemonster under tre olika upstallnings forhallanden—en pilot studie. *Institutionen for husdjurshygien med horslarskalan. Rapport,* **1**, 1–40. Uppsala: Sveriges Lantbruksuniversitet.

Jensen, P. (1980a). Fixeringens effect pa sinsuggors beteende—en etologisk studie. *Institutionen for husdjurshygien med hovslagarskolan. Rapport* **2** pp 66. Uppsala: Sveriges Lantbruksuniversitet.

Jensen, P. (1980b). An ethogram of social interaction patterns in group-housed dry sows. *Appl. Anim. Ethol.* **6**, 341–350.

Jensen, P. (1981). Fixeringens effect pa sinsuggors beteende. *Svensk veterinartidning* **33**, 73–78.

Jensen, P. (1982). An analysis of agonistic interaction patterns in group-housed dry sows—aggression regulation through an 'avoidance order'. *Appl. Anim. Ethol.* **9**, 47–61.

Jensen, P. (1984). Effects of confinement on social interaction patterns in dry sows. *Appl. Anim. Behav. Sci.,* **12**: 93–101.

Jensen, P. (1986). Observations on the maternal behaviour of free ranging domestic pigs. *Appl. Anim. Behav. Sci.,* **16**, 131–142.

Jensen, P. and Algers, B. (1983). An ethogram of piglet vocalisations during suckling. *Appl. Anim. Ethol.* **11**, 237–248.

Jensen, P. and Wood-Gush, D. G. M. (1984). Social interactions in a group of free-ranging sows. *Appl. Anim. Behav. Sci.* **12**, 327–337.

Jensen, P. Algers, B. and Ekesbo, I. (1986). *Methods of Sampling and Analysis of Data in Farm Animal Ethology. Tierhaltung,* **17**. Basel: Birkhauser Verlag.

Jensen, P., Floren, F. and Hobroh, B. (1987). Pre-parturient changes in behaviour in free ranging domestic pigs. *Appl. Anim. Behav. Sci.* **17**, 69–76.

Jeppesen, L. E. (1981). An artificial sow to investigate the behaviour of sucking piglets. *Appl. Ani. Ethol.,* **7**, 359–367.

Jeppesen, L. E. (1982). Teat-order in groups of piglets reared on an artificial sow. I. Formation of teat-order and influence of milk yield on teat preference. *Appl. Anim. Ethol.,* **8**, 335–345.

Johnson, K. G. (1987). Shading behaviour of sheep: preliminary studies of its relation to thermoregulation, feed and water intakes, and metabolic rate. *Aust. J. agric. Res.,* **38**, 587–596.

Johnston, I. D. Obst, J. M. and Deland, M. P. (1979). Field observations of calving behaviour of two year old Hereford and Hereford-cross heifers. In *Behaviour in Relation to Reproduction. Management and Welfare of Farm Animals.* ed. M. Wodzicka-Tomaszewska, T. N. Edey and J. J. Lynch. Armidale: University of New England. pp. 127–132.

Jones, J. E. T. (1966a). Observations on parturition in the sow. I. The pre-partum phase. *Br. vet. J.,* **122**, 420–426.

Jones, J. E. T. (1966b). Observations on parturition in the sow. II. The parturient and post-parturient phases. *Br. vet. J.* **122**, 471–478.

Jones, R. B. (1985). Fear responses of individually-caged laying hens as a function of cage level and aisle. *Appl. Anim. Behav. Sci.* **14**, 63–74.

Jones, R. B. and Faure, J. M. (1984). The technique of jumping a steeplechase fence by competing event-horses. *Appl. Anim. Ethol.* **7**, 15–24.

Jongebreur, A. A. (1983). Housing design and welfare in livestock production. In *Farm Animal*

Housing and Welfare ed. Baxter, S.H., Baxter, M.R. and MacCormack, J.A.C. *Curr. Top. vet. Med. Anim. Sci.,* **24**, 265–269. The Hague: Martinus Nijhoff.

Kaiser, R. and Lippitz, O. (1974). Untersuchungen zum Verhalten von Milchkuhen im Boxen laufstall bei unterschiedlichem Tier-Liegeplatz-Verhaltniss und standig freim Zugang zur reduzierten Krippe. *Tierzucht,* **28**, 187–189.

Kandel, E.R. and Schwartz, J.H. (1981). *Principles of Neural Science,* London: Edward Arnold.

Katz, D. and Revesz, G. (1921). Experimentelle Studien zur vergleichenden Psychologie (Versuche mit Huhnern). *A. angew. Psychol.* **18**, 307.

Kear, J. (1964). Colour preference in young Anatidae. *Ibis* **106**, 361–369.

Kear, J. (1966). The pecking response of young coots *Fulica atra* and moorhens *Gallinula chloropus. Ibis* **108**, 118–122.

Keeling, L.J. and Duncan, I.J.H. (1988). The effect of activity transitions on spacing behaviour in domestic fowl. In *Proceedings of the International Congress on Applied Ethology in Farm Animals Skara 1988* ed. J. Unshelm, G. van Putten, K. Zeeb and I. Ekesbo, 291–296. Darmstadt: K.T.B.L.

Keiper, R.R. and Berger, J. (1982). Refuge-seeking and pest avoidance by feral horses in desert and island environments. *Appl. Anim. Ethol.,* **90**, 111–120.

Kelley, K.W. *et al* (1981). Whole blood leukocyte vs separated mononuclear cell blastogenesis in calves. Time dependent changes after shipping. *Can. J. comp. Med.,* **45**, 249–258.

Kelley, K.W. (1980). Stress and immune function. A bibliographic review. *Ann. Rech. Vet.* **11**, 445–478.

Kelley, K.W. (1983). *Trans. Amer. Soc. Agric. Eng.,* **26**, 834.

Kelley, K.W. (1985). Immunological consequences of changing environmental stimuli. In: *Animal Stress.* pp. 193–223. American Physiological Association.

Kelley, K.W., Greenfield, R.E., Evermann, J.F., Parish, S.M. and Perryman, L.E. (1982). Delayed-type hypersensitivity, contrast sensitivity, and phytohemagglutinin skin-test reponses of heat- and cold-stressed calves. *Amer. J. vet. Res.,* **43**, 775–779.

Kendrick, J.W. (1954). Psychic impotence in bulls. *Cornell Vet.,* **44**, 289–293.

Kennedy, J.M. and Baldwin, B.A. (1972). Taste preferences in pigs for nutritive and non-nutritive sweet solutions. *Anim. Behav.* **20**, 706–718.

Kenny, F.J. and Tarrant, P.V. (1982). Behaviour of cattle during transport and penning before slaughter. In *Transport of Animals Intended for Breeding, Production and Slaughter.* ed. R. Moss, *Curr. Top. vet. Med. Anim. Sci.,* **18**, 87–102. The Hague: Martinus Nijhoff.

Kent, J.E. and Ewbank, R. (1983). Changes in the behaviour of cattle during and after road transportation. *Appl. Anim. Ethol.,* **11**, 85.

Kent, J.E. and Ewbank, R. (1986a). The effect of road transportation on the blood constituents and behaviour of calves. II One to three weeks old. *Br. vet. J.,* **142**, 326–335.

Kent, J.E. and Ewbank, R. (1986b). The effect of road transportation on the blood constituents and behaviour of calves. III Three months old. *Br. vet. J.,* **142**, 326–335.

Kent, J.P. (1984). A note on multiple fostering of calves onto nurse cows at a few days post-partum. *Appl. Anim. Behav. Sci.,* **12**, 183–186.

Keogh, R.G. and Lynch, J.J. (1982). Early feeding experience and subsequent acceptance of feed by sheep. *Proc. N.Z. Soc. Anim. Prod.,* **42**, 73–75.

Keverne, E.B. Levy, F. Poindron, P. *et al* (1983). Vaginal stimulation: an important determinant of maternal bonding in sheep. *Science, N.Y.,* **219**, 81–83.

Key, C. and Maciver, R.M. (1980). The effects of maternal influences on sheep: Breed differences in grazing, resting and courtship behaviour. *Appl. Anim. Ethol.* **6**, 33–48.

Kidwell, J.F., Bohman, V.R. and Hunter, J.E. (1954). Individual and group feeding of experimental beef cattle as influenced by hay maturity. *J. Anim. Sci.* **13**, 543.

Kiel, H. (1963). Die Untugend des Kannibalismus bei Huhnern. *Tierärzlt. Umschau,* **18**, 636–639.

Kiley, M. (1972). The vocalisations of ungulates. *Z. Tierpsychol.,* **31**, 171–222.

Kiley-Worthington, M. (1977). *Behavioural Problems of Farm Animals.* Stocksfield: Oriel Press.

Kiley-Worthington, M. and de la Plain, S. (1983). *The Behaviour of Beef Suckler Cattle.* Basel: Birkhäuser Verlag.

Kiley-Worthington, M. and Savage, P. (1978). Learning in dairy cattle using a device for economical management of behaviour. *Appl. Anim. Ethol.,* **4**, 119–124.

Kilgour, R. (1972). Behaviour of sheep at lambing. *N.Z.J. Agric.,* **125**, 24–27.

Kilgour, R. (1975). The open-field test as an

assessment of the temperament of dairy cows. *Anim. Behav.,* 23, 615–624.

Kilgour, R. (1978). The application of animal behaviour and the humane care of farm animals. *J. Anim. Sci.* 45, 1478–1486.

Kilgour, R. (1987). Learning and the training of farm animals. In: *The Veterinary Clinics of North America, Vol. 3, No. 2, Farm Animal Behavior,* ed. E. O. Price, Philadelphia: Saunders.

Kilgour, R. and Dalton, C. (1984). *Livestock Behaviour : a Practical Guide.* London : Granada.

King, J. and Klingel, H. (1965). The use of the oripavine derivative M99 for the restraint of equine animals, and its antogonism with the related compound M285. *Res. vet. Sci.,* 6, 447–455.

King, J. A. and Millar, R. P. (1980). Comparative aspects of luteinising hormone-releasing hormone structure and function in vetobrate physiology. *Endocrinology* 106, 707–717.

Kite, V. G. (1985). Does a hen require a nest? *Proc. 2nd Eur. Symp. Poult Welfare,* ed. R.-M. Wegner, 118–135. Celle: World Poultry Science Association.

Kittner, M. (1967). Zur Verhinderung des gegenseitigen Besaugens bei der Gruppenhaltung der Kälber. *Tierzucht.,* 21, 584–585.

Klemm, W. R. (1966). Sleep and paradoxical sleep in ruminants. *Proc. Soc. Exp. Biol. Med.* 121, 635–638.

Klemm, W. R., Sherry, C. J., Schake, L. M. and Sis, R. F. (1983). Homosexual behaviour in feedlot steers: an aggression hypothesis. *Appl. Anim. Ethol.* 11, 187–195.

Klemm, W. R., Sherry, C. J., Sis, R. F. Schake, L. M., and Waxman, A. B. (1984). Evidence of a role for the vomeronasal organ in social hierarchy in feedlot cattle. *Appl. Anim. Behav. Sci.,* 12 : 53–62.

Klinghammer, E. (1967). Factors influencing choice of mate in birds. In: *Early Behavior: Comparative and Developmental Approaches* ed. H. W. Stevenson, E. H. Hess and H. L. Rheingold. New York: Wiley.

Knight, T. W. (1973). The effect of androgen status of rams on sexual activity and fructose concentration in the semen. *Aust. J. agric. Res.,* 24, 573–578.

Knowles. T. G. and Broom, D. M. (in press). The handling and transport of broilers and spent hens. *Appl. Anim. Behav. Sci.*

Kondo, S. Kawakami, N. Kohama, H. and Nishino, S. (1983). Changes in activity, spatial pattern and social behaviour in calves after grouping. *Appl. Anim. Ethol.* 11, 217–228.

Konggaard, S. P. (1983). Feeding conditions in relation to welfare for dairy cows in loose-housed conditions. In *Farm Animal Housing and Welfare* ed. S. H. Baxter, M. R. Baxter and J. A. C. MacCormack, *Curr. Top. vet. Med. Anim. Sci.,* 24, 272–278. The Hague: Martinus Nijhoff.

de Koning, R. (1983). Results of a methodical approach with regard to external lesions of sows as an indicator of animal well being. In *Indicators Relevant to Farm Animal Welfare* ed. D. Smidt, *Curr. Top. vet. Med. Anim. Sci.,* 23, 155–162. The Hague: Martinus Nijhoff.

Kraus, H. (1978). Vergleichende Untersuchungen an Legehennen aus Kommerzieller Boden—und Käfighalten unter besonderer Berucktsichtigung der Zerlegeergebnisse. *Tierärztl. Lebensmittel. des Kreises Mettmann.*

Kruijt, J. P. (1964). Ontogeny of social behaviour in Burmese red jungle fowl *(Gallus gallus spadiceus). Behaviour,* Suppl 12.

Kruse, P. E. (1983). The importance of colostral immunoglobulins and their absorption from the intestine of the newborn animals. *Ann. Rech. vét.,* 14, 349–353.

Kuffler, S. W., Nicholls, J. G. (1976). *From Neuron to Brain.* Sunderland Massachusetts: Sinauer.

Kuo, Z. Y. (1967). *The Dynamics of Behaviour Developments.* New York: New York.

Kummer, H. (1968). *Social Organization of Hamadryas Baboons.* Chicago: University of Chicago Press.

Ladewig, J. (1984). The effect of behavioural stress on the episodic release and circadian variation of cortisol in bulls. In *Proc. Int. Cong. Appl. Ethol. Farm Anim.* ed. J. Unshelm, G. van Putten and K. Zeeb. pp. 339–342, Darmstadt: K. T. B. L.

Lagerlof, N. (1951). Hereditary forms of sterility in Swedish cattle breeds. *Fert. Steril.* 2, 230.

Lambert, R. J., Ellis, M. and Rowlinson, P. (1983a). An alternative system of sow housing and feeding based upon a sow activated feeder. *Anim. Prod.,* 36, 532.

Lambert, R. J. Ellis, M. Rowlinson, P. and Saville, C. A. (1983b). Influence of housing/feeding system on sow behaviour. *Anim. Prod.,* 36, 532.

Lambert, R. J., Ellis, M. and Rowlinson, P. (1984). The effect of feeding frequency on the behaviour patterns of group-housed dry sows using an electronic sow-activated feeder. *Anim. Prod.,* 38, 540.

Lambert, R. J., Ellis, M. and Rowlinson, P. (1985). The effect of feeding frequency on levels of aggression and 24th behaviour patterns of large groups of loose-housed dry sows. *Anim. Prod.,* **40**, 546.

Lambert, R. J., Ellis, M. and Rowlinson, P. (1986). An assessment of an electronic feeding system and "dynamic" grouping in loose-housed sows. *Anim. Prod.,* **42**, 468.

Lampkin, G. H., Quarterman, J. and Kidner, M. (1958). Observations on the grazing habits of grada and zebu steers in a high altitude temperature climate. *J. agric. Sci. Camb.* **50**, 211.

Larkin, S. and McFarland, D. (1978). The cost of changing from one activity to another. *Anim. Behav.* **26**, 1237–46.

Leach, D. H. and Ormrod, K. (1984). The technique of jumping a steeplechase fence by competing event-horses. *Appl. Anim. Ethol.* **12**, 15–24.

Leach, D. H., Ormrod, K. and Clayton, H. M. (1984). Standardised terminology for the description and analysis of equine locomotion. *Equine Vet. J.* **16**, 522–528.

Le Denmat, M. Saulnier, J. and Le Muir, D. (1982). *Pointe Elev.* (quoted by Tillon, J. P. and Madec, F. 1984).

Leeson, S., and Morrison, W. E. (1978). Effect of feather cover on feed efficiency in laying birds. *Poult. Sci.,* **57**, 1094–1096.

Le Magnen, J. (1971). Advances in studies on the physiological control and regulation of food intake. In *Progress in Physiological Psychology*, Vol 4, ed. E. Stellar and J. M. Sprague. Academic Press: New York.

Le Neindre, P. and Sourd, C. (1984). Influence of rearing conditions on subsequent social behaviour of Friesian and Salers heifers from birth to six months of age. *Appl. Anim. Behav. Sci.,* **12**, 43–52.

Le Neindre, P. (1989). Influences of rearing conditions and breeds on social behaviour and activity in a novel environment. *Appl. Anim. Behav. Sci.* **23**, 129–140.

Lendfers, L. H. H. M. (1970). De invloed van transport op sterfte en vleeskwaliteit van slachtvarkens. *Tijdschr. Diergeneesk.,* **95** (25): 1331–13342.

Lent, P. C. (1974). Mother-infant relationships in ungulates. In *The Behaviour of Ungulates and its Relationships to Management*, ed. V. Geist and F. Walther. Morges: Int. Union Conservation of Nature.

Levine, S., Goldman, L. and Coover, G. D. (1972). Expectancy and the pituitary-adrenal system. In *Physiology, Emotion and Psychosomatic Illness*, ed. R. Porter and J. Knight. Amsterdam: Elsevier.

Levy, D. M. (1944). On the problem of movement restraint. *Am. J. Orthopsychiat.,* **14**, 644–671.

Levy, F. Poindron, P. and Le Neindre, P. (1983). Attraction and repulsion by amniotic fluids and their olfactory control in the ewe around parturition. *Physiol. Behav.,* **31**, 687–692.

Lewis, C. J. and Oakley, G. A. (1970). Treatment of puerperal psychosis in sows and sedative and anaesthetic drugs. *Vet. Rec.,* **87**, 614.

Lewis, N. J. and Hurnik, J. F. (1985). The development of nursing behaviour in Swine. *Appl. Anim. Behav. Sci.,* **14**, 225–232.

Li, C. H. (1972). Hormones of the adenohypophysis. *Proc. Amer. Physiol. Soc.,* **116**, 365.

Lickliter, R. E. (1982). Effects of a post-partum separation on maternal responsiveness in primiparous and multiparous domestic goats. *Appl. Anim. Ethol.,* **8**, 537–542.

Lickliter, R. E. (1984). Hiding Behaviour in domestic goat kids. *Appl. Anim. Behav. Sci.* **12**, 187–192.

Lickliter, R. E. (1985). Behaviour associated with parturition in the domestic goat. *Appl. Anim. Behav. Sci.,* **13**, 335–3435.

Lickliter, R. E. and Heron, J. R. (1984). Recognition of mother by newborn goats. *Appl. Anim. Behav. Sci.,* **12**, 187–192.

Lill, A. (1968). Spatial organisation in small flocks of domestic fowl. *Behaviour* **32**, 258–290.

Lincoln, G. A. (1971). The seasonal reproductive changes in the Red deer stag *(Cervus elaphus) J. Zool. Lond.,* **163**, 105–123.

Lindahl, I. L. (1964). Time of parturition in ewes. *Anim. Behav.* **12**, 231–234.

Lindsay, D. R. (1965). The importance of olfactory stimuli in the mating behaviour of the ram. *Anim. Behav.* **13**, 75–78.

Lindsay, D. R. (1978). Effect of stimulation by partners on reproduction success (Effect de la stimulation par des partners sur le succes de la reproduction). *Proc. 1st. Wld. Congr. on Ethol. Appl. to Zootechnics,* **1**, 513–523.

Lindsay, D. R. (1985). Reproductive anomalies. In *Ethology of Farm Animals*, World Animal Science, A5, ed. A. F. Fraser, 413–418. Amsterdam: Elseiver.

Lindsay, D. R. and Robinson, T. J. (1964). Oestrogenic and antioestrogenic activity of androgens in the ewe. *J. Reprod. Fert.* **7**, 267–274.

Lindsley, D. B. (1972). Two thousand years of

pondering brain and behaviour. In *Brain Mechanisms and the Control of Behaviour*, ed. H. Messel and S.T. Butler, Sydney: Shakespeare Head Press.

Löliger, H.C., von dem Hagen., and Matthew, S. (1980). Tiergesundheit und klinische parameter als Indiz für die Beurteilung tierschutzelevanter Tatbestande in der Geflügelhaltung. *Arch Gefglügelk.*, 6, 229–236.

Löliger, H.C. von dem Hagen, D. and Matthes, S. (1981). Einfluss der Haltungssysteme auf die Tiergesundheit Bericht über Ergebnisse klinischpathologischer Untersuchungen. *Landbauforschung Völkenrode*, 60, 47–67.

Lorenz, K. (1935). Der Kumpan in der Umwelt des Vogels. *J. Orn., Lpz.* 83, 137–213 and 289–394. (Translated 1937). The companion in the birds' world. *Auk 54*, 245–73.

Lorenz, K. (1939). Vergleichende Verhaltensforschung. *Zool. Anz. Suppl.* 12, 69–102.

Lorenz, K. (1941). Vergleichende Bewegungsstudien an Anatiden. *J. Ornithol.*, 89, 194–293.

Lorenz, K. (1965). *Evolution and Modification of Behavior*. Chicago: University of Chicago Press.

Lorenz, K. (1966). *On Aggression*. London: Methuen.

Low, W.A. Tweedie, R.L. Edwards, C.B.H. Hodder, R.M. Malapant, K.W.J. and Cunningham, R.B. (1981). The influence of environment on daily maintenance behaviour of free-ranging shorthorn cows in central Australia. I. General introduction and decriptive analysis of day-long activities. II. Multivariant analysis of duration and incidence of activities. III. Detailed analysis of sequential behaviour patterns and integrated discussion. *Appl. Anim. Ethol.* 7, 11–26, 27–38, 39–56.

Lustgarten, C., Bottoms, G.D. and Shaskas, J.R. (1973). Experimental adrenalectomy of pigs. *Am. J. vet. Res.* 34, 279–282.

Lynch, J.J. (1980). Behaviour of livestock in relation to their productivity. In: *Handbook of Nutrition and Food* (ed. M. Rechcigl). West Palm Beach, Fla: RC Press.

Lynch, J.J. and Alexander, G. (1977). Sheltering behaviour of lambing Merino sheep in relation to grass hedges and artificial windbreaks. *Aust. J. agric. Res.* 28, 691–701.

MacArthur, R.H. and Pianka, E.R. (1966). On the optimal use of a patchy environment. *Am. Nat.* 102, 381–3.

McBride, G. (1963). The "teat order" and communication in young pigs. *Anim. Behav.*, 11, 53–56.

McBride, G. and Foenander, F. (1962). Territorial behaviour in flocks of domestic fowls. *Nature, Lond.* 194, 102.

McBride, G. Arnold, G.W. Alexander, G. and Lynch, J.J. (1967). Ecological aspects of behaviour of domestic animals. *Proc. ecol. Soc. Aust.* 2, 133–65.

McBride, G., Parer, I.P. and Foenander, F. (1969). The social organisation of the feral domestic fowl. *Anim. Behav. Monogr.* 2: 125–181.

McCann, S.M. (1970). Chemistry and physiological aspects of hypothalamic releasing and inhibiting factors. In *The Hypothalamus*, p. 277. New York: Academic Press.

McCleery, R.H. (1978). Optimal behaviour sequences and decision making. In *Behavioural Ecology an Evolutionary Approach*. ed. J.R. Krebs and N.B. Davies, Oxford: Blackwell.

MacDonald, C.L. Beilharz, R.G. and McCutchen, J.C. (1981). Training cattle to control by electric fences. *Appl. Anim. Ethol.*, 7, 113–121.

McFarland, D.J. (1965). The effect of hunger on thirst motivated behaviour in the Barbary dove. *Anim. Behav.*, 13, 286–300.

McFarland, D.J. (1971). *Feedback Mechanisms in Animal Behaviour*. London: Academic Press.

McFarland, D.J. and Sibly, R.M. (1975). The behavioural final common path. *Phil. Trans. R. Soc.*, B, 270, 265–93.

McFarlane, I. (1976a). Ratonale in the design of housing and handling facilities. In *Beef Cattle Science Handbook*, ed. M.E. Ensminger, 13, 223–227. Clovis, California: Agriservices Foundation.

McFarlane, I. (1976b). A practical approach to animal behaviour. In *Beef Cattle Science Handbook*, ed. M.E. Ensminger, 13, 420–426. Clovis.

McGrath, M.J. and Cohen, D.B. (1978). REM sleep facilitation of adaptive waking behaviour: A review of the literature. *Psychol. Bull.* 85, 24–57.7.

McGlore, J.J. and Curtis, S.E. (1985). Behaviour and performance of weanling pigs in pens equipped with hide areas. *J. Anim. Sci.*, 60, 20–24.

Machlis, L. (1977). An analysis of the temporal patterning of pecking in chicks. *Behaviour*, 63, 1–70.

McKinney, F. (1978). Comparative approaches to social behaviour in closely related species of birds. *Adv. Study Behav.* 8, 1–38.

MacKay, P.C. and Wood-Gush, D.G.M. (1980). The responsiveness of beef calves to novel stimulation: An interaction between exploration and fear. *Appl. Anim. Ethol.,* **6**, 383–384.

Mackintosh, N. J. (1973). Stimulus selection: learning to ignore stimuli that predict no change in reinforcement. In *Constraints on Learning.* eds. R. A. Hinde and J. Stevenson-Hinde. London: Academic Press.

Maclean, C. W. (1969). Observations on noninfectious infertility in sows. *Vet. Rec.,* **85**, 675–682.

MacPhail, E. M. (1982). *Brain and Intelligence in Vertebrates.* Oxford: Clarendon Press.

Madec, F. (1982). *Pig International,* **12**, 28.

Madec, F. (1984). Urinary disorders in intensive pig herds. *Pig News and Information,* **5**, No. 2, 89–93.

Madec, F. (1985). La consommation d'eau chez la truie gestante en élevage intensif. *Journées Rech. Porcine en France,* **17**, 223–236.

Mankovich, N. J. and Banks, E. M. (1982). An analysis of social orientation and the use of space in a flock of domestic fowl. *Appl. Anim. Ethol.* **9**, 177–193.

Manson, F. J. and Leaver, J. D. (1986). Effect of hoof trimming and protein level on lameness in dairy cows. *Anim. Prod.* **42**, 451.

Manson, F. J. and Leaver, J. D. (1989). The effect of concentrate: silage ratio and of hoof-trimming on lameness in dairy cattle. *Anim. Prod.* **49**, 15–22.

Marler, P. R., and Hamilton, W. J. (1966). *Mechanisms of Animal Behavior.* New York: Wiley.

Marler, P. R., and Tamura, M. (1964). Culturally transmitted patterns of vocal behaviour in sparrows. *Science, N. Y.* **146**, 1483–6.

Martin, G. (1975). Über Verhaltenstörungen von Legehennen in Käfig. Ein Beitrag zur Klarung des Problems tierschutzgeschechter Huhnerhaltung. *Angew. Ornithol.,* **4**, 145–176.

Martin, G. (1987). Animal welfare in chicken management: obtaining knowledge and evaluating results. In *Ethical Ethological and Legal Aspects of Intensive Farm Animal Management,* ed. E. von Loeper, G. Martin, J. Muller, A. Nabholz, G. van Putten, H. H. Sambraus, G. M. Teutsch, J. Troxler and B. Tschanz, *Tierhaltung,* **18**, 49–82. Basel: Birkhauser Verlag.

Martin, P. and Bateson, P. P. G. (1986). *Measuring Behaviour* Cambridge: Cambridge University Press.

Marx, D. and Mertz, R. (1987). Behaviour of early weaned piglets in free-choice or forced situations. In *Welfare Aspects of Pig Rearing* ed. D. Marx, A. Grauvogl and D. Smidt, EUR 10776 EN, p. 81–93.

Luxembourg: Commission of the European Communitites.

Marx, D. and Schuster, H. (1980). Ethologische Wahlversuche mit fruhabgesetzten Ferkeln wahrend der Flatdeckhaltung. 1. Mitteilung: Ergebnisse des ersten Abschnitts der Untersuchungen zur tiergerechten Fussbodengestaltung. *Dtsch. tierärztl. Wschr.,* **87**, 365–400.

Marx, D. and Schuster, H. (1982). Ethologische Wahlversuche mit fruhabgesetzten ferkeln wahrend Flatderckhaltung. 2. Mitteilung: Ergebnisse des zweiten Abschnitts der Untersuchungen zur tiergerechten Fussbodengestaltung. *Dtsch. tierärztl. Wschr.,* **89**, 313–352.

Marx, D. and Schuster, H. (1984). Ethologische Wahlversuche mit fruhabgesetzten Ferkeln wahrend der Flatdeckhaltung. 3. Mitteilung: Ergebnisse der Untersuchungen zur tiergerechten flachengrosse. *Dtsch. tierärztl. Wschr.,* **31**, 18–22.

Mason, W. A. (1960). The effects of social restriction on the behavior of rhesus monkeys: I. Free social behavior. *J. comp. physiol. Psychol.* **53**, 582–9.

Mason, W. A. (1961). The effects of social restriction on the behavior of rhesus monkeys: III. Dominance tests. *J. comp. physiol. Psychol.* **54**, 694–9.

Mason, A. S. (1972). Diseases of the Adrenal Cortex. In: *Clinics Endocrinology and Metabolism,* ed. Mason, A. S. Philadephia: W. B. Saunders.

Mason, S. T. (1984). *Catecholamines and Behaviour,* Cambridge: Cambridge University Press.

Massion, J. and Gahery, T. (1979). Diagonal stance in quadrupeds: A postural support for movement. *Prog. Brain Res.* **50**, 219–226.

Mattner, P. E., Braden, A. W. H. and George, J. M. (1973). Studies of flock mating of sheep. 5. Incidence, duration and effect on flock fertility of initial sexual inactivity in young rams. *Aust. J. exp. Agric. Anim. Husb.,* **13**, 35–44.

Mavrogenis, A. P. and Robinson, O. W. (1976). Factors affecting puberty in swine. *J. Anim. Sci.,* **42**, 1251–1255.

Mayes, A. (1983). *Sleep Mechanisms and Functions in Humans and Animals.* Van Nostrand Reinhold.

Maynard Smith, J. (1978). The evolution of sex. In *Behavioural Ecology* ed. J. R. Krebs and N. B. Davies. Oxford: Blackwell.

Maynard Smith, J. (1982). *Evolution and the Theory of Games.* Cambridge: Cambridge University Press.

Meddis, R. (1975). On the function of sleep. *Anim. Behav.,* **23**, 676–691.

Melrose, D. R. Red, H. C. B. and Patterson, R. L. S.

(1971). Androgen steroids associated with boar odour as an aid to the detection of oestrus in pig artificial insemination. *Br. vet. J.,* **127**, 497.

Mench, J.A. (1988). The development of aggressive behaviour in male broiler chicks: a comparison with laying-type males and the effects of feed restriction. *Appl. Anim. Behav. Sci.,* **21**, 233–242.

Menzel, E.W., Davenport, R.K., and Rogers, C.M. (1963). The effects of environmental restriction upon the chimpanzee's responsiveness to objects. *J. comp. physiol. Psychol.* **56**, 78–85.

Meredith, M.J. (1982). Anoestrus in the pig: diagnosis and aetiology. *Irish vet. J.* **36**, 17–24.

Merrick, A.W. and Scharp, D.W. (1971). Electro-encephalography of resting behaviour in cattle with observations on the question of sleep. *Am. J. vet. Res.,* **32**, 1893–1897.

Messent, P.R. and Broom, D.M. (1986) (Eds.) *Encyclopaedia of Domestic Animals.* New York: Grolier.

du Mesnil du Buisson, F. and Signoret, J.P. (1962). Influences de facteur externes sur le dechlenchement de la puberte chez la truie. *An. Zootechn.* **11**, 53–59.

Mess, B., Zanisi, M. and Tima, L. (1970). The hypothalamus as the centre of endocrine feedback mechanisms. In *The Hypothalamus* p. 259. New York: Academic Press.

Metz, J. and Metz, J.H.M. (1987). Behavioural phenomena related to normal and difficult deliveries in dairy cows. *Neth. J. agric. Sci.,* **35**, 87–101.

Metz. J.H.M. (1975). Time patterns of feeding and rumination in domestic cattle. *Meded. Landbhoogesch. Wageningen,* 75–12, 1–66.

Metz, J.H.M. (1981). Social reactions of cows when crowded. *Appl. Anim. Ethol.,* **7**, 384–385.

Metz, J.H.M. (1983). Food competition in cattle. In *Farm Animal Housing and Welfare* ed. S.H. Baxter, M.R. Baxter and J.A.C. MacCormack *Curr. Top. vet. Med. Anim. Sci.,* **24**, 164–170. The Hague: Martinus Nijhoff.

Metz, J.H.M. (1987). The response of farm animals to humans. In *The Role of the Stockman in Livestock Production and Management,* ed. M. Seabrook, 23–37, Brussels: Commission of the European Communities, Report EUR 10982 EN.

Metz J.H.M. and Mekking, P. (1984). Crowding phenomena in dairy cows as related to available idling space in a cubicle housing system. *Appl. Anim. Behav. Sci.,* **12** 63–78.

Metz, J.H.M. and Oosterlee, C.C. (1981).

Immunologische und ethologische Kriterien fur die artgemassehaltung von Sauen und Ferkeln in: *Aktuelle Arbeiten zur artgemassen Tierhaltung KTBL Schrift* **264**, 39–50. Darmstadt: KTBL.

Meunier-Salaun, M.C. and Faure, J.M. (1984). On the feeding and social behaviour of the laying hen. *Appl. Anim. Behav. Sci.* **12**.

Meunier-Salaun, M.C., Vantrimponte, M.N., Raab, A. and Dantzer, R. (1987). Effect of floor area restriction upon performance, behaviour and physiology of growing-finishing pigs. *J. Anim. Sci.,* **64**, 1371–1377.

Meyer, W.A. and Sunde, M.L. (1974). Bone breakages as affected by type of housing or an exercise matching for layers. *Poult. Sci.,* **53**, 878–885.

Meyer-Holzapfel, M. (1968). Abnormal behaviour in zoo animals. In *Abnormal Behavior in Animals,* ed. M.W. Fox, 476–503. Philadelphia: W.B. Saunders.

von Mickwitz, G. (1982). Various transport conditions and their influence on physiological reaction. In: R. Moss (ed.): *Transport of Animals Intended for Breeding, Production and Slaughter,* 45–53. Martinus Nijhoff.

Mill, P.J. (1982). *Comparative Neurobiology.* London: Edward Arnold.

Miller, E.R., Vathana, S., Green, F.F., Black, J.R., Romsos, D.R. and Ullrey, D.E. (1974). Dietary caloric density and caloric intake in the pig. *J. Anim. Sci.* **39**, 980.

Miller, M.G. (1981). Trigeminal deafferentation and ingestive behaviour in rats. *J. comp. Physiol. Psychol.* **95**, 252–269.

Miller, N.E. (1959). Liberalization of basic S-R concepts: extensions to conflict behaviour, motivation and social learning. In *Psychology: a Study of a Science,* Vol. II (S. Koch, ed.). New York: McGraw Hill.

Moberg, G.P. and Wood, V.A. (1982). Effect of differential rearing on the behavioural and adrenocortical response of lambs to a novel environment. *Appl. Anim. Ethol.,* **8**, 269–279.

Mogenson, G.J. and Calaresu, F.R. (1978) In *Hunger Models:* ed. D.A. Booth *et al.* London: Academic Press.

Morgan, P.D. and Arnold, G.W. (1974). Behavioural relationships between Merino ewes and lambs during the four weeks after birth. *Anim. Prod.* **19**, 196.

Morgan, P.D. Boundy, C.A.P. Arnold, G.W. and Lindsay, D.R. (1975). The roles played by the senses of the ewe in the location and recognition of lambs. *Appl. Anim. Ethol.*, **1**, 139–150.

Morisse, J. P. (1982). *Recueils Med. Vét.*, **158**, 307.

Mormède, P., Soissons, J., Bluthé, R., Raoult, J., Legarff, G., Levierax, D. and Dantzer, R. (1982). Effects of transportation on blood serum composition, disease incidence and production traits in young calves. Influence of the journey duration. *Annls Rech. vét.*, **13**, 369–384.

Morrison, S. R. Heitman, H. Jr. and Bond, T. E. (1969). Effect of humidity on swine at temperatures above optimum. *Int. J. Biometeorol.* **13**, 135–139.

Morrow, D. A. (1966). Postpartum ovarian activity and uterine involation in dairy cattle. *J. Am. vet. Med. Ass.*, **149**, 1596.

Morton, D. B. and Griffiths, P. H. M. (1985). Guidelines on the recognition of pain, distress and discomfort in experimental animals and an hypothesis for assessment. *Vet. Rec.*, **116**, 431–436.

Moss, B. W. (1981). The development of a blood profile for stress assessment. In *The Welfare of Pigs*, ed. W. Sybesma. *Curr. Top. vet. Med. Anim. Sci.*, **11**, 112–125. The Hague: Martinus Nijhoff.

Motta, M., Priva, F. and Martini, L. (1970). The hypothalamus as the centre of endocrine feedback mechanisms. In *The Hypothalamus*. p. 463. New York: Academic Press.

Mottershead, B. E. Lynch, J. J. and Alexander, G. (1982). Sheltering behaviour of shorn and unshorn sheep in mixed or separate flocks. *Appl. Anim. Ethol.* **8**, 127–136.

Mount, L. E. (1968). *The Climatic Physiology of the Pig*. London: Edward Arnold. 217pp.

Mount, L. E. (1979). *Adaptation to Thermal Environment*. London: Edward Arnold. 333pp.

Mueller, H. C. and Parker, P. G. (1980). Naive ducklings show different cardiac responses to hawk than to goose models. *Behaviour.* **74**, 101–113.

Müller-Fickenwirth, A. and Fölsch, D. W. (1988). Dustbathing of hens—sequence analysis indicates normal behaviour and welfare. *Proc. Int. Cong. Appl. Ethol. Farm Anim.* ed. J. Unshelm, G. van Putten, K. Zeeb and I. Ekesbo. Darmstadt: K. T. B. L.

Müller-Schwarze, D. (1977). Complex mammalian behaviour and pheromone bioassay in the field. In *Chemical Signals in Vertebrates* ed. D. Muller-Schwarze and M. M. Mozell. New York: Plenum Press.

Murphy, R. M. and Duarte, F. A. M. (1983). Calf control by voice command in a Brazilian dairy. *Appl. Anim. Ethol.*, **11**, 7–18.

Mwanjali, S. Smidt, D. and Ellendorff, F. (1983). A multiple free choice model for pigs. *Appl. Anim. Ethol.* **9**, 263–271.

Naaktgeboren, C. and Slijper, E. J. (1970). *Biologie der Geburt*. Hamburg: Paul Parey.

Newberry, R. C. and Hall, J. W. (1988). Space utilisation by broiler chickens in floor pens. In *Applied Ethology in Farm Animals Skara 1988* ed. J. Unshelm, G. van Putten, K. Zeeb and I. Ekesbo, 305–309. Darmstadt: K. T. B. L.

Nichol, L. (1974). *L'épopée pastorienne et la medicine vétérinaire*. Garches: Nichol.

Nicol, C. J. (1987a). Effect of cage height and area on the behaviour of hens housed in battery cages. *Br. Poult. Sci.*, **28**, 327–335.

Nichol, C. J. (1987b). Behavioural responses of laying hens following a period of spatial restriction. *Anim. Behav.*, **35**, 1709–1719.

Nielsen, B. (1980). Wing bone fractures in laying hens. *Danish vet. J.*, , 981–1016.

Norgaard-Nielsen, G. (1985). Featherpecking and plumage condition in laying hens in an enriched environment in cages and on litter. In *Proc. 2nd Eur. Symp. Poult. Welfare*, ed. R.-M. Wegner 330–332. Celle: World Poultry Science Association.

Nottebohm, F. (1967). The role of sensory feedback in the development of avian vocalisations. *Proc. 14th Ornith. Cong.* Oxford: Blackwell.

Nygaard, A., Austod, D., Lys, A., Kraggerud, H. Standal, N. (1970). Experiments with housing for dry sows. *Agr. Univ. Norway, Dept. Buildg. techn. Rep.*, **56**.

O'Brien, P. H. (1983). Feral goat parturition and laying-out sites: Spatial, physical and meterological characteristics. *Appl. Anim. Ethol.*, **10**, 325–329.

O'Brien, P. H. (1984a). Feral goat home range: Influence of social class and environmental variables. *Appl. Anim. Behav. Sci.* **12**: 373–386.

O'Brien, P. H. (1984b). Leavers and stayers: Maternal postpartum strategies in feral goats. *Appl. Anim. Behav. Sci.*, **12**, 233–243.

O'Brien, P. H. (1988). Feral goat social organisation: a review and comparative analysis. *Appl. Anim. Behav. Sci.*, **21**, 209–221.

Ödberg, F. O. (1978). Abnormal behaviours: stereotypies. *Proc. First Wld. Cong. Ethol. Appl. Zootechnics*, Madrid.

Ödberg, F. O. and Francis-Smith, K. (1976). A study

on eliminative and grazing behaviour—the use of the field by captive horses. *Equine Vet. J.* **8**, 147–149.

Ödberg, F. O. and Francis-Smith, K. (1977). Studies on the formation of ungrazed eliminative areas in fields used by horses. *Appl. Anim. Ethol.* **3**, 27–34.

Oliver, J. E. and Lorenz, M. D. (1983). *Handbook of Veterinary Neurologic Diagnosis*. Philadelphia: Saunders.

Olson, D. P., Papasian, C. J., and Ritter, R. C. (1980). *Canad. J. comp. Med.*, **44**, 19.

Ookawa, T. (1972). Avian wakefulness and sleep on the basis of recent electroencephalographic observations. *Poult. Sci.*, **51**, 1565–1574.

Ooms, L. Degryse, A. and Mostmans, R. (1981). Clinical observations of R51703 in cattle. *Janssen Pharmaceutica*, Beerse Belgium.

Orgeur, P. and Signoret, J. P. (1984). Sexual play and its functional significance in the domestic sheep (*Ovis aries*). *Physiol. Behav.*, **33**, 111–118.

Ortavant, R. and Thibault, C., 1956. Influence de la durée d'éclairement sur les productions spermatiques de belier. *C. R. Séanc. Soc. Biol.*, **2**, 358–361.

Overmier, J. B., Patterson, J. and Wielkiewicz, R. M. (1980). Environmental contingencies as sources of stress in animals. In *Coping and Health*, ed. S. Levine and H. Ursin, 1–38. New York: Plenum Press.

Owen, J. B. and Ridgman, W. J. (1967). The effect of dietary energy content on the voluntary intake of pigs. *Anim. Prod.* **9**, 107–113.

Owens, J. L. Bindon, B. M. Edey, T. N. and Piper, L. R. (1985). Parturient behaviour and calf survival in a herd selected for twinning. *Appl. Anim. Behav. Sci.* **13**, 321–333.

Packer, C. (1977). Reciprocal altruism in *Papio anubis. Nature, Lond.* **265**, 441–3.

Padilla, S. C. (1935). Further studies on the delayed pecking of chicks. *J. comp. Psychol.*, **20**, 413–443.

Pain, B. F. and Broom, D. M. (1978). The effects of injected and surface-spread slurry on the intake and behaviour of dairy cows. *Anim. Prod.* **26**, 75–83.

Pain, B. F., *et al* (1974). Effects of cow slurry on herbage production intake by cattle and grazing behaviour. *J. Br. Grassld. Soc.* **29**, 85–91.

Palmer, A. C. (1976). *Introduction to Animal Neurology*. 2nd edn. Oxford: Blackwell.

Pamment, P. Foenander, F. and McBride, G. (1983). Social and spatial organisation of male behaviour in mated domestic fowl. *Appl. Anim. Ethol.* **9**: 341–349.

Parker, G. A. and Pearson, R. G. (1976). A possible origin and adaptive significance of the mounting behaviour shown by some female mammals in oestrus. *J. nat. Hist.*, **10**, 241–245.

Pasteels, J. L. (1970). Control of prolactin secretion. In *The Hypothalamus*. p. 385. New York: Academic Press.

Patterson, R. L. S. (1968). Identification of 3_a-hydroxy-5_a androst-16-ene as the musk odour component of boar submaxillary salivary gland and its relationship to the sex odour taint in pork meat. *J. Sci. Fd. Agric.* **19**, 43.

Pearson, A. J. and Kilgour, R. (1980). The transport of stock—an assessment of its effects. In: M. Wodzicka-Tomaszewska, T. N. Edey and J. J. Lynch (eds.): *Behaviour in Relation to Reproduction, Management and Health of Farm Animals*. Reviews in Rural Science, No. IV.

Penning, P. D. (1983). A technique to record automatically some aspects of grazing and ruminating behaviour in sheep. *Grass For. Sci.* **38**, 89–96.

Penning, P. D., Steel, G. L. and Johnson, R. H. (1984). Further development and use of an automatic recording system in sheep grazing studies. *Grass For. Sci.*, **39**, 345–351.

Penny, R. H. C., Osborne. A. D., Wright, A. I. and Stephens, T. R. (1965). Foot rot in pigs: observations on the clinical diseases. *Vet. Rec.*, **77**, 1101–1108.

Perkins, N. A. and Westfall, T. C. (1978). The effect of prolactin on dopamine release from rat striatum and medial basal hypothalamus. *Neurosci.* **3**, 59.

Perry, G. C. Patterson, R. L. S. and Stinson, G. C. (1972). Submaxillary salivary gland involvement in procine mating behaviour. *Proc. VII. Int. Cong. Anim. Reprod. Artif. Insem.*, Munich. 395–399.

Perry, G. C. Patterson, R. L. S. Stinson, G. CC. and Macfie, H. J. (1980). Pig courtship behaviour: Phermonal property of androstene steroids in male submaxillary secretion. *Anim. Prod.* **31**, 191–199.

Petherick, J. C. (1982). A note on the space use for excretory behaviour of suckling piglets. *Appl. Anim. Ethol.* **9**, 367–371.

Petherick, J. C. (1983a). A biological basis for the design of space in livestock housing. In *Farm Animal Housing and Welfare* ed. S. H. Baxter, M. R. Baxter and J. A. C.

MacCormack. *Curr. Top. vet. Med. Anim. Sci.,* **24**, 103–120. The Hague: Martinus Nijhoff.

Petherick, J.C. (1983b). A note on nursing termination and resting behaviour of suckling piglets. *Appl. Anim. Ethol.* **9**, 359–365.

Petre-Quadens, O. and Schlag, J.D. (1974). *Basic Sleep Mechanisms*. New York: Academic Press.

Pinel, J.P.J. and Wilkie, D.M. (1983). Conditional defensive burying: a biological and cognitive approach to avoidance learning. In *Animal Cognition and Behaviour*, ed. R.L. Mellgren, 285–318. Amsterdam: North Holland.

Ploog, D. (1970). Social communication among animals. In: *The Neurosciences: Second Study Program*. F.O. Schmitt (ed), pp. 349–361. New York: The Rockefeller University Press.

Poindron, P. and Schmidt, P. (1985). Distance recognition in ewes and lambs kept permanently indoors or at pasture. *Appl. Anim. Behav. Sci.,* **13**, 267–273.

Pollard, J.S., Baldock, M.D. and Lewis, R.F.V. (1971). Learning rates and visual information in five animal species. *Aust. J. Psychol.,* **23**, 29–34.

Pollock, J. (1980). Behavioural ecology and body condition changes in New Forest ponies. *Scientific Publication No. 6*, RSPCA, Horsham, Sussex, UK.

Potter, M.J. and Broom, D.M. (1987). The behaviour and welfare of cows in relation to cubicle house design. In *Cattle Housing Systems, Lameness and Behaviour*, ed. H.K. Wierenga and D.J. Peterse, *Curr. Top. vet. Med. Anim. Sci.,* **40**, 129–147. Dordrecht: Martinus Nijhoff.

Preston, A.P. (1987). Location in the cage and diurnal distribution of feather pecking by caged layers. *Br. Poult. Sci.,* **28**, 653–658.

Price, E.O. (1985). Sexual behaviour of large domestic farm animals: an overview. *J. Anim. Sci.,* **61**, Suppl. 3, 62.

Price, E.O. Dunbar, M. and Dally, M. (1984a). Behaviour of ewes and lambs subjected to restraint fostering. *J. Anim. Sci.* **58**, 1084–1089.

Price, E.O. Dunn, G.C. Talbot, J.A. *et al* (1984b). Fostering lambs by odour transfer: the substitution experiment *J. Anim. Sci.* **59**, 301–307.

Price, E.O. Smith, V.M. and Katz, L.S. (1984c). Sexual stimulation of male dairy goats. *Appl. Anim. Behav. Sci.* **13**, 83.

Price, E.O. Martinez, C.L. and Coe, B.L. (1985). The effects of twinning on mother-offspring behaviour in range beef cattle. *Appl. Anim.*

Behav. Sci. **13**, 309–320.

Price, E.O. and Smith, V.M. (1984). The relationship of male-male mounting to mate choice and sexual performance in male dairy goats. *Appl. Anim. Behav. Sci.,* **13**, 71–82.

Provine, R.R. (1980). Development of between-limb movement synchronisation in the chick embryo. *Develop. Psychobiol.* **13**, 151–163.

Provine, R.R. (1984). Wing-flapping during development and evolution. *Amer. Sci.* **72**, 448–455.

van Putten, G. (1977). Comfort behaviour in pigs and its significance regarding their well being. In *European Association for Animal Production 28th Annual Meeting*.

van Putten, G. (1978). Schweine. In *Nutztierethologie* ed. Sambraus, H.H. Berlin: Paul Parey.

van Putten, G. (1980). Objective observations on the behaviour of fattening pigs. *Anim. Regul. Stud.,* **3**, 105–118.

van Putten, G. (1982). Handling of slaughter pigs prior to loading and during loading on a lorry. In *Transport of Animals Intended for Breeding, Production and Slaughter*, ed. R. Moss. *Curr. Top. vet. Med. Anim. Sci.,* **18**, 15–25. The Hague: Martinus Nijhoff.

van Putten, G. and Dammers, J. (1976). A comparative study of the well-being of piglets reared conventionally and in cages. *Appl. Anim. Ethol.* **2**, 339–356.

van Putten, G. and Elshof, W.J. (1978). Observations on the effect of transport on the well being and lean quality of slaughter pigs. *Anim. Regul. Stud.,* **1**, 247–271.

Rathore, A.K. (1978). Order of cow entry for milk and its relationship with milk yield in dairy cows. *1st Wld Cong. Ethol. Appl. Zootechnics. Madrid, Spain*. 53–57.

Rathore, A.K. (1982). Order of cow entry at milking and its relationship with milk yield and consistency of the order. *Appl. Anim. Ethol.* **8**, 45–52.

Ratner, S.C. and Thompson, R.W. (1960). Immobility functions (fear) of domestic fowl as a function of age and prior experience. *Anim. Behav.,* **8**, 186–191.

Rauch, W. and Wegner, R.-M. (1984). Legehennenhaltung in Volierensystem—Ergebnisse aus sechs Versuchen. *Vortryagstagung Gesellschaft der Forderer und Freunde des Instituts für Kleintierzucht Celle der Bundesforschungsanstallt für Landwirtschaft Braunschweig-Völkenrode*, 22 March 1984.

Reinhardt, V. (1973). Social rank order and milking

order in cows. *Z. Tierpsychol.* **32**, 281–292.

Reinhardt, V. and Reinhardt, A. (1982). Mock fighting in cattle. *Behaviour,* **81**, 1–13.7

Reinhardt, V. and Flood, P.F. (1983). Behavioural assessment in musk-ox calves. *Behaviour,* **87**, 1–21.

Reinhardt, V., Mutiso, F.M. and Reinhardt, A. (1978). Social behaviour and social relationships between female and male prepubertal bovine calves *(Bos indicus). Appl. Anim. Ethol.* **4**, 43–54.

Rheingold, H.L. (1963). *Maternal Behaviour in Mammals.* New York: Wiley.

Richter, J. (1933). Die geburtschilfich-gynäkologische Tierklinik der Universität Leipsig in den Jahren 1927–1931. *Berliner Tierärzt Wochenschr.,* **49**, 517–521.

Rickard, W.H., Uresk, D.W. and Cline, J.F. (1975). Impact of cattle grazing on three perennial grasses in south-cental Washington. *J. Rang. Mgmt.* **28**, 108–112.

Riese, G., Klee, G. and Sambraus, H.H. (1977). Das Verhalten vol Kälbern in verschiedenen Haltungs formen. *Dtsch. Tierärtzl. Wschr.,* **84**, 388–394.

Robinson, D.W. (1975). Food intake regulation in pigs: IV. The influence of dietary threonine imbalance on food intake, dietary choice and plasma acid patterns. *Br. Vet. J.* **131**, 595–600.

van Rooijen, J. (1980). Wahlversuche, eine ethologische Methode zum Sammeln von Messwerten, un Haltungseinflusse zu erfassen und zu beurteilen. *Aktuelle Arbeiten zur artgemässen Tierhaltung, K.T.B.L. – Schrift,* **264**, 165–185.

van Rooijen, J. (1981). Die Anpassungsfahigkeit von Schweinen an einstreulose Buchten. *Aktuelle Arbeiten zur artgemässen Tierhaltung, K.T.B.L. – Schrift,* **281**, 174–185.

van Rooijen, J. (1982). Operant preference test with pigs. *Appl. Anim. Ethol.,* **9**, 83–100.

Rose, R.M., Wodzicka-Tomaszewska, M. and Cumming, R.B. (1985). Agonistic behaviour, responses to a novel object and some aspects of maintenance behaviour in feral-strain and domestic chickens. *Appl. Anim. Behav. Sci.,* **13**, 283–294.

Rosen, J. and Hart, F.M. (1963). Effects of experience on sexual behaviour in male cats. In *Sex and Behaviour* (F.A. Beach, ed.). New York: Wiley.

Ross, P.A. and Hurnik, J.F. (1983). Drinking behaviour of broiler chickens. *Appl. Anim. Ethol.* **11**, 25–31.

Rossdale, P.D. (1968). Perinatal behaviour in the thoroughbred horse. In *Abnormal Behavior in Animals* ed. M.W. Fox, p 563. St. Louis, Missouri Washington University.

Rossdale, P.D. (1970). Perinatal behaviour in the thoroughbred horse. *Br. vet. J.* **126**, 656.

Rossdale, P.D. and Short, R.V. (1967). The time of foaling of thoroughbred mares. *J. Reprod. Fert.* **13**, 341–343.

Rossi, P.J. (1968). Adaption and negative after effect to lateral optical displacement in newly hatched chicks. *Science, N.Y.* **160**, 430–2.

Rottensten, K. and Touchberry, R.W. (1957). Observations on the degree of expression of oestrus in cattle. *J. dairy Sci.* **40**, 1457–1465.

Rowell, C.H.F. (1961). Displacement grooming in the chaffinch. *Anim. Behav.,* **9**, 38–63.

Rozin, P. (1968). Specific aversions and neophobia as a consequence of vitamin deficiency and/or poisoning in half-wild and domestic rats. *J. comp. Physiol. Psychol.* **66**, 82.

Rozin, P. (1976). The selection of foods by rats, humans and other animals. *Adv Study Behav.* **6**, 21–76.

Ruckebusch, Y. (1972a). Development of sleep and wakefulness in the foetal lamb. *Electroenceph. Clin. Neurophysiol.* **32**, 119–128.

Ruckebusch, Y. (1972b). The relevance of drowsiness in farm animals. *Anim. Behav.* **20**, 637–643.

Ruckebusch, Y. (1974). Sleep deprivation in cattle. *Brain Res.* **78**, 495–499.

Ruckebusch, Y. and Bell, F.R. (1970). Étude electropolygraphique et comportementale des états de veille et de sommeil chez la vache. *(Bos taurus). Ann. Rech. vét.* **1**, 41–62.

Ruckebusch, Y. and Bueno, L. (1978). An analysis of ingestive behaviour and activity of cattle under field conditions. *Appl. Anim. Ethol.* **4**, 301–313. 77

Ruckebusch, Y. Dougherty, R.W. and Cook, H.M. (1974). Jaw movements and rumen motility as criteria for measurement of deep sleep in cattle. *Amer. J. vet. Res.* **35**, (10) 1309–1312.

Rushen, J. (1983). The development of sexual relationships in the domestic chicken. *Appl. Anim. Ethol.* **11**, 55–66.

Rushen, J. (1984a). How peck orders of chickens are measured: a critical review. *Appl. Anim. Ethol.,* **11**, 255–264.

Rushen, J. (1984b). Stereotyped behaviour, adjunctive drinking and the feeding periods of tethered sows. *Anim. Behav.,* **32**, 1059–1067.

Rushen, J. (1986). Aversion of sheep for handling

treatments: paired choice experiments. *Appl. Anim. Behav. Sci.,* 16, 363–370.

Russel, E.M. and Pearce, G.A. (1971). Exploration of novel objects by marsupials. *Behaviour* 40, 312–22.

Sachs, D.B. and Harris, V.S. (1978). Sex differences and development changes in selected juvenile activities (play) of domestic lambs. *Anim. Behav.* 26, 678–684.

Sainsbury, D.W.B. (1974). *Proceedings 1st International Liverstock—Environment Symposium*, 4, St.Joseph Missouri: American Society of Agricultural Engineers.

Sainsbury, D. (1980). *Poultry Health and Management.* London: Granada.

Sainsbury, D. (1981). The covered straw yard. In *Alternatives to Intensive Husbandry Systems*, 37–40. Potters Bar: Universities Federation for Animal Welfare.

Sainsbury, D.W.B. (1984). Animal welfare, husbandry and disease, with particular reference to the galliform species. In *Priorities in Animal Welfare.* ed. L. Bagnall, 43–56. London: British Veterinary Association Animal Welfare Foundation.

Sainsbury, D.W.B. (1986). *Farm Animal Welfare.* London: Collins.

Sainsbury, D.W.B. and Sainsbury, P. (1988). *Livestock Health and Housing.* London: Bailliere Tindall.

Salter, R.E. and Hudson, R.J. (1982). Social organisation of feral horses in Western Canada. *Appl. Anim. Ethol.* 8, 207–223.

Salzinger, K. and Waller, M.B. (1962). The operant control of vocalisation in the dog. *J. exp. Animal. Behav.,* 5, 383–389.

Sambraus, H.H. (1971). Zum-Mutter—Kind—Verhalten der Wiederkauer., *Berl. Münch. Tierärztl. Wochenschr.* 84, 24–27.

Sambraus, H.H. (1976). Kronismus bein Schweinen. *Dtsch. tierärzlt. Wschr.* 83, 17–19.

Sambraus, H.H. (1979). A review of historically significant publications from German speaking countries concerning the behaviour of domestic farm animals. *Appl. Anim. Ethol.* 5, 5–13.

Sambraus, H.H. (1985). Abnormal behaviour as an indication of immaterial suffering. *Int. J. Stud. Anim. Prob.,* 2, 245–248.

Sambraus, H.H. (1985). Mouth-based anomalous syndromes, In: *Ethology of Farm Animals, World Animal Science, A5*, ed. A.F. Fraser, 381–411. Amsterdam: Elsevier.

Sanford, J., Ewbank, R., Maloney, V., Tavernor, W.D. and Uvarov, O. (1986). Guidelines for the recognition and assessment of pain in animals. *Vet. Rec.,* 118, 334–338.

Satinoff, E. and Teitelbaum, P. (1983). *Handbook of Behavioural Neurobiology*, Vol. 6, Motivation. New York: Plenum Press.

Sato, S. (1982). Leadership during actual grazing in a small herd of cattle. *Appl. Anim. Ethol.* 8, 53–65.

Sato, S. (1984). Social licking pattern and its relationships to social dominance and live weight gain in weaned calves. *Appl. Anim. Behav. Sci.* 12, 25–32.

Savory, C.J. (1980). Diurnal feeding patterns in domestic fowls: a review. *Appl. Anim. Ethol.* 6, 71–82.

Savory, C.J., Gentle, M.J., Hodgkiss, J.P. and Kueznel, W. (1982). Voluntary regulation of food intake of poultry. *App. Anim. Ethol.* 6, 71–82.

Schafer, M. (1975). In *The Language of the Horse.* pp. 142–158. Transl. by D.M. Goodall, New York: Arco. Publ. Co.

Schake, L.M., Dietrich, R.A., Thomas, M.L., Vermedahl, L.D. and Bliss, R.L. (1979). Performance of feedlot steers reimplanted with DES or Synovex-S. *J. Anim. Sci.,* 49, 324–329.

Schaller, G.B. (1963). *The Mountain Gorilla: Ecology and Behavior.* Chicago: University of Chicago Press.

Schein, M.W. (1963). On the irreversibility of imprinting. *Z. Tierpsychol.* 20, 462–7.

Schein, M.W. and Fohrman, M.H. (1955). Social dominance relationships in a herd of dairy cattle. *Br. J. Anim. Behav.* 3, 45–55.

Schein, M.W. and Hale, E.B. (1965). Stimuli eliciting sexual behaviour. In *Sex and Behavior* ed. F.A. Beach 440–482. New York: Wiley.

Schenk, P.M., Meysser, F.M. and Limpens, H.J.G.A.M. (1984). Gakeln als Indicator für Frustration beim Legehennen. In *K.T.B.L. Schrift*, 299. Darmstadt: K.T.B.L.

Scheurmann, E. (1974). Ursachen und Verhutung des gegenseitigen Besaugens bei Kälbern. *Tierarztl. Prax.,* 2, 389–394.

Schjelderup-Ebbe, T. (1922). Beiträge zur Sozialpsychologie des Haushuhns. *Z. Psychol.,* 88, 225–252.

Schleidt, W.M. (1961). Reaktionen von Truthuhnern auf fliegende Raubvögel und Versuche zur Analyse ihrer AAM's *Z. Tiersychol.* 18, 534–60.

Schleidt, W.M. (1970). Precocial sexual strutting behaviour in turkeys (*Meleagris gallopavo* L.) *Anim. Behav.* 18, 760–761.

Schlichting, M.C. and Smidt, D. (1987). (Eds). *Welfare Aspects of Housing Systems for Veal Calves and Fattening Bulls.* Luxembourg: Commission of the European Communities, EUR 10777 EN.

Schloeth, R. (1961). Das Socialleben des Camargues-Rindes. *Z. Tierpsychol.* 18, 574–627.

Schmidt, M. (1982). Abnormal oral behaviour in pigs. *Disturbed Behaviour in Farm Animals* ed. W. Bessei, *Hohenheimer Arbeiten,* 121, 115–132. Stuttgart: Eugen Ulmer.

Schmidtmann, E.T. and Valla, M.E. (1982). Face-fly pest intensity, fly-avoidance behaviour (bunching) and grazing time in Holstein heifers. *Appl. Anim. Ethol.* 8, 429–438.

Schneider, K.M. (1930). Das Flehmen. *Zool. Gart. Lpz.* 4, 183–198.

Schneirla, T.C. (1965). Approach/withdrawal and behaviour. In *Advances in the Study of Behaviour,* D.S. Lenrman, R.A. Hinde and E. Shaw (eds) 1, 1–74. New York: Academic Press.

Schoen, A.M.S. Banks, E.M. and Curtis, S.E. (1976). Behaviour of young Shetland and Welsh ponies (Equus caballus). *Biol of Behav.* 1, 192–216.

Schouten, W.G.P. (1986). *Rearing conditions and behaviour in pigs.* Ph.D. thesis, University of Wageningen.

Schutz, F. (1965). Sexuelle Prägung bei Anatiden. *Z. Tierpsychol.* 22, 50–103.

Scoglund, W.C. and Palmer, D.H. (1961). Light intensity studies with broilers. *Poult. Sci.,* 40, 1458–1460.

Scott, J.P. and Fuller, J.L. (1965). *Dog behavior: the genetic basis.* Chicago: University of Chicago Press.

Seabrook, M.F. (1977). Cowmanship. *Fmrs' Wkly Extra,* Dec. 23, 26pp.

Seabrook, M.F. (1984). The psychological interaction between the stockman and his animals and its influence on performance of pigs and dairy cows. *Vet. Rec.* 115, 84–87.

Seabrook, M.F. (1987). The role of the stockman in livestock productivity and management. In *The role of the stockman in livestock production and management.* ed. M. Seabrook, 39–51. Brussels: Commission of the European Communities, Report EUR 10982 EN.

Sedgwick, C.J. (1979). Field anaesthesia in stressed animals. *Mod. Vet. Practice.* July, 531–537.

Selman, I.E. McEwan, A.D. and Fisher, E.W. (1970a). Studies on natural suckling in cattle during the first eight hours post partum. I.

Behavioural studies (Dams). *Anim. Behav.* 18, 276–283.

Selman, I.E. McEwan, A.D. and Fisher, E.W. (1970b). Studies on natural suckling in cattle during the first eight hours post partum. II. Behavioural studies (Calves). *Anim. Behav.* 18, 284–289.

Selman, I.E. McEwan, A.D. and Fisher, E.W. (1971). Studies on dairy calves allowed to suckle their dams at fixed times post-partum. *Res. vet. Sci.,* 12, 1.

Sharman, D.F. and Stephens, D.B. (1974). The effect of apomorphine on the behaviour of farm animals. *J. Physiol.,* 242, 259.

Shelley, L. (1970). Interrelationships between the duration of parturition postnatal behaviour of ewes and lambs, and the incidence of neonatal mortality. *Proc. Aust. Soc. Anim. Prod.,* 8, 348–352.

Sherwin, C.M. and Johnson, K.G. (1987). The influence of social factors on the use of shade by sheep. *Appl. Anim. Behav. Sci.* 18, 143–155.

Shettleworth, S.J. (1972). Constraints on learning. *Adv. Study Behav.,* 4, 1–68.

Shillito, E. (1975). A comparison of the role of vision and hearing in lambs finding their own dams. *Appl. Anim. Ethol.* 1, 369–377.

Shillito-Walser, E. (1980). Maternal recognition and breed identity in lambs living in a mixed flock of Jacob, Clun Forest and Dalesbred sheep. *Appl. Anim. Ethol.* 6, 221–231.

Shillito-Walser, E. (1985a). Neonatal sensory development and exploratory behaviour. In *Ethology of Farm Animals, World Animal Science,* Vol A5, 121–125. Amsterdam: Elsevier.

Shillito-Walser, E. (1985b). Neonatal nursing progress. In: *Ethology of Farm Animals, World Animal Science* A5, ed. A.F. Fraser, 143–148. Amsterdam: Elsevier.

Shillito-Walser, E. Walters, E. and Hague, P. (1981a). Vocal recognition of recorded lambs voices by ewes of three breeds of sheep. *Behav.* 78, 260–272.

Shillito-Walser, E. Willadsen, S. and Hague, P. (1981b). Pair association between lambs of different breeds born to Jacob and Dalsbred ewes after embryo transplantation. *Appl. Anim. Ethol.* 7, 351–358.

Shillito-Walser, E. Hague, P. and Yeomans, M. (1983). Variations in the strength of maternal behaviour and its conflict with flocking behaviour in Dalesbred, Jacob and Soay ewes. *Appl. Anim. Ethol.* 10, 245–250.

Shimizu, M. Shimizu, Y. and Kodama, Y. (1978).

Infections and Immunology, **21**, 747.

Shorten, M. (1954). The reaction of the brown rat towards changes in its environment. In *Control of Rats and Mice,* Vol. 2. Rats (D. Chitty, ed.) Oxford: Oxford University Press

Shreffler, C. and Hohenboken, W. (1980). Circadian behaviour, including thermoregulatory activities, in feedlot lambs. *Appl. Anim. Ethol.* **6**, 241–246.

Sibly, R. (1975). How incentive and deficit determines feeding tendency. *Anim. Behav.* **23**, 437–46.

Sibly, R. and McCleery, R. H. (1976). The dominance boundary method of determining motivational state, *Anim. Behav.* **24**, 108–24.

Shutt, D. A., Fell, L. R., Cornell, R., Bell, A. K., Wallace, C. A. and Smith, A. I. (1987). Stress-induced changes in plasma concentrations of immunoreactive β endorphin and cortisol in response to routine surgical procedures in lambs. *Aust. J. biol. Sci.,* **40**, 97–103.

Sibly, R. and McFarland, D. (1976). On the fitness of behaviour sequences. *Am. Nat.* **110**, 601–17.

Siegel, H. S. (1985). *World Poultry Science Journal,* **41**, 36–43.

Siegel, H. S. (1987). Effects of behavioural and physical stressors on immune responses. In: *Biology of Stress in Farm Animals* ed. P. R. Wiepkema and P. W. M. van Adrichem, *Curr. Top. vet. Med. Anim. Sci.,* **42**, 39–54. Dordrecht: Martinus Nijhoff.

Signoret, J. P. (1970). Reproductive behaviour in pigs. *J. Reprod. Fert. Suppl.* **11**, 105.

Signoret, J. P. (1975). Influence of the sexual receptivity of a teaser ewe on the mating preference in the ram. *Appl. Anim. Ethol.* **1**, 229–232.

Signoret, J. P., Baldwin, B. A., Fraser, D. and Hafex, E. S. E. (1975). The behaviour of swine. In *The Behaviour of Domestic Animals.* 3rd, ed., p. 41. London: Balliere Tindall.

Signoret, J. P. Fulkerson, W. J. and Lindsay, D. R. (1982). Effectiveness of testosterone-treated wethers and ewes as teasers. *Appl. Anim. Ethol.* **9**, 37–45.

Silver, G. V. and Price, E. O. (1986). Effects of individual vs. group-rearing on the sexual behaviour of pre-puberal beef bulls: mount orientation and sexual responsiveness. *Appl. Anim. Behav. Sci.,* **15**, 287–

Simonsen, H. B. (1983). Ingestive behaviour and wing-flapping in assessing welfare of laying hens. In *Indicators Relevant to Farm Animal Welfare,* ed. D. Smidt, *Curr. Top. vet. Med. Anim. Sci.,* **23**, 89–95. The Hague: Martinus Nijhoff.

Simonsen, H. B., Vestergaard, K. and Willeby, P. (1980). Effect of floor type and density on the integument of egg layers. *Poult. Sci.,* **59**, 2202–2206.

Slater, P. J. B. (1975). Temporal patterning and the causation of bird behaviour. In *Neural and Endocrine Aspects of Behaviour in Birds* ed. P. Wright, P. C. Caryl and D. M. Vowles. Amsterdam: Elsevier.

Sly, J. and Bell, F. R. (1979). Experimental analysis of the seeking behaviour observed in ruminants when they are sodium deficient. *Physiol. Behav.* **22**, 499–

Smidt, D. ed. (1983). *Indicators Relevant to Farm Animal Welfare.* Curr. Top. vet. Med. Anim. Sci., **23**. The Hague: Martinus Nijhoff.

Smith, F. V. (1962). Perceptual aspects of imprinting. *Symp. zool. Soc. Lond.* **8**, 171–91.

Smith, W. J. and Robertson, A. M. (1971). Observations on injuries to sows confined in part slatted stalls. *Vet. Rec.,* **89**, 531–533.

Sokolov, E. N. (1960). Neuronal models and the orienting reflex. In *The Central Nervous System and Behaviour,* ed. M. A. Brazier. New York: Macy Foundation.

Sommer, B. (1979). Zuchtsauen in Kastenstand – und in Gruppenhaltung – Rauschverhalten, Gerburten, Fruchbarkeit und Schaden am Bewegungsapparat. Inaugural dissertation Ludwig-Maximilians Universität, München, pp 1–203.

Sommer, B., Sambraus, H. H., Osterkorn, K. and Krausslich, H. (1982). Heat behaviour, birth reproduction performance and reasons for losses of sows in cage and group housing. *Zuchtungskunde,* **54**, 138–154.

Squires, V. R. and Daws, G. T. (1975). Leadership and dominance relationships in Merino and Border Leicester sheep. *Appl. Anim. Ethol.* **1**, 263–274.

Squires, V. R. Wilson. A. D. and Daws, G. T. (1972). Comparison of walking behaviour of some Australian sheep. *Proc. of Aust. Soc. Anim. Prod.* **9**, 376–380.

Stafford-Smith, D. M. Noble, I. R. and Jones, G. K. (1985). A heat balance model for sheep and its use to predict shade-seeking behaviour in hot conditions. *J. appl. Ecol.* **22**, 753–774.

Stark, L. (1968). *Neurological Control Systems* New York: Plenum Press. pp. 428.

Stephens, D. B. (1974). Studies on the effect of social environment on the behaviour and growth rates of artifically-reared British Friesian male calves. *Anim. Prod.* **18**, 23–24.

Stephens, D. B. and Toner, J. N. (1975). Husbandry influences on some physiological parameters of emotional responses in calves. *Appl. Anim. Ethol.*, **1**, 233–243.

Stevens, D. Alexander, G. and Lynch, J. J. (1981). Do Merino ewes seek isolation or shelter at lambing? *Appl. Anim. Ethol.* **7**, 149–155.

Stevens, D., Alexander, G. and Lynch, J. J. (1982). Lamb mortality due to inadequate care of twins by Merino ewes. *Appl. Anim. Ethol.*, **8**, 243–252.

Stobbs, T. H. (1973). The effect of plant structure on the intake of tropical pastures. I. Variation in the bite size of grazing cattle. *Aust. J. agric. Res.* **24**, 809–19.

Stobbs, T. H. (1974). Components of grazing behaviour of dairy cows on some tropical and temperate pastures. *Proc. Aust. Soc. Anim. Prod.* **10**, 299–301.

Stolba, A. (1982). A family system of pig housing. *Proc. Symp. Alternatives to Intensive Husbandry Systems.* Potters Bar: Universities Federation for Animal Welfare.

Stolba, A., Baker, N. and Wood-Gush, D. G. M. (1983). The characterisation of stereotyped behaviour in stalled sows by informational redundancy. *Behaviour,* **87**, 157–182.

Stone, C. C., Brown, M. S. and Waring, G. H. (1974). An ethological means to improve swine production. *J. Anim. Sci.* **39**, 137.

Stricklin, W. R. (1976). Spatial and temporal dimensions of bovine behaviour and social organisation. *Dissertation Abstracts International,* B **36**, (7), 31–39.

Stricklin, W. R. (1978). Knowledge of animal behaviour can reduce livestock handling and management problems. *Proc. 62nd Ann. Mtg. Livestock Conservation Inst.* 83–86. Oak Brook, Illinois.

Stricklin, W. R. and Gonyou, H. W. (1981). Dominance and eating behaviour of beef cattle fed from a single stall. *Appl. Anim. Ethol.* **7**, 135–140.

Stricklin, W. R. Wilson, L. L. and Graves, H. B. (1976). Feeding behaviour of Angus and Charolais-Angus cows during summer and winter. *J. Anim. Sci.* **43**, (3), 721–732.

Stricklin, W. R. Graves, H. B. and Wilson, L. L. (1979). Some theoretical and observed relationships of fixed and portable spacing behaviour of animals. *Appl. Anim. Ethol.,* **5**, 201–214.

Stricklin, W. R. and Kautz-Scanavy, C. C. (1984). The role of behaviour in cattle production: a review of research. *Appl. Anim. Ethol.,* **11**, 359–390.

Stokols, D. (1972). On the distinction between density and crowding: some implications for future research. *Psychol Rev.,* **79**, 275–7.

Susmel, P. (1987). The veal production in the EEC countries. In *Welfare Aspects of Housing Systems for Veal Calves and Fattening Bulls,* ed. M. C. Schlichting and D. Smidt, 5–7. Luxembourg: Commission of the European Communities, EUR 10777. EN.

Sybesma, W., Westerink, N. G., Cortiaesen, G. P. and van Logestijn, J. G. (1978). Kongressdokumentation I. **24**, 1–7. Europäischer Fleischforscherkongress. Kulmbach.

Syme, G. J. (1974). Competitive orders as measures of social dominance. *Anim. Behav.* **22**, 931.

Syme, G. J. and Syme, L. A. (1979). *Social structure in farm animals.* Elsevier: Amsterdam.

Syme, L. A. and Elphick, G. R. (1982). Heart-rate and the behaviour of sheep in yards. *Appl. Anim. Ethol.,* **9**, 31–35.

Syme, L. A., Syme, G. J., Waite, T. G. and Pearson, A. J. (1975). Spatial distribution and social status in a small herd of dairy cows. *Anim. Behav.* **23**, 609–614.

Tallarico, R. B. (1961). Studies of visual depth perception: choice behaviour of newly hatched chicks on a visual cliff. *Percept. Mot. Skills* **12**, 259–62.

Tarrant, P. V. (1981). The occurrence, causes and economic consequences of dark-cutting in beef – a survey of current information. In: D. E. Hood and P. V. Tarrant (eds.) *The Problem of Dark-Cutting in Beef.* Martinus Nijhoff.

Tauson, R. (1977). The influence of different technical environment on the performance of laying hens. *Report 49, Department of Animal Husbandry.* Uppsala: Swedish Agricultural University.

Tauson, R. (1978). Reactions of laying hens to different technical environments (I–III). *Report 64, Department of Animal Husbandry.* Uppsala: Swedish Agricultural University.

Tauson, R. (1980). Cages: could they be improved? In *The Laying Hen and its Environment,* ed. R. Moss, *Curr. Top. vet. Med. Anim. Sci.,* **8**, 269–299. The Hague: Martinus Nijhoff.

Tauson, R. (1984a). Plumage conditions in SCWL laying hens kept in conventional cages of different designs. *Acta Agric. Scand.,* **34**, 221–230.

Tauson, R. (1984b). Effects of a perch in conventional cages for laying hens. *Acta Agric. Scand.,* **34**, 193–209.

Tauson, R. (1985). Mortality in laying hens caused by

differences in cage design. *Acta Agric. Scand.*, **34**, 193–209.

Tauson, R. (1986). Avoiding excessive growth of claws in caged laying hens. *Acta Agric. Scand.*, **35**, 165–174.

Tauson, R. (1988). Effects of redesign. In *Cages for the Future*, Proceedings of Cambridge Poultry Conference, 42–69. London: A.D.A.S.

Tauson, R., and Svensson, S.A. (1980). Influence of plumage condition on the hen's feed requirement. *Swedish J. agric. Res*, **10**, 35–39.

Tannenbaum, J. (1989). *Veterinary Ethics*. Baltimore: Williams and Wilkins.

Taylor, I.A. Widowski, T.M. and Cortis, S.E. (1986). Sows use toys with increasing intensity as farrowing approaches. *J. Anim. Sci.*, **61**, Suppl, 83–84.

Tennessen, T. (1983). An ethological investigation into the husbandry of bulls. Ph.D. Thesis, University of Alberta, Canada.

Tennessen, T. Price, M.A. and Berg, R.T. (1985). The social interactions of young bulls and steers after re-grouping. *Appl. Anim. Behav. Sci.* **14**, 37–48.

Teutsch, G.M. (1978). Soziologie und Ethik der Lebewesen. Eine materialsamlung. *Europaische Hochschulschriften*, **23/54**, 2 Aufl. Frankfurt.

Teutsch, G.M. (1987). Intensive farm animal management seen from an ethical standpoint. *In Ethical, Ethological and Legal Aspects of Intensive Farm Animal Management*. ed. E. von Loeper, G. Martin, J. Müller et al. *Tierhaltung*, **18**, 9–40. Basel: Birkhäuser.

Thomas, C. and Signoret, J.P. (1989). Apprentissage de l'utilisation d'un systeme de libre-service alimentaire par un groupe de truies gestantes: roles des facteurs individuels et sociaux. *Journées Rech. France*, **21**, 297–300.

Thompson, D.L., Elgert, K.D., Gross and Siegel, P.B. (1980). Cell mediated immunity in Mareks disease virus-infected chickens genetically selected for high and low concentrations of plasma corticosterone. *Amer. J. Vet. Res.*, **41**, 91–96.

Thompson, W. (1984). Kliba-Voletage, das neueste Modelle einer Voliere für Legetiere. *Schweiz. Geflügl-Zeitung*, **20**, 11 October 1984.

Thorpe, W.H. (1958). The learning of song patterns by birds, with especial reference to the song of the chaffinch. *Fringilla coelebs. Ibis.* **100**, 535–70.

Tilbrook, A.J. (1987). Physical and behavioural factors affecting sexual ''attractiveness'' of the ewe. *Appl. Anim. Behav. Sci.* **17**, 109–115.

Tillon, J.P. and Madec, F. (1984). Diseases affecting confined sows. Data from epidemiological observations. *Ann. Rech. vét.*, **15**, 195–199.

Tinbergen, N. (1940). Die Übersprungsbewegung. *Z. Tierpsychol*, **4**, 1–10.

Toates, F. (1982). Exploration as a motivational and learning system: A (tentative) cognitive-incentive model. In *Exploration in Animals and Humans*, ed. J. Archer and L. Birke London: Van Nostrand Reinhold.

Toates, F. (1986). *Motivational Systems*. Cambridge: Cambridge University Press.

Toates, F. (1987). The relevance of models of motivation and learning to animal welfare. In *Biology of Stress in Farm Animals: an Integrative Approach*, ed. P.R. Wiepkema and P.W.M. van Adrichem. *Curr. Top. vet. Med. Anim. Sci.* **42**, 153–186. Dordrecht: Martinus Nijhoff.

Tolman, C.W. and Wilson, G.F. (1965). Social feeding in domestic chicks. *Anim. Behav.* **13**, 134–142.

Tomlinson, K.A. Price, E.O. and Torell, D.T. (1982). Responses of tranquilised post-partum ewes to alien lambs. *Appl. Anim. Ethol.*, **8**, 109–117.

Tribe, D. (1950). The composition of a sheep's natural diet. *J. Br. Grassl. Soc.* **5**, 81.

Trunkfield, H.R. and Broom, D.M. (in press). The welfare of calves during handling and transport. *Appl. Anim. Behav. Sci.*

Tsuyoshi, I. Akemi, M. Nasoshige, A. Hirotoshi, T. Masahiro, O. and Kayoko, K. (1981). Grazing behaviour of dairy beef steers, IV. Fights and social order. *Jap. J. Livestock Mgmt.* **16** (3), 1–13.

Tucker, J.E. Walker, P.M. and Winter, J.R. (1985). Relationship between cow feeding time and time of parturition. *J. Anim. Sci.*, **61**, Suppl. 1, 83–84.

Tyler, S.J. (1972). The behaviour and social organisation of the New Forest ponies. *Anim. Behav. Monog.*, Part 5, 87–196.

Vandenbergh, J.C. (ed.) (1983). *Pheromones and Reproduction in Mammals*. London: Academic Press, 298pp.

Vannier, P., Tillon, J.P., Madec, F. and Morisse, J.P. (1983). *Ann. Rech. vet.*, **14**, 450–455.

Veissier, I., Le Neindre, P. and Trillat, G. (1989). The use of circadian behaviour to measure adaptation of calves to changes in their environment. *Appl. Anim. Behav. Sci.*, **22**, 1–12.

Vermeer, H.M. Wierenga, H.K. Metz, J.H.M. Mekking, P. and Smits, A.C. (1988). De invloed van een waterspeen ophet preputium suigen bij vleeskalveren. *Rapport* B-323, ppl-45.

Zeist: Instituut voor Veeteelkundig Onderzoek "Schoonoord".

Vestergaard, K. (1980). The regulation of dustbathing and other behaviour patterns in the laying hen: a Lorenzian approach. In *The Laying Hen and its Environment*, ed. R. Moss, *Curr. Top. vet. Med. Anim. Sci.*, **8**, 101–113. The Hague: Martinus Nijhoff.

Vestergaard, K. (1982). Dust-bathing in the domestic fowl—diurnal rhythm and dust deprivation. *Appl. Anim. Ethol.*, **8**, 487–495.

Vestergaard, K. (1989). Environmental influences on the development of behaviour and their relation to welfare. In *Proc. 3rd Env. Symp. Poult. Welfare*, ed J.M. Faure and A.D. Mills. Tours: World Poultry Science Association.

Vestergaard, K., Hansen, L.L. (1984). Tethered versus loose sows: ethological observations and measures of productivity. *Ann. Rech. vét.*, **15**, 245–256.

Vince, M.A. (1964). Social facilitation of hatching in the bobwhite quail. *Anim. Behav.* **12**, 531–534.

Vince, M.A. (1966). Artificial acceleration of hatching in quail embryos. *Anim. Behav.*, **14**, 389–394.

Vince, M.A. (1973). Effects of external stimulation on the onset of lung ventilation and the time of hatching in the fowl, duck and goose. *Br. Poult. Sci.* **14**, 389–401.

Vince, M.A. (1983). Sensory factors involved in the newly born lamb's initial search for the teat. *J. Physiol.*, 343:2.

Vince, M.A. (1984). Teat-seeking or pre-sucking behaviour in newly born lambs: Possible effects of maternal skin temperature. *Anim. Behav.* **32**, 249–254.

Vince, M.A. and Armitage, S. (1980). Sound stimulation available to the sheep foetus. *Reprod. Nutr. Develop.* **20**, (38): 801–806.

Vince, M.A. Armitage, S.E. Baldwin, B.A. Toner, J. and Moore, B.C.J. (1982). The sound environment of the foetal sheep. *Behav.* **81**, 296–315.

Vincent, J.F.V. (1982). The mechanical design of grass. *J. Materials Sci.* **17**, 856–860.

Vincent, J.F.V. (1983). The influence of water content on the stiffness and fracture properties of grass leaves. *Grass For. Sci.* **38**, 107–114.

Wagnon, K.A. (1963). Behaviour of beef cows on a Californian range. *Calif. Agric. Exp. Stn. Bull.*, **799**, 58pp.

Wagnon, K.A. (1965). Social dominance in range cows and its effects on supplemental feeding. *Calif. Agric. exp. Station Bull.*, **819**, pp 31.

Wagnon, K.A. Guilbert, H.R. and Hart, G.H. (1959). Beef cattle investigation on the San Joaquin Exp. Range. *Calif. Agric. exp. Stn. Bull.*, **765**, 71pp.

Wagnon, K.A., Loy, R.G., Rollins, W.C. and Carroll, F.D. (1966). Social dominance in a herd of Angus, Hereford and Shorthorn cows. *Anim. Behav.* **14**, 474–479.

Wald, G. (1958). *Introduction to the Fitness of the Environment*, Boston: Beacon Press.

Wallace, L.R. (1949). Observations of lambing behaviour in ewes. *Proceedings of the New Zealand Society of Animal Production* **9**, 85–96.

Walther, F.R. (1977). Sex and activity dependence of distances between Thomson's gazelles (*Gasella thomsoni* Gunther 1884). *Anim. Behav.* **25**, 713–19.

Waring, G.H. (1983). Horse Behavior. New Jersey: Noyes Publications, 292pp.

Waring, G.H. Wierzbowski, S. and Hafez, E.S.E. (1975). The behaviour of horses. In *The Behaviour of Domestic Animals*, 3rd edn., ed. E.S.E. Hafez, pp 330–369. London: Ballière Tindall.

Waterhouse, A. (1978). The effects of pen conditions on the development of calf behaviour. *Appl. Anim. Ethol.* **4**, 285–286.

Waterhouse, A. (1979). The effects of rearing conditions on the behaviour and growth of dairy calves. Ph.D. thesis, University of Reading.

Wathes, D.C.M. (1976). The efforts of feathering on the heat loss of a laying fowl. *Glead thorpe Experimental Husbandry Farm Booklet. No. 2224*. London: Ministry of Agriculture Fisheries and Food.

Watkin, B.R. and Clements, R.J. (1978). The effect of grazing animals on pastures. In *Plant Relations in Pastures* ed. J.R. Wilson. Melbourne: CSIRO.

Webb, W.B. (1969). Partial and differential sleep deprivation. In A. Kales (ed.). Sleep: Physiology and Pathology. Lippincot, Philadelphia, Pa., pp. 221–231.

Webster, A.J.F. (1988). The welfare requirements of sick farm animals. In *Animal Disease—a Welfare Problem*, ed. T.E. Gibson, 56–61. London: British Veterinary Association Animal Welfare Foundation.

Webster, A.J.F. Smith, J.S. and Brockway, J.M. (1972). Effects of isolation, confinement and competition for feed on energy exchanges of growing lambs. *Anim. Prod.* 15, 189–201.

Webster, A. J. F., Saville, C., Church, B. M., Gnanastakthy, A. and Moss R. (1985a). The effect of different rearing conditions on the development of calf behaviour. *Br. vet. J.,* 141, 249–264.

Webster, A. J. F., Saville, C., Church, B. M., Gnanasakthy, A. and Moss, R. (1985b). Some effects of different rearing systems on health, cleanliness and injury in calves. *Br. vet. J.,* 141, 472–483.

Webster, J., Saville, C. and Welchman, D. (1986). *Improved Husbandry Systems for Veal Calves.* London: Farm Animal Care Trust, p 26.

Wegner, R-M. (1980). Measurement of essential and behavioural needs as provided by present husbandry systems: battery, 'get-away' cage, aviary. In *The Laying Hen and its Environment,* ed. R. Moss, *Curr. Top. vet. Med. Anim. Sci.,* 8, 195–202. The Hague: Martinus Nijhoff.

Wegner, R-M. Rauch, H-W. and Torges, H-G. (1981). Vergleichende Versuche mit Legehennen in Bodenhaltung mit und ohne Auslauf und in Käfigen: Planung, Ablauf und leistungsbezogene Ergebnisse. *Landbauforchung Völkenrode,* 60, 23–38.

Weiss, J. M. (1971). Effects of coping behaviour in different warning signal conditions on stress pathology in rats. *J. comp. physiol. Psychol,* 77, 1–13.

Welch, R. A. S. and Kilgour, R. (1970). Mismothering among Romneys. *N. Z. J. Agric.,* 121, 26–27.

Wells, G. A. H. (1984). Locomotor disorders of the pig. *Vet. Rec.,* 114, 43–53.

Welsh, D. A. (1975). Population, behavioural and grazing ecology of the horses of Sable Island, Nova Scotia, D. Phil. thesis, Dalhousie University, Nova Scotia.

Wemelsfelder, F. and van Putten, G. (1985). Behaviour as a possible indicator for pain in piglets. *I. V. O. Report B-260.* Zeist: Institut voor Veeteelkundig Onderzoek.

Wennrich, G. (1975a). Untersuchungen über die Bewegungsaktivität von Haushennen. *Arch Geflügelkd,* 39, 113–121.

Wennrich, G. (1975b). Studium zum Verhalten verschiedener Hybrid-Herkunfte von Haushuhnern (*Gallus domesticus*) in Bodenintensivhaltung mit besonderer Berucksichtigung aggressiven Verhaltens sowie des Federpickens und des kannibalismus. 5. Mitteilung: Verhaltensweisen des Federpickens, *Arch. f. Geflügelkd.,* 39, 37–43.

Wennrich, G. (1977). Zum Nachweis eines "Trieb staus" bei Haushennen. In *K. T. B. L. Schrift,* 223, Darmstadt: K. T. B. L.

Wentink, G. (1978). Biokinetical analysis of the movements of the pelvic limb of the horse and the role of the muscles in the walk and the trot. *Anat. Embryol.* 152, 261–272.

Westoby, M. (1974). An analysis of diet selection by large generalist herbivores. *Am. Nat.* 108, 290–304.

Westly, H. J. and Kelley, K. W. (1984). *Proc. Soc. exp. Biol. Med.,* 117, 156–164.

Whatson, T. S. (1978). The development of dunging preference in piglets. *Appl. Anim. Ethol.* 4, 293.

Whitten, W. K. (1956). Modifications of the oestrus cycle of the mouse by external stimuli associated with the male. *J. Endocr.* 13, 399.

Whitten, W. K. and Champlin, A. K. (1972). Phermones and olfaction in mammalian reproduction. *Biblphy. Reprod.* 19, (2) 149.

Whittemore, C. T. and Fraser, D. (1974). The nursing and suckling behaviour of pigs. II Vocalisations of the sow in relation to suckling behaviour and milk ejection. *Br. vet. J.,* 130, 346–356.

Wiepkema, P. R. (1985). Abnormal behaviour in farm animals: ethological implications. *Neth. J. Zool.* 35, 279–289.

Wiepkema, P. R. (1987). Behavioural aspects of stress. In *Biology of Stress in Farm Animals: an Integrative Approach* ed. P. R. Wiepkema and P. W. M. van Adrichem. *Curr. Top. vet. Med. Anim. Sci.* 42, 113–183. Dordrecht: Martinus Nijhoff.

Wiepkema, P. R., Broom, D. M., Duncan, I. J. H. and van Putten, G. (1983). *Abnormal Behaviours in Farm Animals.* Brussels: Commission of the European Communities:

Wiepkema, P. R., Cronin, G. M. and van Ree, J. M. (1984). Stereotypies and endorphins: functional significance of developing stereotypies in tethered sows. In: J. Unshelm, G. van Putten and K. Zeeb (eds.) *Proc. Int. Cong. Appl. Ethol. Farm Anim.,* pp. 93–96. Darmstadt: K. T. B. L.

Wierenga, H. K. (1983). The influence of space for walking and lying in a cubicle system on the behaviour of dairy cattle. In *Farm Animal Housing and Welfare* ed. S. H. Baxter, M. R. Baxter and S. H. MacCormack. *Curr. Top. vet.*

Med. Anim. Sci., **24**, 171–180. Martinus Nijhoff: The Hague.

Wierenga, H. K. (1987). Behavioural problems in fattening bulls. In *Welfare Aspects of Housing Systems for Veal Calves and Fattening Bulls,* ed. M. C. Schlichting and D. Smidt., 105–122. Luxembourg: Commission of the European Communities, EUR 10777. EN.

Wierenga, H. K. (in press). Adaptation of automatic feeding systems for dairy cows. *Appl. Anim. Behav. Sci.*

Wierenga, H. K. and van der Burg, A. (ed.) (1989). *Krachtvoeropname en Gedrag van Melkkoeien bij Geprogrammeerde Krachtvoerverstrekking.* (English summary) Concentrate intake and behaviour of dairy cows with programmed concentrate distribution (pp. 7–10). Wageningen: Pudoc.

Wierenga, H. K. and Peterse, D. J. (1987). (eds). *Cattle Housing Systems, Lameness and Behaviour. Curr. Top. vet. Med. Anim. Sci.,* **40**. Dordrecht: Martinus Nijhoff.

Wierzbowski, S. (1959). The sexual reflexes of stallions. *Roczn. Nank. Roln.* **73**, 753.

Wierzbowski, S. (1966). The scheme of sexual behaviour in bulls, rams and stallions. *World Rev. Anim. Prod.* **2** (2) 66–74.

Wierzbowski, S. (1975). The sexual behaviour in experimentally underfed bulls. *Appl. Anim. Ethol.,* **1**, 203 (Abstract).

Williams, R. (ed.) (1974). *Textbook on Endocrinology,* Philadelphia: Saunders.

Wilson, E. O. (1975). *Sociobiology.* Cambridge Mass: Belknap Press.

Wilson, J. (1929). Merit essay in herding a hill hersel. *The Scottish Farmer and Farming World and Household,* pp. 51–55, Glasgow: Scottish Agricultural Publishing Co. Ltd.

de Wilt, J. G. (1985). Behaviour and welfare of veal calves in relation to husbandry systems. Doctoral thesis, University of Wageningen.

Winfield, C. G. (1970). The effect of stocking intensity at lambing on lamb survival and ewe and lamb behaviour. *Proc. Aust. Anim. Prod.,* **32**, 115–122.

Winfield, C. and Kilgour, R. (1976). A study of following behaviour in young lambs. *Appl. Anim. Ethol.,* **2**, 235–243.

Winfield, C. G., Syme, G. J. and Pearson, A. J. (1981). Effect of familiarity with each other and breed on the spatial behaviour of sheep in an open field. *Appl. Anim. Ethol.,* **7**, 67–75.

Wisniewski, E. W. and Albright, J. L. (1978). Parlor entrance behavior of dairy cattle trained to enter a herringbone parlor with conditioning methods. *Proc. Int. Symp. Machine Milking, Louisville Kentucky U. S. A.,* 460–6.

Wodzicka-Tomaszewska. M., Kilgour, R. and Ryan, M. (1981). "Libido" in the larger farm animals: A review. *Appl. Anim. Ethol.,* **7**, 203–238.

Wolski, T. Houpt, K. and Alonson, R. (1980). The role of the senses in mare–foal recognition. *Appl. Anim. Ethol.* **6**, 121–138.

Wood, P. D. P., Smith, G. F. and Lisle, M. F. (1967). A survey of intersucking in dairy herds in England and Wales. *Vet. Rec.,* **81**, 396–398.

Wood-Gush, D. G. M. (1954). Observations on the nesting habits of Brown Leghorn hens, *Wld. Poult. Congr.,* **10**, 187–192.

Wood-Gush, D. G. M. (1969). Laying in battery cages. *Wld. Poult. Sci. J.,* **25**, 145.

Wood-Gush, D. G. M. (1971). *The Behaviour of the Domestic Fowl.* London: Heinemann.

Wood-Gush, D. G. M. (1972). Strain differences in response to sub optimal stimuli in the fowl. *Anim. Behav.,* **20**, 72–76.

Wood-Gush, D. G. M. (1983). *Elements of Ethology.* London: Chapman and Hall.

Wood-Gush, D. G. M. (1988). The relevance of the knowledge of free ranging domesticated animals for animal husbandry. *Proc. Int. Cong. Appl. Ethol. Farm Animals,* Skara, ed. G. van Putten, J. Unshelm and K. Zeeb. Darmstadt: K. T. B. L.

Wood-Gush, D. G. M. and Beilharz, R. G. (1983). The enrichment of a bare environment for animals in confined conditions. *Appl. Anim. Ethol.* **10**, 209–217.

Wood-Gush, D. G. M. and Gilbert, A. B. (1969). Observations on the laying behaviour of hens in battery cages, *Br. Poult. Sci.,* **10**, 29–36.

Wood-Gush, D. G. M., Duncan, I. J. H., and Savory, C. J. (1978). Observations on the social behaviour of domestic fowl in the wild. *Biol. Behav.,* **3**, 193–205.

Wurtman, R. J. (1970). The role of brain and pineal indoles in neuro-endocrine mechanisms. In *The Hypothalamus,* p. 153. New York: Academic Press.

Yang, T. S., Howard, B. and Macfarlane, W. V. (1981). Effects of food on drinking behaviour of growing pigs. *Appl. Anim. Ethol.* **7**, 259–270.

Yarney, T. A. Rahnefeld, G. W. and Konefal, G. (1979). Time of day of parturition in beef cows. *Can. J. Anim. Sci.,* **59**, 836.

Yeates, N.T.M. (1963). The activity pattern in poultry in relation to photo-period. *Anim. Behav.* **11**, 287–289.

Younis, A.A. and El-Gaboory, I.A.H. (1978). On the diurnal variation in lambing and time for placenta expulsion in Awassi ewes. *J. agric. Sci. Cambs.*, **91**, 757–760.

Zahorik, D.M. and Houpt, K.A. (1981). Species differences in feeding strategies, food hazards and the ability to learn food aversions. In *Foraging Behavior*, ed. A.C. Kamil and T.D. Sargent, pp. 289–310. New York: Garland Press.

Zeeb, K. (1959). Verhaltensforschung beim Pferd. *Tierärztl. Umsch.*, **14**, 334–341.

Zeeb, K. (1961). Der Freie Herdensprung bei Pferden. *Wien Tierärztl. Msch.* **48**, 90–102.

Zenchak, J., and Anderson, C.C. (1980). Sexual performance levels of rams (*Ovis aries*) as affected by social experiences during rearing. *J. Anim. Sci.*, **50**, 167–174.

Zimmermann, M. (1984). Ethical considerations in relation to pain in animal experimentation. In *Biomedical Research Involving Animals* ed. Z. Bankowski and N. Howard Jones, 132–139. Genf: Council for International Organisations of Medical Sciences.

Zimmermann, M. (1985). Behavioral investigations of pain in animals. In. *Proc. 2nd. Eur. Symp. Poult. Welfare*, ed. R.-M. Wegner. Celle: World Poultry Science Association.

Zito, C.A., Wilson, L.L., and Graves, H.B. (1977). Some effects of social deprivation on behavioural development of lambs. *Appl. Anim. Ethol.*, **3**, 367–377.

Zwolinski, J. and Sindinski. (1965). Dobowy rozklad wysrebiern u klasczy. *Medyncyna Weterynaryjna.* **21**, 614–616.

Index

Glossary page references, where appropriate, are listed first.